AF333849

Visualization and Processing of Tensor F

Joachim Weickert   Hans Hagen (Editors)

Visualization and Processing of Tensor Fields

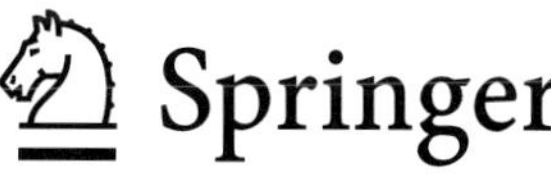 Springer

Professor Joachim Weickert
Faculty of Mathematics and
Computer Science
Saarland University, Building 27
66041 Saarbrücken
Germany
E-mail: weickert@mia.uni-saarland.de

Professor Hans Hagen
Computer Graphics and Visualization Group
Technical University of Kaiserslautern
PO Box 3049
67653 Kaiserslautern
Germany
E-mail: hagen@informatik.uni-kl.de

Library of Congress Control Number: 2005931221

Mathematics Subject Classification Numbers (2000)   15A48, 15A72, 35J60, 35K55, 53-02, 53-06, 54-06, 62-07, 65D05, 65D17, 65D18, 68T45, 68U10, 65K10, 83-08, 86-08

ISBN-10   3-540-25032-8 Springer Berlin Heidelberg New York
ISBN-13   978-3-540-25032-6 Springer Berlin Heidelberg New York

Springer is a part of Springer Science+Business Media
springeronline.com
© Springer-Verlag Berlin Heidelberg 2006
Printed in The Netherlands

Typesetting: by the authors and TechBooks using a Springer LaTeX macro package

Cover design: *design & production* GmbH, Heidelberg

Printed on acid-free paper   SPIN: 11307570   46/TechBooks   5 4 3 2 1 0

Preface

Matrix-valued data sets – so-called tensor fields – have gained significant importance in the fields of scientific visualization and image processing. The tensor concept is a common physical description of anisotropic behaviour, especially in solid mechanics and civil engineering. It arises e.g. in the measurements of stress and strain, inertia, permeability and diffusion. In the field of medical imaging, diffusion tensor magnetic resonance imaging (DT-MRI) has become widespread in order to gain valuable insights into connectivity properties of the brain. Tensors have also shown their use as feature descriptors in image analysis, segmentation and grouping.

These recent developments have created the need for appropriate tools for visualizing and processing tensor fields. Due to the multivariate structure of the data and their multidimensional variation in space, tensor field visualization belongs to the most challenging topics in the area of scientific visualization. Moreover, most signal and image processing methods have been developed for scalar- and vector-valued data sets, and only recently researchers have tried to investigate how they can be extended to tensor fields. In this case one has to take into account a number of additional constraints such as an appropriate coupling of the different channels, and preservation of properties such as positive semidefiniteness during the filtering process.

Unfortunately the results in the field of tensor-valued visualization and image processing are scattered in the literature, and often researchers in one application area are not aware of recent progress in another area. In order to address this problem, the editors of this book organized a perspective workshop that took place at Schloss Dagstuhl, Germany from April 18 to 23, 2004. In that week 30 invited scientists, representing many of the world-wide leading experts in tensor field visualization and processing, had the opportunity to exchange ideas in a highly inspiring atmosphere. Since many of them met for the first time, this exchange proved to be particularly fruitful.

One of these fruits was the wish of all participants to compile their knowledge in a single edited volume. The present book – which is the first of its kind in this field – is the result of these efforts. Its goal is to present the state-of-the-art in the visualization and processing of tensor fields, both as an overview for the inquiring scientist, and as a basic foundation for developers and practitioners. The book contains some longer chapters dedicated to surveys and tutorials of specific topics, as well as a great deal of original work not previously published. In all cases the emphasis has been on presenting the details necessary for others to reproduce the techniques and algorithms. Another goal of this book is to provide the basic material for teaching state-of-the-art techniques in tensor field visualization and processing. It can therefore also serve as a textbook for specialized classes and seminars for graduate and doctoral students. An extended bibliography is included at the end of each chapter pointing out where to obtain further information.

Organization of the Book

This volume consists of 25 chapters. Each of them has been reviewed by two experts and carefully revised according to their suggestions. The chapters are arranged in five thematic areas. Color plates can be found in the Appendix.

The book starts with an introductory chapter by Hagen and Garth. It gives the mathematical background from linear algebra and differential geometry that is necessary for understanding the concept of tensor fields.

Part I of the book is devoted to feature detection using tensors. Here one typically starts with scalar- or vector-valued images and creates tensor-valued features that are suitable for corner detection, texture analysis or optic flow estimation. Structure tensors are the most prominent representatives of these concepts. Chapter 2 by Brox et al. is a survey chapter on adaptive structure tensors, while Chap. 3 by Nagel analyzes closed form solutions for a structure tensor concept in image sequence analysis. An alternative framework for tensor-valued feature detection is presented in Chap. 4 by Köthe who shows that the so-called boundary tensor may overcome some problems of more traditional approaches.

Part II deals with the currently most important technique for creating tensor-valued images, namely Diffusion Tensor Magnetic Resonance Imaging (DT-MRI), often simply called Diffusion Tensor Imaging (DTI). This technique measures the diffusion properties of water molecules and has gained significant popularity in medical imaging of the brain. Chapter 5 by Alexander gives a general overview of the principles of biomedical diffusion MRI and algorithms for reconstructing the diffusion tensor fields, while the subsequent chapter by Hahn et al. describes the empirical origin of noise and analyzes its influence on the DT-MRI variables. After having understood the formation of DT-MR images their adequate visualization remains a challenging task. This is the topic of the survey chapter by Vilanova et al. that also sketches the clinical impact of DT-MR imaging. A more specific medical application is treated in Chap. 8 by Gee et al. who study anatomical labeling of cerebral white matter in DT-MR images. For conventional DT-MR imaging, the identification and analysis of fibre crossings constitutes a severe difficulty. In Chap. 9, Pasternak et al. introduce a variational image processing framework for resolving these ambiguities. An alternative strategy is investigated in Chap. 10 by Özarslan et al. They reconstruct higher-order tensors from the MR measurements. These allow to encode a richer orientational heterogeneity.

In the third part, general visualization strategies for tensor fields are explored. This part starts with a review chapter by Benger and Hege who also consider applications in relativity theory. Kindlmann's chapter is concerned with visualizing discontinuities in tensor fields by computing the gradients of invariants. The subsequent Chaps. 13–16 investigate different strategies for understanding the complex nature of tensor fields by extracting suitable differential geometric information. While Chap. 13 by Tricoche et al. deals with the topology and simplification of static and time-variant 2-D tensor fields, Chap. 14 by Zheng et al. is concerned with a novel and numerically stable analysis of degerated tensors in 3-D fields. In Chap. 15, Wischgoll and Meyer investigate the detection of alternative topological features, namely closed hyperstreamlines. The third part is concluded with a chapter by Hotz et al. who introduce specific visualization concepts for stress and strain tensor fields by interpreting them as distortions of a flat metric.

Part IV of the book is concerned with transformations of tensor fields, in particular interpolation and registration strategies. In Chap. 17, Moakher and Batchelor perform a differential geometric analysis of the space of positive definite tensors in order to derive appropriate interpolation methods. The next chapter by Pajevic et al. deals with non-uniform rational B-splines (NURBS) as a flexible interpolation tool, while in Chap. 19 Weickert and Welk introduce a rotationally invariant framework for tensor field approximation, interpolation and inpainting. It is based on partial differential equations (PDEs). Finally, Chap. 20 by Gee and Alexander treats the problem of diffusion tensor registration. Compared to scalar-valued registration approaches, incorporating the orientation information provides additional challenges.

The fifth part is a collection of contributions on signal and image processing methods that are specifically developed to deal with tensor fields. Chapter 21 by Welk et al. as well as Chap. 22 by Burgeth et al. show that seemingly simple ideas like median filtering and morphological image processing can create substantial difficulties when one wants to generalize them to tensor fields. Since tensor lack a full ordering, many straightforward concepts cannot be applied and alternative generalizations become necessary. In Chap. 23, Suárez-Santana et al. review adaptive local filters for tensor field regularization and interpolation that are steered by a structure tensor, while Chap. 24 by Westin et al. is concerned with two other regularization techniques for tensor fields: normalized convolution and Markov random fields. These ideas a complemented by Chap. 25 where Weickert et al. survey the most important PDE approaches for discontinuity-preserving smoothing and segmentation of tensor fields.

Acknowledgements

It is a pleasure to thank all authors for their excellent contributions. We are very grateful to Reinhard Wilhelm and the Scientific Directorate for accepting our proposal for a Dagstuhl Perspective Workshop on Visualization and Processing of Tensor Fields, and the local team at Schloss Dagstuhl for providing a very pleasant atmosphere that allowed all participants to enjoy this workshop with real scientific benefits. Moreover, we thank the editors of the Springer book series *Mathematics and Visualization* as well as Martin Peters and Ute McCrory (Springer, Heidelberg) for their support to publish this edited volume in their series. Last but not least, we are greatly indebted to Martin Welk (Saarland University) who was of substantial help in the final compilation of all chapters to a coherent, single volume.

<table>
<tr><td>Saarbrücken and Kaiserslautern,
June 2005</td><td align="right">Joachim Weickert
Hans Hagen</td></tr>
</table>

Contents

Part IV Tensor Field Transformations

Part V Image Processing Methods for Tensor Fields

Appendix

Introduction

1

An Introduction to Tensors

Hans Hagen and Christoph Garth

Computer Graphics and Visualization Group, Technical University of
Kaiserslautern, PO Box 3049, 67653 Kaiserslautern, Germany
{hagen,garth}@informatik.uni-kl.de

Summary. This chapter is a short introduction into tensor fields, some basic techniques from linear algebra, differential geometry and the mathematical concept of tensor fields are presented. The main goal of this chapter is to give readers from different backgrounds some fundamentals to access the research papers in the following chapters.

1.1 Some Linear Algebra

Remark: Since we are only able to sketch out some of the basic facts of linear algebra, the reader is referred to a comprehensive body of literature on the topic. For example, the book by Fuhrmann [1] provides an introduction in a modern language.

1.1.1 Bases and Basis Transforms

Let U a vector space over a field $\mathbb{F}$ (e.g. $\mathbb{F} = \mathbb{R}$ or $\mathbb{F} = \mathbb{C}$). A set of elements $\{a_1, \ldots, a_n\} \subset U$, $n \in \mathbb{N}$, is called a basis if every $u \in U$ admits a unique non-trivial linear combination of the a_i over $\mathbb{F}$:

$$u = u_1 a_1 + \cdots + u_n a_n$$

The coefficients u_i give rise to the vector notation of $u \in U$ with respect to this basis as

$$u = \begin{pmatrix} u_1 \\ \vdots \\ u_n \end{pmatrix}.$$

We say that U has dimension n, since every basis has exactly n elements and every $u \in U$ can be described by n elements of $\mathbb{F}$ (coordinates).

Let V a vector space over $\mathbb{F}$ with basis $(b_1, \ldots, b_m)$, $m \in \mathbb{N}$. Hence, $\dim V = m$. A linear map $L : U \to V$ is a map satisfying

$$L(\alpha u + \beta u') \;=\; \alpha L(u) + \beta L(u') \qquad\qquad \forall u, u' \in U, \forall \alpha, \beta \in \mathbb{F} \ .$$

We can observe

$$L(u) = L\left(\sum_{i=1}^{n} u_i a_i\right) = \sum_{i=1}^{n} u_i L(a_i) = \sum_{i=1}^{n} u_i \sum_{j=1}^{m} l_{ij} b_j \ ,$$

where l_{ij} denotes the j-th coefficient of $L(a_i)$ w.r.t. the basis $(b_1, \ldots, b_n)$. Hence, L can be represented as $L = (L_{ij})$, $i \in \{1, \ldots, m\}$, $j \in \{1, \ldots, n\}$, leading to matrix notation

$$v \;=\; L(u) = L \cdot u \ .$$

In this form, L and its matrix representation are identified. The dot represents the matrix-vector product

$$(L \cdot u)_i = \sum_{j=1}^{m} l_{ij} u_j \ .$$

The space of all linear maps from U to V is denoted by $\mathrm{Hom}(U, V)$. It can be shown that, given a basis for each U and V, every $L \in \mathrm{Hom}(U, V)$ can be written in the form of an $(m \times n)$-matrix. The algebraic structure of $\mathrm{Hom}(U, V)$ is reflected by the rules of matrix algebra.

We next consider the effect of a basis change on the vector representation of $u \in U$. Let $(\tilde{a}_1, \ldots, \tilde{a}_n)$ another basis of U, then

$$a_i = \sum_{j=1}^{n} p_{ij} \tilde{a}_j \qquad\qquad \forall i \in \{1, \ldots, m\} \ .$$

Hence, the representation $\tilde{u}$ of u w.r.t. $\{\tilde{a}_1, \ldots, \tilde{a}_n\}$ is given through

$$u \;=\; \sum_{i=1}^{n} u_i a_i \;=: \sum_{i=1}^{n} u_i \sum_{j=1}^{n} p_{ij} \tilde{a}_j \ ,$$

or equivalently,

$$\tilde{u}_j = \sum_{i=1}^{n} p_{ij} u_i \ .$$

In other words, the (p_{ij}) represent a linear transform $P \in \mathrm{Hom}(U, U)$. P is called a basis transform, and

$$\tilde{u} = P \cdot u \ .$$

Since $\{a_1, \ldots, a_n\}$ and $\{\tilde{a}_1, \ldots, \tilde{a}_n\}$ can be exchanged in the above calculation, the transformation is invertible, and we easily see that

$$P \cdot P^{-1} = P^{-1} \cdot P = I \,,$$

with the identity map I. The linear map L can be transformed to another basis in a similar fashion as the elements of U (and V). Let $\{\tilde{b}_1, \ldots, \tilde{b}_m\}$ another basis of V and Q the corresponding basis change matrix, then

$$\tilde{L} = Q \cdot L \cdot P^{-1}$$

denotes L w.r.t. the bases $\{\tilde{a}_i\}$ and $\{\tilde{b}_j\}$. As a special case, if $U = V$, it is

$$\tilde{L} = P \cdot L \cdot P^{-1} \,.$$

1.1.2 Dual Spaces

Let U an n-dimensional vector space. A linear map

$$\alpha : \ U \to \mathbb{F}$$

is called a *linear form* on U. The set of all linear forms on U is called the *dual space* and noted U^*. As $\mathbb{F}$ is implicitly a vector space, any $\alpha \in U^*$ possesses a representation as a $(1 \times n)$-matrix. For a given basis $\{a_1, \ldots, a_n\}$ of U and the notation from above, linearity mandates

$$\alpha(u) = \sum_{i=1}^{m} \alpha_i \left(a_i u_i \right) \,.$$

It can be shown that U^* is again an n-dimensional vector space, and there exists a *dual basis* $\{a^1, \ldots, a^n\}$ of U^* with the property

$$a^i \left(a_j \right) = \delta_{ij}$$

where δ_{ij} is the Kronecker symbol. If U is equipped with a symmetric (hermitean in the complex case) and positive inner product $< \cdot, \cdot >$, then the *Riesz representation theorem* guarantees to every $\alpha \in U^*$ the existence of $u_\alpha \in U$ such that

$$\alpha(u) = < u_\alpha \,, u > \qquad \text{for any } u \in U \,.$$

Similarly, for arbitrary $u \in U$, $\alpha_u := < u \,, \cdot >$ is an element of U^*. Hence, the two spaces are isomorphic. Furthermore, it is easily seen that $V^{**} = (V^*)^*$ is also isomorphic to V. Commonly, elements of the dual space are written as row vectors.

A linear map $A : U \to V$ between vector spaces gives rise to the *adjoint map* $A^* : V^* \to U^*$ that is defined via

$$(A^*\alpha)(u) := \alpha(Au) \qquad \text{for all } \alpha \in U^*, u \in U \,.$$

A^* is obviously linear, and in the dual bases of U^* and V^* its matrix representation is given as

$$(A^*)_{ij} = (A_{ji})^* \,,$$

where the star on the right hand side denotes complex conjugation. In other words, the matrix representation of A^* is the conjugate transpose of the matrix of A. In the special case $U = V$, A is called self-adjoint if the matrix representations of A and A^* coincide. In tensor calculus, the concept of dual spaces is found in the occurrence of upper and lower indices, referring to dual or primal properties of a tensor, respectively. These considerations are detailed in Sect. 1.3.

1.1.3 Eigenvalues and Eigenvectors

Let U an n-dimensional vector space and $L \in \mathrm{Hom}(U, U)$ a linear map on U. A vector $u \in U$ is called an *eigenvector* of L to the *eigenvalue* $\lambda \in \mathbb{F}$ if

$$L(u) = \lambda u$$

holds true. Clearly, any scalar multiple of u is also an eigenvector of L to λ, and the eigenvectors to λ form a linear subspace of U, the *eigenspace* E_λ to U. It can be shown that the eigenvalues of any linear map are the roots of its *characteristic polynomial*

$$\chi_L(\lambda) := \det(L - \lambda I) \,,$$

where $I \in Hom(U, U)$ is again the identity map. The characteristic polynomial is of degree n, which implies that there are at most n eigenvalues of L. If an eigenvalue λ is known, E_λ can be determined as the set of solutions v to the equation

$$(L - \lambda I)(v) = 0 \,.$$

In the case $\mathbb{F} = \mathbb{R}$, the characteristic polynomial has n real roots $\lambda_1, \ldots, \lambda_n$ already if the matrix representation of L in some basis is symmetric, i.e. if $l_{ij} = l_{ji}$ for $i, j \in \{1, \ldots, n\}$. We then say that L is *diagonalizable*, because U can be decomposed into an orthogonal sum of eigenspaces

$$U = E_{\lambda_1} \oplus \cdots \oplus E_{\lambda_n} \,,$$

giving rise to an orthonormal basis $\{u_1, \ldots u_n\}$ of eigenvectors of U. If P is the corresponding basis transform matrix, then L takes the very simple diagonal matrix representation

$$P \cdot L \cdot P^{-1} = \mathrm{diag}(\lambda_1, \ldots, \lambda_n) \,.$$

In this basis, the properties of the map L are most easily comprehended.

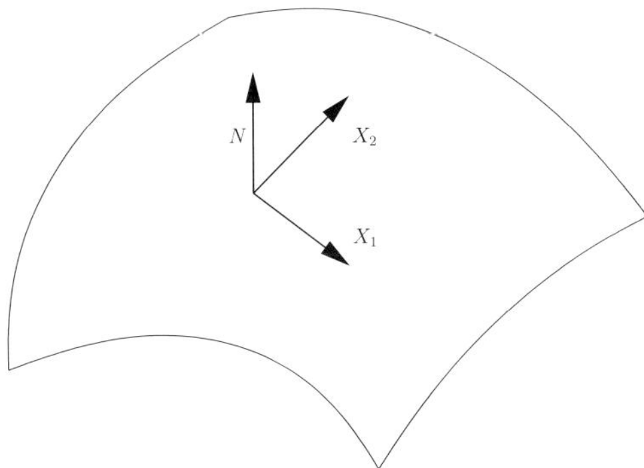

Fig. 1.1. The Gauss frame of a surface

1.2 Fundamentals of Differential Geometry

Definition 1. *A parametrized C^r-surface is a C^r-differential map $X : U \to \mathbb{E}^3$ of an open domain $U \subset \mathbb{R}^2$ into the Euclidean space $\mathbb{E}^3$, whose differential dX is one-to-one for each $u \in U$.*

Remarks.   1. Let $X : U \to \mathbb{E}^3$ be a parametrized surface. A change of variables of X is a diffeomorphism $\tau : \tilde{U} \to U$, where $\tilde{U}$ is an open domain in $\mathbb{R}^2$, such that $d\tau$ has always rank 2. If $\det(\tau^*) > 0$, τ is orientation-preserving (τ^* is the Jacobian matrix of τ). Relationship by change of variables defines an equivalence relation on the class of all parametrized surfaces. A corresponding equivalence class of parametrized surfaces is called a surface in $\mathbb{E}^3$.

  2. In this context, the differential dX is a linear map from the tangent space (introduced below) at a point u into $\mathbb{R}$. It is one-to-one if and only if $\partial X/\partial u^1$ and $\partial X/\partial u^2$ are linearly independent at p.

Definition 2. *The two-dimensional subspace $T_u X$ of $\mathbb{E}^3$ generated by* $\mathrm{span}(X_1, X_2)$ *is called the* tangent space *of X at u ($X_i := \frac{\partial X}{\partial u^i}$; $i = 1, 2$). Elements of $T_u X$ are called* tangent vectors. *The vector field $N := \frac{[X_1, X_2]}{||X_1|| \cdot ||X_2||}$ is called* unit normal field *($[\cdot, \cdot] : \mathbb{E}^3 \times \mathbb{E}^3 \to \mathbb{E}^3$ is the vector product of $\mathbb{E}^3$). The map N from U to the unit sphere S^2 is called Gauss map and the moving frame is called the Gauss frame of the surface in $\mathbb{E}^3$.*

Remarks.   1. The Gauss frame is in general not an orthogonal frame.

  2. Every tangential vector field Y along the surface $X : U \to \mathbb{E}^3$ can be represented in the following form:

$$Y(s) = \lambda^2(s) X_1(u^1(s), u^2(s)) + \lambda^2(s) X_2(u^1(s), u^2(s))$$

Definition 3. *Let $X : U \to \mathbb{E}^3$ be a surface and $u \in U$. The bilinear form I_u on $T_u X$ induced by the inner product of $\mathbb{E}^3$ by restriction is called the* first fundamental form *of the surface.*

Remarks.   1. The matrix representation of the first fundamental form with respect to the basis $\{X_1, X_2\}$ of $T_u X$ is given by

$$\begin{bmatrix} g_{11} & g_{12} \\ g_{21} & g_{22} \end{bmatrix} = \begin{bmatrix} \langle X_1, X_1 \rangle & \langle X_1, X_2 \rangle \\ \langle X_2, X_1 \rangle & \langle X_2, X_2 \rangle \end{bmatrix}.$$

Here, $\langle \cdot, \cdot \rangle : I\!\!E^3 \times I\!\!E^3 \to I\!\!R$ is the scalar product.

2. The first fundamental form is symmetric, positive definite and a geometric invariant.

3. Geometrically, the first fundamental form allows us to make measurements on the surface (lengths of curves, angles of tangent vectors, areas of regions) without referring back to the ambient space $I\!\!E^3$.

Definition 4. *(a) Let $X : U \to I\!\!E^3$ be a surface and $u \in U$. The linear map $L : T_u X \to T_u X$ defined by*

$$L := -dN_u \cdot dX_u^{-1}$$

is called the Weingarten map.
(b) The bilinear form II_u defined by

$$II_u(A, B) := \langle L(A), B \rangle$$

for each $A, B \in T_u X$ is called the second fundamental form *of the surface.*

Remarks.   1. The matrix representation of II_u with respect to the canonical basis of $T_u I\!\!R^2$ (identified with $I\!\!E^2$) and the associated basis $\{X_1, X_2\}$ of $T_u X$ is given by

$$h_{ij} := \langle -N_i, X_j \rangle = \langle N, X_{ij} \rangle \qquad i, j \in \{1, 2\}.$$

2. The second fundamental form is invariant under congruences of $I\!\!E^3$ and orientation-preserving changes of variables.

Proposition and Definition 1. Let $X : U \to I\!\!E^3$ be a surface.

(a) The Weingarten map L is self-adjoint. The eigenvalues k_1, k_2 are therefore real and the corresponding eigenvectors are orthogonal.
(b) k_1, k_2 are called the *principal curvatures* of the surface.
(c) The quantity

$$K := k_1 \cdot k_2 = \det(L) = \frac{\det II}{\det I}$$

is called the *Gauss curvature* and

$$H := \frac{1}{2} \operatorname{trace}(L) = \frac{1}{2}(k_1 + k_2)$$

is called the *mean curvature.*

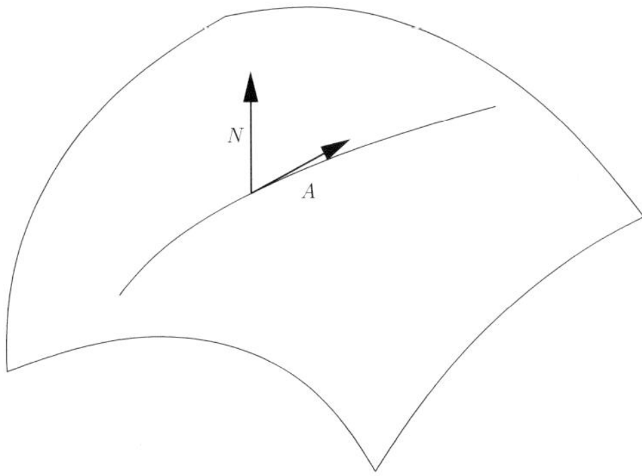

Fig. 1.2. A normal section curve on a surface

Considering surface curves we get to know the geometric interpretations of the second fundamental form: Let $A := \lambda^1 X_1 + \lambda^2 X_2$ be a tangent vector with $\|A\| = 1$. Intersecting the surface with the plane given by N and A, we get an intersection curve $y(s)$ with the properties

$$y'(s) = A \qquad \text{and} \qquad e_2 = \pm N \, .$$

(e_2 is the principal normal vector of the space curve y). The implicit function theorem implies the existence of this so-called normal section curve. To calculate the extreme values of the curvature of a normal section curve (the so-called normal section curvature) we can use the method of Lagrange multipliers, because we are looking for the extreme values of the normal section curvature k_N under the condition

$$\sum_{i,j=1}^{2} g_{ij}\lambda^i\lambda^j = \|y'(s)\| = 1 \, .$$

As the result of these considerations we get:

Proposition 1. Let $X : U \to \mathbb{E}^3$ be a surface and for a tangent vector $A := \lambda^1 X_1 + \lambda^2 X_2$ let $k_N(\lambda^1, \lambda^2)$ be the normal section curvature.

(a)

$$k_N(\lambda^1, \lambda^2) = \sum_{i,j} \frac{h_{ij}\lambda^i\lambda^j}{g_{ij}\lambda^i\lambda^j}$$

(b) Unless the normal section curvature is the same for all directions, there are two perpendicular directions A_1 and A_2 in which k_N attains its absolute maximum and its absolute minimum. These directions and the corresponding normal section curvatures are k_1 and k_2, the *principal curvatures* of the surface.

Proposition and Definition 2. Let $X : U \to \mathbb{E}^3$ be a surface. If $I \subset \mathbb{R}$ is an interval on the real line, let $y : I \to \mathbb{E}^3$ be a surface curve. We denote by $\hat{y}(t)$ the orthogonal projection of $y(t)$ on the tangent plane to X at (an arbitrary) point p.

(a) The *geodesic curvature* k_g of y at p is defined to be the curvature of the projected curve $\hat{y}(t)$ at p.

(b) A curve $y(t)$ on a surface X is called a geodesic curve or simply geodesic if its geodesic curvature k_g vanishes identically.

(c)
$$k_g := \det(y', y'', N) \, ,$$

where the dots denote derivatives with respect to the arc length s of y.

The great importance of tensor fields is totally obvious by just looking briefly on these facts and results from differential geometry. This motivates to have closer look on tensors in general.

For question no touched upon here, the book by do Carmo [2] provides an detailed introductory-level treatment of differential geometry. For a more comprehensive overview, see [3].

1.3 Tensor Fields – A Mathematical Concept

Tensor fields are invariant under parameter transformation and therefore an appropriate tool to describe certain 'geometric invariant situations'. We are using Einstein's summation convention for simplicity (if an index occurs more than once in the same expression, the expression is implicitly summed over all possible values for that index).

Definition 5 ((r, s)-tensor).

(a) V is an n-dimensional vector space and V^* is its dual space. A multilinear map

$$T : \underbrace{V \times \cdots \times V}_{r} \times \underbrace{V^* \times \cdots \times V^*}_{s} \to \mathbb{R}$$

is called an (r, s)-tensor.

(b) $E_1, \ldots, E_n$ is the basis of V, and $E^1, \ldots, E^n$ is the dual basis of V^*. Then

$$
\begin{aligned}
&T(A_1, \ldots, A_r, B^1, \ldots, B^s) \\
&= T(a_1^{i_1} E_{i_1}, \ldots, a_r^{i_r} E_{i_r}, b_{j_1}^1 E^{j_1}, \ldots, b_{j_s}^s E^{j_s}) \\
&= T(E_{i_1}, \ldots, E_{i_r}, E^{j_1}, \ldots, E^{j_s}) \, a_1^{i_1} \cdots a_r^{i_r} \cdot b_{j_1}^1 \cdots b_{j_s}^s \\
&= t_{i_1 \ldots i_r}{}^{j_1 \cdots j_s} \cdot a_1^{i_1} \cdots a_r^{i_r} \cdot b_{j_1}^1 \cdots b_{j_s}^s .
\end{aligned}
$$

The n^{r+s} real numbers are called components of the (r, s)-tensor T.

Under a change of basis

$$\bar{E}_i = \alpha_i{}^j\, E_j \qquad \text{and} \qquad \bar{E}^i = \bar{\alpha}^i{}_j\, E^j$$

an (r,s)-tensor transforms in this way:

$$t_{i_1\ldots i_r}{}^{j_1\ldots j_s} = t_{l_1\ldots l_r}{}^{k_1\ldots k_s} \cdot \alpha_{i_1}{}^{l_1}\cdots\alpha_{i_r}{}^{l_r} \cdot \bar{\alpha}_{k_1}{}^{j_1}\cdots\bar{\alpha}_{k_s}{}^{j_s}\ .$$

Remarks.   1. The elements of $\mathbb{R}$ are tensors of type $(0,0)$.
2. The elements of V^* are tensors of type $(1,0)$.
3. The elements of V can be identified with tensors of type $(0,1)$, since V^{**} and V are canonically isomorphic.
4. The determinant on V as a multilinear map from V^n to $\mathbb{R}$ is a prototypical example of a $(n,0)$-tensor.

Tensor operations:

1. Tensors of the same type can be added and scaled like vectors.

2. **Tensor product:**

   Let T an (r,s)-tensor and $\tilde{T}$ a $(\tilde{r},\tilde{s})$-tensor. Then

   $$T \circ \tilde{T}(A_1,\ldots,A_{r+\tilde{r}},B^1,\ldots,B^{s+\tilde{s}}) \quad :=$$
   $$T(A_1,\ldots,A_r,B^1,\ldots,B^s) \cdot \tilde{T}(A_{r+1},\ldots,A_{r+\tilde{r}},B^{s+1},\ldots,B^{s+\tilde{s}})$$

   is called the tensor product of T and $\tilde{T}$. In components:

   $$(t\tilde{t})_{i_1\ldots i_{r+\tilde{r}}}{}^{j_1\ldots j_{s+\tilde{s}}} := t_{i_1\ldots i_r}{}^{j_1\ldots j_s} \cdot t_{i_{r+1}\ldots i_{r+\tilde{r}}}{}^{j_{s+1}\ldots j_{s+\tilde{s}}}\ .$$

   Clearly, $T \circ \tilde{T}$ is a $(r+\tilde{r}, s+\tilde{s})$-tensor.

3. **Contraction of a tensor:**

   $$(r,s)\text{-tensor} \quad \left|\ \begin{array}{ccc} T & \to & \tilde{T} \\ t_{i_1\ldots i_r}{}^{j_1\ldots j_s} & \mapsto & t_{i\, i_2\ldots i_r}{}^{i\, j_2\ldots j_s} \end{array}\ \right| \quad (r-1, s-1)\text{-tensor}$$

   Example: $\{g_{ij}\}$ and $\{h_{ij}\}$ are the components of the first and second fundamental forms of a surface and H is the mean curvature.

   $$g_{ij}, h_{rs} \xrightarrow[\text{tensor product}]{} g^{ij}h_{rs} \xrightarrow[\text{contraction}]{} g^{ij}h_{is} \xrightarrow[\text{contraction}]{} g^{ij}h_{ij} = 2H$$

4. Inner multiplication with a metric tensor: $\{g_{ij}\}$ are the components of a non-degenerate metric tensor.

   $$g^{ij}\, t_{j\, i_2\ldots i_r}{}^{j_1\ldots j_s} =: t^i{}_{i_2\ldots i_r}{}^{j_1\ldots j_s}$$
   $$g_{ik}\, t_{i_1\ldots i_r}{}^{k\, j_2\ldots j_s} =: t_{i_1\ldots i_r\, k}{}^{j_2\ldots j_s}$$

   Example: the Weingarten map $h_i{}^j = h_{ir}g^{rs}$.

The tensor concept is by no means restricted to differential geometry.

Examples.   1. In the context of physics, the fundamental characteristic that affects the deformation of materials is called *stress*. Since the behavior of a material does not depend on the coordinates used in its description, stress can be described by the *stress tensor T*. The name 'tensor' originates in this context since it was first used to describe tension (stress).

Considering an infinitesimal volume element of a certain material, the stress tensor describes the force that is necessary to establish an equilibrium condition in the material. It depends linearly on the normal of the surface on which the force acts. In turn, force is given as vector, hence the stress tensor can be written in the form of a matrix, which is a tensor of order 2.

In three dimensions of space, given an orthogonal coordinate system e_x, e_y, e_z, the stress tensor components are given with respect to the planes normal to the coordinate axes. For each plane, three scalars describe the required force. Therefore, the tension t with respect to a plane normal to n is given as

$$t = T(n) = \begin{pmatrix} \sigma_{xx} & \sigma_{xy} & \sigma_{xz} \\ \sigma_{yx} & \sigma_{yy} & \sigma_{yz} \\ \sigma_{zx} & \sigma_{zy} & \sigma_{zz} \end{pmatrix} \cdot n$$

Here, for example, σ_{xz} denotes the stress on the plane normal to e_x in direction of e_z.

In many applications, T is a symmetric tensor and therefore possesses an orthogonal system of eigenvectors. They are called *principal stress directions*. In this coordinate system, the off-diagonal components of T vanish, and the volume can be held in equilibrium by forces parallel to the principal directions.

2. In medical applications, Diffusion Tensor Imaging is playing an important role. Using Magnetic Resonance Imaging (MRI), it is possible to record the directional diffusion behavior of water in the brain. This allows to deduce information about structures of interest. Again, the diffusion properties are independent of the reference frame used to describe them.

Mathematically speaking, the diffusion tensor T is a second-order 3×3-tensor that maps a direction d to the directional diffusion coefficient c via

$$c(d) = d^T T d \qquad \text{with} \qquad T = \begin{pmatrix} t_{xx} & t_{xy} & t_{xz} \\ t_{yx} & t_{yy} & t_{yz} \\ t_{zx} & t_{zy} & t_{zz} \end{pmatrix} .$$

The diffusion tensor is symmetric and positive semidefinite, which implies that its eigenvalues are real and non-negative. Roughly speaking, the homogeneity of the eigenvalues is a measure of the isotropy of the material with respect to diffusion. If one of the eigenvalues is essentially larger than the others, the corresponding eigenvector indicates the preferred diffusion direction. Looking for locations with anisotropic diffusion tensors, it is possible to identify the direction of certain structures (mostly fibers) in the brain.

We refer the reader to the books by Borisenko and Tarpov [4] and Abraham, Marsden and Ratiu [5] for more detailed introductions and examples to the general topic of tensor calculus and analysis.

References

1. Fuhrmann, P.A.: A Polynomial Approach to Linear Algebra. Springer, Berlin (2002)
2. do Carmo, M.P.: Differential Geometry of Curves and Surfaces. Prentice-Hall, Englewood Cliffs, N.J. (1976)
3. Spivak, M.: Differential Geometry. Publish or Perish, Berkeley (1979)
4. Borisenko, A.I., Tarpov, I.E.: Vector and Tensor Analysis with Applications. Dover, New York (1980)
5. Abraham, R., Marsden, J.E., and Ratiu, T.S.: Manifolds, Tensor Analysis, and Applications, 2nd ed. Springer, New York (1991)

Part I

Feature Detection with Tensors

2

Adaptive Structure Tensors
and their Applications

Thomas Brox[1], Rein van den Boomgaard[2], François Lauze[3], Joost van de Weijer[2], Joachim Weickert[1], Pavel Mrázek[1], and Pierre Kornprobst[4]

[1] Mathematical Image Analysis Group, Faculty of Mathematics and Computer Science, Building 27, Saarland University, 66041 Saarbrücken, Germany
`{brox,weickert,mrazek}@mia.uni-saarland.de`
[2] Intelligent Sensory Information Systems Group, Informatics Institute, University of Amsterdam, Kruislaan 403, 1098 SJ Amsterdam, The Netherlands
`rein@science.uva.nl`
[3] IT University of Copenhagen, Glentevej 67, DK-2400 Copenhagen, Denmark
`francois@itu.dk`
[4] Odyssée Project, INRIA Sophia-Antipolis, 2004 Route des Lucioles, 06902 Sophia Antipolis, France
`Pierre.Kornprobst@sophia.inria.fr`

Summary. The structure tensor, also known as second moment matrix or Förstner interest operator, is a very popular tool in image processing. Its purpose is the estimation of orientation and the local analysis of structure in general. It is based on the integration of data from a local neighborhood. Normally, this neighborhood is defined by a Gaussian window function and the structure tensor is computed by the weighted sum within this window. Some recently proposed methods, however, adapt the computation of the structure tensor to the image data. There are several ways how to do that. This chapter wants to give an overview of the different approaches, whereas the focus lies on the methods based on robust statistics and nonlinear diffusion. Furthermore, the data-adaptive structure tensors are evaluated in some applications. Here the main focus lies on optic flow estimation, but also texture analysis and corner detection are considered.

2.1 Introduction

Orientation estimation and local structure analysis are tasks that can be found in many image processing and early vision applications, e.g. in fingerprint analysis, texture analysis, optic flow estimation, and in geo-physical analysis of soil layers. The classical technique to estimate orientation is to look at the set of luminance gradient vectors in a local neighborhood. This leads to a very popular operator for orientation estimation, the matrix field of the so-called *structure tensor* [4, 10, 16, 20, 38].

The concept of the structure tensor is a consequence of the fact that one can only describe the local structure at a point by considering also the data of its neighborhood. For instance, from the gradient at a single position, it is not possible to distinguish a corner from an edge, while the integration of the gradient information in the neighborhood of the pixel gives evidence about whether the pixel is occupied by an edge or a corner. Further on, the consideration of a local neighborhood becomes even more important as soon as the data is corrupted by noise or other disturbing artifacts, so that the structure has to be estimated before the background of unreliable data.

The structure tensor therefore extends the structure information of each pixel, which is described in a first order approximation by the gradient at that pixel, by the structure information of its surroundings weighted with a Gaussian window function. This comes down to the convolution of the structure data with a Gaussian kernel, i.e. Gaussian smoothing.

Note however, that the smoothing of gradients can lead to cancellation effects. Consider, for example, a thin line. At one side of the line there appears a positive gradient, while at the other side the gradient is negative. Smoothing the gradients will cause them to mutually cancel out. This is the reason why in the structure tensor, the gradient is considered in form of its outer product. The outer product turns the gradient vector ∇I of an image I into a symmetric positive semi-definite matrix, which we will refer to as the *initial matrix field*

$$J_0 := \nabla I \nabla I^\top = \begin{pmatrix} I_x^2 & I_x I_y \\ I_x I_y & I_y^2 \end{pmatrix} . \tag{2.1}$$

Subscripts thereby denote partial derivatives. The structure tensor can be easily generalized from scalar-valued data to vector-valued data. As with the matrix representation it is possible to sum up gradient information, the structure information from all channels of a vector-valued image $\mathbf{I} = (I_1, \ldots, I_N)$ can be integrated by taking the sum of all matrices [8]:

$$J_0 := \sum_{i=1}^{N} \nabla I_i \nabla I_i^\top . \tag{2.2}$$

The structure tensor for a certain neighborhood of scale ρ is then computed by convolution of the components of J_0 with a Gaussian kernel K_ρ:

$$J_\rho = K_\rho * J_0 . \tag{2.3}$$

The smoothing, i.e. the integration of neighborhood information, has two positive effects on orientation estimation. Firstly, it makes the structure tensor robust against noise or other artifacts, and therefore allows a more reliable estimation of orientation in real-world data. Secondly, it distributes the information about the orientation into the areas between edges. This is a very important effect, as it allows to estimate the dominant orientation also at those points in the image where the gradient is close to zero. The dominant orientation can be obtained from the structure tensor as the eigenvector to the largest eigenvalue. An operator which is closely related to the structure tensor is the boundary tensor discussed in Chap. 4 by Köthe.

There are many applications for the structure tensor in the field of image processing. One popular application is optic flow estimation based on the local approach of Lucas and Kanade [21]. In optic flow estimation one searches for the spatio-temporal direction with least change in the image, which is the eigenvector to the *smallest* eigenvalue of the structure tensor [4, 15].

Another application for orientation estimation is texture analysis. Here the dominant orientation extracted from the structure tensor can serve as a feature to discriminate textures [4, 28]. The dominant local orientation is also used in order to drive anisotropic diffusion processes, which enhance the coherence of structures [39]. Often the structure tensor is also used as a feature detector for edges or corners [10]. An application apart from image processing is a structure analysis for grid optimization in the scope of fluid dynamics [34].

Although the classic structure tensor has proven its value in all these applications, it also holds a drawback. This becomes apparent as soon as the orientation in the local neighborhood is not homogeneous like near the boundary of two different textures or two differently moving objects. In these areas, the local neighborhood induced by the Gaussian kernel integrates ambiguous structure information that actually does not belong together and therefore leads to inaccurate estimations.

There are two alternatives to remedy this problem. One is to adapt the neighborhood to the data. A classical way of doing so is the Kuwahara-Nagao operator [2, 18, 25]. At a certain position in an image this operator searches for a nearby neighborhood where the response (the orientation) is more homogeneous than it is at the border. That response is then used at the point of interest. In this way the neighborhoods are not allowed to cross the borders of the differently oriented regions. In [36] it was shown that the classic Kuwahara-Nagao operator can be interpreted as a 'macroscopic' version of a PDE image evolution that combines linear diffusion (smoothing) with morphological sharpening (a shock filter in PDE terms). A very similar approach is to use adaptive Gaussian windows [23, 26] for choosing the local neighborhood. Also by nonlinear diffusion one can perform data-adaptive smoothing that avoids the integration of ambiguous data [7, 41].

A second possibility to enhance local orientation estimation is to keep the non-adaptive window, but to clearly choose one of the ambiguous orientations by means of robust statistics [37]. This chapter will describe both approaches and will show their performance in the most common applications also in comparison to the conventional structure tensor. Note that for a data-adaptive structure tensor to reveal any advantages, discontinuities or mixed data must play a role for the application. Some applications where this is the case are optic flow estimation, texture discrimination, and corner detection.

Chapter organization. The chapter is organized as follows. In the next section we give an overview on data-adaptive structure tensors. The approaches using robust statistics and nonlinear diffusion are described in detail and relations between methods are examined. In Sect. 2.3 – Sect. 2.5 the structure tensor is applied to optic flow estimation, texture analysis, and corner detection. Some experiments show the superiority of adaptive structure tensors in comparison to the classic structure tensor and differences between the methods. The chapter is concluded by a brief summary in Sect. 2.6.

2.2 Data-adaptive Structure Tensors

An early approach to data-adaptive structure tensors is the *gray value local structure tensor* of Nagel and Gehrke [26], which has been designed for its use in spatio-temporal optic flow estimation. Instead of using a fixed isotropic Gaussian kernel K_ρ for smoothing the structure tensor, a space-dependent Gaussian

$$G(x) = \frac{1}{\sqrt{(2\pi)^3 |\Sigma(x)|}} e^{-\frac{1}{2} x^\top \Sigma(x)^{-1} x} \tag{2.4}$$

is employed, which is parameterized by the covariance matrix $\Sigma(x)$. This covariance matrix is locally adapted to the image by setting

$$\Sigma(x) = U(x) \begin{pmatrix} \sigma_{min} + \frac{\sigma_{max}^2}{1+\sigma_{max}^2 \lambda_1(x)} & 0 & 0 \\ 0 & \sigma_{min} + \frac{\sigma_{max}^2}{1+\sigma_{max}^2 \lambda_2(x)} & 0 \\ 0 & 0 & \sigma_{min} + \frac{\sigma_{max}^2}{1+\sigma_{max}^2 \lambda_3(x)} \end{pmatrix} U^\top(x) \tag{2.5}$$

where $\lambda_i(x), i \in \{1, 2, 3\}$ are the eigenvalues of the resulting structure tensor and U holds its eigenvectors. Initially, $\Sigma(x)$ is set to an arbitrary diagonal matrix. The parameters σ_{min} and σ_{max} are for restricting the anisotropy and the size of the Gaussian. This concept of using a data-adaptive Gaussian for the convolution with the structure tensor has been further investigated in the works of Middendorf and Nagel [22, 23]. See also Chap. 3 by Nagel for the estimation of an adaptive Gaussian.

Another data-adaptive structure tensor has been proposed by Köthe [17] for the purpose of corner detection. For corner detection one uses the fact that the coherence of the orientation measured by the structure tensor becomes small when two edges meet. To achieve an accurate localization of these points, it is favorable to smooth the structure tensor mainly along edges in the image. Köthe has therefore proposed to use an hourglass-shaped filter for the convolution with the structure tensor. The orientation of the filter is thereby adapted to the orientation of the edges, so it is a data-adaptive smoothing.

Note that though the two previous structure tensors are data-adaptive, they are still linear operators, as they imply a convolution operation (which is linear) based on the initial image data. The adaptation quality can be further improved by nonlinear operators, which use the updated data in a kind of feedback loop for the adaptation. Two such nonlinear operators have been proposed for the structure tensor, firstly the concept based on robust statistics by van den Boomgaard and van de Weijer [37], and secondly the techniques based on nonlinear diffusion, proposed by Weickert and Brox [7, 41]. These methods will now be explained in more detail.

2.2.1 Structure Tensors Based on Robust Statistics

Before describing data-adaptive structure tensors based on robust statistics it will be shown that the classic structure tensor is the result of least squares estimation procedures for local orientation. For illustration consider also the texture in Fig. 2.1(a). The histogram of the gradient vectors in this texture patch is shown in Fig. 2.1(b). Let $\mathbf{v}$ be the true orientation vector of the patch, i.e. the vector perpendicular to the stripes. In an ideal image patch every gradient vector should be parallel to the orientation $\mathbf{v}$. In practice they will not be parallel. The error of a gradient vector $\mathbf{g}(\mathbf{y}) := \nabla I(\mathbf{y})$ observed in a point $\mathbf{y}$ with respect to the orientation $\mathbf{v}(\mathbf{x})$ of an image patch centered at location $\mathbf{x}$ is defined as:

$$e(\mathbf{x}, \mathbf{y}) = \|\mathbf{g}(\mathbf{y}) - (\mathbf{g}(\mathbf{y})^\top \mathbf{v}(\mathbf{x}))\mathbf{v}(\mathbf{x})\|$$

The difference $\mathbf{g}(\mathbf{y}) - (\mathbf{g}(\mathbf{y})^\top \mathbf{v}(\mathbf{x}))\mathbf{v}(\mathbf{x})$ is the projection of $\mathbf{g}$ on the normal to $\mathbf{v}$. The error $e(\mathbf{x}, \mathbf{y})$ thus measures the perpendicular distance from the gradient vector $\mathbf{g}(\mathbf{y})$ to the orientation vector $\mathbf{v}(\mathbf{x})$. Integrating the squared error over all positions $\mathbf{y}$ using a soft Gaussian aperture for the neighborhood definition we define the total error:

$$\epsilon(\mathbf{x}) = \int_\Omega e^2(\mathbf{x}, \mathbf{y}) K_\rho(\mathbf{x} - \mathbf{y}) d\mathbf{y} \tag{2.6}$$

The error measure can be rewritten as

$$\epsilon = \int_\Omega \mathbf{g}^\top \mathbf{g} K_\rho d\mathbf{y} - \int_\Omega \mathbf{v}^\top (\mathbf{g}\mathbf{g}^\top) \mathbf{v} K_\rho d\mathbf{y} \ .$$

where we have omitted the arguments of the functions. Minimizing the error thus is equivalent with maximizing

$$\int_\Omega \mathbf{v}^\top (\mathbf{g}\mathbf{g}^\top) \mathbf{v} K_\rho d\mathbf{y} \ ,$$

subject to the constraint that $\mathbf{v}^\top \mathbf{v} = 1$. Note that $\mathbf{v}$ is not dependent on $\mathbf{y}$ so that we have to maximize:

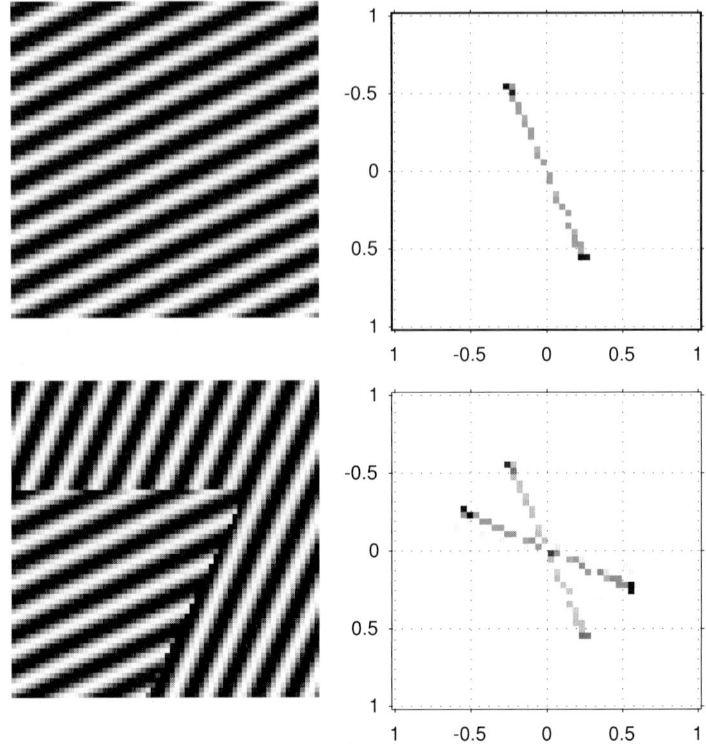

Fig. 2.1. Histograms of gradient vector space. In (**a**) an image (64×64) is shown with in (**b**) the histogram of all gradient vectors (where darker shades indicate that those gradient vectors occur more often in the image. In (**c**) a composition of two differently oriented patterns is shown with the corresponding histogram in (**d**)

$$\mathbf{v}^\top \left(\int_\Omega (\mathbf{g}\mathbf{g}^\top) K_\rho d\mathbf{y} \right) \mathbf{v} = \mathbf{v}^\top J_\rho \mathbf{v}$$

where J_ρ is the structure tensor.

Using the method of Lagrange multipliers to maximize $\mathbf{v}^\top J_\rho \mathbf{v}$ subject to the constraint that $\mathbf{v}^\top \mathbf{v} = 1$, we need to find an extremum of

$$\lambda(1 - \mathbf{v}^\top \mathbf{v}) + \mathbf{v}^\top J_\rho \mathbf{v} \ .$$

Differentiating with respect to $\mathbf{v}$ (remember that $\frac{d}{d\mathbf{v}}(\mathbf{v}^\top A \mathbf{v}) = 2A\mathbf{v}$ in case $A = A^\top$) and setting the derivative equal to zero results in:

$$J_\rho \mathbf{v} = \lambda \mathbf{v} \ . \tag{2.7}$$

The 'best' orientation thus is an eigenvector of the structure tensor J_ρ. Substitution in the quadratic form then shows that we need the eigenvector corresponding to the largest eigenvalue.

The least squares orientation estimation works well in case all gradients in the set of vectors in an image neighborhood all belong to the same oriented pattern. In case the image patch shows two oriented patterns the least squares estimate will mix the two orientations and give a wrong result.

A robust estimator is constructed by introducing the Gaussian error norm:

$$\psi(e) = 1 - \exp\left(\frac{e^2}{2m^2}\right)$$

as depicted in Fig. 2.2. In a robust estimator large deviations from the model (what is considered 'large' is determined by the value of m) are not taken into account very heavily. In our application large deviations from the model are probably due to the mixing of two different linear textures (see Fig. 2.1(c-d)).

The error, (2.6), can now be rewritten as (we will omit the spatial arguments):

$$\epsilon = \int_\Omega \psi\left(\sqrt{\mathbf{g}^\top\mathbf{g} - \mathbf{v}^\top(\mathbf{g}\mathbf{g}^\top)\mathbf{v}}\right) K_\rho d\mathbf{y}\ .$$

Again we use a Lagrange multiplier method to minimize the error subject to the constraint that $\mathbf{v}^\top\mathbf{v} = 1$:

$$\frac{d}{d\mathbf{v}}\left(\lambda(1 - \mathbf{v}^\top\mathbf{v}) + \int_\Omega \psi\left(\sqrt{\mathbf{g}^\top\mathbf{g} - \mathbf{v}^\top(\mathbf{g}\mathbf{g}^\top)\mathbf{v}}\right) K_\rho d\mathbf{y}\right) = 0\ .$$

This leads to

$$J_\rho^m(\mathbf{v})\mathbf{v} = \lambda\mathbf{v} \tag{2.8}$$

where

$$J_\rho^m(\mathbf{v}) = \int_\Omega \mathbf{g}\mathbf{g}^\top K_m(\mathbf{g}^\top\mathbf{g} - \mathbf{v}^\top(\mathbf{g}\mathbf{g}^\top)\mathbf{v})K_\rho d\mathbf{y} \tag{2.9}$$

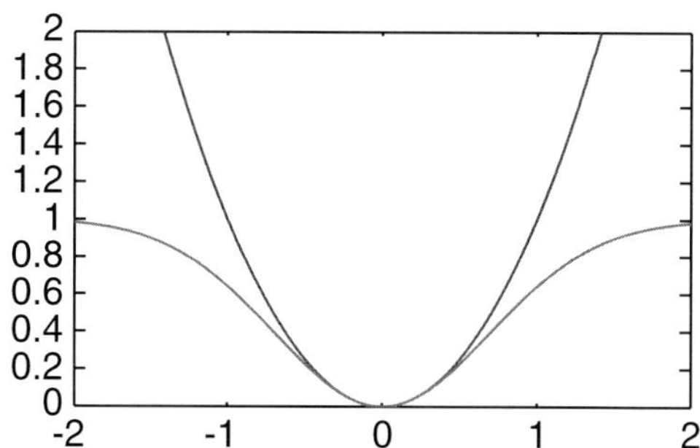

Fig. 2.2. Quadratic versus (robust) Gaussian error norm. The Gaussian error norm is of 'scale' $m = 0.7$

with $K_m(e^2) = \exp\left(e^2/2m^2\right)$. The big difference with the least squares estimator is that now the matrix $J_\rho^m(\mathbf{v})$ is dependent on $\mathbf{v}$ (and on $\mathbf{x}$ as well). Note that $J_\rho^m(\mathbf{v})$ can be called a *'robustified' structure tensor* in which the contribution of each gradient vector is weighted not only by its distance to the center point of the neighborhood, but also weighted according to its 'distance' to the orientation model.

Note that the 'robustification' of the structure tensor is dependent on the model that is fitted to the data, so there is no unique robust structure tensor. The structure tensor is a local averaging of the gradient product $\mathbf{g}\mathbf{g}^\top$, but whereas in the classical case each point in the neighborhood contributes in an equal amount to this average, in the robust formulation the weight is dependent on the plausibility of the gradient observation $\mathbf{g}$ given the model.

A *fixed point* iteration scheme is used to find a solution. Let $\mathbf{v}^i$ be the orientation vector estimate after i iterations. The estimate is then updated as the eigenvector $\mathbf{v}^{i+1}$ of the matrix $J_\rho^m(\mathbf{v}^i)$ corresponding to the largest eigenvalue, i.e. one solves:

$$J_\rho^m(\mathbf{v}^i)\mathbf{v}^{i+1} = \lambda\mathbf{v}^{i+1}$$

The proposed scheme is a generalization of the well-known fixed point scheme (also called *functional iteration*) to find a solution of the equation $v = F(v)$.

Note that the iterative scheme does not necessarily lead to the *global* minimum of the error. In fact one is often not even interested in that global minimum. Consider for instance the situation of a point in region A (with orientation α) that is surrounded by many points in region B (with orientation β). It is not too difficult to imagine a situation where the points of region B outnumber those in region A. Nevertheless the algorithm is to find the orientation α whereas the global minimum would correspond with orientation β. Because the algorithm starts in the initial orientation estimate and then finds the local minimum nearest to the starting point it hopefully ends up in the desired *local* minimum: orientation α. The choice for an initial estimate of the orientation vector is thus crucial in a robust estimator in case the image patch shows two (or more) orientations.

2.2.2 Structure Tensors Based on Nonlinear Diffusion

In the preceding subsection it has been shown that a least squares estimate of the local orientation comes down to solving an eigenvalue problem of the structure tensor smoothed with the Gaussian kernel K_ρ which determines the local neighborhood. We have also seen a more general technique than least squares that introduces an additional weighting dependent on the data. Now the question may arise if there is on the other hand also a more general smoothing approach than Gaussian convolution, and indeed there is one.

The generalization of Gaussian smoothing, which is equivalent to diffusion with a constant diffusivity, is nonlinear diffusion. In contrast to Gaussian convolution, nonlinear diffusion reduces the amount of smoothing in the presence of discontinuities in the data, so it is a data-adaptive smoothing method. Being a nonlinear approach, discontinuities are determined iteratively in the updated, smoothed data and therefore one can integrate data from an arbitrarily shaped neighborhood, as illustrated in Fig. 2.3. Thus nonlinear diffusion seems very appropriate to replace the Gaussian convolution of the classic structure tensor in order to bring in data-adaptive neighborhoods for the integration.

Nonlinear diffusion has been introduced by Perona and Malik [27]. With the initial condition $u(t = 0) = I$, the PDE

$$\partial_t u = \mathrm{div}\left(g(|\nabla u|^2)\nabla u\right) \tag{2.10}$$

evolves a scalar-valued data set, such as a gray value image, where I is the initial image. The so-called *diffusivity function* g correlates the amount of smoothing to the gradient magnitude and thereby prevents smoothing across edges. For smoothing the structure tensor, a good choice for this diffusivity function is

$$g(|\nabla u|) = \frac{1}{\sqrt{|\nabla u|^2 + \epsilon^2}} \tag{2.11}$$

where ϵ is a small positive constant only introduced in order to prevent unlimited diffusivities. Diffusion with this diffusivity is called *total variation (TV) flow* [1], which is the diffusion filter corresponding to TV regularization [32].

Since the structure tensor is not a scalar-valued but a matrix-valued data set, one needs an extension of (2.10) to matrix-valued data. Such an extension has been provided in [35]:

$$\partial_t u_{ij} = \mathrm{div}\left(g\left(\sum_{k,l=1}^{N} |\nabla u_{kl}|^2\right)\nabla u_{ij}\right) \qquad i,j = 1,\ldots,N \ . \tag{2.12}$$

Details can also be found in Chap. 25 by Weickert et al. When setting the initial condition to $u_{ij}(t = 0) = J_{0,ij}$ (cf. (2.1) and (2.2)), this PDE provides the nonlinear structure tensor J_t for some diffusion time t. Here, N is the

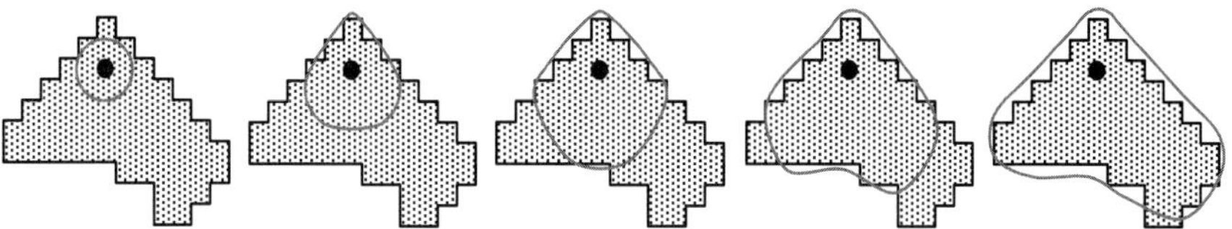

Fig. 2.3. Illustration of how the local neighborhood is adapted by an increasing amount of nonlinear diffusion

number of rows/columns of the structure tensor (which is symmetric), i.e. $N = 2$ for the spatial structure tensor and $N = 3$ for its spatio-temporal version. Note that all matrix channels are coupled in this scheme. They are smoothed with a joint diffusivity taking into account the edges of all channels. Consequently, a discontinuity in one matrix channel inhibits also smoothing in the others.

There exists also an anisotropic counterpart to this scheme, which has been introduced in [7, 41]. In the anisotropic case not only the *amount* of diffusion is adapted locally to the data but also the *direction* of smoothing. This has positive effects for instance in the application of corner detection where one is interested in smoothing mainly along edges in the image.

$$\partial_t u_{ij} = \mathrm{div} \left(D \left(\sum_{k,l=1}^{N} \nabla u_{kl} \nabla u_{kl}^{\top} \right) \nabla u_{ij} \right) \qquad i,j = 1,\ldots,N \qquad (2.13)$$

The matrix D is the so-called *diffusion tensor* that replaces the scalar-valued diffusivity g and which we define in the spatial case, where $N = 2$, as

$$D = U \begin{pmatrix} g(\lambda_1) & 0 \\ 0 & 1 \end{pmatrix} U^{\top} \qquad (2.14)$$

The diffusivity function g is the same as in the isotropic setting and λ_1 denotes the larger eigenvalue of the matrix $\sum_{i,j=1}^{N} \nabla u_{ij} \nabla u_{ij}^{\top}$ while U holds its eigenvectors. Simply speaking, the diffusion tensor reduces the amount of smoothing in gradient direction depending on the gradient magnitude, while it employs the full amount of smoothing in the direction perpendicular to the gradient. For detailed information about anisotropic diffusion in general, we refer to [38]. Anisotropic nonlinear matrix diffusion is also a topic of Chap. 25 by Weickert et al.

By applying a Gaussian convolution with a kernel K_ρ to the matrix $\sum_{k,l=1}^{N} \nabla u_{kl} \nabla u_{kl}^{\top}$ that determines the diffusion tensor D, one can even emphasize the smoothing along discontinuities in the data [40]. With such a nonlinear diffusion process, one obtains the anisotropic structure tensor $J_{t,\rho}$.

2.2.3 Relations

After the description of these approaches to data-adaptive structure tensors, one might wonder how they are related. Are they basically all the same, or are there significant differences?

Let us first consider the gray value local structure tensor of Nagel and Gehrke and the nonlinear structure tensor based on diffusion. Both methods perform a smoothing operation on the structure tensor, using a neighborhood that is adapted to the data, so one would expect that both methods do approximately the same. However, despite the similarities, there are some significant differences.

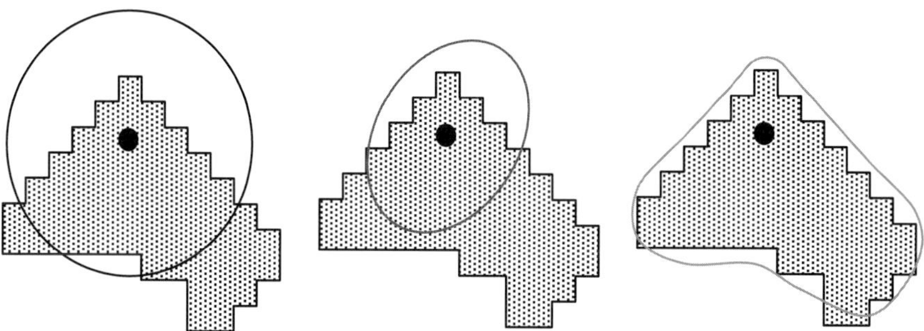

Fig. 2.4. *Left*: Neighborhood of a non-adaptive isotropic Gaussian *Center*: Neighborhood of a data-adaptive anisotropic Gaussian. *Right*: Neighborhood obtained with an iterative diffusion process

Figure 2.4 visualizes these differences between the approach of Nagel and Gehrke and the classic as well as the nonlinear structure tensor. The classic structure tensor uses a fixed isotropic Gaussian kernel for smoothing the data, thus it is not data-adaptive at all. The method proposed by Nagel and Gehrke parameterizes the neighborhood by an anisotropic Gaussian and adapts the parameters locally to the data. Although this approach is more precise than the classic structure tensor, one can see that in many situations the Gaussian cannot fully cover the region of interest without also integrating ambiguous information. The iterative diffusion process involved in the nonlinear structure tensor is more flexible and can therefore cover a neighborhood with arbitrary shape.

Furthermore, the nonlinear structure tensor is based on a nonlinear smoothing operation, i.e. the operation works on the *updated* data, while the method of Nagel and Gehrke is still a linear operation as it smooths the *initial* data.

The robust structure tensor described in Sect. 2.2.1 is also based on a nonlinear process, so let us consider its relations to the nonlinear structure tensor. From (2.9) one can see that dependent on how well the values fit to the currently estimated orientation, their influence is decreased. This is similar to the concept of the nonlinear structure tensor, where the further expansion of the local neighborhood is reduced if the new values do not fit well to the values of the current neighborhood. Note that the weighting function $\psi'(s^2)$ in (2.9) is one of the diffusivity functions used by Perona and Malik when they introduced nonlinear diffusion (cf. [27]). Thus both the nonlinear structure tensor and the robust structure tensor make the integration of further data dependent on whether it fits to the already gathered data. One can even choose the same weighting function for this selection process.

The difference between both approaches is that the nonlinear structure tensor applies this selection process in order to determine the local neighborhood and then uses a simple least squares approach within this neighborhood, while the structure tensor based on robust statistics first gathers the data from the simple fixed Gaussian neighborhood K_ρ and applies the nonlinear weighting process afterwards. Thus the nonlinear structure tensor assumes that the values needed for a good estimation are connected, whereas the robust statistics ignore the aspect of connectivity. Consequently, it can be expected that in situations where the assumption of connected data holds, the nonlinear structure tensor is better suited, while in situations where the assumption is false, robust statistics should be advantageous.

Relations between robust statistics, nonlinear diffusion, and other data-adaptive smoothing approaches are also dealt with in [24].

2.3 Optic Flow Estimation

A well-known application of the structure tensor is optic flow estimation. In optic flow estimation one searches for the displacement field $(u(x,y), v(x,y))$ that says for each pixel (x,y) of one image $I(x,y,t)$ to which position it has moved in a second image $I(x,y,t+1)$.

In Bigün et al. [4] optic flow estimation has been regarded as the search for the spatio-temporal orientation where there is the least change in the image sequence. This immediately leads to an orientation estimation problem that can be solved by computing the eigenvector $\mathbf{w} = (w_1, w_2, w_3)$ to the smallest eigenvalue of the structure tensor. The optic flow vector can then be computed by normalizing the last component of $\mathbf{w}$ to 1, which leads to $u = w_1/w_2$ and $v = w_2/w_3$.

Although this has been the first explicit usage of the structure tensor for optic flow estimation, the structure tensor is also implicitly present in the early method of Lucas and Kanade [21]. In this method the assumptions of the optic flow estimation problem become more explicit. Furthermore, the method of Lucas-Kanade is an ordinary least squares approach, while the method of Bigün estimates the flow vector by means of total least squares. For optic flow estimation in practice, it turns out that a simple least squares approach is more robust, so we will stick here to the method of Lucas-Kanade.

2.3.1 Lucas-Kanade with the Conventional Structure Tensor

The assumption that is most frequently used in optic flow estimation is the assumption that the displacement of pixels does not alter their gray values. This can be expressed by the well-known optic flow constraint (OFC) [14]

$$I_x u + I_y v + I_z = 0 . \tag{2.15}$$

The optic flow is not uniquely determined by this constraint, since this is only one equation for two flow components. This is also called the *aperture problem*. In order to obtain a unique solution, Lucas and Kanade proposed to assume the optic flow vector to be constant within some neighborhood, e.g. a Gaussian window K_ρ.

With this second assumption, it is possible to estimate the optic flow at each point by the minimizer of the local energy function

$$E(u, v) = \frac{1}{2} K_\rho * \left((I_x u + I_y v + I_z)^2 \right) . \tag{2.16}$$

A minimum (u, v) of E must satisfy $\partial_u E = 0$ and $\partial_v E = 0$, what leads to the 2×2 linear system

$$\begin{pmatrix} K_\rho * I_x^2 & K_\rho * I_x I_y \\ K_\rho * I_x I_y & K_\rho * I_y^2 \end{pmatrix} \begin{pmatrix} u \\ v \end{pmatrix} = \begin{pmatrix} -K_\rho * I_x I_z \\ -K_\rho * I_y I_z \end{pmatrix} . \tag{2.17}$$

Note that it is possible to use instead of a purely spatial neighborhood also a spatio-temporal neighborhood where the assumption of constant flow is extended to hold also over time. Since the spatio-temporal version has access to more data, it leads in general to more accurate results. However, for simplicity we considered only spatial neighborhoods in the experiments.

2.3.2 Lucas-Kanade with the Nonlinear Structure Tensor

One can easily observe that the entries of this linear system are five of the six different components of the spatio-temporal structure tensor

$$J_\rho = K_\rho * \left(\nabla I \nabla I^\top \right) = K_\rho * \begin{pmatrix} I_x^2 & I_x I_y & I_x I_z \\ I_x I_y & I_y^2 & I_y I_z \\ I_x I_z & I_y I_z & I_z^2 \end{pmatrix} . \tag{2.18}$$

Thus it is possible to replace these entries by the components of one of the data-adaptive structure tensors. Such a replacement means that the fixed neighborhood of the original method is replaced by an adaptive neighborhood which prefers those pixels that fit the assumption of constant optic flow.

As already discussed in Sect. 2.2, one can obtain a good adaptation of the neighborhood by nonlinear diffusion. Thus with the nonlinear structure tensor [7, 41] described in Sect. 2.2.2 and determined by the nonlinear diffusion process given by (2.12), the assumption of constant flow holds much more often than in the case of the conventional structure tensor. Consequently, there are less estimation errors, in particular near motion boundaries.

2.3.3 Robust Structure Tensor for Optic Flow Estimation

Compared to Sect. 2.2.1, with optic flow estimation the orientation estimation task has changed a bit. We now search for the orientation with *least* change in a *spatio-temporal* space. Since the robustified structure tensor selects the data according to how well it fits to the model, a new robust structure tensor has to be derived due to the change of the model. In order to see the relations to the derivation in Sect. 2.2.1 we adapt to the same notation and write $\mathbf{g} = \nabla I$. The optic flow vector (u, v) will be written as the estimated orientation $\mathbf{v}$. Further on, the Lucas-Kanade approach will be interpreted as a least squares estimation procedure first, before the generalized robust estimation procedure is described.

Least squares estimation. As stated above, the optic flow constraint (2.15) has two unknowns: the two components of the optic flow vector $\mathbf{v}$, and a way to get an expression for a unique solution for $\mathbf{v}$ is to come up with more equations each describing the same vector $\mathbf{v}$. This is achieved with the assumption of Lucas-Kanade that within a local neighborhood of a point $\mathbf{x}$ the optical flow vector is constant. Like in Sect. 2.2.1 a Gaussian aperture is selected to define the local neighborhood. Let $\mathbf{v}(\mathbf{x})$ be the optical flow vector at $\mathbf{x}$ then the error towards the optic flow constraint is given as:

$$\epsilon(\mathbf{x}) = \int_\Omega \left(I_z(\mathbf{y}) + \mathbf{v}(\mathbf{x}) \cdot \mathbf{g}(\mathbf{y})\right)^2 K_\rho(\mathbf{x} - \mathbf{y}) d\mathbf{y} \qquad (2.19)$$

If we now select the vector $\mathbf{v}^*$ that minimizes the above expression then the OFC expression $I_z + \mathbf{v} \cdot \mathbf{g}$ is minimized on average in the local neighborhood of a point $\mathbf{x}$:

$$\mathbf{v}^* = \mathrm{argmin}_{\mathbf{v}} \epsilon(\mathbf{x})$$

The optimal value is found by solving for $\mathrm{d}_v \epsilon = 0$:

$$\mathrm{d}_v \epsilon = 2 \int_\Omega \left(I_z(\mathbf{y}) + \mathbf{v}(\mathbf{x}) \cdot \mathbf{g}(\mathbf{y})\right) \mathbf{g}(\mathbf{y}) K_\rho(\mathbf{x} - \mathbf{y}) d\mathbf{y}$$

Here we use the convention used throughout this chapter that the integration of a matrix/vector equation is to be done for each of the matrix/vector components individually. Consider the term $(\mathbf{v} \cdot \mathbf{g})\mathbf{g}$, where we have omitted the spatial arguments for clarity. This can be rewritten as $(\mathbf{g}\mathbf{g}^\top)\mathbf{v}$. Note that $\mathbf{g}\mathbf{g}^\top$ is a 2×2 matrix which, when integrated over a spatial neighborhood, is the structure tensor $J(\mathbf{x})$. Using this we can rewrite the above equation as:

$$\left(\int_\Omega \mathbf{g}(\mathbf{y})\mathbf{g}^\top(\mathbf{y}) \, K_\rho(\mathbf{x} - \mathbf{y}) d\mathbf{y}\right) \mathbf{v}(\mathbf{x}) = - \int_\Omega I_z(\mathbf{y}) \, \mathbf{g}(\mathbf{y}) \, K_\rho(\mathbf{x} - \mathbf{y}) d\mathbf{y} \quad (2.20)$$

or

$$J(\mathbf{x})\mathbf{v}(\mathbf{x}) = - \int_\Omega I_z(\mathbf{y}) \, \mathbf{g}(\mathbf{y}) \, K_\rho(\mathbf{x} - \mathbf{y}) d\mathbf{y}$$

After integration the structure tensor can be assumed to be non-singular and thus:

$$\mathbf{v}(\mathbf{x}) = -J^{-1}(\mathbf{x}) \int_\Omega I_z(\mathbf{y}) \, \mathbf{g}(\mathbf{y}) \, K_\rho(\mathbf{x} - \mathbf{y}) d\mathbf{y}$$

This is the well-known linear least squares estimator of the optical flow vector. Like many local structure calculations it suffers from the fact that *all* points in the neighborhood are used in the calculation. At motion boundaries the above expression is known to give the wrong answers.

Robust estimation. Robustifying optical flow calculations can be found e.g. in [5]. Here we emphasize that a robust estimator of the optical flow vector nicely fits into the framework for robust local structure calculations as set up in this chapter.

The squared error of (2.19) is replaced with a robust error measure:

$$\epsilon(\mathbf{x}) = \int_{\Omega} \psi\left(I_z(\mathbf{y}) + \mathbf{v}(\mathbf{x}) \cdot \mathbf{g}(\mathbf{y})\right) K_\rho(\mathbf{x} - \mathbf{y})d\mathbf{y} \qquad (2.21)$$

leading to the following expression for the derivative $\mathrm{d}_{\mathbf{v}}\epsilon$:

$$\mathrm{d}_{\mathbf{v}}\epsilon = \int_{\Omega} \psi'\left(I_z(\mathbf{y}) + \mathbf{v}(\mathbf{x})\,\mathbf{g}(\mathbf{y})\right) \mathbf{g}(\mathbf{y})\, K_\rho(\mathbf{x} - \mathbf{y})d\mathbf{y}$$

Like in Sect. 2.2.1 we select the Gaussian error norm for ψ, leading to:

$$\mathrm{d}_{\mathbf{v}}\epsilon = \int_{\Omega} \frac{I_z(\mathbf{y}) + \mathbf{v}(\mathbf{x}) \cdot \mathbf{g}(\mathbf{y})}{m^2} \exp\left(-\frac{(I_z(\mathbf{y}) + \mathbf{v}(\mathbf{x}) \cdot \mathbf{g}(\mathbf{y}))^2}{2m^2}\right) \mathbf{g}(\mathbf{y}) K_\rho(\mathbf{x}-\mathbf{y})d\mathbf{y}$$

This can be rewritten as:

$$\mathrm{d}_{\mathbf{v}}\epsilon = \int_{\Omega} \left(I_z(\mathbf{y}) + \mathbf{v}(\mathbf{x}) \cdot \mathbf{g}(\mathbf{y})\right)\mathbf{g}(\mathbf{y})K_m(I_z(\mathbf{y}) + \mathbf{v}(\mathbf{x}) \cdot \mathbf{g}(\mathbf{y}))K_\rho(\mathbf{x} - \mathbf{y})d\mathbf{y}$$

Solving for $\mathrm{d}_{\mathbf{v}}\epsilon = 0$ we obtain:

$$\left(\int_{\Omega} \mathbf{g}(\mathbf{y})\mathbf{g}(\mathbf{y})^\top K_m(\ldots)K_\rho(\mathbf{x} - \mathbf{y})d\mathbf{y}\right) \mathbf{v}$$

$$= -\int_{\Omega} I_z(\mathbf{y})\,\mathbf{g}(\mathbf{y})K_m(\ldots)K_\rho(\mathbf{x} - \mathbf{y})d\mathbf{y}$$

Compared with the linear least squares estimator, a new term $K_m(\ldots)$ has been added that can be interpreted as the *model error penalty*. This equation is the 'robustified' equivalent of 2.20.

Again we obtain a 'robustified' structure tensor. Carefully note that the model error penalty term is different from the one we have derived in a previous section where we looked for the local orientation of *maximum* change in a purely *spatial* neighborhood. Here we arrive at the equation

$$J_\rho^m(\mathbf{v})\mathbf{v} = \mathbf{l}(\mathbf{v})$$

where

$$J_\rho^m(\mathbf{v}) = \int_{\Omega} \mathbf{g}(\mathbf{y})\mathbf{g}(\mathbf{y})^\top K_m(I_z(\mathbf{y}) + \mathbf{v}(\mathbf{x}) \cdot \mathbf{g}(\mathbf{y}))K_\rho(\mathbf{x} - \mathbf{y})d\mathbf{y}$$

and

$$\mathbf{l}(\mathbf{v}) = - \int_\Omega I_z(\mathbf{y})\, \mathbf{g}(\mathbf{y}) K_m(\dots) K_\rho(\mathbf{x} - \mathbf{y}) d\mathbf{y} \ .$$

And again we can solve this through a fixed point procedure:

$$\mathbf{v}^{i+1} = - \left(J_\rho^m\right)^{-1}(\mathbf{v}^i)\mathbf{l}(v^i)$$

with $\mathbf{v}^0$ some initial estimate of the optical flow vector (the linear least squares estimate is an obvious choice for this).

2.3.4 Adapting the Neighborhood with a Coherence Measure

As stated above, the assumption of constant flow field over a neighborhood is used in order to disambiguate the optic flow constraint equation. This leads to the idea that diffusion should be reduced at those areas where the aperture problem is already reasonably solved [19]. In regions with non-constant smooth motion fields, this will avoid oversmoothing the tensor field and then preserve small motion differences. The aperture problem is solved as soon as the two larger eigenvalues of the structure tensor are large enough compared to the smallest one, i.e. that the ellipsoid associated to the tensor is flat. In order to quantify the flatness of a tensor, we use a slightly changed version of the *coherence* or *corner* measure proposed in [13]:

$$c_m(J) = \left(\frac{\lambda_1 - \lambda_3}{\lambda_1 + \lambda_3 + \epsilon}\right)^2 - \left(\frac{\lambda_1 - \lambda_2}{\lambda_1 + \lambda_2 + \epsilon}\right)^2 \tag{2.22}$$

where $\lambda_1 \geq \lambda_2 \geq \lambda_3 \geq 0$ are the eigenvalues of the structure tensor J and ϵ is a small positive constant for regularization purposes. If $\lambda_2 \approx \lambda_3$, this measure yields a value close to 0, while if $\lambda_1 \approx \lambda_2 > \lambda_3$, the value is close to 1. This measure can be use to steer the diffusion of the structure tensor through a matrix-valued nonlinear diffusion scheme, written in a continuous formulation as

$$\partial_t J_{ij} = \text{div}\ (g(c_m)\nabla J_{ij}) \tag{2.23}$$

where g is decreasing, $g(0) = 1$, $g(1) = 0$. Note that the continuous formulation is problematic if g is not smooth. However, an associated discrete scheme will be generally well defined. It can be written as

$$J_s^{n+1} = J_s^n + \tau \sum_{r \in N(s)} \beta_r g\left(c_m(J_r^n + J_s^n)\right)\left(J_r^n - J_s^n\right) \tag{2.24}$$

where $s = (i, j)$ denotes a image location (and not the tensor component), $N(s)$ a discrete neighborhood, τ an evolution step and the β_r are positive values that depend on the neighborhood (but not on the tensors), with reflecting boundary conditions. The diffusivity function used here

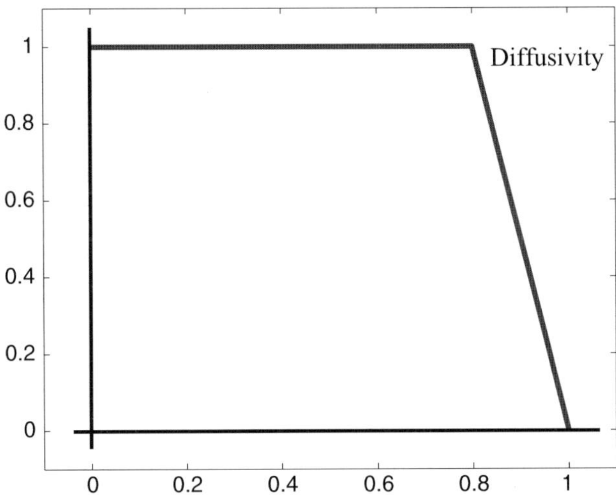

Fig. 2.5. The diffusivity function $g(c_m)$

$$g(c_m) = \begin{cases} 1 & \text{if } c_m < \alpha - \eta \\ (\alpha + \eta - c_m)/2\eta & \text{if } \alpha - \eta \leq c_m < \alpha - \eta \\ 0 & \text{if } c_m \geq \alpha - \eta \end{cases} \qquad (2.25)$$

is depicted in Fig. 2.5. The thresholds α and η have been set respectively to 0.9 and 0.1 in the experiments. This diffusion is an alteration of the linear diffusion and possesses the same stability properties. It behaves well in presence of small structures with high curvatures, but has the same drawback that the linear diffusion with respect to motion discontinuities. Indeed, as it can be seen from the discrete formulation (2.24), if J_s and J_r are neighboring tensors with different orientations, their sum will become isotropic and their coherence measure small, so a maximal diffusivity of 1 will be assigned in the corresponding term of (2.24).

2.3.5 Comparison

Figures 2.6–2.8 shows three well-known test sequences for optic flow estimation and the results obtained with the methods described above[1]. The visualization of both the orientation and the magnitude of the flow vector is achieved by using color plots where the hue is determined by the orientation and the intensity corresponds to the magnitude of the flow vector.

---

[1] The Yosemite sequence with clouds was created by Lynn Quam and is available at `ftp://ftp.csd.uwo.ca/pub/vision`. The version without clouds is available at `http://www.cs.brown.edu/people/black/images.html`. The original, uncropped, street sequence has been published in [11] and is available at `http://www.cs.otago.ac.nz/research/vision`.

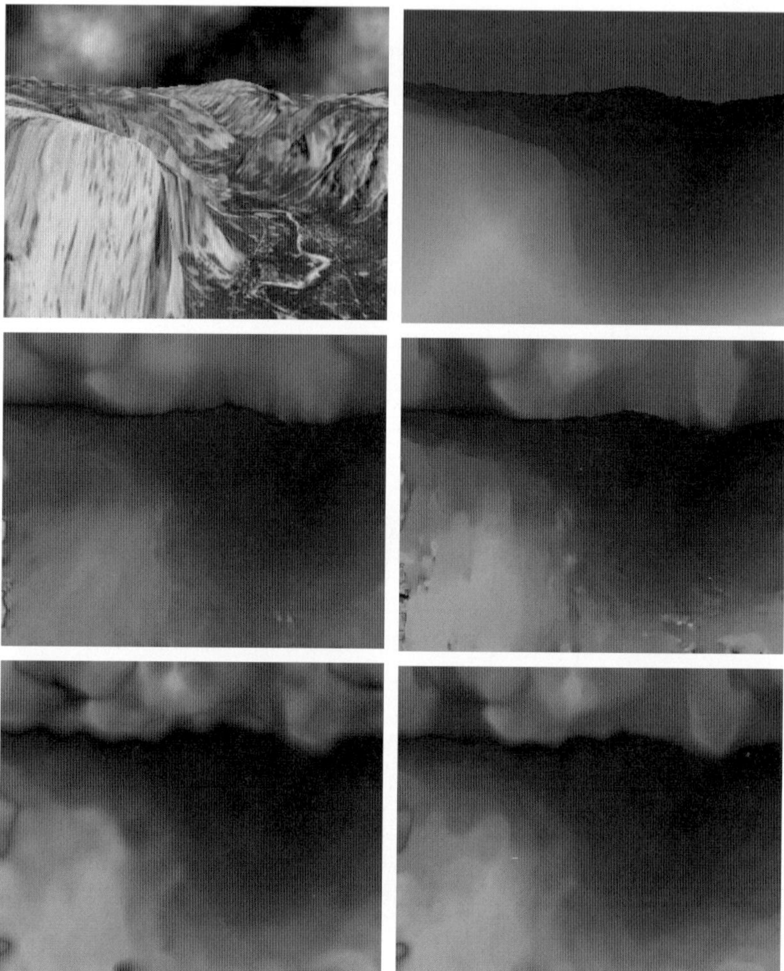

Fig. 2.6. Yosemite sequence ($316 \times 252 \times 15$). From *Left* to *Right*, *Top* to *Bottom*: (**a**) Frame 8. (**b**) Ground truth. (**c**) Classic structure tensor. (**d**) Nonlinear structure tensor. (**e**) Robust structure tensor. (**f**) Coherence based smoothing. See colour plates

In all sequences, one can see a clear qualitative difference between the Lucas-Kanade method based on the classical structure tensor and the methods based on its data-adaptive versions. While the classic structure tensor causes blurring artifacts at motion discontinuities, leading to bad estimates in these areas, the data-adaptive structure tensors avoid mixing the data from the different regions and therefore yield much more accurate results.

For the test sequences used here, there is also the ground truth available, so it becomes possible to compare the methods by a quantitative measure. The standard measure used in the literature is the average angular error (AAE)

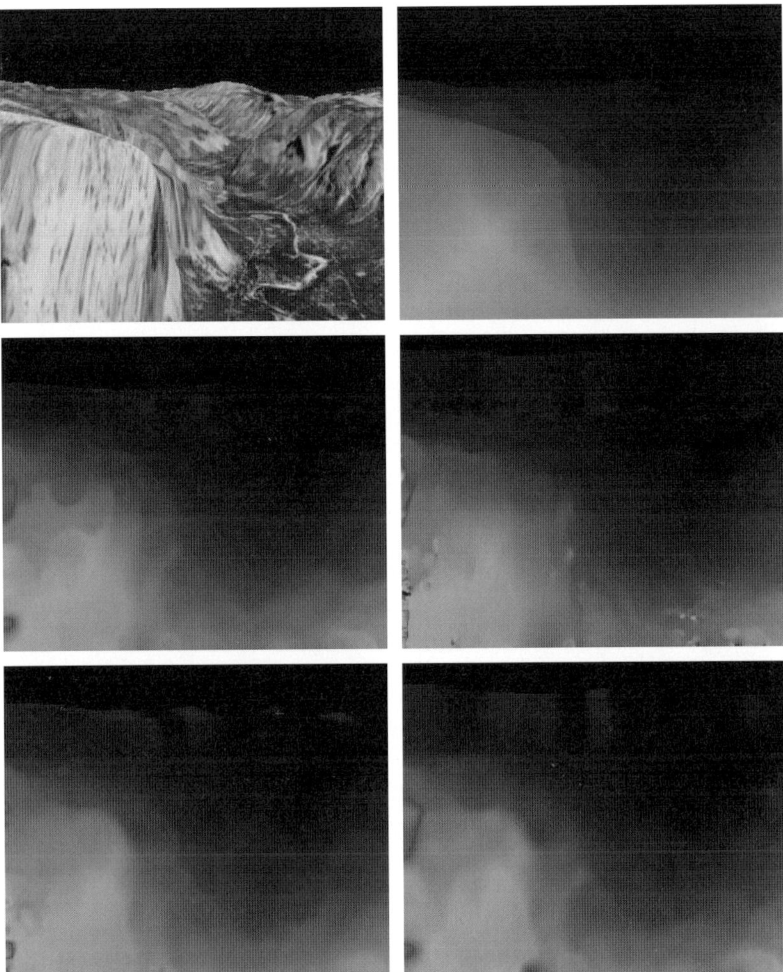

Fig. 2.7. Yosemite sequence without clouds ($316 \times 252 \times 15$). From *Left* to *Right*, *Top* to *Bottom*: (**a**) Frame 8. (**b**) Ground truth. (**c**) Classic structure tensor. (**d**) Nonlinear structure tensor. (**e**) Robust structure tensor. (**f**) Coherence based smoothing. See colour plates

introduced in [3]. Given the estimated flow field (u_e, v_e) and ground truth (u_c, v_c), the AAE is defined as

$$
aae = \frac{1}{N} \sum_{i=1}^{N} \arccos \left(\frac{u_{ci} u_{ei} + v_{ci} v_{ei} + 1}{\sqrt{(u_{ci}^2 + v_{ci}^2 + 1)(u_{ei}^2 + v_{ei}^2 + 1)}} \right) \qquad (2.26)
$$

where N is the total number of pixels. Against its indication, this quality measure not only measures the angular error between the estimated flow vector

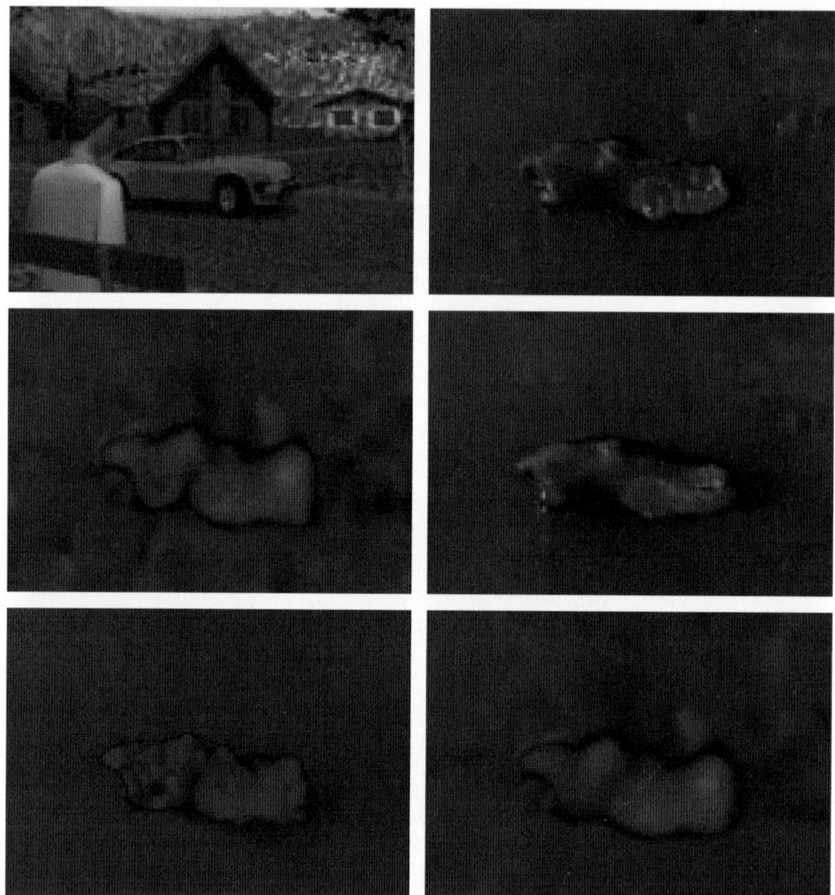

Fig. 2.8. Street sequence (cropped) ($145 \times 100 \times 20$). From *Left* to *Right*, *Top* to *Bottom*: (**a**) Frame 10. (**b**) Ground truth. (**c**) Classic structure tensor. (**d**) Nonlinear structure tensor. (**e**) Robust structure tensor. (**f**) Coherence based smoothing. See colour plates

and the correct vector, but also differences in the magnitude of both vectors, since it measures the angular error of the *spatio-temporal* vector $(u, v, 1)$.

Table 2.1 compares the errors of the different methods. It can be observed that all data-adaptive approaches show a higher performance than the conventional method in all sequences. Between the data-adaptive methods there are some differences, however, there is no clear winner.

Table 2.1. Comparison between results. In all cases the flow fields are dense. AAE = average angular error

Yosemite sequence without clouds.

Technique	AAE
Classic structure tensor	$3.80°$
Nonlinear structure tensor	$3.74°$
Robust structure tensor	$3.21°$
Coherence based structure tensor	$3.43°$

Yosemite sequence with clouds.

Technique	AAE
Classic structure tensor	$8.78°$
Nonlinear structure tensor	$7.67°$
Robust structure tensor	$8.01°$
Coherence based structure tensor	$8.21°$

Street sequence.

Technique	AAE
Classic structure tensor	$10.54°$
Nonlinear structure tensor	$7.75°$
Robust structure tensor	$7.08°$
Coherence based structure tensor	$9.79°$

2.4 Texture Analysis

2.4.1 Robust Orientation Estimation

An important property of texture is its dominant orientation. In Sect. 2.2.1 it was shown that the dominant orientation of an line pattern can be estimated using a linear least squares estimator. The resulting orientation turns out to be the eigenvector of the structure tensor belonging to the largest eigenvalue.

In Fig. 2.9(a) an oriented pattern is shown and in (b) the scatter diagram of the gradient vectors observed at small scale in a neighborhood in the image at the border of the two differently oriented regions. It is evident that a least squares estimator cannot distinguish between the two oriented patterns and will 'smooth' the orientation.

A robust estimation of orientation greatly improves this. We start again with the estimator for the orientation that is based on the error measure as given in (2.6):

$$\epsilon = \int_{\Omega} K_\rho \, \psi(\sqrt{\mathbf{g} - (\mathbf{g}^\top \mathbf{v})\mathbf{v}})d\mathbf{x}$$

where we have replaced the quadratic error norm with a robust error norm ψ. The local orientation is then found by minimizing the above error measure for $\mathbf{v}$ under the constraint that $\mathbf{v}^\top \mathbf{v} = 1$. Using a Lagrange multiplier we have to minimize $\epsilon + \lambda(1 - \mathbf{v}^\top \mathbf{v})$. Setting $\partial \epsilon / \partial \mathbf{v} = 0$ and solving for $\mathbf{v}$ we arrive at:

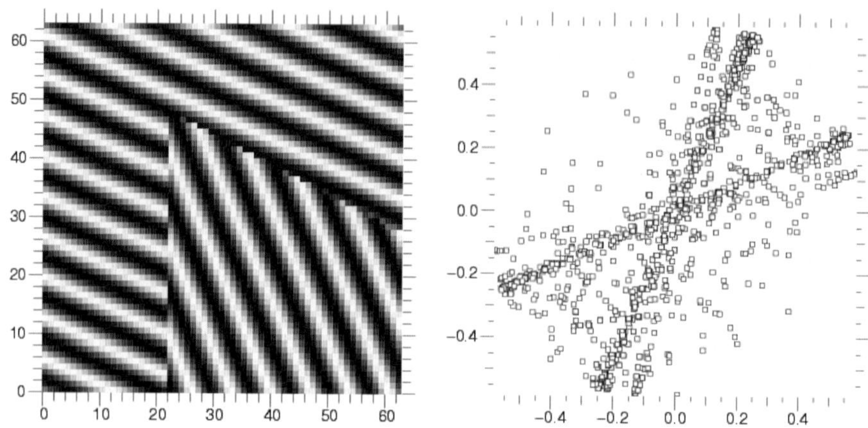

Fig. 2.9. Gradient histogram with two differently oriented textures

$$J_\rho^m(\mathbf{v})\mathbf{v} = \lambda\mathbf{v}$$

where

$$J_\rho^m(\mathbf{v}) = \int_\Omega \mathbf{g}\mathbf{g}^\top K_m(\mathbf{g} - (\mathbf{g}^\top\mathbf{v})\mathbf{v})K_\rho d\mathbf{x}$$

is the 'robustified' structure tensor. Note that the structure tensor $J_\rho^m(\mathbf{v})$ depends on the orientation $\mathbf{v}$ and thus we have to solve for the optimal orientation in an iterative fixed point manner. Starting with an initial estimate $\mathbf{v}^0$, calculate the structure tensor $J_\rho^m(\mathbf{v}^0)$ and calculate a new orientation estimate as the eigenvector of largest eigenvalue. This iterative procedure in practice needs very few iterations to converge (typically 3 to 5 iterations).

In Fig. 2.10 the robust orientation estimation is compared with the linear least squares estimation. It can be clearly observed that whereas the linear estimator 'gently' changes from the one orientation to the second, the robust estimator shows a sharp transition. A pattern with only slight variation in orientation is shown in Fig. 2.11. Again the robust estimator is capable of clearly detecting the edges between areas of different orientation.

2.4.2 Texture Segmentation

The three different components of the structure tensor can also directly be integrated as features into a segmentation method, like the one proposed in [6, 31]. This segmentation framework computes a two region segmentation given a suitable feature vector. In our case this is the vector composed of the three different components of the structure tensor and the image gray value. The components of the structure tensor are normalized to the same range as the image gray value in order to ensure a fair weighting between the

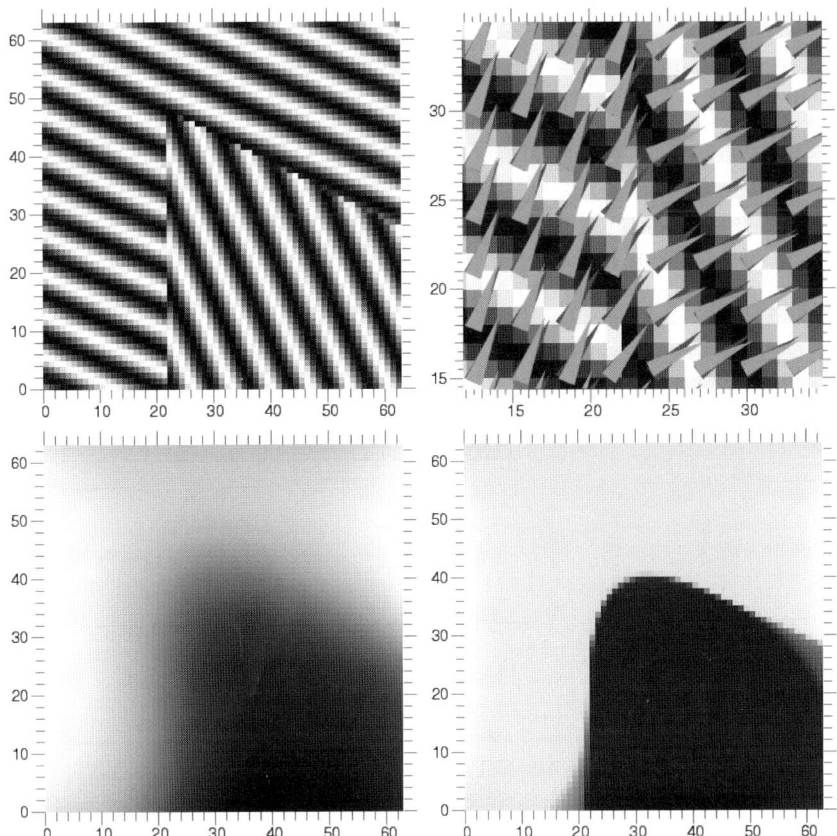

Fig. 2.10. Comparison between least squares and robust orientation estimation. See also colour plates

channels. Figure 2.12 reveals that with a data-adaptive approach, the segmentation can benefit from the reduced blurring effects in the feature channels and yields a higher accuracy at region boundaries. Note that although the components of the nonlinear structure tensor look almost unsmoothed, there is some smoothing that provides the dominant orientation also in the gaps between the stripes. For comparison, the segmentation result obtained with the unsmoothed structure tensor J_0 is depicted in Fig. 2.13.

2.5 Corner Detection

When looking for some important, distinguished locations of an image, one often considers points where two or more edges meet. Such locations have been named *corners* or *interest points*, and a range of possible approaches

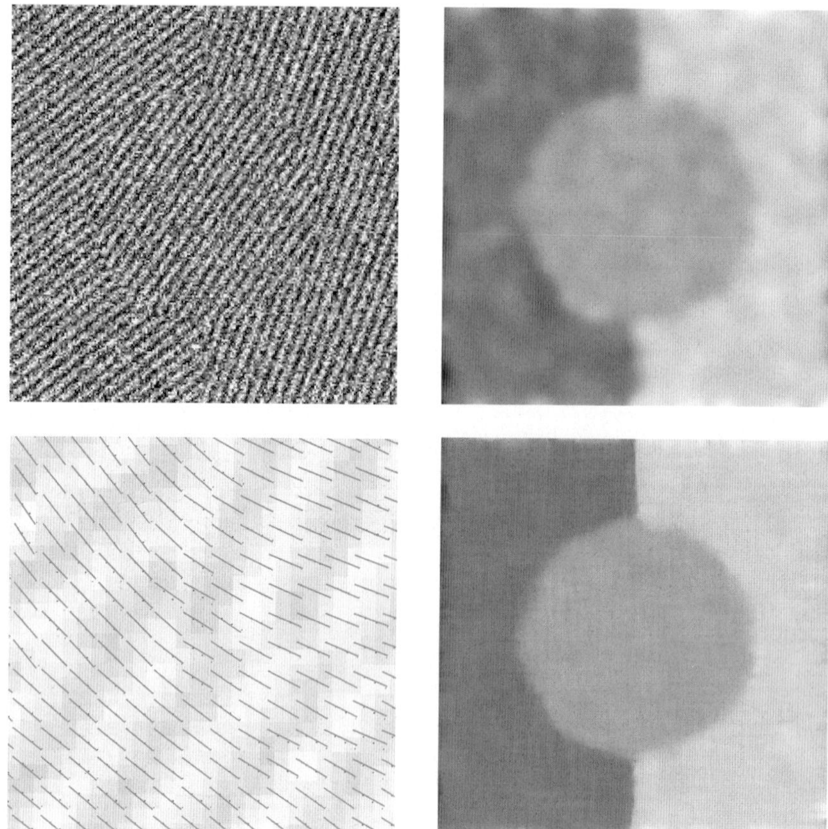

Fig. 2.11. Comparison between least squares and robust orientation estimation. See also colour plates

exists to detect them in an image, see e.g. the reviews in [30, 33]. Methods based on the structure tensor are well established in this field.

For detecting corners, the coherence information present in the structure tensor after integration is exploited. At zero integration scale, the structure tensor J_0 as introduced in (2.1) or (2.2) contains information on intrinsically 1-dimensional features of the image, i.e. edges. For gray-scale images, only one eigenvalue of the structure tensor J_0 may attain nonzero values (equal to the squared gradient magnitude), while its corresponding eigenvector represents the gradient direction.

Two-dimensional features of an image (corners) can be detected after integrating the local 1-D information of J_0 within some neighborhood, since the consideration of a local neighborhood makes additional information: that of the homogeneity, or coherence, of the surrounding orientation. If two differently oriented edges appear in the neighborhood, the smoothed structure

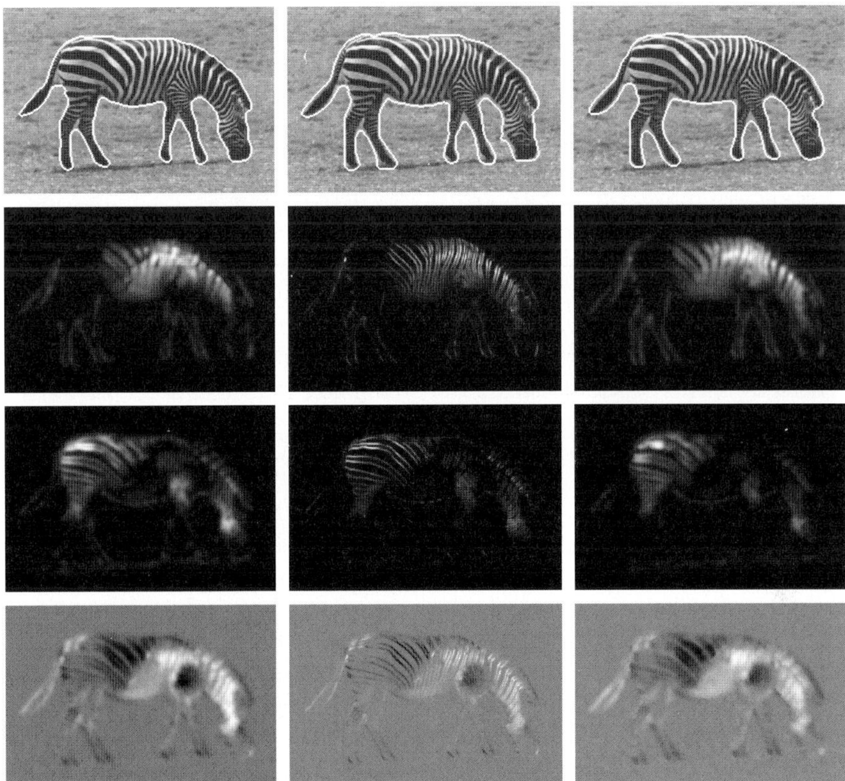

Fig. 2.12. *Left Column:* Segmentation with the classic structure tensor ($\rho = 2$). *Center Column:* Segmentation with the nonlinear structure tensor ($t = 25$). *Right Column:* Segmentation with the robust structure tensor ($\rho = 3$, $m = 0.05$). *From Top to Bottom.* (**a**) Segmented image (250×167). (**b**) Tensor component J_{11} based on I_x^2. (**c**) J_{22} based on I_y^2. (**d**) J_{12} based on $I_x I_y$

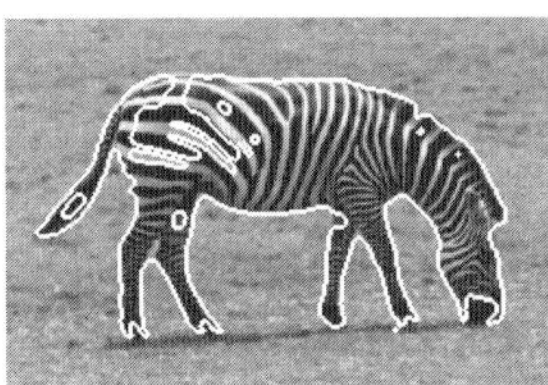

Fig. 2.13. Segmentation with the unsmoothed structure tensor J_0

tensor J will possess two nonzero eigenvalues λ_1, λ_2. An analysis of the eigenvalues can serve as a measure for the coherence of the surrounding structure. Three cases can be distinguished when regarding the eigenvalues $\lambda_1 \geq \lambda_2$ of the matrix:

- $\lambda_1 \approx \lambda_2 \approx 0$: homogeneous areas, almost no structure present

42   T. Brox et al.

- $\lambda_1 > 0, \lambda_2 \approx 0$: edges, one dominant orientation
- $\lambda_1 > 0, \lambda_2 > 0$: corners, structure with ambiguous orientation

Several possibilities have been proposed to convert this information into a coherence measure or a measure of 'cornerness', e.g. by Förstner [9], Harris and Stephens [12], Rohr [29], or Köthe [17]. In our experiments on corner detection we employ the last approach, and detect corners at local maxima of the smaller eigenvalue of the smoothed structure tensor.

One should note that for this application of the structure tensor, it is necessary to allow the integration of ambiguous orientation, because one searches for exactly the points where these ambiguities attain a maximum. This is completely contrary to orientation estimation where ambiguities are to be avoided. It therefore seems contradictive on the first glance that a data-adaptive structure tensor could perform better than the classic one on this task. Indeed, the structure tensor based on robust statistics is not applicable here, since it uses the same neighborhood as the classic structure tensor but selects the weighting of the pixels in order to *minimize* the ambiguities.

With the nonlinear structure tensor, however, the situation is a bit different. The nonlinear diffusion process does not select the pixels in order to minimize the ambiguities, but it selects the neighborhood. Thus ambiguities in the orientation, though they are reduced, can still appear. Since the neighborhood is better adapted to the structures in the image, this even leads to advantages in comparison to the classic structure tensor, see Fig. 2.15 and Fig. 2.16. Corners remain well localized even for higher diffusion times when any possible noise or small-scale features would have been removed.

The better concept of data-adaptive smoothing in the case of corner detection, however, is the nonlinear diffusion process stated in (2.13). The anisotropic diffusion process propagates information along the edges. This leads to a very precise maximum in the second eigenvalue of the structure tensor at the position where two edges meet, see Fig. 2.15. A small diffusion time already suffices to produce significant corner features which are well localized. In Fig. 2.16 it can be observed that this kind of smoothing leads to the best performance.

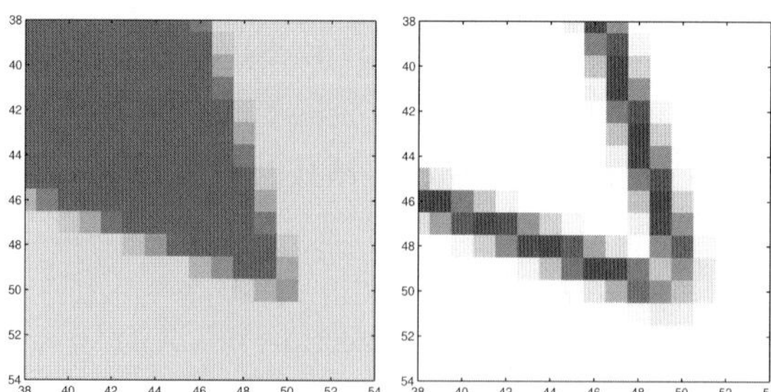

Fig. 2.14. *Left*: Detail of a test image with ideal corner position $(50, 50)$. *Right*: Larger eigenvalue of the unsmoothed structure tensor J_0

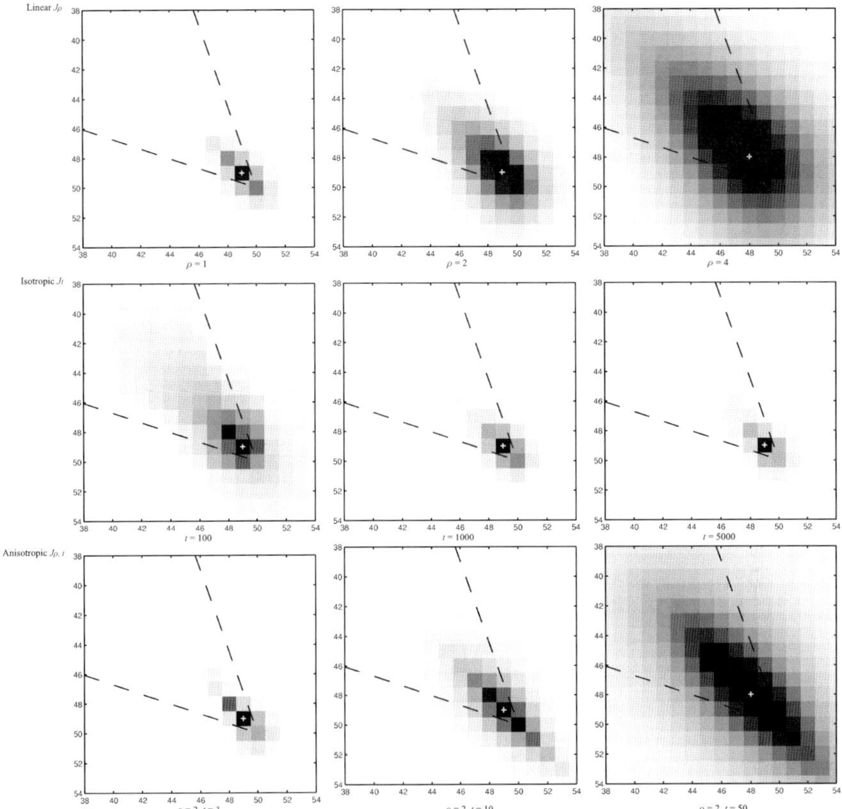

Fig. 2.15. Cornerness measured by the smaller eigenvalue of a smoothed structure tensor J, and the detected corner. *Top*: Linear smoothing. *Center*: Isotropic nonlinear diffusion with TV diffusivity. *Bottom*: Anisotropic nonlinear diffusion

It is also very closely related to the data-adaptive structure tensor proposed by Köthe [17]. In order to detect corners, Köthe also smoothes along edges, in his case using a linear, hourglass-shaped filter. This filter as well propagates information along edges and leads to a maximum in the second eigenvalue of the structure tensor at the position where edges meet.

2.6 Summary

In this chapter, we have juxtaposed several concepts for data-adaptive structure tensors. It has emerged that though the different techniques have the same basic motivation, there are quite important differences in detail. All data-adaptive structure tensors discussed here are to deal with the inaccuracies and blurring artifacts caused by the Gaussian neighborhood of the

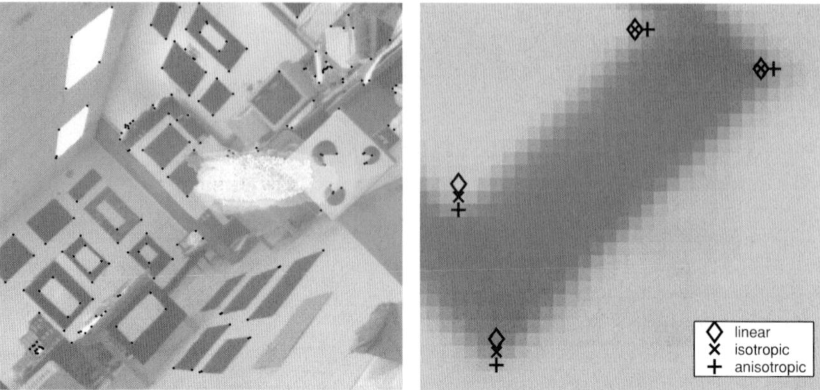

Fig. 2.16. *Left*: Corners detected in the 'lab' test image using the nonlinear structure tensor with anisotropic diffusion. *Right*: Comparison of the corners detected by the classic linear structure tensor and the nonlinear structure tensor with an underlying isotropic and anisotropic diffusion process, respectively

conventional structure tensor. However, the strategies how to choose an adaptive neighborhood are different. In some typical applications of the structure tensor, the data-adaptive structure tensors have shown their beneficial properties in comparison to the classic structure tensor. The differences between the data-adaptive structure tensors have been sometimes marginal, sometimes larger, depending on the application. This yields two messages: firstly, compared to the conventional structure tensor, the data-adaptive methods are in many cases worth the additional effort. Secondly, it is wise to choose a data-adaptive technique depending on the application. There is no clear winner that always performs better than the other techniques.

Acknowledgements

Our research was partly funded by the DFG project WE 2602/1-1 and the project *Relations between Nonlinear Filters in Digital Image Processing* within the DFG Priority Program 1114. This is gratefully acknowledged.

References

1. F. Andreu, C. Ballester, V. Caselles, and J. M. Mazón. Minimizing total variation flow. *Differential and Integral Equations*, 14(3):321–360, March 2001.
2. P. Bakker, L.J. van Vliet, and P.W. Verbeek. Edge preserving orientation adaptive filtering. In M. Boasson, J.A. Kaandorp, J.F.M. Tonino, and M.G. Vosselman, editors, *ASCI'99, Proc. 5th Annual Conference of the Advanced School for Computing and Imaging*, pp. 207–213, 1999.

3. J. L. Barron, D. J. Fleet, and S. S. Beauchemin. Performance of optical flow techniques. *International Journal of Computer Vision*, 12(1):43–77, February 1994.
4. J. Bigün, G. H. Granlund, and J. Wiklund. Multidimensional orientation estimation with applications to texture analysis and optical flow. *IEEE Transactions on Pattern Analysis and Machine Intelligence*, 13(8):775–790, August 1991.
5. M. J. Black and P. Anandan. The robust estimation of multiple motions: parametric and piecewise smooth flow fields. *Computer Vision and Image Understanding*, 63(1):75–104, January 1996.
6. T. Brox, M. Rousson, R. Deriche, and J. Weickert. Unsupervised segmentation incorporating colour, texture, and motion. Technical Report 4760, INRIA Sophia-Antipolis, France, March 2003.
7. T. Brox, J. Weickert, B. Burgeth, and P. Mrázek. Nonlinear structure tensors. Technical report, Dept. of Mathematics, Saarland University, Saarbrücken, Germany, July 2004.
8. S. Di Zenzo. A note on the gradient of a multi-image. *Computer Vision, Graphics and Image Processing*, 33:116–125, 1986.
9. W. Förstner. A feature based corresponding algorithm for image matching. *International Archive of Photogrammetry and Remote Sensing*, 26:150–166, 1986.
10. W. Förstner and E. Gülch. A fast operator for detection and precise location of distinct points, corners and centres of circular features. In *Proc. ISPRS Intercommission Conference on Fast Processing of Photogrammetric Data*, pp. 281–305, Interlaken, Switzerland, June 1987.
11. B. Galvin, B. McCane, K. Novins, D. Mason, and S. Mills. Recovering motion fields: an analysis of eight optical flow algorithms. In *Proc. 1998 British Machine Vision Conference*, Southampton, England, September 1998.
12. C. G. Harris and M. Stephens. A combined corner and edge detector. In *Proc. Fouth Alvey Vision Conference*, pp. 147–152, Manchester, England, August 1988.
13. H. Haußecker and H. Spies. Motion. In B. Jähne, H. Haußecker, and P. Geißler, editors, *Handbook on Computer Vision and Applications. Vol. 2: Signal Processing and Pattern Recognition*, pp. 309–396. Academic Press, San Diego, 1999.
14. B. Horn and B. Schunck. Determining optical flow. *Artificial Intelligence*, 17:185–203, 1981.
15. B. Jähne. *Spatio-Temporal Image Processing*, volume 751 of *Lecture Notes in Computer Science*. Springer, Berlin, 1993.
16. M. Kass and A. Witkin. Analyzing oriented patterns. *Computer Graphics and Image Processing*, 37:363–385, 1987.
17. U. Köthe. Edge and junction detection with an improved structure tensor. In B. Michaelis and G. Krell, editors, *Pattern Recognition. 25th DAGM Symposium*, number 2781 in Lecture Notes in Computer Science, pp. 25–32, Berlin, 2003. Springer.
18. M. Kuwahara, K. Hachimura, S. Eiho, and M. Kinoshita. Processing of ri-angiocardiographic images. In K. Preston and M. Onoe, editors, *Digital Processing of Biomedical Images*, pp. 187–202, 1976.
19. F. Lauze, P. Kornprobst, C. Lenglet, R. Deriche, and M. Nielsen. About some optical flow methods from structure tensors: review and contribution. In *RFIA 2004, Actes du 14e Congrès Francophone AFRIF-AFIA*, volume 1, pp. 283–292, Toulouse, January 2004. LAAS-CNRS. In French.

20. T. Lindeberg and J. Garding. Shape from texture from a multi-scale perspective. In *Proc. 4th International Conference on Computer Vision*, pp. 683–691, Berlin, Germany, May 1993.

21. B. Lucas and T. Kanade. An iterative image registration technique with an application to stereo vision. In *Proc. Seventh International Joint Conference on Artificial Intelligence*, pp. 674–679, Vancouver, Canada, August 1981.

22. M. Middendorf and H.-H. Nagel. Estimation and interpretation of discontinuities in optical flow fields. In *Proc. Eighth International Conference on Computer Vision*, volume 1, pp. 178–183, Vancouver, Canada, July 2001. IEEE Computer Society Press.

23. M. Middendorf and H.-H. Nagel. Empirically convergent adaptive estimation of grayvalue structure tensors. In L. van Gool, editor, *Proc. 24th DAGM Symposium*, volume 2449 of *Lecture Notes in Computer Science*, pp. 66–74, Zürich, Switzerland, September 2002. Springer.

24. P. Mrázek, J. Weickert, and A. Bruhn. On robust estimation and smoothing with spatial and tonal kernels. Technical Report 51, Series SPP-1114, Department of Mathematics, University of Bremen, Germany, June 2004.

25. M. Nagao and T. Matsuyama. Edge preserving smoothing. *Computer Graphics and Image Processing*, 9(4):394–407, April 1979.

26. H.-H. Nagel and A. Gehrke. Spatiotemporally adaptive estimation and segmentation of OF-fields. In H. Burkhardt and B. Neumann, editors, *Computer Vision – ECCV '98*, volume 1407 of *Lecture Notes in Computer Science*, pp. 86–102. Springer, Berlin, 1998.

27. P. Perona and J. Malik. Scale space and edge detection using anisotropic diffusion. *IEEE Transactions on Pattern Analysis and Machine Intelligence*, 12:629–639, 1990.

28. A. R. Rao and B. G. Schunck. Computing oriented texture fields. *CVGIP: Graphical Models and Image Processing*, 53:157–185, 1991.

29. K. Rohr. Modelling and identification of characteristic intensity variations. *Image and Vision Computing*, 10(2):66–76, 1992.

30. K. Rohr. Localization properties of direct corner detectors. *Journal of Mathematical Imaging and Vision*, 4:139–150, 1994.

31. M. Rousson, T. Brox, and R. Deriche. Active unsupervised texture segmentation on a diffusion based feature space. In *Proc. 2003 IEEE Computer Society Conference on Computer Vision and Pattern Recognition*, pp. 699–704, Madison, WI, June 2003.

32. L. I. Rudin, S. Osher, and E. Fatemi. Nonlinear total variation based noise removal algorithms. *Physica D*, 60:259–268, 1992.

33. S. M. Smith and J. M. Brady. SUSAN – a new approach to low level image processing. *International Journal of Computer Vision*, 23(1):45–78, May 1997.

34. I. Thomas. Anisotropic adaptation and structure detection. Technical Report F11, Institute for Applied Mathematics, University of Hamburg, Germany, August 1999.

35. D. Tschumperlé and R. Deriche. Diffusion tensor regularization with contraints preservation. In *Proc. 2001 IEEE Computer Society Conference on Computer Vision and Pattern Recognition*, volume 1, pp. 948–953, Kauai, HI, December 2001. IEEE Computer Society Press.

36. R. van den Boomgaard. The Kuwahara-Nagao operator decomposed in terms of a linear smoothing and a morphological sharpening. In H. Talbot and R. Beare,

editors, *Mathematical Morphology, Proceedings of the 6th International Symposium on Mathematical Morphology*, pp. 283–292, Sydney, Australia, April 2002. CSIRO Publishing.

37. R. van den Boomgaard and J. van de Weijer. Robust estimation of orientation for texture analysis. In *Proc. Texture 2002, 2nd International Workshop on Texture Analysis and Synthesis*, Copenhagen, June 2002.

38. J. Weickert. *Anisotropic Diffusion in Image Processing*. Teubner, Stuttgart, 1998.

39. J. Weickert. Coherence-enhancing diffusion filtering. *International Journal of Computer Vision*, 31(2/3):111–127, April 1999.

40. J. Weickert. Coherence-enhancing diffusion of colour images. *Image and Vision Computing*, 17(3–4):199–210, March 1999.

41. J. Weickert and T. Brox. Diffusion and regularization of vector- and matrix-valued images. In M. Z. Nashed and O. Scherzer, editors, *Inverse Problems, Image Analysis, and Medical Imaging*, volume 313 of *Contemporary Mathematics*, pp. 251–268. AMS, Providence, 2002.

On the Concept of a *Local* Greyvalue Distribution and the *Adaptive* Estimation of a Structure Tensor

Hans–Hellmut Nagel

Institut für Algorithmen und Kognitive Systeme, Fakultät für Informatik der Universität Karlsruhe (TH), 76128 Karlsruhe, Germany
`nagel@iaks.uni-karlsruhe.de`

Summary. As a step towards a *local* analysis of local image features, the position, peak value, and covariance matrix of an isolated, noise-free multivariate Gaussian are determined *in closed form* from four 'observables', computed by gaussian-weighted averaging first and second powers of (up to second order) partial derivatives of a digitized greyvalue distribution.

3.1 Introduction

Spatiotemporal greyvalue variations in an image sequence encode information about status and change of a depicted scene. The segmentation and tracking of characteristic *greyvalue* structures constitute, therefore, basic processing steps in any attempt to infer the *scene* structure and its temporal development from an image sequence.

3.1.1 Optical Flow (OF) and the *Greyvalue Structure Tensor*

Let $g(\mathbf{x}) = g(x, y, t)$ with $g \geq 0$ define a digitized image sequence where the argument specifies a point $\mathbf{x} = (x, y, t)^T$ at location $(x, y)^T$ in the image plane at time t. Optical Flow (OF) will be denoted by the three-dimensional vector $\mathbf{u} = (u_1, u_2, 1)^T$ in the (x,y,t)-space. OF is usually estimated based on the assumption that a local greyvalue distribution moves in the image plane without changes, i.e. the total variation $dg(x, y, t) = 0$ should vanish.

A *local* estimation approach determines the OF-vector $\mathbf{u}$ by the following requirement (an overbar indicates – unweighted or weighted – averaging):

$$\overline{\left((\nabla g)^T \mathbf{u}\right)^2} \overset{!}{=} \min_{\mathbf{u}} \ . \tag{3.1}$$

In order to exclude the trivial solution $\mathbf{u} = \mathbf{0}$, a unit-vector $\mathbf{e} = (e_1,\ e_2,\ e_3)^T$ is introduced. The boundary condition $u_3 = 1$ is replaced by $\|\mathbf{e}\| = 1$. This allows to transform the determination of $\mathbf{u}$ into an eigenvector problem for $\mathbf{e}$:

$$\overline{\nabla g (\nabla g)^T} \mathbf{e} \;=\; \lambda \, \mathbf{e} \; . \tag{3.2}$$

The solution is given by the eigenvector $\mathbf{e}_{min}(\mathbf{x})$ associated with the smallest eigenvalue λ_{min} of the tensor $\overline{\nabla g (\nabla g)^T}$: the local greyvalue distribution around $\mathbf{x}$ changes the *least* along the direction given by $\mathbf{e}_{min}(\mathbf{x})$ from which one can recover (provided $\mathbf{e}_{min,3} \neq 0$) the corresponding OF-vector

$$\mathbf{u} = (u_1, \; u_2, \; 1)^T \;=\; \left(\frac{\mathbf{e}_{min,1}}{\mathbf{e}_{min,3}}, \; \frac{\mathbf{e}_{min,2}}{\mathbf{e}_{min,3}}, \; 1 \right)^T . \tag{3.3}$$

3.1.2 The Concept of a '*Characteristic* Greyvalue Structure'

The concept of a '*characteristic* greyvalue structure' thus deserves closer attention – see, e.g., [2, 7, 12]. Koenderink [8] (see also [9]) suggested that a Gaussian intensity distribution should be considered to represent the *most elementary* characteristic greyvalue structure:

$$\mathrm{g}(\boldsymbol{x}) \;=\; g_0 \, e^{-\frac{1}{2}(\boldsymbol{x}-\boldsymbol{x}_0)^T \Sigma_0^{-1}(\boldsymbol{x}-\boldsymbol{x}_0)} \tag{3.4}$$

where g_0 denotes the maximum greyvalue at the center-position $\boldsymbol{x}_0$ of a multivariate, bell-like Gaussian greyvalue distribution and the covariance matrix $\Sigma_{0_{3\times3}}$ specifies its extent and shape. The notion of an elementary characteristic greyvalue structure may gain additional support if it becomes possible to estimate the parameters g_0, $\boldsymbol{x}_0$, and $\Sigma_{0_{3\times3}}$ from real-world image sequences.

In principle, these parameters can be estimated easily provided one can assume that the Gaussian to be determined is the *only* function which differs significantly from zero in the entire image plane at all times. This assumption, however, will in general be grossly violated within an image sequence with many different *local* spatio-temporal greyvalue structures. It thus will be useful to estimate the parameters of a 3D *Gaussian Bell* (3D-GB) by *using only local evidence.*

A procedure will be presented in the sequel which allows – at least in principle – to determine the parameters of a 3D-GB in a closed-form solution. This solution approach combines four 'observables' which are obtained by averaging up to second order partial derivatives of the greyvalue distribution within a *local* Gaussian bell-like 'probing environment'. This weighted averaging is expected to compensate to some extent a potential noise-sensitivity caused by the use of partial derivatives (see, e.g., [5]).

3.2 Greyvalue Structure Tensor of a Gaussian Bell

Let a 'probing environment' be defined by a Gaussian weighting function centered at the origin of the coordinate system with known covariance matrix

$\Sigma_{3\times3}$ – see (3.5). Eventually, the unknown parameters of a 3D-GB according to (3.4) have to be determined from noisy image data. It appears natural, therefore, to reduce the influence of noise on parameter estimation by lowpass–filtering. In order to keep the number of system parameters small, lowpass–filtering is performed by convolving the given greyvalue distribution with a Gaussian which has the same covariance matrix as the one defining the probing environment:

$$\text{gauß}(\boldsymbol{x}) \;=\; \frac{1}{\sqrt{(2\pi)^3|\Sigma|}}\, \mathrm{e}^{-\frac{1}{2}\boldsymbol{x}^T\Sigma^{-1}\boldsymbol{x}} \tag{3.5}$$

where $|\Sigma|$ denotes the determinant of Σ. Somewhat tedious, but otherwise straightforward manipulations yield (to save space, triple integrals are represented by a single integral symbol in the remainder of this contribution)

$$g_{LP}(\boldsymbol{x},\boldsymbol{x}_0) \;=\; \frac{1}{\sqrt{(2\pi)^3|\Sigma|}} \int_{-\infty}^{+\infty} \mathrm{d}\boldsymbol{\xi}\, g(\boldsymbol{\xi}) \cdot \mathrm{e}^{-\frac{1}{2}(\boldsymbol{\xi}-\boldsymbol{x})^T\Sigma^{-1}(\boldsymbol{\xi}-\boldsymbol{x})}$$

$$=\; \frac{1}{\sqrt{(2\pi)^3|\Sigma|}} \int_{-\infty}^{+\infty} \mathrm{d}\boldsymbol{\xi}\, g_0\, \mathrm{e}^{-\frac{1}{2}(\boldsymbol{\xi}-\boldsymbol{x}_0)^T\Sigma_0^{-1}(\boldsymbol{\xi}-\boldsymbol{x}_0)} \mathrm{e}^{-\frac{1}{2}(\boldsymbol{\xi}-\boldsymbol{x})^T\Sigma^{-1}(\boldsymbol{\xi}-\boldsymbol{x})}$$

$$=\; \frac{g_0\, \mathrm{e}^{-\frac{1}{2}(\boldsymbol{x}-\boldsymbol{x}_0)^T(\Sigma+\Sigma_0)^{-1}(\boldsymbol{x}-\boldsymbol{x}_0)}}{\sqrt{\left|\Sigma^{\frac{1}{2}}\left(\Sigma_0^{-1}+\Sigma^{-1}\right)\Sigma^{\frac{1}{2}}\right|}}\;. \tag{3.6}$$

3.2.1 Determination of $\overline{g_{LP}^2}(\boldsymbol{x}_0)$, a First Observable

The weighted squared greyvalue of the lowpass–filtered greyvalue distribution within the probing environment constitutes the first observable to be derived:

$$\overline{g_{LP}^2}(\boldsymbol{x}_0) \;=\; \frac{1}{\sqrt{(2\pi)^3|\Sigma|}} \int_{-\infty}^{+\infty} \mathrm{d}\boldsymbol{x}\, \left(g_{LP}(\boldsymbol{x},\boldsymbol{x}_0)\right)^2 \mathrm{e}^{-\frac{1}{2}\boldsymbol{x}^T\Sigma^{-1}\boldsymbol{x}}$$

$$=\; \frac{g_0^2 \int_{-\infty}^{+\infty} \mathrm{d}\boldsymbol{x}\, \left(\mathrm{e}^{-\frac{1}{2}(\boldsymbol{x}-\boldsymbol{x}_0)^T(\Sigma_0+\Sigma)^{-1}(\boldsymbol{x}-\boldsymbol{x}_0)}\right)^2 \mathrm{e}^{-\frac{1}{2}\boldsymbol{x}^T\Sigma^{-1}\boldsymbol{x}}}{\left|\Sigma^{\frac{1}{2}}\left(\Sigma_0^{-1}+\Sigma^{-1}\right)\Sigma^{\frac{1}{2}}\right|\sqrt{(2\pi)^3|\Sigma|}}$$

$$=\; \frac{g_0^2 \int_{-\infty}^{+\infty} \mathrm{d}\boldsymbol{x}\, \mathrm{e}^{-\frac{1}{2}(\boldsymbol{x}-\boldsymbol{x}_0)^T 2(\Sigma_0+\Sigma)^{-1}(\boldsymbol{x}-\boldsymbol{x}_0)}\, \mathrm{e}^{-\frac{1}{2}\boldsymbol{x}^T\Sigma^{-1}\boldsymbol{x}}}{\left|I+\Gamma^{-1}\right|\sqrt{(2\pi)^3|\Sigma|}}\;. \tag{3.7}$$

The last equation uses the abbreviation $\Gamma = \Sigma^{-\frac{1}{2}}\Sigma_0\,\Sigma^{-\frac{1}{2}}$ with I denoting the (3×3)-identity matrix $diag(1,1,1)$. Similar manipulations as in the case of lowpass–filtering eventually lead to

$$\overline{g_{LP}^2}(\boldsymbol{x}_0) \;=\; \frac{g_0^2\, e^{-\,\boldsymbol{x}_0^T\,(\Sigma_0 + 3\,\Sigma)^{-1}\,\boldsymbol{x}_0}}{|\Gamma^{-1}|\,\sqrt{|\Gamma\,+\,I|\times|\Gamma\,+\,3\,I|}}\,. \tag{3.8}$$

3.2.2 The Grayvalue Structure Tensor, a Second Observable

As usual, the gradient of a greyvalue distribution $g(\boldsymbol{x})$ is obtained by convolving $g(\boldsymbol{x})$ with the derivative of a Gaussian lowpass–filter:

$$\nabla g_{LP}(\boldsymbol{x}) \;=\; \Big(\nabla\text{gauß} * g\Big)(\boldsymbol{x})\,. \tag{3.9}$$

According to (3.4 + 3.6), this results for the case of a 3D-GB in

$$\nabla g_{LP}(\boldsymbol{x},\boldsymbol{x}_0) = \frac{g_0\Big(-(\Sigma_0 + \Sigma)^{-1}(\boldsymbol{x}-\boldsymbol{x}_0)\Big)}{\sqrt{|I\,+\,\Gamma^{-1}|}}\; e^{-\frac{1}{2}(\boldsymbol{x}-\boldsymbol{x}_0)^T(\Sigma_0+\Sigma)^{-1}(\boldsymbol{x}-\boldsymbol{x}_0)}. \tag{3.10}$$

The Greyvalue Structure Tensor (GST) for the 3D-GB is defined as

$$\text{GST}(\boldsymbol{x}_0) \;=\; \int d\boldsymbol{x}\,\Big\{\,\nabla g_{LP}(\boldsymbol{x},\boldsymbol{x}_0)\,\big(\nabla g_{LP}(\boldsymbol{x},\boldsymbol{x}_0)\big)^T\,\text{gauß}(\boldsymbol{x})\,\Big\} \tag{3.11}$$

which – after insertion of $\nabla g_{LP}(\boldsymbol{x},\boldsymbol{x}_0)$ from (3.10) – can be written in the form

$$\text{GST}(\boldsymbol{x}_0) \;=\; \frac{g_0^2}{|I\,+\,\Gamma^{-1}|}$$

$$\times \int_{-\infty}^{+\infty} d\boldsymbol{x}\,\Big((\Sigma_0 + \Sigma)^{-1}(\boldsymbol{x}-\boldsymbol{x}_0)\Big)\Big((\boldsymbol{x}-\boldsymbol{x}_0)^T(\Sigma_0 + \Sigma)^{-1}\Big)$$

$$\times \Big(e^{-\frac{1}{2}(\boldsymbol{x}-\boldsymbol{x}_0)^T(\Sigma_0+\Sigma)^{-1}(\boldsymbol{x}-\boldsymbol{x}_0)}\Big)^2\,\frac{1}{\sqrt{(2\pi)^3|\Sigma|}}e^{-\frac{1}{2}\boldsymbol{x}^T\Sigma^{-1}\boldsymbol{x}}$$

$$=\; \frac{g_0^2}{|I\,+\,\Gamma^{-1}|\,\sqrt{(2\pi)^3|\Sigma|}}\int_{-\infty}^{+\infty} d\boldsymbol{x}\,(\Sigma_0 + \Sigma)^{-1}(\boldsymbol{x}-\boldsymbol{x}_0)(\boldsymbol{x}-\boldsymbol{x}_0)^T$$

$$e^{-\frac{1}{2}\big\{(\boldsymbol{x}-\boldsymbol{x}_0)^T 2\,(\Sigma_0+\Sigma)^{-1}(\boldsymbol{x}-\boldsymbol{x}_0)\,+\,\boldsymbol{x}^T\Sigma^{-1}\boldsymbol{x}\big\}}\,(\Sigma_0 + \Sigma)^{-1}\,. \tag{3.12}$$

In order to evaluate the integral, the integration variable is changed to

$$\boldsymbol{\eta} = \Big(\Sigma^{-1} + 2\,(\Sigma_0 + \Sigma)^{-1}\Big)^{\frac{1}{2}}\boldsymbol{x} - \Big(\Sigma^{-1} + 2\,(\Sigma_0 + \Sigma)^{-1}\Big)^{-\frac{1}{2}} 2\,(\Sigma_0 + \Sigma)^{-1}\boldsymbol{x}_0$$

with

$$\mathrm{d}\boldsymbol{\eta} \;=\; \left|\left(\varSigma^{-1} + 2\,(\varSigma_0 + \varSigma)^{-1}\right)^{\frac{1}{2}}\right| \mathrm{d}\boldsymbol{x} \;=\; \left|\varSigma^{-1} + 2\,(\varSigma_0 + \varSigma)^{-1}\right|^{\frac{1}{2}} \mathrm{d}\boldsymbol{x}\,.$$

The vector difference $\boldsymbol{x} - \boldsymbol{x}_0$ can then be expressed in the form

$$\boldsymbol{x} - \boldsymbol{x}_0 = \left(\varSigma^{-1} + 2\,(\varSigma_0 + \varSigma)^{-1}\right)^{-\frac{1}{2}} \boldsymbol{\eta}$$

$$+ \left(\left(\varSigma^{-1} + 2\,(\varSigma_0 + \varSigma)^{-1}\right)^{-1} 2\,(\varSigma_0 + \varSigma)^{-1} - I\right)\boldsymbol{x}_0\,.$$

Upon insertion, the integral will comprise outer products $\boldsymbol{\eta}\,\boldsymbol{\eta}^T$, $\boldsymbol{\eta}\,\boldsymbol{x}_0^T$, $\boldsymbol{x}_0\,\boldsymbol{\eta}^T$, and $\boldsymbol{x}_0\,\boldsymbol{x}_0^T$. Since the outer products $\boldsymbol{\eta}\,\boldsymbol{x}_0^T$ and $\boldsymbol{x}_0\,\boldsymbol{\eta}^T$ are antisymmetric with respect to a sign inversion of the integration variable $\boldsymbol{\eta}$, the integrals containing these factors vanish due to symmetry considerations. A gradual reduction of the resulting expressions eventually leads to

$$\mathrm{GST}(\boldsymbol{x}_0) = \frac{g_0^2\,\mathrm{e}^{-\boldsymbol{x}_0^T (\varSigma_0 + 3\varSigma)^{-1}\boldsymbol{x}_0}\,|\varGamma|}{\sqrt{|\varGamma + I|\,|\varGamma + 3\,I|}}$$

$$\times \varSigma^{-\frac{1}{2}}\left((\varGamma + I)^{-\frac{1}{2}} \times \left(\varGamma + 3\,I\right)^{-1} \times (\varGamma + I)^{-\frac{1}{2}}\right.$$

$$\left. + (\varGamma + 3\,I)^{-1} \times \varSigma^{-\frac{1}{2}}\,\boldsymbol{x}_0\,\boldsymbol{x}_0^T\,\varSigma^{-\frac{1}{2}} \times (\varGamma + 3\,I)^{-1}\right)\varSigma^{-\frac{1}{2}}\,.$$

$$(3.13)$$

The expression for the 3×3-tensor GST given by (3.13) relates an 'observable' computed according to (3.11) with the unknown peak greyvalue g_0, three unknown position parameters $\boldsymbol{x}_0$ and six parameters of the unknown covariance matrix $\varSigma_0$. The scalar factor in front of the sum of matrix products can be completely replaced by $\overline{g_{LP}^2}(\boldsymbol{x}_0)$. Since matrices on both sides are symmetric, they can be diagonalized simultaneously, yielding one equation for each of the three eigenvalues. So far, we are thus left with three equations for six remaining unknowns, namely the components of $\boldsymbol{x}_0$ and the eigenvalues of $\varGamma$, i.e. $\varSigma_0$, because the covariance matrix $\varSigma$ for the 'Gaussian probe' is known.

3.3 Weighted Average of the Hessian

The considerations at the end of the preceding section suggest to search for another independent matrix equation. As will be shown in the sequel, a weighted average of the tensor of second partial derivatives – the Hessian[1] of the GB – can provide the desired equations after suitable normalization. This

---

[1] As used, e.g., in [3, p. 488]; occasionally, the term 'Hessian' denotes the *determinant* of the matrix of second partial derivatives, see [6, p. 22]

tensor, however, is a *linear* function of the (lowpass–filtered) input greyvalues whereas the GST comprises the *square* of these lowpass–filtered greyvalues and, thereby, indirectly some product of the lowpass–filter with itself. In order to obtain results compatible with (3.13), lowpass–filtering prior to the computation of the *second* partial derivatives will thus be performed based on a Gaussian with *twice* the covariance matrix as the one given in (3.5):

$$g_{LP,2\Sigma}(\boldsymbol{x}, \boldsymbol{x}_0) \;=\; \frac{g_0 \, e^{-\frac{1}{2}(\boldsymbol{x}-\boldsymbol{x}_0)^T(\Sigma_0+2\,\Sigma)^{-1}(\boldsymbol{x}-\boldsymbol{x}_0)}}{\sqrt{|2\,\Sigma| \times \left|\Sigma_0^{-1} + (2\,\Sigma)^{-1}\right|}} \;. \tag{3.14}$$

The tensor of second partial derivatives of a twice lowpass–filtered 3D-GB thus can be written as

$$\nabla\nabla g_{LP,2\Sigma}(\boldsymbol{x}, \boldsymbol{x}_0) \;=\; \left[(\Sigma_0 + 2\Sigma)^{-1}(\boldsymbol{x}-\boldsymbol{x}_0)(\boldsymbol{x}-\boldsymbol{x}_0)^T(\Sigma_0+2\Sigma)^{-1} \right.$$
$$\left. - (\Sigma_0 + 2\Sigma)^{-1} \right] g_{LP,2\Sigma}(\boldsymbol{x}) \;. \tag{3.15}$$

3.3.1 Weighted Average of the Tensor of Second Partial Derivatives

Using the expression for $\nabla\nabla g_{LP,2\Sigma}(\boldsymbol{x}, \boldsymbol{x}_0)$ given by the last equation of the preceding section, the computation of its weighted average requires to evaluate

$$\overline{\nabla\nabla g_{LP,2\Sigma}}(\boldsymbol{x}_0) = \frac{g_0}{\sqrt{(2\,\pi)^3\,|\Sigma|\,|2\,\Sigma| \times \left|\Sigma_0^{-1} + (2\,\Sigma)^{-1}\right|}}$$

$$\times \int_{-\infty}^{+\infty} d\boldsymbol{x} \left\{ \left[(\Sigma_0 + 2\,\Sigma)^{-1}(\boldsymbol{x}-\boldsymbol{x}_0)(\boldsymbol{x}-\boldsymbol{x}_0)^T(\Sigma_0+2\,\Sigma)^{-1} - (\Sigma_0+2\,\Sigma)^{-1} \right] \right.$$
$$\left. \times e^{-\frac{1}{2}(\boldsymbol{x}-\boldsymbol{x}_0)^T(\Sigma_0+2\,\Sigma)^{-1}(\boldsymbol{x}-\boldsymbol{x}_0)} \times e^{-\frac{1}{2}\boldsymbol{x}^T\Sigma^{-1}\boldsymbol{x}} \right\} \;. \tag{3.16}$$

A lengthy, but otherwise elementary computation eventually yields the following compact result:

$$\overline{\nabla\nabla g_{LP,2\Sigma}}(\boldsymbol{x}_0) = \frac{g_0 \, e^{-\frac{1}{2}\boldsymbol{x}_0^T(\Sigma_0+3\,\Sigma)^{-1}\boldsymbol{x}_0} \sqrt{|\Gamma|}}{\sqrt{|\Gamma + 3\,I|}}$$
$$\left[\left(\Sigma_0 + 3\,\Sigma\right)^{-1}\boldsymbol{x}_0\,\boldsymbol{x}_0^T\left(\Sigma_0+3\,\Sigma\right)^{-1} - \left(\Sigma_0+3\,\Sigma\right)^{-1} \right] \;. \tag{3.17}$$

3.3.2 Weighted Average of a Twice Lowpass–Filtered 3D-GB

The determination of the unknown covariance matrix Σ_0 will be greatly simplified if the scalar factor in front of the matrix difference in (3.17) can be compensated, too, by a suitable normalization. The experience from the preceding section suggests to compute the weighted average of the *twice* lowpass–filtered 3D-GB greyvalue distribution given in (3.14):

$$\overline{g_{LP,2\Sigma}}(\boldsymbol{x}_0) = \int_{-\infty}^{+\infty} d\boldsymbol{x} \; \frac{g_0 \, e^{-\frac{1}{2}(\boldsymbol{x}-\boldsymbol{x}_0)^T(\Sigma_0+2\,\Sigma)^{-1}(\boldsymbol{x}-\boldsymbol{x}_0)}}{\sqrt{|2\,\Sigma| \times \left|\Sigma_0^{-1}+(2\,\Sigma)^{-1}\right|}} \times \frac{e^{-\frac{1}{2}\boldsymbol{x}^T\Sigma^{-1}\boldsymbol{x}}}{\sqrt{(2\,\pi)^3\,|\Sigma|}} \, . \quad (3.18)$$

Similar, but much simpler manipulations as in the case of the preceding integrals result in

$$\overline{g_{LP,2\Sigma}}(\boldsymbol{x}_0) = \frac{g_0 \, e^{-\frac{1}{2}\boldsymbol{x}_0^T(\Sigma_0+3\,\Sigma)^{-1}\boldsymbol{x}_0}\sqrt{|\Gamma|}}{\sqrt{|\Gamma+3\,I|}} \, . \quad (3.19)$$

3.4 Determination of Parameters of a Gaussian Bell

Using the result of the preceding section, the difference of matrix products in the expression for the averaged tensor of second partial derivatives from (3.17) can be rewritten in the form

$$\frac{\overline{\nabla\nabla g_{LP,2\Sigma}}(\boldsymbol{x}_0)}{\overline{g_{LP,2\Sigma}}(\boldsymbol{x}_0)} = \left[\left(\Sigma_0+3\,\Sigma\right)^{-1}\boldsymbol{x}_0\,\boldsymbol{x}_0^T\left(\Sigma_0+3\,\Sigma\right)^{-1} - \left(\Sigma_0+3\,\Sigma\right)^{-1}\right] \, .$$

$$(3.20)$$

Simultaneous extraction of the known factor $\Sigma^{\frac{1}{2}}$ from the expressions $(\Sigma_0+3\,\Sigma)$ – once to the left and once to the right – allows to isolate the difference of matrix products in a form suitable for further evaluation:

$$\frac{\Sigma^{\frac{1}{2}}\,\overline{GST}(\boldsymbol{x}_0)\,\Sigma^{\frac{1}{2}}}{g_{LP}^2(\boldsymbol{x}_0)} = \Big((\Gamma+I)^{-\frac{1}{2}} \times (\Gamma+3\,I)^{-1} \times (\Gamma+I)^{-\frac{1}{2}}$$

$$+ \, (\Gamma+3\,I)^{-1} \times \, \Sigma^{-\frac{1}{2}}\boldsymbol{x}_0\,\boldsymbol{x}_0^T\,\Sigma^{-\frac{1}{2}}$$

$$\times \, (\Gamma+3\,I)^{-1}\Big) \, , \quad (3.21)$$

$$\frac{\Sigma^{\frac{1}{2}}\,\overline{\nabla\nabla g_{LP,2\Sigma}}(\boldsymbol{x}_0)\,\Sigma^{\frac{1}{2}}}{\overline{g_{LP,2\Sigma}}(\boldsymbol{x}_0)} = \left[\left(\Gamma+3\,I\right)^{-1} \times \, \Sigma^{-\frac{1}{2}}\boldsymbol{x}_0\,\boldsymbol{x}_0^T\,\Sigma^{-\frac{1}{2}}\right.$$

$$\left. \times \left(\Gamma+3\,I\right)^{-1} - \left(\Gamma+3\,I\right)^{-1}\right] \, . \quad (3.22)$$

Subtraction of the second matrix equation from the first one – obtained from (3.13) – removes the terms which depend on the unknown 3D-GB center position $\boldsymbol{x}_0$:

$$\frac{\Sigma^{\frac{1}{2}}\, GST(\boldsymbol{x}_0)\, \Sigma^{\frac{1}{2}}}{\overline{g^2_{LP}}(\boldsymbol{x}_0)} - \frac{\Sigma^{\frac{1}{2}}\, \overline{\nabla\nabla g_{LP,2\Sigma}}(\boldsymbol{x}_0)\, \Sigma^{\frac{1}{2}}}{\overline{g_{LP,2\Sigma}}(\boldsymbol{x}_0)}$$

$$= (\varGamma + I)^{-\frac{1}{2}} \times \left(\varGamma + 3\,I\right)^{-1} \times (\varGamma + I)^{-\frac{1}{2}} + \left(\varGamma + 3\,I\right)^{-1} . \qquad (3.23)$$

Note that the left-hand side has been constructed entirely from previously derived 'observables' in combination with the known covariance matrix Σ of the 'Gaussian probe'. Using the abbreviation $\varPhi = \varGamma + 2\,I$, the right-hand side can be transformed into $\left(\varPhi - \varPhi^{-1}\right)^{-1}$. Let $\lambda_i, i = 1, 2, 3$ denote the eigenvalues of the *inverse* of the observable expression on the left-hand side and correspondingly $\lambda_{\varPhi_i}, i = 1, 2, 3$ the eigenvalues of the matrix $\varPhi$. One thus obtains three quadratic equations $\lambda_i = \lambda_{\varPhi_i} - \lambda_{\varPhi_i}^{-1}$ with the solutions

$$\lambda_{\varPhi_i} = \frac{\lambda_i}{2} \pm \sqrt{\frac{\lambda_i^2}{4} + 1} \ , \quad i = 1, 2, 3 . \qquad (3.24)$$

The positive root has to be taken because $\varPhi$ represents a positive-definite matrix. Since both sides of the matrix equation (3.23) share the same eigenvectors, $\varPhi$ has been determined which implies that $\varGamma = \varPhi - 2\,I$ is known and thus $\Sigma_0 = \Sigma^{\frac{1}{2}}\, \varGamma\, \Sigma^{\frac{1}{2}}$. The known $\varGamma$ can now be exploited in order to extract the unknown vector $\boldsymbol{x}_0$ from the *sum* of the two component-equations (3.21 + 3.22):

$$\frac{\Sigma^{\frac{1}{2}}\, GST(\boldsymbol{x}_0)\, \Sigma^{\frac{1}{2}}}{\overline{g^2_{LP}}(\boldsymbol{x}_0)} + \frac{\Sigma^{\frac{1}{2}}\, \overline{\nabla\nabla g_{LP,2\Sigma}}(\boldsymbol{x}_0)\, \Sigma^{\frac{1}{2}}}{\overline{g_{LP,2\Sigma}}(\boldsymbol{x}_0)}$$

$$- (\varGamma + I)^{-\frac{1}{2}} \left(\varGamma + 3\,I\right)^{-1} (\varGamma + I)^{-\frac{1}{2}} + \left(\varGamma + 3\,I\right)^{-1}$$

$$= 2 \times \left(\varGamma + 3\,I\right)^{-1} \times \Sigma^{-\frac{1}{2}}\, \boldsymbol{x}_0\, \boldsymbol{x}_0^T\, \Sigma^{-\frac{1}{2}} \times \left(\varGamma + 3\,I\right)^{-1} . \qquad (3.25)$$

The right-hand side represents the outer product of a vector $\sqrt{2}\,(\varGamma + 3\,I)^{-1} \times \Sigma^{-\frac{1}{2}}\, \boldsymbol{x}_0$ with itself, i.e. $\boldsymbol{x}_0$ can be determined from the eigenvector related to the – in general uniquely defined – non-zero eigenvalue of this matrix. The sign to be used is fixed by selecting the alternative which points towards the center, i.e. the eigenvector should point into the same direction as the gradient vector – unless the corresponding eigenvalue is zero, too, because the probe happens to be already positioned 'on top' of the GB to be determined.

3.5 Discussion

The preceding exposition outlines an algorithm to determine all unknown parameters of an isolated 'Gaussian Bell (3D-GB)' from a *noise-free* greyvalue distribution.

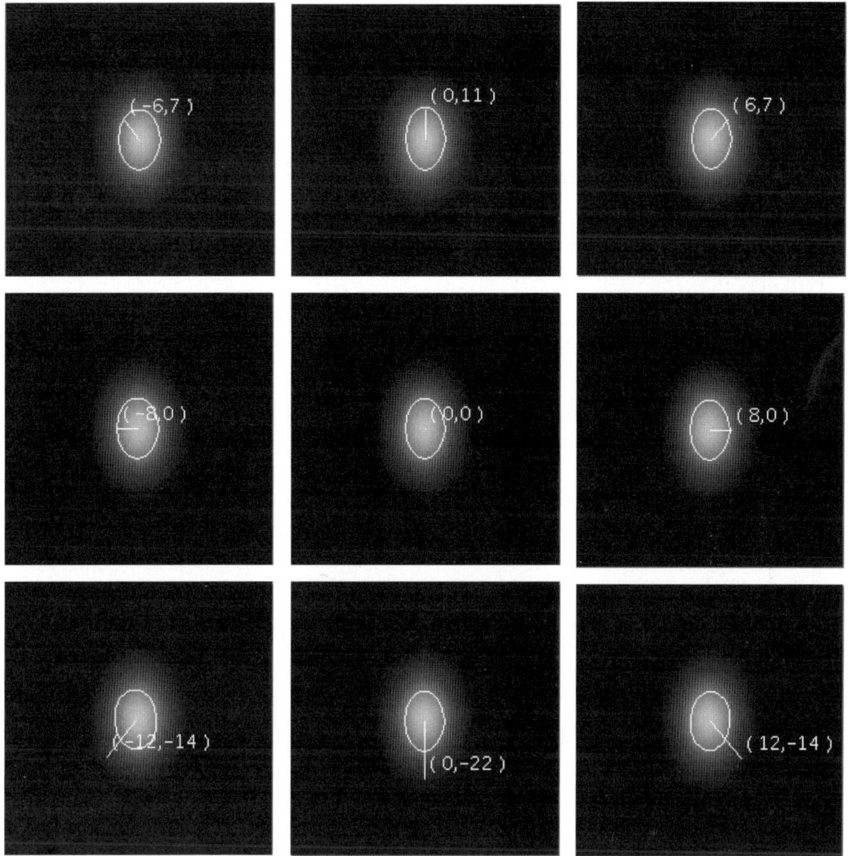

Fig. 3.1. A bivariate 'Gaussian Bell' GB_{input} with $\Sigma_0 = diag(64, 128)$ (in pixel units) is intensity-coded (brightest pixel = peak value). The center of the 'probe' Gaussian GB_{probe} is given in parentheses relative to the center of GB_{input}. The (1 s.d.) ellipse indicates the *estimated* center and covariance matrix (see text)

Figure 3.1 illustrates results obtained by this approach. To simplify comparisons across panels, the 'input' GB with $\Sigma_0 = diag(64, 128)$ (in pixel units) is centered at the origin, whereas the *'probe'* Gaussian Bell GB_{probe} is centered at different locations given in parentheses, with the same covariance matrix $\Sigma_{probe} = diag(2, 2)$ used for all tests. The 'footprint' for the discretized GB_{probe} has been extended automatically such that neglected contributions outside the footprint remain below 0.1 %, see [14]. In the center panel, the estimated center and 1 standard deviation (s.d.) ellipse – superimposed onto the greyvalue-coded GB_{input} – agrees well with expectations. The panels surrounding the center one show the *estimated* center location and 1 s.d. ellipse when the GB_{probe} is shifted away from the origin by (roughly, caused by the probe center being quantized to integer pixel units) 1 s.d. of Σ_0 up and to

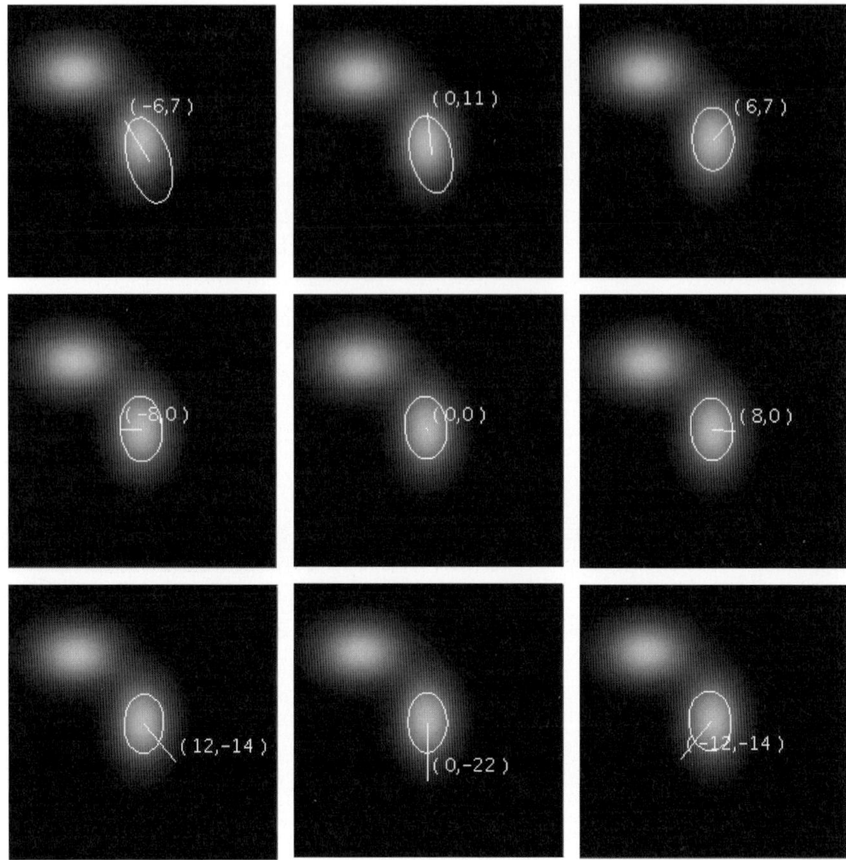

Fig. 3.2. Analogously to Fig. 3.1, but with another GB added, centered at $(-25, +25)$ with a covariance matrix $\Sigma_{0_2} = diag(128, 64)$. In comparison with Fig. 3.1, the effect of this second GB on the estimation results becomes the more prominent the closer the GB_{probe} is located to the second GB (see text). Note, however, the comparatively quick decay of this effect

the left, vertical upwards, and sloping up and to the right, respectively. The line segment connects the center of GB_{probe} with the *estimated* center for GB_{input}. The bottom row shows results for shifts by roughly 2 s.d. in the opposite direction as in the top row, respectively. Even with a probe center having been shifted up to 2 s.d. away from the center of GB_{input}, the estimates agree acceptably with the corresponding parameters of GB_{input}. This reminds of findings reported for a low-level feature extraction approach with some formal similarities (see [4, Sect. 3.1]).

Figure 3.2 illustrates results if another Gaussian Bell is added at location $(-25, +25)$ with a covariance matrix $\Sigma_{0_2} = diag(128, 64)$. The probe centers have been chosen identically to those in the corresponding panels of Fig. 3.1.

The closer the GB_{probe} is located to the second GB, the stronger is the effect on the estimates. At the origin, the effect can be just noticed, however, and it becomes almost unnoticeable further away (bottom row, center and right panel). Inspection of the result for the GST in (3.13) and for the tensor of averaged second partial derivatives in (3.17) shows that the influence of a 3D-GB centered at $\boldsymbol{x}_0$ decays exponentially with the Mahalanobis distance from the center of the 'probing environment' (the origin *for these equations*). Additional characteristic greyvalue distributions which are compatible with a 3D-GB model and are positioned at greater Mahalanobis distances from the current 'probing center' are thus expected to quickly loose their influence upon the estimates for a 'locally dominant' 3D-GB. It remains to be investigated how sensitive this procedure will be to noise and possible related numerical problems like, for example, in analogous studies on self-adaptive GST and OF estimation [14, 15, 16]. When applied to OF-estimation, this approach assumes that a delayed evaluation can delimit non-causal effects (see, e.g., [10, 13]) reasonably well.

An advantage of this contribution is seen in the fact that the concept of a characteristic local greyvalue structure has been operationalized by a *direct local* computation – at least for the 'ideal' case of GBs not corrupted by noise. This suggests an (at most) three-step estimation approach: (i) choose an isotropic GB_{probe}, a 'test' lattice with a unit size commensurate with Σ_{probe}, and apply this approach. (ii) Pick those lattice positions where the estimate for $\boldsymbol{x}_0$ attains a local minimum, i.e. at locations where an 'input GB' appears to have been localized. (iii) Possibly re-estimate with GB_{probe} located at these locations *once* if $\|\boldsymbol{x}_0\|$ exceeds some multiple of the s.d. of GB_{probe}.

Another reason for a re-estimation could be that Σ_{probe} differs too much from the estimated Σ_0 – or if it is suspected that a strongly localized grey-value structure happens to be on top of a substantially more extended one. It should be noted, though, that such a procedure *does not iterate* for a solution, but searches for two substantially different structures in the same area. In essence, the approach 'adapts' in a single step in the sense that it estimates *non-iteratively* the (structure) parameters of the assumed underlying GB. The structure-estimation problem is thus approached in a more *model-based* manner in comparison with the adaptive approaches reviewed in Chap. 2 [1]. In particular, it does not require a Laplacian-Pyramid search – potentially necessitating fine-graded steps – as discussed in Chap. 4 [11] where, however, more complex structures such as corners have to be localized.

It may be conceivable to study this closed-form solution approach as a tool for *analytical* investigations of structure estimation. Obviously, it appears interesting to study it for estimating the parameters of Gaussian mixture distributions. An extension towards more general local greyvalue structures appears attractive although initial attempts in this direction quickly lead to nonlinear equations for which I did not yet find solutions as in the case presented above. This experience does not imply, however, that closed solutions cannot be found.

Acknowledgements

Help by M. Middendorf and M. Arens in creating the figures as well as discussions with M. Middendorf and Ch. Plagemann are gratefully acknowledged, likewise comments of the anonymous reviewers which helped me to clarify the presentation. This research has been supported partially by the European Union through the project CogViSys (IST-2000-29404).

References

1. Brox Th., van den Boomgaard R., Lauze F., van de Weijer J., Weickert J., Mrázek P., Kornprobst P. (2004) Adaptive Structure Tensors and their Applications. (This volume)
2. Chomat O., Colin de Verdière V., Hall D., Crowley J.L. (2000) Local Scale Selection for Gaussian Based Description Techniques. In: Vernon D. (Ed.) Proc. ECCV-2000 (Part I) at Dublin, Ireland, June 26–July 1, 2000. LNCS 1842 Springer, Berlin Heidelberg, 117–133
3. Duda R.O., Hart P.E., Storck D.G. (2001) Pattern Classification. 2nd edn. John Wiley & Sons, New York
4. Förstner W.A. (1994) A Framework for Low–Level Feature Extraction. In: Eklundh J.-O. (Ed.), Proc. ECCV-1994 (Part II) at Stockholm, Sweden, May 2–6, 1994. LNCS 801 Springer, Berlin Heidelberg, 383–394
5. Förstner W.A., Gülch E. (1987) A Fast Operator for Detection and Precise Location of Distinct Points, Corners and Centers of Circular Features. In: Proc. Workshop of the Intern. Soc. for Photogrammetry & Remote Sensing at Interlaken, Switzerland, June 1987, 281–305
6. Gelb, A. (Ed.) (1974) Applied Optimal Estimation. The MIT Press, Cambridge and London
7. Kadir T., Brady M. (2001) Saliency, Scale and Image Description. Intern. J. Computer Vision 45(2):83–105
8. Koenderink J.J. (1984) The Structure of Images. Biolog. Cybernetics 50:363–370.
9. Koenderink J.J., van Doorn A.J. (1992) Generic Neighborhood Operators. IEEE Trans. Pattern Analysis Machine Intelligence PAMI-14(6):597–605.
10. Koenderink J.J., van Doorn A.J. (2002) Image Processing Done Right. In: Heyden A., Sparr G., Nielsen M., Johansen P. (Eds.) Proc. ECCV-2002 (Part I) at Copenhagen, Denmark, May 28–31, 2002. LNCS 2350 Springer, Berlin Heidelberg, 158–172
11. Köthe U. (2004) Low-Level Feature Detection Using the Boundary Tensor. (This volume)
12. Lindeberg T. (1998) Feature Detection with Automatic Scale Selection. Intern. J. Computer Vision 30(2):79–116
13. Lindeberg T. (2002) Time–Recursive Velocity–Adapted Spatio–Temporal Scale–Space Filters. In: Heyden A., Sparr G., Nielsen M., Johansen P. (Eds.) Proc. ECCV-2002 (Part I) at Copenhagen, Denmark, May 28–31, 2002. LNCS 2350 Springer, Berlin Heidelberg, 52–67

14. Middendorf M. (2003) Zur Auswertung lokaler Grauwertstrukturen (in German). Dissertation, Fakultät für Informatik der Universität Karlsruhe (TH), Juli 2003. Norderstedt, ISBN 3-8334-1175-9
15. Middendorf M., Nagel H.-H. (2002) Empirically Convergent Adaptive Estimation of Greyvalue Structure Tensors. In: Van Gool L. (Ed.) Proc. 24th DAGM Symposium 2002 at Zurich, Switzerland, September 16–20, 2002. LNCS 2449 Springer, Berlin Heidelberg, 66–74
16. Spies H., Scharr H. (2001) Accurate Optical Flow in Noisy Image Sequences. In: Proc. ICCV-2001 (Vol. I) at Vancouver, BC, July 9–12, 2001. 587–592.

4

Low-level Feature Detection Using the Boundary Tensor

Ullrich Köthe

Cognitive Systems Group, University of Hamburg, Vogt-Kölln-Str. 30, 22527 Hamburg, Germany
`koethe@informatik.uni-hamburg.de`

Summary. Tensors are a useful tool for the detection of low-level features such as edges, lines, corners, and junctions because they can represent feature strength and orientation in a way that is easy to work with. However, traditional approaches to define feature tensors have a number of disadvantages. By means of the first and second order *Riesz transforms*, we propose a new approach called the *boundary tensor*. Using quadratic convolution equations, we show that the boundary tensor overcomes some problems of the older tensor definitions. When the Riesz transform is combined with the Laplacian of Gaussian, the boundary tensor can be efficiently computed in the spatial domain. The usefulness of the new method is demonstrated for a number of application examples.[1]

4.1 Introduction

Even when the raw image data are not tensor-valued, tensor-based methods have been found useful in image analysis because tensors describe local image properties in a way that is invariant under Euclidean transformations of the space. The two main applications so far are feature extraction and optical flow computation. Historically, the latter one has been investigated first. The optical flow problem can be formulated as the task of finding the main local orientation at every point of the 3-dimensional spatio-temporal domain that is formed by interpreting an image sequence as a 3-dimensional data set with two spatial and one temporal dimensions. One can then define the spatio-temporal gradient of the sequence f_3 as:

$$\nabla f_3 = \left(\frac{\partial f_3}{\partial x}, \frac{\partial f_3}{\partial y}, \frac{\partial f_3}{\partial t} \right)^T \tag{4.1}$$

---

[1] This work was performed during a visit at the Computer Vision Lab of the University of Linköping, Sweden. I'd like to thank G. Granlund, M. Felsberg and K. Nordberg for many valuable discussions, and the Informatics Department of the University of Hamburg for their generous support of this visit.

Under the assumption of constant optical flow in a neighborhood of the current point, the flow vector $\mathbf{v}$ can be determined from the null-space of the *structure tensor* $\mathbf{S}_3$ [2, 11], cf. Chaps. 2 by Brox et al. and 3 by Nagel in this volume:

$$\mathbf{S}_3\mathbf{v} = 0 \qquad \text{with} \qquad \mathbf{S}_3 = g_\sigma \star (\nabla f_3 \nabla f_3^T) \qquad (4.2)$$

The structure tensor is the averaged outer product of the spatio-temporal gradient with itself, where the averaging filter g_σ (usually a Gaussian) is chosen according to the size of the neighborhood where the flow is assumed constant. The flow vector is only uniquely determined if the null space of the 3-dimensional structure tensor is 1-dimensional, i.e. if the structure tensor has rank 2. If it has lower rank, there is no unique flow vector, which is known as the *aperture problem*. This problem naturally leads to the definition of the 2D structure tensor as the averaged outer product of just the spatial gradient:

$$\mathbf{S}_2 = g_\sigma \star (\nabla f_2 \nabla f_2^T) \qquad \text{with} \qquad \nabla f_2 = \left(\frac{\partial f_2}{\partial x}, \frac{\partial f_2}{\partial y}\right)^T \qquad (4.3)$$

This 2-dimensional tensor must have full rank for a unique flow vector to exist, which is the case if the local image structure is neither flat (as in homogeneous regions) nor 1-dimensional (as at edges), but has high variation in all directions. Points of maximal variation are called *spatial interest points* and correspond to important structural features such as gray level corners, junctions, and extrema. They can for example be found as the local maxima of the corner strength measures proposed by *Förstner* [6] and *Harris* [8]:

$$c_{\text{Förstner}} = \frac{\det(\mathbf{S}_2)}{\text{tr}(\mathbf{S}_2)} \qquad c_{\text{Harris}} = \det(\mathbf{S}_2) - \kappa \, \text{tr}^2(\mathbf{S}_2) \qquad (4.4)$$

where κ is usually set to 0.04. In addition, Förstner [6] and Nagel [11] used the structure tensor to define a contrast independent measure of local isotropy:

$$c_{\text{roundness}} = \frac{4 \det(\mathbf{S}_2)}{(\text{tr}(\mathbf{S}_2))^2} \qquad (4.5)$$

A completely different approach to tensor-based feature detection was proposed by Granlund and Knutsson [9]. They were interested in the characterization of locally 1-dimensional image structures, i.e. edges and lines, which they call *simple structures*. Formally, simple structures are defined by the fact that the image is locally reduced to a 1-dimensional function that varies only along a certain direction $\mathbf{n}$ and is constant perpendicular to that direction:

$$f_2(\mathbf{x}) \approx f_1(\mathbf{x}^T \mathbf{n}) \qquad (4.6)$$

Then the local signal energy and orientation can be represented by an *orientation tensor* as

$$\mathbf{T} = \lambda \mathbf{n}\mathbf{n}^T \qquad (4.7)$$

Since in [9] the authors are interested in arbitrary 1-dimensional features, the estimation procedure for $\mathbf{T}$ must react uniformely to edges and lines. This property is called *phase invariance* because edges and lines can be understood as superpositions of trigonometric (complex exponential) basis functions at different phase (namely phase 0 or π for lines and $\pm\pi/2$ for edges). Phase invariance can be achieved by estimating the tensor with oriented quadrature filters [9] or with a local [4]. *Quadrature filter pairs* were originally invented to estimate the instantaneous energy and phase of a 1-dimensional signal. A quadrature pair $(h_{\text{even}}, h_{\text{odd}})$ consists of an even and an odd symmetric filter, and the instantaneous (edge or line) energy can be calculated as the sum of squares of the filter responses:

$$E(x) = (h_{\text{even}} \star f_1)^2 + (h_{\text{odd}} \star f_1)^2 \tag{4.8}$$

To actually form a quadrature pair, the filters must be related by the Hilbert transform $\mathcal{H}$, which is defined in the Fourier domain by

$$H_{\text{odd}}(u) = \mathcal{H}[H_{\text{even}}(u)] = j\frac{u}{|u|}H_{\text{even}}(u) = j\,\text{sign}(u)H_{\text{even}}(u) \tag{4.9}$$

(slanted capitals denote the Fourier transforms of the corresponding lower-case functions). To apply these filters in 2D, it is conventional to rotate them into some orientation of interest. In order to estimate $\mathbf{T}$ on a 2D image, at least 3 orientations are necessary [9]. When the local image structure is indeed 1-dimensional and the orientations $\theta_i = [0, \pi/3, 2\pi/3]$ are used, we get

$$\mathbf{T} = \sum_i (\mathbf{m}_i \mathbf{m}_i^T - \mathbf{I}/4)\, E_i \tag{4.10}$$

where E_i is the energy computed for orientation i, $\mathbf{m}_i = (\cos\theta_i, \sin\theta_i)^T$ and $\mathbf{I}$ is the unit tensor. A second order *polynomial approximation* of the image structure around $\mathbf{x}_0$ is defined by the local model

$$f_{\text{model}}(\mathbf{x}_0 + \dot{\mathbf{x}}) = c + \mathbf{x}^T\mathbf{b} + \mathbf{x}^T\mathbf{A}\mathbf{x} \tag{4.11}$$

An in-depth discussion of how to estimate $\mathbf{A}, \mathbf{b}, c$ can be found in [4]. Possibilities include local polynomial fits, facet models, moment filters, and Gaussian derivative filters. The orientation tensor is then defined as

$$\mathbf{T} = \mathbf{A}\mathbf{A}^T + \gamma\mathbf{b}\mathbf{b}^T \tag{4.12}$$

However, with the common estimation methods for $\mathbf{A}$ and $\mathbf{b}$ this tensor is only phase invariant for a single frequency determined by γ, which is therefore considered as an algorithm tuning parameter.

The existing methods have a number of shortcomings. The structure tensor approach is not phase invariant, because, being based on the image gradient, it reacts differently to edges and lines. Furthermore, due to averaging over a neighborhood, nearby features (e.g. the corners of a small triangle) will blend into only a single response and cannot be resolved separately. In the quadrature filter approach, definite statements about the properties of $\mathbf{T}$ can only be made if the local image structure is indeed 1-dimensional. It is unclear exactly what happens at 2-dimensional configurations. Finally, when the tensor is based on a polynomial approximation, the choice of the parameter γ is problematic. Usually it is impossible to find a single γ that works well on the entire image, and a procedure to choose it locally is not known. Consequently, the response is not phase invariant at most locations, and multiple responses near a single line are common.

In this contribution I am discussing the *boundary tensor* introduced in [10] as a method designed to overcome these shortcomings. It will be based on a new generalization of quadrature filters to 2 dimensions using the *Riesz transform*. The boundary tensor will turn out to be structurally equivalent to the polymial-based tensor definition, but with a uniquely determined parameter $\gamma = 1$. It will exhibit phase invariance for all frequencies in the same way as the quadrature filter approach. By analysing the new method in the framework of quadratic convolution, we can also show that it reacts in a useful way to locally 2-dimensional configurations. An efficient spatial domain algorithm and a number of feature analysis examples conclude the chapter.

4.2 The Boundary Tensor

Before we go on to define the boundary tensor, we recall that (Cartesian) tensors are in general characterized by the fact that the tensor elements in a rotated coordinate system can be calculated as linear combinations of the tensor elements in the original coordinate system (cf. Chap. 1 in this book):

$$\tilde{T}_{i_1\ldots i_p} = \sum_{l_1=1}^{N} \cdots \sum_{l_p=1}^{N} r_{i_1 l_1} \ldots r_{i_p l_p} T_{l_1\ldots l_p} \tag{4.13}$$

where $T_{l_1\ldots l_p}$ are the elements of a pth-order tensor, and r_{il} are the elements of the N-dimensional rotation matrix. These transformation rules ensure that the properties represented by the tensor as a whole remain invariant under Euclidean transformations of the space, even when the individual tensor elements do not. New tensors can be created from existing ones by linear combinations, by means of the Cartesian (outer) product and by contraction. A tensor of order zero is a rotationally invariant scalar. Therefore, we can interpret every pixel of the original image or an image obtained by a rotationally symmetric filter as a 0th-order tensor.

We can define a tensor-based generalization of quadrature filtering by replacing the 1-dimensional Hilbert transform with the N-dimensional *Riesz transform* [5] which is defined as:

$$\text{Fourier domain:} \quad \mathcal{H}_N[H(\mathbf{u})] = j\frac{\mathbf{u}}{|\mathbf{u}|}H(\mathbf{u}) \tag{4.14}$$

$$\text{spatial domain:} \quad \mathcal{H}_N[h(\mathbf{x})] = \frac{\Gamma((N+1)/2)}{\pi^{(N+1)/2}}\left(\frac{-\mathbf{x}}{|\mathbf{x}|^{N+1}} \star h(\mathbf{x})\right) \tag{4.15}$$

where Γ is the gamma function. In essence, the scalar-valued frequency coordinate u of the Hilbert transform is simply replaced by an N-dimensional frequency vector $\mathbf{u}$. The Riesz transform can be interpreted as a first-order tensor operator because it turns a scalar valued function into a first order tensor-valued one. This can be easily seen by observing that the ratio $\frac{\mathbf{u}}{|\mathbf{u}|}$ defines the first order spherical harmonics (i.e. $(\cos\theta,\sin\theta)^T$ in 2D, $(\cos\theta\cos\phi,\sin\theta\cos\phi,\sin\phi)^T$ in 3D etc.), and polar separable functions with this angular behavior conform exactly to (4.13) with $p = 1$. Spherical harmonics are preserved by inverse Fourier transformation, so that the spatial domain version (4.15) of the Riesz transform has the same angular behavior and the tensor requirements are still satisfied. The Riesz transform is closely related to the gradient and acts in a qualitatively similar way, as can be seen by defining the latter in terms of the former:

$$\nabla_N h(\mathbf{x}) \quad \circ\!\!-\!\!\bullet \quad \mathcal{H}_N[|\mathbf{u}|\,H(\mathbf{u})] \tag{4.16}$$

where $\circ\!\!-\!\!\bullet$ denotes Fourier correspondence. Both operators have the same angular behavior, but the gradient in addition changes the radial part of the spectrum. This difference is of crucial importance for the definition of phase-invariant operators. Another important observation concerns the difference between the 1-dimensional Hilbert transform and the multi-dimensional Riesz transform: while applying the former transform twice just reproduces the original signal (with reversed sign), multiple applications of the Riesz transform create tensors of higher and higher orders. This is again similar to the gradient operator, where twofold application results in the Hessian matrix etc.

However, applying the Riesz transform to the original image makes little sense in practice, because its spatial domain kernel decreases only as $|\mathbf{x}|^{-N}$, so that feature localization would be bad. Instead, one combines it with a radially symmetric band-pass. In contrast to derivative filters, where the band-pass changes with the derivative order, the band-pass is kept the same for all orders of the Riesz transform. We define the first and second order band-pass Riesz transforms $\mathbf{b}$ and $\mathbf{A}$ of an image F in the Fourier domain as

$$\mathbf{b} \quad \circ\!\!-\!\!\bullet \quad \mathcal{H}_N[K(|\mathbf{u}|)F(\mathbf{u})] = j\frac{\mathbf{u}}{|\mathbf{u}|}K(|\mathbf{u}|)F(\mathbf{u}) \tag{4.17}$$

$$\mathbf{A} \quad \circ\!\!-\!\!\bullet \quad \mathcal{H}_N^2[K(|\mathbf{u}|)F(\mathbf{u})] = -\frac{\mathbf{u}\mathbf{u}^T}{|\mathbf{u}|^2}K(|\mathbf{u}|)F(\mathbf{u}) \tag{4.18}$$

where $K(|\mathbf{u}|)$ is the band-pass. It should be noted that these definitions are valid for all dimensions $N \geq 2$. The boundary tensor is now defined as

$$\mathbf{B} = \mathbf{b}\mathbf{b}^T + \mathbf{A}\mathbf{A}^T \qquad (4.19)$$

This definition is structurally equivalent to (4.12), but the parameter γ is no longer needed, because the boundary tensor is phase invariant for all frequencies (see below). Since $\mathbf{A}$ and $\mathbf{b}$ are both real, it follows that $\mathbf{B}$ is always positive semi-definite. Therefore, the trace of the tensor can be interpreted as a measure of local signal energy, which will be called *boundary energy*. The choice of this name stems from the fact that the tensor indeed detects important boundary features, as is shown below.

4.3 Analysis of the Boundary Tensor as a Quadratic Filter

In order to analyse the properties of the boundary tensor, we follow the proposal of [12] and formulate the tensor as a quadratic filter [13]. Quadratic convolution is defined as

$$\tilde{f}(\mathbf{x}) = \iint h(\mathbf{x} - \mathbf{x_1}, \mathbf{x} - \mathbf{x_2}) f(\mathbf{x_1}) f(\mathbf{x_2}) \, d\mathbf{x_1} \, d\mathbf{x_2} \qquad (4.20)$$

where $h(.,.)$ is the kernel, and the method is termed 'quadratic' because the original image f appears twice in the integral. Let $g_i(\mathbf{x})$ denote the ith component $(i = 1...N)$ of the first order band-pass Riesz transform kernel. Then

$$(\mathbf{b}\mathbf{b}^T)_{il} = \mathbf{b}_i\mathbf{b}_l = (g_i \star f)(g_l \star f)$$
$$= \int g_i(\mathbf{x} - \mathbf{x_1}) f(\mathbf{x_1}) \, d\mathbf{x_1} \int g_l(\mathbf{x} - \mathbf{x_2}) f(\mathbf{x_2}) \, d\mathbf{x_2}$$
$$= \iint g_i(\mathbf{x} - \mathbf{x_1}) g_l(\mathbf{x} - \mathbf{x_2}) f(\mathbf{x_1}) f(\mathbf{x_2}) \, d\mathbf{x_1} \, d\mathbf{x_2} \qquad (4.21)$$

Similarly, let $g_{il}(\mathbf{x})$ represent component il $(i, l = 1...N)$ of the kernel for the second order band-pass Riesz transform. This leads to

$$(\mathbf{A}\mathbf{A}^T)_{il} = \sum_k \mathbf{A}_{ik}\mathbf{A}_{kl} = \sum_k (g_{ik} \star f)(g_{kl} \star f)$$
$$= \iint \left(\sum_k g_{ik}(\mathbf{x} - \mathbf{x_1}) g_{kl}(\mathbf{x} - \mathbf{x_2}) \right) f(\mathbf{x_1}) f(\mathbf{x_2}) \, d\mathbf{x_1} \, d\mathbf{x_2} \qquad (4.22)$$

We can combine both equations into a single quadratic convolution with

$$h_{il}(\mathbf{x_1}, \mathbf{x_2}) = g_i(\mathbf{x_1}) g_l(\mathbf{x_2}) + \sum_k g_{ik}(\mathbf{x_1}) g_{kl}(\mathbf{x_2}) \qquad (4.23)$$

Then the components of the boundary tensor can be written as

$$\text{spatial domain: } \mathbf{B}_{il}(\mathbf{x}) \quad = \quad \iint h_{il}(\mathbf{x} - \mathbf{x_1}, \mathbf{x} - \mathbf{x_2}) f(\mathbf{x_1}) f(\mathbf{x_2}) \, d\mathbf{x_1} \, d\mathbf{x_2}$$

$$\text{Fourier domain: } \mathbf{B}_{il}(\mathbf{x}) \ \circ\!\!\!-\!\!\!\bullet \ \iint H_{il}(\mathbf{u}, \mathbf{v}) F(\mathbf{u}) F(\mathbf{v}) e^{j(\mathbf{u}+\mathbf{v})^T \mathbf{x}} \, d\mathbf{u} \, d\mathbf{v} \quad (4.24)$$

where F is the N-dimensional Fourier transform of f, H_{il} is the $2N$-dimensional Fourier transform of h_{il}, and $e^{j(\mathbf{u}+\mathbf{v})^T \mathbf{x}}$ translates f so that the current point $\mathbf{x}$ becomes the origin. Inserting the Fourier representation of the band-pass Riesz transform, H_{il} gets a simple functional form:

$$H_{il}(\mathbf{u}, \mathbf{v}) = -\frac{\mathbf{u}_i}{|\mathbf{u}|} \frac{\mathbf{v}_l}{|\mathbf{v}|} K(|\mathbf{u}|) K(|\mathbf{v}|) + \sum_k \left(\frac{\mathbf{u}_i \mathbf{u}_k}{|\mathbf{u}|^2} \frac{\mathbf{v}_k \mathbf{v}_l}{|\mathbf{v}|^2} \right) K(|\mathbf{u}|) K(|\mathbf{v}|)$$

$$= \frac{\mathbf{u}_i \mathbf{v}_l}{|\mathbf{u}||\mathbf{v}|} \left(-1 + \frac{\mathbf{u}^T \mathbf{v}}{|\mathbf{u}||\mathbf{v}|} \right) K(|\mathbf{u}|) K(|\mathbf{v}|) \quad (4.25)$$

In order for $\mathbf{B}_{il}$ to be real for real images f, it is required that $H_{il}(-\mathbf{u}, -\mathbf{v}) = \overline{H_{il}(\mathbf{u}, \mathbf{v})}$, which is easily verified. Conditions for an N-dimensional tensor operator to behave like a 1-D quadrature filter for simple images (i.e. images where $f(\mathbf{x}) = \hat{f}(\mathbf{x}^T \mathbf{n})$ for some unit vector $\mathbf{n}$ giving the signal orientation) are derived in [12]. If the signal is simple, the spectrum of $F(\mathbf{u})$ vanishes for all $\mathbf{u} \neq t\mathbf{n}$, and the restriction of the kernel to this line must reduce to

$$H_{il}(t\mathbf{n}, \tau\mathbf{n}) = \mathbf{n}_i \mathbf{n}_l \hat{H}(t, \tau) \quad (4.26)$$

Furthermore, in order for the signal energy to be phase invariant $\hat{H}(t, t) = 0$ must hold for all t. Both conditions are fulfilled, because $\mathbf{u}_i = t\mathbf{n}_i$ and $\mathbf{v}_i = \tau\mathbf{n}_i$, and thus

$$H_{il}(t\mathbf{n}, \tau\mathbf{n}) = \frac{t\tau \mathbf{n}_i \mathbf{n}_l}{|t||\tau|} \left(-1 + \frac{t\tau \mathbf{n}^T \mathbf{n}}{|t||\tau|} \right) K(|t|) K(|\tau|)$$

$$= \mathbf{n}_i \mathbf{n}_l \left(-\operatorname{sign}(t\tau) + 1 \right) K(|t|) K(|\tau|) \quad (4.27)$$

In fact, this is precisely 4 times the expression which [12] derived for the quadrature filter method according to [9], cf. 4.10), so that both approaches behave identically for simple signals. For simple signals the signal energy $\operatorname{tr}(\mathbf{B}) = \sum_k \mathbf{B}_{kk}$ reduces exactly to the 1-dimensional quadrature energy (4.8):

$$\operatorname{tr}(\mathbf{B}) = \sum_k \iint \mathbf{n}_k^2 (-\operatorname{sign}(t\tau) + 1) K(|t|) K(|\tau|) \hat{F}(t\mathbf{n}) \hat{F}(\tau\mathbf{n}) \, e^{j(t+\tau)\mathbf{n}^T \mathbf{x}} \, dt \, d\tau$$

$$= \left(\mathcal{H}_1[k_1] \star \hat{f} \right)^2 + \left(k_1 \star \hat{f} \right)^2 \quad (4.28)$$

where k_1 is the 1-dimensional inverse Fourier transform of K and $\mathcal{H}_1[k_1]$ its Hilbert transform (derivation see appendix).

H_{il} is also a useful tool to analyse the behavior of the boundary tensor for intrinsically 2-dimensional features. To simplify matters, we consider points

$\mathbf{x}$ where the spectrum $F(\mathbf{u})$ computed with $\mathbf{x}$ as coordinate origin is polar separable within the pass-band of the tensor filter $K(|\mathbf{u}|)$. At many structures of interest this is at least approximately true. Then the product $K(|\mathbf{u}|)F(\mathbf{u})$ can be written as $K(|\mathbf{u}|)F_r(|\mathbf{u}|)F_a(\phi)$. After inserting this and (4.25) into the boundary tensor expression (4.24), the latter can be transformed into polar coordinates and simplifies into a product of two integrals:

$$
\begin{aligned}
\mathbf{B}_{il} &= \iint \frac{u_i v_l}{|\mathbf{u}||\mathbf{v}|}\left(-1 + \frac{\mathbf{u}^T \mathbf{v}}{|\mathbf{u}||\mathbf{v}|}\right) K(|\mathbf{u}|)K(|\mathbf{v}|)F(\mathbf{u})F(\mathbf{v})\, d\mathbf{u}\, d\mathbf{v} \\
&= \left(\iint \mathbf{n}_i(\phi)\mathbf{n}_l(\psi)\left(-1 + \mathbf{n}^T(\phi)\,\mathbf{n}(\psi)\right) F_a(\phi)F_a(\psi)\, d\phi\, d\psi\right) \\
&\quad \left(\iint K(\rho_1)K(\rho_2)F_r(\rho_1)F_r(\rho_2)\,\rho_1\, d\rho_1\,\rho_2\, d\rho_2\right) \\
&= \mathbf{B}_{a,il}\, tensor\, B_r
\end{aligned}
\tag{4.29}
$$

with $\mathbf{u} = \rho_1\mathbf{n}(\phi) = \rho_1(\cos(\phi),\sin(\phi))^T$ and $\mathbf{v} = \rho_2\mathbf{n}(\psi) = \rho_2(\cos(\psi),\sin(\psi))^T$. It should be noted that this is a major advantage of using the Riesz transform: Otherwise, the first and second order filter kernels would have had different radial parts, and the separation of angular and radial behavior were impossible. The angular integral $\mathbf{B}_{a,il}$ in (4.29) can be further simplified in terms of the Fourier coefficients of F_a:

$$
\alpha_n = \int \cos(n\phi)F_a(\phi)\, d\phi \qquad \beta_n = \int \sin(n\phi)F_a(\phi)\, d\phi
\tag{4.30}
$$

It turns out that only the Fourier coefficients up to second order are relevant (the others drop out due to orthogonality of trigonometric functions), and the boundary tensor components can be written as (see appendix):

$$
\begin{aligned}
\mathbf{B}_{11} &= (\alpha_1^2 + \tfrac{1}{4}(\alpha_0 + \alpha_2)^2 + \tfrac{1}{4}\beta_2^2)\, \mathbf{B}_r \\
\mathbf{B}_{22} &= (\beta_1^2 + \tfrac{1}{4}(\alpha_0 - \alpha_2)^2 + \tfrac{1}{4}\beta_2^2)\, \mathbf{B}_r \\
\mathbf{B}_{12} &= (\alpha_1\beta_1 + \tfrac{1}{2}\alpha_0\beta_2)\, \mathbf{B}_r
\end{aligned}
\tag{4.31}
$$

where $\mathbf{B}_r$ is the radial part of (4.29). These equations give us a qualitative understanding of how the boundary tensor reacts to 2D features: At (approximately) polar separable locations, its components are products of radial and angular expressions. The former measure the contrast of the local structure at the scale of the bandpass filter, and the latter determine how well the angular shape can be represented with circular harmonics up to order 2. Since many important structures (edges, lines, saddles, corners) are covered by this model, the boundary tensor reacts reasonably at many locations where for example the gradient (which solely relies on first-order circular harmonics) fails. We illustrate this with two examples: parameterized step and line edges. In the spatial domain the angular parts of these features can be written as

$$
f_{a,\mathrm{edge}}(\phi) = \Theta(\phi+\phi_0)-\Theta(\phi-\phi_0) \qquad f_{a,\mathrm{line}}(\phi) = \delta(\phi+\phi_0)-\delta(\phi-\phi_0)
\tag{4.32}
$$

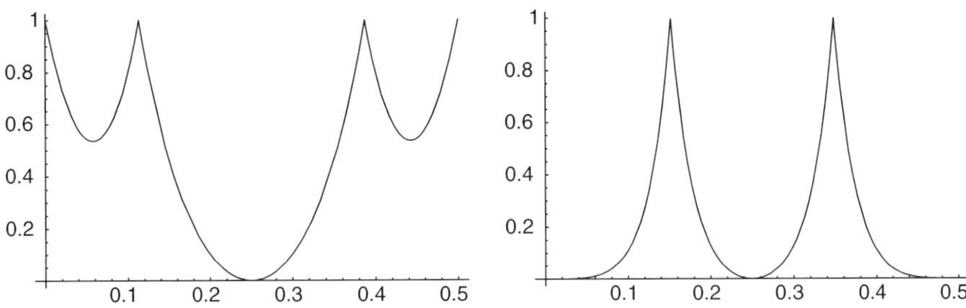

Fig. 4.1. Eigenvalue ratios $\mu = \min(\mathbf{B}_{11}, \mathbf{B}_{22})/\max(\mathbf{B}_{11}, \mathbf{B}_{22})$ for a parameterized edge (*left*) and line (*right*) as a function of $l_0 = \phi_0/(2\pi)$

where Θ is the step function and δ the impulse function. The parameter $\phi_0 \in [0, \pi]$ determines the angle of the corner, and $\phi_0 = \pi/2$ results in a straight edge or line. Due to symmetry, $\mathbf{B}_{12}$ is always zero at the center of these configurations, and $\mathbf{B}_{11}$, $\mathbf{B}_{22}$ are the tensor eigenvalues. The ratio of the eigenvalues is a measure that distinguishes locally 1-dimensional and 2-dimensional configurations – it is near 0 in the former and near 1 in the latter case. Figure 4.1 shows these ratios as a function of ϕ_0. It can be seen that we get indeed $\mu = 0$ for $\phi_0 = \pi/2$ (straight edge/line) and $\mu = 1$ for $\phi_0 = \pi/4$ and $\phi_0 = 3\pi/4$ (90 degree corners). For $\phi_0 = 0$ the edge disappears, and $\mu = 1$ indicates that the remaining homogenuous region is interpreted as a 2D configuration, whereas in case of the line, $\phi_0 = 0$ results in a half-line which the boundary tensor cannot distinguish from a straight line, hence $\mu = 0$. Since more complex junction configurations can be expressed as combinations of multiple edge and/or line corners, they can be analysed in essentially the same way. All junctions that can be approximated well with an angular second-order Fourier series (e.g. saddle points, crossings of two straight lines) will be characterized correctly by the boundary tensor.

4.4 Efficient Computation of the Boundary Tensor

In order to compute the boundary tensor in practice we have to choose a suitable band-pass K. Filters based on Gaussian or exponential transfer functions and log-normal filters are obvious choices. If implemented in the Fourier domain, all these filters are equally easy to compute. However, we have only been able to find an efficient *spatial* domain implementation of the boundary tensor (or actually a close approximation of it) if the band-pass equals the magnitude of the Laplacian of Gaussian

$$K(|\mathbf{u}|, \sigma) = |\mathbf{u}|^2 e^{-\frac{|\mathbf{u}|^2 \sigma^2}{2}} \tag{4.33}$$

Moreover, we have experimentally found that this band-pass gives better feature resolution (less blending of nearby features into each other) than other choices, which is probably due to the Gaussian's optimal localization in both the spatial and frequency domains. The spectra of the filters are the product of the bandpass with first and second order Riesz transforms:

$$G_i(\mathbf{u}) = j\mathbf{u}_i|\mathbf{u}|e^{-\frac{|\mathbf{u}|^2\sigma^2}{2}} \tag{4.34}$$

$$G_{il}(\mathbf{x}) = -\mathbf{u}_i\mathbf{u}_l e^{-\frac{|\mathbf{u}|^2\sigma^2}{2}} \tag{4.35}$$

It can be seen that the second order spectra are exactly those of the second derivative of the Gaussian. Therefore, the spatial filter function is:

$$g_{il}(\mathbf{x}) = \frac{\mathbf{x}_i\mathbf{x}_l - 2\sigma^2\delta_{il}}{2\pi\sigma^6} e^{-\frac{|\mathbf{x}|^2}{2\sigma^2}} \tag{4.36}$$

and the resulting tensor $\mathbf{A}$ is the Hessian of Gaussian, which can be efficiently computed by separable convolutions. Inverse Fourier transform of the first order filters is more complicated (see appendix). The result is

$$g_i(\mathbf{x}) = \frac{\mathbf{x}_i}{4\sqrt{2\pi}\sigma^7} e^{-\frac{|\mathbf{x}|^2}{4\sigma^2}} \left((|\mathbf{x}|^2 - 3\sigma^2)I_0\left(\frac{|\mathbf{x}|^2}{4\sigma^2}\right) - (|\mathbf{x}|^2 - \sigma^2)I_1\left(\frac{|\mathbf{x}|^2}{4\sigma^2}\right) \right) \tag{4.37}$$

where I_0 and I_1 are modified Bessel functions of the first kind. Figure 4.2 left depicts the shape of g_1 and g_{11} along the $\mathbf{x}_1$ axis. Unfortunately, the first order kernels are unsuitable for practical applications because their asymptotic decay is only $\mathcal{O}(|\mathbf{x}|^{-4})$ and they are not Cartesian separable. This means that large 2-dimensional filter masks are needed, which makes computation of g_i very slow. Therefore, we apply a design technique similar to the one used for steerable quadrature filters [7] to approximate g_i with filters $\tilde{g}_i$ that can be computed separably and decay exponentially. The idea is to realize $\tilde{g}_i$ as sums of filters that are third order polynomials times a Gaussian. The polynomials-times-Gaussian are defined so that they together form a supersymmetric third order tensor filter $\tilde{g}_{ijk}$ (a supersymmetric tensor has the property that its

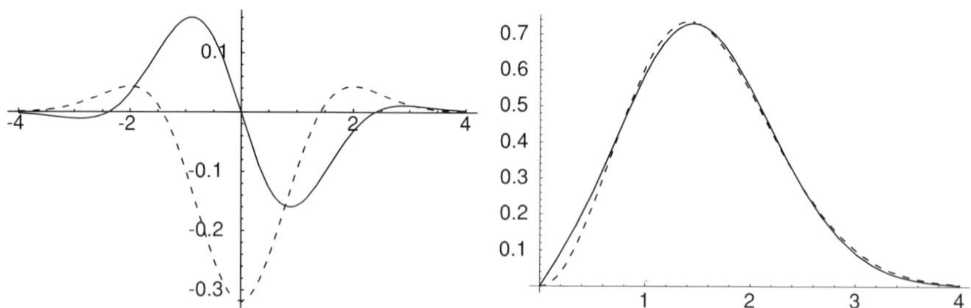

Fig. 4.2. *Left*: g_1 (*solid*) and g_{11} (*dashed*) along the $\mathbf{x}_1$ axis when the band-pass is the Laplacian of Gaussian at $\sigma = 1$ (g_1 and its approximation $\tilde{g}_1$ according to (4.39) and (4.41) are almost indistinguishable in the depicted 4σ interval). *Right*: spectra of K (*dashed*) and its approximation $\tilde{G}_1 = \mathcal{F}[\tilde{g}_1]$ (*solid*) at $\sigma = 1$

components don't change under permutation of indices, i.e. $\tilde{g}_{112} = \tilde{g}_{121} = \tilde{g}_{211}$ etc.). Then the first order tensor filter can be obtained by contraction over any pair of indices, i.e. $\tilde{g}_i = \sum_k \tilde{g}_{ikk}$. We make the following ansatz:

$$\tilde{g}_{iii}(\mathbf{x}, \sigma') = \left(\frac{a\mathbf{x}_i^3}{\sigma'^5} + \frac{b\mathbf{x}_i}{\sigma'^3} \right) g(\mathbf{x}, \sigma')$$

$$\tilde{g}_{ill}(\mathbf{x}, \sigma') = \frac{\mathbf{x}_i}{\sigma'^2} \left(\frac{a\mathbf{x}_l^2}{\sigma'^3} + \frac{b}{3\sigma'} \right) g(\mathbf{x}, \sigma') \qquad (i \neq l) \tag{4.38}$$

$$\tilde{g}_{ilk}(\mathbf{x}, \sigma') = \frac{a}{\sigma'^5} \mathbf{x}_i \mathbf{x}_l \mathbf{x}_k \, g(\mathbf{x}, \sigma') \qquad (i \neq l \neq k)$$

where $g(\mathbf{x}, \sigma')$ is an N-dimensional Gaussian, and the last function is only required if $N > 2$ (for $N = 2$, the condition $i \neq l \neq k$ is never satisfied). By expressing these functions in a rotated coordinate system, it is easy (if tedious) to verify that (4.13) is fulfilled with $p = 3$. The spectrum of $\tilde{g}_i$ is

$$\tilde{g}_i = \sum_k \tilde{g}_{ikk} \quad \circ\!\!-\!\!\bullet \quad \tilde{G}_i(\mathbf{u}, \sigma') = \frac{\mathbf{u}_i}{\sigma'} \left(a(4 - |\mathbf{u}|^2\sigma'^2) + \frac{4b}{3} \right) e^{-|\mathbf{u}|^2\sigma'^2/2} \tag{4.39}$$

We now formulate a least squares problem to choose a, b, σ' so that the radial part of $\tilde{G}_i(\mathbf{u}, \sigma')$ becomes as similar to $K(\mathbf{u}, \sigma)$ as possible:

$$\text{minimize w.r.t. } a, b, \sigma' : \quad \int \left(\tilde{G}(|\mathbf{u}|, \sigma') - K(|\mathbf{u}|, \sigma) \right)^2 d\mathbf{u} \tag{4.40}$$

where $\tilde{G}(|\mathbf{u}|, \sigma')$ is obtained from $\tilde{G}_i(\mathbf{u}, \sigma')$ by replacing $\mathbf{u}_i$ with $|\mathbf{u}|$. The optimum depends on the dimension N of the space. For $N = 2, 3$ we get

$$a_{2D} = -0.5589, \qquad b_{2D} = 2.0425, \qquad \sigma'_{2D} = 1.0818\,\sigma$$

$$a_{3D} = -0.5086, \qquad b_{3D} = 1.8562, \qquad \sigma'_{3D} = 1.0683\,\sigma \tag{4.41}$$

Figure 4.2 right depicts $\tilde{G}$ and K for the 2D case. It should be noted that it is important to include the filter scale in the optimization because this significantly improves the fit. To conclude, we can compute the boundary tensor by using 7 separable, exponentially decaying filters in 2D, and 15 such filters in 3D. This can be compared with the structure tensor, where N filters are used to compute the gradients, but then $N(N + 1)/2$ filters at a larger (typically doubled) scale are applied to integrate the gradient tensors over a neighborhood. Thus, the number of filters is lower, but larger windows are required, making the overall computational effort about equal.

4.5 Applications

The boundary tensor can be used much like the structure tensor, e.g. as an integrated detector for low-level image features such as edges, lines, corners,

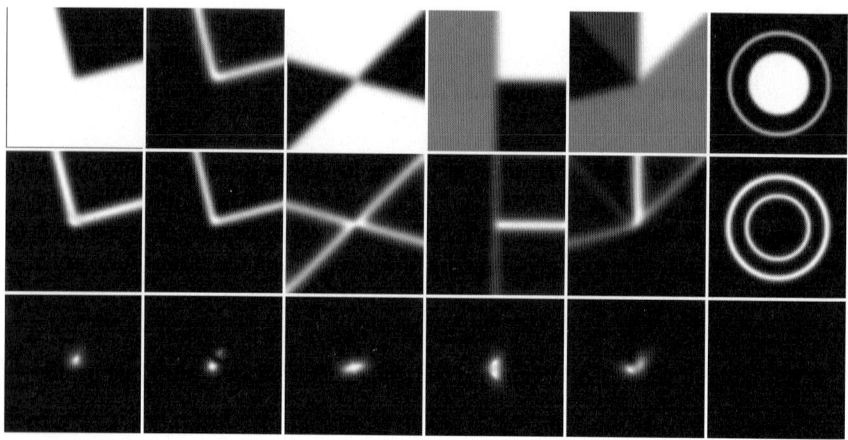

Fig. 4.3. *Top*: test patterns, *center*: boundary energy tr($\mathbf{B}$), *bottom*: junction energy tr($\mathbf{B}_{\text{junction}}$)

and junctions (in 3D additionally surfaces), and to estimate local orientation. For feature analysis it is advantageous to consider the eigensystem of the boundary tensor. Using the eigenvalues $\mu_1 \geq \mu_2 \geq 0$ and the eigenvector $\mathbf{n}$ corresponding to μ_1 (cf. Chap. 1 by Hagen and Garth), one can decompose the boundary tensor into its 1D and 2D (edge/line and corner/junction) contributions:

$$\mathbf{B} = \mathbf{B}_{\text{edge}} + \mathbf{B}_{\text{junction}} = (\mu_1 - \mu_2)\mathbf{n}\mathbf{n}^T + \mu_2\mathbf{I} \tag{4.42}$$

Figure 4.3 demonstrates this for a number of test patterns. The angle ψ between $\mathbf{n} = (\cos(\psi), \sin(\psi))^T$ and the x-axis is given as

$$\psi = \frac{1}{2}\arctan\left(\frac{2\mathbf{B}_{12}}{\mathbf{B}_{11} - \mathbf{B}_{22}}\right) \tag{4.43}$$

Local maxima of the 2D energy tr($\mathbf{B}_{\text{junction}}$) = $2\mu_2$ are a good corner and junction detector. Its localization error is only half as big as the errors of the Förstner and Harris detectors (4.4), Fig. 4.4 left. Moreover, it does not give multiple responses at saddle-like junctions, Fig. 4.4 right. An edge detector can be defined by reducing the edge part of the tensor to a vector

$$\mathbf{g} = \sqrt{\mu_1 - \mu_2}\,\mathbf{n} \tag{4.44}$$

which can be used instead of the gradient vector in Canny's algorithm [3]. This algorithm can then detect lines as well as edges, and sub-pixel accurate localization is still possible, although we have found the noise sensitivity of edge position to be somewhat higher than for the standard Canny algorithm. Edge/line detection can also be integrated with corner/junction detection, because both feature types are derived from the same tensor representation. In this way, a complicated integration step of edge and corner responses into a unified boundary representation is avoided. This is illustrated in Fig. 4.5.

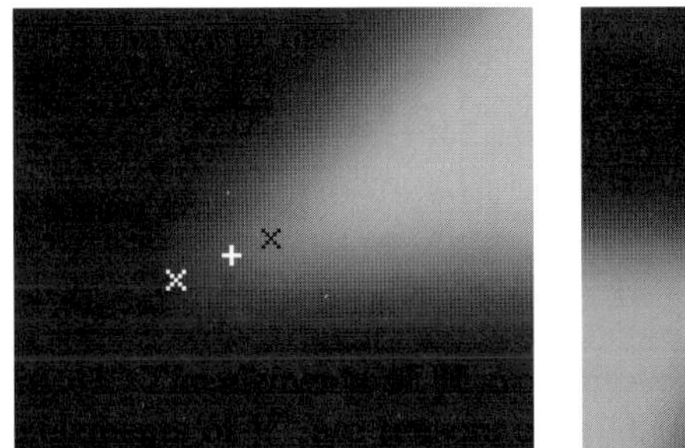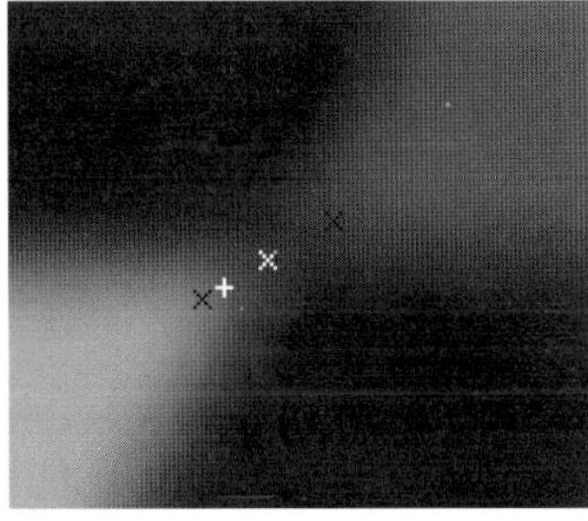

Fig. 4.4. Corner localization of the boundary tensor (white +) and Förstner detector (black ×) relative to exact corner location (white ×). Note the double response of the Förstner detector in the right image. Had the contrast of the two wings of the saddle been equal, the boundary tensor response would have been exact. Harris detector results are very close to Förstner's

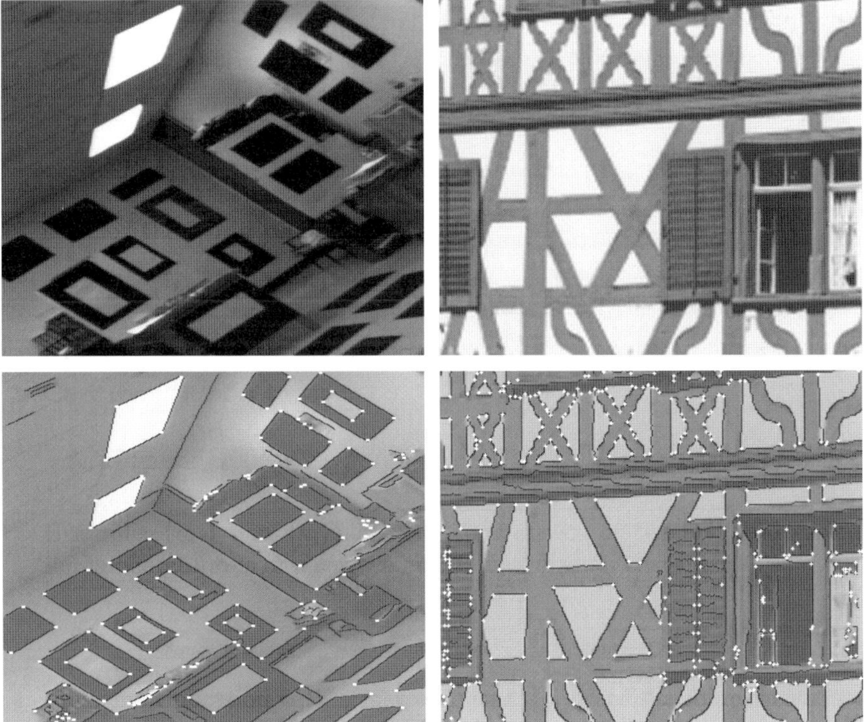

Fig. 4.5. *Top*: original image. *bottom*: integrated edge (*black lines*) and junction (*white crosses*) detection

4.6 Conclusions

In this chapter we discussed the *boundary tensor* as a new way to represent low-level feature strength and orientation. It combines many good properties of existing tensor-based approaches and avoids a number of problems. The key insight is that the filters used to compute the boundary tensors should be defined in terms of the *Riesz transform* which determines the angular filter sensitivity, combined with a band-pass which controls scale sensitivity. In this way, the tensor components become products of an angular part that characterizes the feature type, and a radial part that determines feature strength at a given scale. Since the tensor definition does not depend on the dimension of the image, it can readily be used for 3D (volume or space-time) and 4D (volume-time) data sets.

We have shown that a tensor defined with Riesz transform filters reacts like a quadrature filter to locally 1-dimensional configurations. We used filters up to second order, so the boundary tensor also reacts in a predictable and useful way to 2-dimensional configurations that are well approximated by a second-order angular Fourier series, e.g. corners, saddle junctions and crossings of straight lines. If more complex junction configurations have to be analysed, it is possible to extend the boundary tensor definition towards third and higher order Riesz transforms by including terms of the form $\sum_{k,m} T_{ikm} T_{lkm}$ etc. However, higher order filters can no longer be used at small scales due to angular aliasing, so the best trade-off will be application dependent. By choosing the band-pass as the Laplacian of Gaussian, we were able to derive an efficient and accurate spatial domain implementation. In a number of examples we illustrated the good performance of the new method. Further illustrations can be found in [10].

Appendix

Derivation of (4.28): We want to show that in case of a simple signal the trace of the boundary tensor is exactly the 1-dimensional signal energy. Observe that $-\operatorname{sign}(t\tau) = j\operatorname{sign}(t)j\operatorname{sign}(\tau)$ and $\sum_k \mathbf{n}_k^2 = 1$:

$$\operatorname{tr}(\mathbf{B}) = \sum_k \iint \mathbf{n}_k^2 (-\operatorname{sign}(t\tau) + 1) K(|t|) K(|\tau|) \hat{F}(t\mathbf{n}) \hat{F}(\tau\mathbf{n})\, e^{j(t+\tau)\mathbf{n}^T\mathbf{x}}\, dt\, d\tau$$

$$= \sum_k \mathbf{n}_k^2 \left(\iint -\operatorname{sign}(t\tau) K(|t|) K(|\tau|) \hat{F}(t\mathbf{n}) \hat{F}(\tau\mathbf{n})\, e^{j(t+\tau)\mathbf{n}^T\mathbf{x}}\, dt\, d\tau \right.$$

$$\left. + \iint K(|t|) K(|\tau|) \hat{F}(t\mathbf{n}) \hat{F}(\tau\mathbf{n})\, e^{j(t+\tau)\mathbf{n}^T\mathbf{x}}\, dt\, d\tau \right)$$

$$= \left(\int j\operatorname{sign}(t) K(|t|) \hat{F}(t\mathbf{n})\, e^{jt\mathbf{n}^T\mathbf{x}}\, dt \right)^2 + \left(\int K(|t|) \hat{F}(t\mathbf{n})\, e^{jt\mathbf{n}^T\mathbf{x}}\, dt \right)^2$$

$$= \left(\mathcal{H}_1[k_1] \star \hat{f} \right)^2 + \left(k_1 \star \hat{f} \right)^2$$

The last transition is simply based on recognizing the integrals as the Fourier domain correspondents of the respective spatial convolutions.

Derivation of (4.31): We show that the boundary tensor components can be expressed in terms of the Fourier coefficients of the angular function F_a when the spectrum $F(\mathbf{u})$ is polar separable. The Fourier series of F_a is:

$$F_a(\phi) = \frac{\alpha_0}{2\pi} + \sum_{n=1}^{\infty} \frac{j^n}{\pi} \left(\alpha_n \cos(n\phi) + \beta_n \sin(n\phi) \right) \tag{4.45}$$

where α_n and β_n are the Fourier coefficients according to (4.30). Note that the odd order terms are imaginary, because the spatial domain image is real. We perform the derivation for $\mathbf{B}_{a,11}$, the procedure for the other components is analogous.

$$\mathbf{B}_{a,11} = \int_0^{2\pi} \int_0^{2\pi} \mathbf{n}_1(\phi)\mathbf{n}_1(\psi) \left(-1 + \mathbf{n}^T(\phi)\,\mathbf{n}(\psi) \right) F_a(\phi) F_a(\psi)\, d\phi\, d\psi$$

$$= \iint \cos(\phi)\cos(\psi)\left(-1 + \cos(\phi)\cos(\psi) + \sin(\phi)\sin(\psi) \right) F_a(\phi) F_a(\psi)\, d\phi\, d\psi$$

$$= -\left(\int \cos(\phi) F_a(\phi)\, d\phi \right)^2 + \left(\int \cos^2(\phi) F_a(\phi)\, d\phi \right)^2 + \left(\int \cos(\phi)\sin(\phi) F_a(\phi)\, d\phi \right)^2$$

$$= -\left(\int \cos(\phi) F_a(\phi)\, d\phi \right)^2 + \left(\int \frac{1 + \cos(2\phi)}{2} F_a(\phi)\, d\phi \right)^2 + \left(\int \frac{\sin(2\phi)}{2} F_a(\phi)\, d\phi \right)^2$$

Now we insert the Fourier series for F_a. Due to orthogonality, all integrals involving a product of different trigonometric functions are zero. Only terms containing the square of a single trigonometric are nonzero, reproducing a Fourier coefficient, e.g.:

$$\int_0^{2\pi} \cos(\phi) F_a(\phi)\, d\phi = \frac{j}{\pi}\,\alpha_1 \int_0^{2\pi} \cos(\phi)\cos(\phi)\, d\phi = j\,\alpha_1$$

Collecting all 'surviving' terms, we get the desired result:

$$\mathbf{B}_{a,11} = \alpha_1^2 + \frac{1}{4}(\alpha_0 + \alpha_2)^2 + \frac{1}{4}\beta_2^2$$

Derivation of (4.37): We want to calculate the two spatial filter functions (i.e. inverse Fourier transforms) of the first order band-pass Riesz kernels $j u_i |\mathbf{u}| e^{-\frac{|\mathbf{u}|^2 \sigma^2}{2}}$. In this context, it is advantageous to interpret the pair of real valued filters as a complex valued function $g(\mathbf{x}) = g_1(\mathbf{x}) + j\,g_2(\mathbf{x})$. Then the inverse Fourier transform of both filters can be written as a single integral:

$$g(\mathbf{x}) = g_1(\mathbf{x}) + j\,g_2(\mathbf{x}) = \frac{1}{4\pi^2} \iint j\,(\mathbf{u}_1 + j\mathbf{u}_2)|\mathbf{u}| e^{-\frac{|\mathbf{u}|^2 \sigma^2}{2}} e^{j\mathbf{u}^T \mathbf{x}}\, d\mathbf{u}$$

We turn to the polar representations $\mathbf{u} = \rho e^{j\phi}$ and $\mathbf{x} = r e^{j\psi}$ and get:

$$g(re^{j\psi}) = \frac{1}{4\pi^2} \iint j\, e^{j\phi}\, \rho^2 e^{-\frac{\rho^2\sigma^2}{2}}\, e^{jr\rho\cos(\phi-\psi)}\, d\phi\, \rho\, d\rho$$

By means of the substitution $\phi' = \phi - \psi$, we can rearrange terms as follows:

$$g(re^{j\psi}) = \frac{1}{4\pi^2}\, e^{j\psi} \int_0^\infty j\rho^2 e^{-\frac{\rho^2\sigma^2}{2}} \left(\int_0^{2\pi} e^{j(r\rho\cos(\phi')+\phi')}\, d\phi' \right) \rho\, d\rho$$

The inner integral is a well-known representation of the first-order Bessel function of the first kind: $J_1(t) = \frac{1}{2\pi j} \int_0^{2\pi} e^{j(t\cos(\phi')+\phi')}\, d\phi'$. The outer integral is called the *first-order Hankel transform* of the kernel. It can be computed by means of a symbolic mathematics program such as *Mathematica* or, more traditionally, by using [1], formulas 11.4.28, 13.4.2-5, and 13.6.3:

$$\mathcal{Hankel}[\rho^2 e^{-\frac{\rho^2\sigma^2}{2}}] = 2\pi \int_0^\infty \rho^2 e^{-\frac{\rho^2\sigma^2}{2}} J_1(r\rho)\rho\, d\rho$$

$$= \frac{\pi^{3/2}}{\sqrt{2}\sigma^7}\, r\, e^{-\frac{r^2}{4\sigma^2}} \left((3\sigma^2 - r^2)I_0\left(\frac{r^2}{4\sigma^2}\right) + (r^2 - \sigma^2)I_1\left(\frac{r^2}{4\sigma^2}\right) \right)$$

where I_0 and I_1 are modified Bessel functions. Inserting this into the previous equation and going back to Cartesian coordinates, we arrive at the result:

$$g_i(\mathbf{x}) = \frac{\mathbf{x}_i}{4\sqrt{2\pi}\sigma^7}\, e^{-\frac{|\mathbf{x}|^2}{4\sigma^2}} \left((|\mathbf{x}|^2 - 3\sigma^2)I_0\left(\frac{|\mathbf{x}|^2}{4\sigma^2}\right) - (|\mathbf{x}|^2 - \sigma^2)I_1\left(\frac{|\mathbf{x}|^2}{4\sigma^2}\right) \right)$$

During the above calculations, the expression $g(re^{j\psi}) \sim rM(\frac{5}{2}, 2, \frac{-r^2}{4\sigma^2})$ occurs as an intermediate result, where M is a confluent hypergeometric function. Using this together with [1], 13.1.5, we obtain the filters' asymptotic behavior for large r as $\mathcal{O}(r^{-4})$.

References

1. M. Abramowitz, I. Stegun: *Handbook of Mathematical Functions*, Dover: 1972
2. J. Bigün, G. Granlund, J. Wiklund: *Multidimensional Orientation Estimation with Applications to Texture Analysis and Optic Flow*, IEEE Trans. Pattern Analysis and Machine Intelligence, 13(8):775–790, 1991
3. J. Canny: *A Computational Approach to Edge Detection*, IEEE Trans. Pattern Analysis and Machine Intelligence, 8(6):679–698, 1986
4. G. Farnebäck: *Polynomial Expansion for Orientation and Motion Estimation*, PhD thesis, Linköping University, Dissertation No. 790, 2002
5. M. Felsberg, G. Sommer: *The Monogenic Signal*, IEEE Trans. Image Processing, 49(12):3136–3144, 2001
6. W. Förstner: *A Feature Based Correspondence Algorithm for Image Matching*, Intl. Arch. of Photogrammetry and Remote Sensing, vol. 26, pp. 150–166, 1986

7. W. Freeman, E. Adelson: *The design and use of steerable filters*, IEEE Trans. Pattern Analysis Machine Intelligence, 13(9):891–906, 1991

8. C.G. Harris, M.J. Stevens: *A Combined Corner and Edge Detector*, Proc. of 4th Alvey Vision Conference, pp. 147–151, 1988

9. G. Granlund, H. Knutsson: *Signal Processing for Computer Vision*, Kluwer Academic Publishers, 1995

10. U. Köthe: *Integrated Edge and Junction Detection with the Boundary Tensor*, in: ICCV 03, Proc. of 9th Intl. Conf. on Computer Vision, Nice 2003, vol. 1, pp. 424–431, Los Alamitos: IEEE Computer Society, 2003

11. H.H. Nagel: *Analyse und Interpretation von Bildfolgen II*, Informatik-Spektrum, 8(6):312–327, 1985

12. K. Nordberg, G. Farnebäck: *A Framework for Estimation of Orientation and Velocity*, Proc. IEEE Intl. Conf. on Image Processing, vol. 3:57–60, 2003

13. G. Sicuranza: *Quadratic Filters for Signal Processing*, Proc. of the IEEE, 80(8):1263–1285, 1992

Part II

Diffusion Tensor Imaging

5

An Introduction to Computational Diffusion MRI: the Diffusion Tensor and Beyond

Daniel C. Alexander

Department of Computer Science, University College London, Gower Street, London, WC1E 6BT, UK
D.Alexander@cs.ucl.ac.uk

Summary. This chapter gives an introduction to the principles of diffusion magnetic resonance imaging (MRI) with emphasis on the computational aspects. It introduces the philosophies underlying the technique and shows how to sensitize MRI measurements to the motion of particles within a sample material. The main body of the chapter is a technical review of diffusion MRI reconstruction algorithms, which determine features of the material microstructure from diffusion MRI measurements. The focus is on techniques developed for biomedical diffusion MRI, but most of the methods discussed are applicable beyond this domain. The review begins by showing how the standard reconstruction algorithms in biomedical diffusion MRI, diffusion-tensor MRI and diffusion spectrum imaging, arise from the principles of the measurement process. The discussion highlights the weaknesses of the standard approaches to motivate the development of a new generation of reconstruction algorithms and reviews the current state-of-the-art. The chapter concludes with a brief discussion of diffusion MRI applications, in particular fibre tracking, followed by a summary and a glimpse into the future of diffusion MRI acquisition and reconstruction.

5.1 Introduction

Diffusion magnetic resonance imaging (MRI) provides a unique probe into the microstructure of materials. The method observes the displacements of particles that are subject to Brownian motion within a sample material. Specifically, it measures the probability density function p of particle displacements $\mathbf{x}$ over a fixed time t. The microstructure of the material determines the mobility of the particles within and thus determines p. Conversely, features of p provide information about the material microstructure.

In biomedical diffusion MRI, the particles of interest are usually water molecules. Water is a major constituent of biological tissue. Water molecules within tissue undergo random motion due to thermal fluctuations. Currently, brain imaging is the most common application of biomedical diffusion MRI.

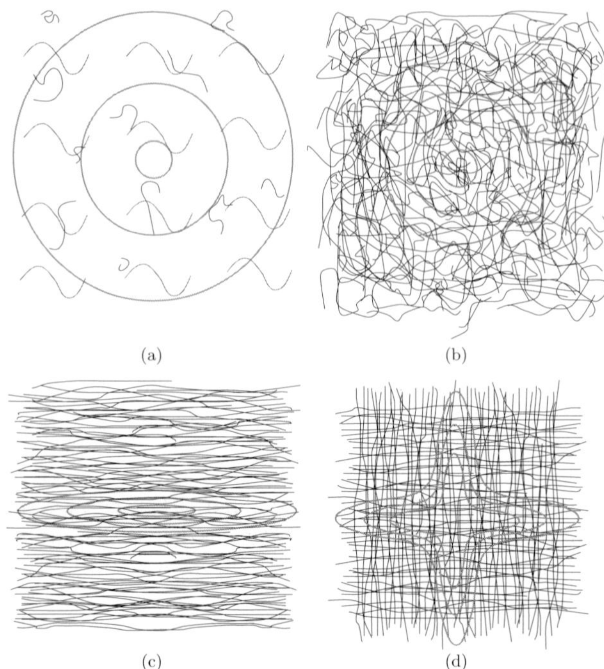

(a)

(b)

(c)

(d)

Fig. 5.1. See colour plates. Schematic diagrams four microstructures found in the brain. The *black* lines are barriers to the movement of water molecules. The *red* contours show the expected shape of p in each tissue. Panel (**a**) shows a fluid-filled region. Panel (**b**) shows isotropic grey matter. Panels (**c**) and (**d**) show white matter with one and two dominant fibre orientations, respectively

The brain has a complex architecture of grey-matter areas connected by white-matter fibres. Diffusion MRI allows non-invasive mapping of the connectivity of the brain.

Figure 5.1 shows schematic diagrams of four different microstructures that appear in brain tissue together with contours of the p that we expect to observe within each kind of tissue. The diagrams do not aim to reproduce true brain-tissue microstructure, but merely to show how different shapes of p can arise from different configurations of barriers to water mobility. Some regions of the brain, such as the ventricles, contain mostly cerebro-spinal fluid (CSF) and Fig. 5.1(a) depicts such a fluid-filled region. Microstructural barriers to water mobility are sparse in these regions, although a few membranes may be present. The function p is isotropic, since displacements are equally likely in all directions. Figure 5.1(b) depicts grey-matter microstructure. Grey matter is dense tissue containing many barriers to water mobility, such as cell walls and membranes. However, the barriers in grey matter often, as in the picture, have no preferred orientation and so hinder the water movement equally in all directions. The function p thus remains isotropic, but is less spread out than in the CSF region, since the average length of displacements is smaller. Figure 5.1(c) depicts the microstructure in a white-matter fibre bundle. White matter contains bundles of parallel axon fibres that connect different regions of the brain. The orientations of the cell walls that form barriers to water mobility have much greater consistency in white matter than in grey matter. The microstructure hinders movement more in directions perpendicular to the fibre than along the fibre axis. Displacements along the fibre are larger on average than displacements across it and p is anisotropic with a ridge in the direction of the fibre. More complex microstructure also appears in white matter. Figure 5.1(d) depicts the microstructure at an orthogonal fibre crossing. Displacements are largest on average in the fibre directions and p has ridges in the directions of each fibre. Other configurations of white matter fibres also occur in the brain.

If we can determine the orientations of the ridges of p, we can infer the dominant orientations of the microstructural fibres. With fibre-orientation estimates in each voxel of a three-dimensional MR image volume, we can follow fibres through the image, using so-called 'tractography' algorithms, see Chap. 7 by Vilanova et al., and construct a connectivity map of the imaged sample.

The following length scales of brain tissue and the measuring process help appreciation of the discussion in the rest of the chapter:

- The voxel volume in biomedical MRI is of order $10^{-9}\,\mathrm{m}^3$.
- The diffusion time, t, in biomedical diffusion MRI is of order $10^{-2}\,\mathrm{s}$ and, over this time, the root-mean-squared displacement of water molecules is in the micrometer range.
- The diameters of axon fibres in human white matter can reach $2.50 \times 10^{-5}\,\mathrm{m}$, but most axon-fibre diameters are less than $10^{-6}\,\mathrm{m}$ [1, 2, 3].
- Coherent white-matter fibre-bundles vary widely in size from several centimetres across down to a few axons.
- The packing density of axon fibres in white matter is of order $10^{11}\,\mathrm{m}^{-2}$ [1, 2, 3].

The next section introduces the basic diffusion MRI measurement and its relationship to the function p. Section 5.3 reviews diffusion MRI reconstruction algorithms, which determine features of the microstructure from diffusion MRI measurements. Section 5.4 gives a brief review of diffusion MRI applications that concentrates on fibre-tracking and connectivity-mapping methods. We conclude in Sect. 5.5 with a summary of the field and some pointers for future research in diffusion MRI methods.

5.2 Diffusion-Weighted MRI

Diffusion-weighted MRI acquires measurements that are sensitive to the motion of nuclei possessing a net spin ('spins'), most commonly hydrogen nuclei.

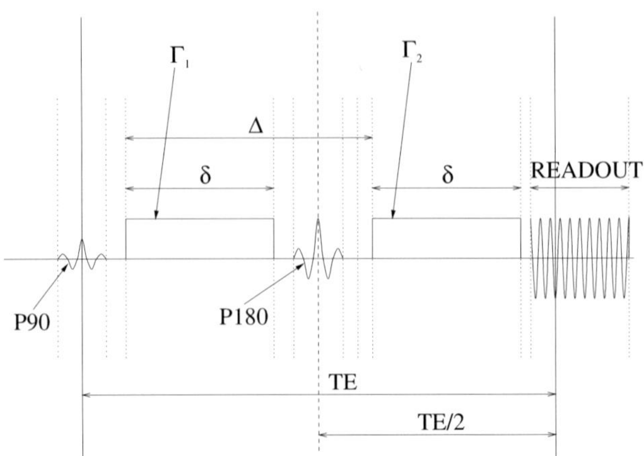

Fig. 5.2. Shows the pulsed-gradient spin-echo sequence

We can sensitize the MRI measurement to spin displacements by introducing magnetic-gradient pulses to the standard spin-echo sequence (or other standard sequences, such as the stimulated-echo sequence). Figure 5.2 shows the pulsed-gradient spin-echo (PGSE) sequence [4], which is the most common pulse sequence for diffusion-weighted MRI. The scanner maintains a constant and approximately homogeneous magnetic field $\mathbf{H}_0$ over the sample. The spins align with $\mathbf{H}_0$ and have a slightly higher probability of having spin up state than spin down, which causes a non-zero net magnetization of the material. The 90° radio-frequency (RF) pulse P90, centred at time $\tau = 0$, tips the spins into the 'transverse' plane perpendicular to $\mathbf{H}_0$. The spins then precess about $\mathbf{H}_0$ at the Larmor frequency, which is proportional to $|\mathbf{H}_0|$. Immediately after P90, the spins precess in phase so that the net magnetization rotates about $\mathbf{H}_0$. Inhomogeneities in $\mathbf{H}_0$ cause the spin precessions to dephase gradually so that the net magnetization decays. The 180° RF pulse P180, centred at time $\tau = \mathrm{TE}/2$ where TE is the 'echo time', negates the phase of each spin. In the absence of the gradient pulses $\boldsymbol{\Gamma}_1$ and $\boldsymbol{\Gamma}_2$, the rate of dephasing is the same before and after P180 so the spins come back into phase at time TE. The 'spin echo' occurs when the spins come back into phase and recover their net magnetization, which is the MR signal.

The spatially homogeneous diffusion-weighting gradient offsets the phase of each spin by a linear function of the spin position. A gradient pulse $\boldsymbol{\Gamma}$ offsets the phase of a spin at position $\mathbf{r}$ by $\mathbf{r} \cdot \mathbf{q}$, where

$$\mathbf{q} = \gamma \int_0^\infty \boldsymbol{\Gamma}(\tau)\mathrm{d}\tau \ ,$$

$\boldsymbol{\Gamma}(\tau)$ is the component of the magnetic-field gradient parallel to $\mathbf{H}_0$ (i.e. $(\nabla \mathbf{H}_0)\,\hat{\mathbf{H}}_0$) at time τ and γ is the gyromagnetic ratio of the spins. The gyromagnetic ratio for protons in water, which are usually the spins in biomedical diffusion MRI, is $2.675 \times 10^8\,\mathrm{s}^{-1}\mathrm{T}^{-1}$. In practice, the pulses are usually approximately rectangular (with brief rise and fall times) so that $\mathbf{\Gamma}_1$ and $\mathbf{\Gamma}_2$ have constant value $\mathbf{g}$ over the pulse duration δ and $\mathbf{q} = \gamma \delta \mathbf{g}$. Since P180 negates the phase of each spin, $\mathbf{\Gamma}_2$ cancels the phase offset from $\mathbf{\Gamma}_1$ for a stationary spin. However, if a spin moves from position $\mathbf{r}_1$ to $\mathbf{r}_2$ between the two pulses, it retains a residual phase offset of $\mathbf{q} \cdot (\mathbf{r}_2 - \mathbf{r}_1) = \mathbf{q} \cdot \mathbf{x}$, where $\mathbf{x}$ is the spin displacement. The magnetic moment of the spin at the spin echo is thus $\mathcal{M} \exp(\mathrm{i} \mathbf{q} \cdot \mathbf{x})$, where $\mathcal{M}$ is the magnitude of the magnetic moment. The MRI signal $A^\star(\mathbf{q})$ is the magnetization of all contributing spins. If we sum over all possible spin displacements, we see that

$$A^\star(\mathbf{q}) = A^\star(\mathbf{0}) \int p(\mathbf{x}) \exp(\mathrm{i} \mathbf{q} \cdot \mathbf{x}) \mathrm{d}\mathbf{x} \;,$$

where $A^\star(\mathbf{0})$ is the signal with no diffusion-weighting gradients and the integral is over three-dimensional space. Diffusion MRI usually assumes that the local advection velocity is zero (no net motion of the spin population), so that $p(\mathbf{x}) = p(-\mathbf{x})$ and $A^\star(\mathbf{q})$ is real valued in the absence of noise. Moreover, we use the normalized signal

$$A(\mathbf{q}) = (A^\star(\mathbf{0}))^{-1} A^\star(\mathbf{q}) = \int p(\mathbf{x}) \cos(\mathbf{q} \cdot \mathbf{x}) \mathrm{d}\mathbf{x} \;, \tag{5.1}$$

which is the Fourier transform of the function p at wavenumber $\mathbf{q}$. A measurement $A(\mathbf{q})$ thus provides the *apparent diffusion coefficient* (ADC) $d = -b^{-1} \log(A(\mathbf{q}))$, where $b = t|\mathbf{q}|^2$ is the *diffusion-weighting factor*, on the assumption that p is an isotropic zero-mean Gaussian function [4, 5]. Researchers in the 1980s [6, 7] combined the basic diffusion-weighted NMR measurement described above with MRI to obtain image maps of the ADC.

The derivation of equation (5.1) assumes that the movement of particles during the gradient pulses is negligible. This assumption is justified if δ is small compared with the pulse separation Δ, which is then the diffusion time $t = \Delta$. In practice however, δ and Δ usually have similar magnitude, as in Fig. 5.2. When δ is non-negligible, the phase offset of a spin depends on its trajectory during $\mathbf{\Gamma}_1$ and $\mathbf{\Gamma}_2$ rather than just its displacement, which complicates the model relating the measurements to p; see discussions in [5, 8, 9]. With some assumptions, we can model the effects of non-negligible δ analytically. For example, if p is Gaussian and the gradient pulses are rectangular, then non-negligible δ reduces t to an effective diffusion time of $\Delta - \delta/3$, see [4, 5]. The effective diffusion time reduces still further for higher moments of p [10]. Mitra and Halperin [9] show that, if p is the displacement density of the centres of mass (COM) of particle trajectories over time δ, rather than the displacements of particles themselves, equation (5.1) holds with $t = \Delta$ even with non-negligible δ. The COM displacement density has similar shape to the particle displacement density (though somewhat blurred) and, in particular, indicates fibre directions in the same way. Thus, although non-negligible δ

confounds absolute measurements of the particle displacement density, the features of p of interest in brain imaging are relatively unaffected. Lori et al. [8] and Brihuega-Moreno et al. [11] provide some further analysis of the non-negligible Δ problem.

The MRI measurement is complex-valued, since the magnetization has magnitude and phase. Often the phase of the measurements is discarded, since inhomogeneities in $\mathbf{H}_0$ and movement of the sample make it unstable. In practice, it is common to take the modulus of $A^\star(\mathbf{q})$ as the real-valued MR signal. An additive Gaussian noise model is common in MRI. With this model, the real and imaginary parts of the signal are independent and identically distributed with distribution $N(0, \sigma^2)$. Noise on the modulus of the signal thus follows a Rician distribution [12], which tends to a Gaussian distribution as the signal-to-noise ratio increases. A common measurement of quality of diffusion MRI data sets is the signal-to-noise ratio $S = A^\star(\mathbf{0})/\sigma$ of the measurement with $\mathbf{q} = \mathbf{0}$, where $A^\star$ is the noise-free signal.

5.3 Diffusion MRI Reconstruction Algorithms

This section reviews diffusion MRI reconstruction algorithms. We focus here on reconstructing fibre orientations, but note that some diffusion MRI techniques aim to estimate other features of the microstructure, such as the ratio of intracellular to extracellular water [13], by targeting other features of p. For this discussion, a diffusion MRI reconstruction algorithm inputs a set of diffusion-weighted MRI measurements from one voxel and outputs, at least, i) the number n of dominant fibre directions and ii) an estimate of each dominant fibre direction. Most of these algorithms determine a feature of p that highlights fibre orientations. In addition to fibre-orientation estimates, these features of p usually provide scalar indices of shape that discriminate different kinds of material and can indicate the reliability of the fibre-orientation estimates.

5.3.1 Diffusion Tensor MRI

Diffusion-tensor (DT) MRI [14] computes the *apparent diffusion tensor* on the assumption that p is a zero-mean trivariate Gaussian distribution:

$$p(\mathbf{x}) = G(\mathbf{x}; \mathsf{D}, t) \,, \tag{5.2}$$

where

$$G(\mathbf{x}; \mathsf{D}, t) = ((4\pi t)^3 \det(\mathsf{D}))^{-\frac{1}{2}} \exp\left(-\frac{\mathbf{x}^T \mathsf{D}^{-1} \mathbf{x}}{4t}\right) \,,$$

D is the diffusion tensor and t is the diffusion time. Since the Gaussian function has a single ridge, DT-MRI assumes $n = 1$. Substitution of (5.2) into (5.1) gives

$$A(\mathbf{q}) = \exp(-t\mathbf{q}^T \mathbf{D}\mathbf{q}) \ . \tag{5.3}$$

If we take the logarithm of (5.3), we see that each $A(\mathbf{q})$ provides a linear constraint on the elements of $\mathbf{D}$. The Gaussian model has six free parameters, which are the elements of the symmetric three-by-three matrix $\mathbf{D}$. To fit the six free parameters, we need a minimum of six $A(\mathbf{q})$ with independent $\mathbf{q}$, although many more are often acquired. Note that six $A(\mathbf{q})$ requires a minimum of seven $A^\star(\mathbf{q})$ including one for normalization. Practitioners most often use the linear least-squares fit of $\mathbf{D}$ to the log measurements. However, fitting directly using equation (5.3), as in [15], can improve results, since the error distribution is closer to normal on $A(\mathbf{q})$ than on $\log(A(\mathbf{q}))$. When fitting directly to $A(\mathbf{q})$, we can include constraints on the diffusion tensor, such as positive definiteness, using the Cholesky decomposition as in [15], or cylindrical symmetry, by writing

$$\mathbf{D} = \alpha\mathbf{n}\mathbf{n}^T + \beta\mathbf{I} \ , \tag{5.4}$$

where $\mathbf{n}$ is the principal direction of the diffusion tensor, $\mathbf{I}$ is the identity tensor and $\mathbf{D}$ has eigenvalues $\alpha + \beta$, β and β.

Diffusion-tensor MRI generalizes the ADC calculation from simple diffusion-weighted MRI to three dimensions. It provides two extra insights into the material microstructure over simple diffusion-weighted MRI. First, it provides rotationally invariant statistics of the anisotropy of p, which reflect the anisotropy of the microstructure. Second, it provides an estimate of the dominant orientation of microstructural fibres. The eigenvalues $\lambda_1 \geq \lambda_2 \geq \lambda_3$ of $\mathbf{D}$ determine the shape of p. The Gaussian function has ellipsoidal contours and the relative lengths of the major axes of the ellipsoids have the same proportions as the $(\lambda_i)^{\frac{1}{2}}$. Statistics of anisotropy come from the distribution of eigenvalues. A common statistic is the *fractional anisotropy* [16]

$$\nu = \left(\frac{3}{2}\sum_{i=1}^{3}\left(\lambda_i - \frac{1}{3}\mathrm{Tr}(\mathbf{D})\right)^2\right)^{\frac{1}{2}} \left(\sum_{i=1}^{3}\lambda_i^2\right)^{-\frac{1}{2}} , \tag{5.5}$$

which is the normalized standard deviation of the eigenvalues. Figure 5.3(a) shows ν over a coronal slice through a healthy human brain. The highest values of ν are in regions of dense white matter, such as the corpus callosum, where the fibres are packed most densely and have consistent orientation. Other common scalar statistics derived from the diffusion tensor are $\mathrm{Tr}(\mathbf{D})$ and the skewness μ. The trace of the diffusion tensor $\mathrm{Tr}(\mathbf{D}) = \sum_{i=1}^{3}\lambda_i$ is proportional to the mean squared displacement of water molecules and thus indicates the mobility of water molecules within each voxel, which reflects the density of microstructural barriers. The skewness

$$\mu = \left(\frac{9}{2}\sum_{i=1}^{3}\left(\lambda_i - \frac{1}{3}\mathrm{Tr}(\mathbf{D})\right)^3\right)^{\frac{1}{3}} \left(\sum_{i=1}^{3}\lambda_i^3\right)^{-\frac{1}{3}} , \tag{5.6}$$

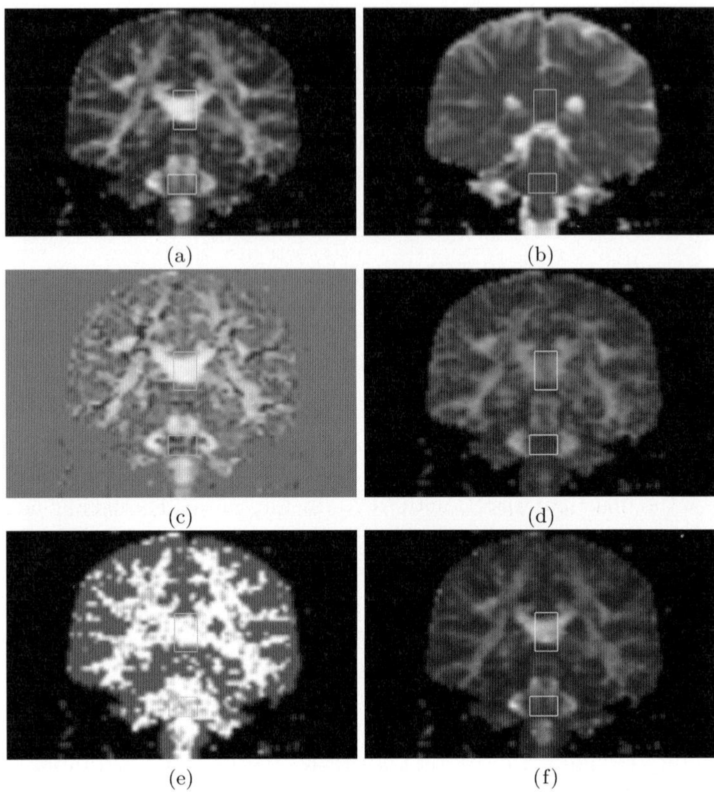

Fig. 5.3. See colour plates. Shows various features of p plotted over a coronal slice through a healthy human brain. Panel (**a**) shows the fractional anisotropy, ν. Panel (**b**) shows Tr(D). Panels (**c**) shows the skewness, μ. Panel (**d**) shows the colour coded principal direction, $\mathbf{e}_1$. Panel (**e**) shows the output of Alexander's voxel classification algorithm (Sect. 5.3.2); black is background, blue is order 0, white is order 2 and pink is order 4. Panel (**f**) shows the spherical-harmonic anisotropy (Sect. 5.3.2). In each panel, the upper region of interest contains some grey matter (*top*), part of the corpus callosum (*middle*) and some CSF (*bottom*). The lower region contains the fibre crossing in the pons

is close to zero for isotropic diffusion tensors with near spherical contours ($\lambda_1 \approx \lambda_2 \approx \lambda_3$), positive for prolate diffusion tensors with cigar-shaped contours ($\lambda_1 \gg \lambda_2 \approx \lambda_3$) and negative for oblate diffusion tensors with pancake-shaped contours ($\lambda_1 \approx \lambda_2 \gg \lambda_3$). Figures 5.3(b) and 5.3(c) show Tr(D) and μ, respectively, over the coronal slice in Fig. 5.3(a). The highest values of Tr(D) are in the ventricles and other regions of cerebro-spinal fluid, where the density of barriers to water mobility is low. The skewness is positive in most white-matter regions. In some white-matter regions, such as the pons, the skewness is negative showing oblate diffusion tensors. Oblate diffusion tensors arise in regions contain orthogonally crossing fibres, as depicted in Fig. 5.1(d), where the best-fit Gaussian model has oblate contours. Many other configurations of fibres or microstructures can also give rise to oblate diffusion tensors.

The eigenvectors $\mathbf{e}_1$, $\mathbf{e}_2$ and $\mathbf{e}_3$ of D determine the orientation of p. In regions of prolate diffusion tensors, the principal eigenvector $\mathbf{e}_1$ (that with eigenvalue λ_1) provides an estimate of the single fibre orientation. At fibre crossings where the diffusion tensor is oblate, $\mathbf{e}_1$ and $\mathbf{e}_2$ span the plane of the crossing fibres. Pajevic and Pierpaoli [17] use colour for a compact visualization of fibre orientations. A popular choice is to use RGB vectors proportional to $\nu^{1/2}\mathbf{e}_1$. Figure 5.3(d) uses this colour orientation-encoding for the coronal slice in Fig. 5.3(a); red indicates left-right orientation, green indicates anterior-posterior (front to back of the head) and blue indicates inferior-superior (top to bottom of the head).

Diffusion-tensor MRI requires a minimum of seven MRI measurements. Most diffusion-tensor MRI sequences acquire more than the minimum seven measurements to reduce the effects of noise. The standard approach [18] is to acquire M measurements with $\mathbf{q} = \mathbf{0}$ and N measurements with non-zero wavenumbers $\mathbf{q}_i$, $i = 1, \ldots, N$. The $|\mathbf{q}_i|$ are all equal and the diffusion time, t, and hence b, is fixed for all the $A(\mathbf{q}_i)$. The directions $\hat{\mathbf{q}}_i$ are unique and distributed uniformly over the sphere. This kind of scheme gives less rotational dependence of the fibre-orientation estimates and shape statistics than schemes that acquire repeated measurements at a smaller number of $\mathbf{q}_i$ [19]. The images in Fig. 5.3 come from a data set with $M = 6$, $N = 54$, $\delta = 0.034\,\mathrm{s}$, $\Delta = 0.040\,\mathrm{s}$ and $|\mathbf{g}| = 0.022\,\mathrm{Tm}^{-1}$. Thus $|\mathbf{q}_i| = 2.0 \times 10^5\mathrm{m}^{-1}$ and $b = 1150\,\mathrm{s}\,\mathrm{m}^2$ using $t = \Delta - \delta/3$. This scheme is typical for whole-brain clinical DT-MRI and requires around 20 minutes scan time on standard hardware. In white-matter regions, the signal to noise ratio at $\mathbf{q} = 0$, S, is around 16 on average.

Diffusion-tensor MRI is the most popular diffusion MRI reconstruction algorithm by far. It is the simplest technique that provides anisotropy statistics and fibre-orientation estimates. The computational and data requirements of the technique are modest. Modern scanners come with built-in acquisition sequences for DT-MRI and the post-processing is simple to implement and fast to run on modern desktop computers. However, a major drawback of DT-MRI is that the Gaussian model is often a poor fit to the data. Diffusion-tensor MRI provides only one fibre-orientation estimate in each voxel. In regions where fibres cross within one voxel, p has multiple ridges, as Fig. 5.1(d) depicts. The Gaussian model of p in Fig. 5.1(d) has oblate ellipsoidal contours. When the Gaussian model is poor the two major selling-points of DT-MRI fail. First, indices of anisotropy derived from the diffusion tensor, such as ν, underestimate the true directional variability of p. The Gaussian model for p in Fig. 5.1(d) smoothes out the ridges in the plane of the page. Second, fibre-orientation estimates are incorrect. For a perfectly oblate Gaussian distribution, D has no unique principal eigenvector. In regions with the microstructure depicted in Fig. 5.1(d), measurement noise will ensure that $\mathbf{e}_1$ is randomly oriented in the plane of the crossing fibres. Non-orthogonally intersecting fibres are potentially more dangerous. The single fibre-orientation estimate from DT-MRI then lies consistently between the two true fibre directions; see [20] for an example.

5.3.2 Modelling the 'ADC Profile'

Equation (5.3) shows that, with no noise, $\log(A)$ is quadratic in $\mathbf{q}$ when p is Gaussian. Several authors model $\log(A)$ with higher-order polynomials both to detect departures from the Gaussian model and to obtain more reliable indices of anisotropy.

Frank [21] and Alexander et al. [22] both fit the spherical-harmonic series to $\log(A)$ at a fixed $|\mathbf{q}|$. In the literature, the term 'ADC profile' refers to $-b^{-1}\log(A)$ as a function of $\hat{\mathbf{x}}$ with fixed $|\mathbf{q}|$. The spherical harmonics Y_{lm}, $l = 0, \ldots, \infty$, $m = -l, \ldots, l$, form a basis for complex-valued functions on the unit sphere in three dimensions $\mathcal{S}^2$. Thus we can write any complex-valued function f of the sphere as

$$f = \sum_{l=0}^{\infty} \sum_{m=-l}^{l} a_{lm} Y_{lm} \, .$$

Each spherical-harmonic series containing only terms up to order $l = L$ is the restriction to $\mathcal{S}^2$ of an order L polynomial, and vice versa. Series with only even-order terms are symmetric, so that $f(\hat{\mathbf{x}}) = f(-\hat{\mathbf{x}})$, and constraining both $\mathrm{Im}(a_{l0}) = 0$ and $a_{lm} = (-1)^m a_{l(-m)}^{\star}$ for all l and m ensures that f is real-valued [22]. Reference [22] shows how to compute the least-squares-fit symmetric real-valued spherical-harmonic series to $\log(A(\mathbf{q}_i))$, $i = 1, \ldots, N$, robustly via a single matrix multiplication.

If $\log(A)$ is quadratic, its spherical-harmonic series contains only terms up to order 2. If the fitted spherical-harmonic series contains significant higher-order terms, the Gaussian model for p is poor. Frank [21] observes significant fourth-order terms in the spherical-harmonic series in various white-matter regions in the human brain. Alexander [22] uses the analysis of variance (ANOVA) test for deletion of variables, the 'F-test' [23], to choose the lowest-order series that fits the data. This simple voxel-classification algorithm classifies each voxel as isotropic (order 0), anisotropic Gaussian (order 2), or non-Gaussian (order 4 or above). Results show clusters of order 4 voxels in several fibre-crossing regions in human-brain data similar to that used for Fig. 5.3. Figure 5.3(e) shows Alexander's voxel classification over the coronal slice in Fig. 5.3(a). Order 4 voxels appear consistently in the pons and other fibre crossings showing failure of the Gaussian model.

Spherical-harmonic models of $\log(A)$ provide anisotropy indices that are robust to departures from the Gaussian model. The moments of a spherical function f are

$$\omega_n[f] = (4\pi)^{n/2} \int f^n(\hat{\mathbf{x}}) \mathrm{d}\hat{\mathbf{x}} \, .$$

A general index of anisotropy of f is $(\omega_1[f])^{-1}(\omega_2[f] - (\omega_1[f])^2)^{1/2}$. For a real-valued symmetric spherical-harmonic series, $\omega_1[f] = 4\pi a_{00}$ and $\omega_2[f] = 4\pi \sum_{l=0}^{\infty} \sum_{m=-2l}^{2l} |a_{(2l)m}|^2$. Figure 5.3(f) shows the spherical-harmonic anisotropy from series including terms up to order 4. Differences between the spherical-harmonic anisotropy and ν are more noticeable at higher b. Other moments may also provide useful shape indices.

Ozarslan et al. [24] use a higher-order tensor model of $\log(A)$ so that

$$\log(A(\mathbf{q})) = -t\mathbf{q}^{(j)}\mathsf{D}^{(2j)}\mathbf{q}^j \, , \tag{5.7}$$

where the term on the right contains the contraction of the order $2j$ tensor $\mathsf{D}^{(2j)}$ by $\mathbf{q}^{(j)}$, which is the outer product of $\mathbf{q}^{(1)} = \mathbf{q}$ and $\mathbf{q}^{(j-1)}$. The tensors $\mathsf{D}^{(2j)}$ are real valued and have symmetry ensuring that $\log(A(\mathbf{q})) = \log(A(-\mathbf{q}))$. It is straightforward to demonstrate that the unique elements of the tensor model in (5.7) with order $2j$ are a linear transformation of the real and imaginary parts of the coefficients of the real symmetric spherical-harmonic model including terms up to order $2j$. In this sense, the two methods are equivalent, both theoretically and computationally. Liu et al. [10] model $\log(A(\mathbf{q}))$ by a sequence of higher-order tensors, which includes both odd and even-order tensors. The inclusion of odd-order tensors allows the model to capture non-symmetric spin displacements.

Neither the spherical-harmonic nor the higher-order-tensor models provide fibre-orientation estimates. Both model $\log(A)$ rather than p and the peaks of $\log(A)$ at a fixed radius are not in the directions of the ridges of p in general. The scalar anisotropy of $\log(A)$ correlates with that of p, so we can compute anisotropy indices from $\log(A)$. Also when p is Gaussian, A is Gaussian, so we can infer departures from the Gaussian model of p from departures of the $A(\mathbf{q}_i)$ from the best-fit Gaussian. To estimate fibre orientations, however, we must invert the Fourier transform in (5.1) and reconstruct directional features of p.

5.3.3 Multi-Compartment Models

A simple generalization of DT-MRI replaces the Gaussian model for p with a mixture of Gaussian densities:

$$p(\mathbf{x}) = \sum_{i=1}^{n} a_i G(\mathbf{x}; \mathsf{D}_i, t) \, , \tag{5.8}$$

where each $a_i \in [0, 1]$ and $\sum_i a_i = 1$. Particle displacements in media containing n distinct compartments, between which no exchange of particles occurs, follow the distribution in equation (5.8) if the displacement density in the i-th compartment, which has volume fraction a_i, is $G(\mathbf{x}; \mathsf{D}_i, t)$.

We take the Fourier transform of (5.8) and substitute into (5.1) to relate the measurement values to the model parameters (D_i and a_i, $i = 1, \ldots, n$):

$$A(\mathbf{q}) = \sum_{i=1}^{n} a_i \exp(-t\mathbf{q}^T \mathbf{D}_i \mathbf{q}) .$$

The constraint on the model parameters from each measurement is non-linear so we must fit the model to the data by non-linear optimization using, for example, a Levenberg–Marquardt algorithm [25]. The principal eigenvector of each $\mathbf{D}_i$ provides a fibre-orientation estimate. The multi-compartment model assumes n is fixed. Practical considerations, such as the number of MRI measurements and the measurement noise level, limit the number of orientations the method can resolve reliably. Most work to date uses a maximum n of 2.

Two problems accompany the use of multi-compartment models. First, the choice of n presents a model-selection problem. Second, the non-linear fitting procedure is unstable and starting-point dependent, because of local minima in the objective function. Parker and Alexander [26] and Blyth et al. [27] use Alexander's voxel classification algorithm [22] to solve the model-selection problem. They use $n = 2$ in order 4 voxels, where DT-MRI fails, and $n = 1$ elsewhere. This method does not extend naturally above $n = 2$, however. Although a fourth-order polynomial is a good approximation to $\log(A)$ from a mixture of two Gaussian densities [21], a mixture of three Gaussians does not necessarily require a sixth-order polynomial. Tuch [28] thresholds the correlation of the measurements with their predictions from a single-component model to decide whether to use one or two components. Constraints on the diffusion tensors in the multi-compartment model can help stabilize the fitting procedure. For example, we can enforce positive definiteness on the $\mathbf{D}_i$, using the Cholesky decomposition [29], or cylindrical symmetry on $\mathbf{D}_i$ using equation (5.4), or specific eigenvalues as in [28]. Spatial regularization techniques also help overcome the fitting problem by ensuring voxel to voxel coherence, see [29] and Chap. 9 by Pasternak et al.

5.3.4 Fibre Models

A similar model-based approach [30] assumes that particles belong to one of two populations: a restricted population within or around microstructural fibres and a free population that are unaffected by microstructural barriers. With negligible exchange between the populations, $p = ap_f + (1-a)p_r$, where p_f is the spin-displacement density for the free population, p_r that for the restricted population, and a is the fraction of particles in the free population. Behrens et al. [30] use an isotropic Gaussian model for p_f. They use a Gaussian model for p_r in which the diffusion tensor has only one non-zero eigenvalue so that particle displacement is restricted to a line. Assaf et al. [31] describe a similar approach. They model p_r with Neuman's model for restricted diffusion in a cylinder [32]. The fitted p_r provides the fibre-orientation estimate. For p_f, which they call the 'hindered compartment', they use an anisotropic Gaussian model.

Both approaches extend naturally to the multiple-fibre case by including multiple restricted populations in the model, which gives a more physically-based mixture model than the multi-compartment models in Sect. 5.3.3. In the multiple-fibre case, fibre-model approaches have the same model-selection and fitting problems as multi-compartment models. Assaf et al. [31] show promising results in the two-fibre case in simulation.

5.3.5 Diffusion Spectrum Imaging

Diffusion spectrum imaging [33], unlike the approaches discussed earlier in this section, does not use a parametric model for p. Instead, DSI reconstructs a discrete representation of p directly from measurements on a regular grid of wavenumbers via a fast Fourier transform. The reconstruction gives values of p on a grid of displacements.

The orientation distribution function (ODF)

$$\phi(\hat{\mathbf{x}}) = \int_0^\infty p(\alpha\hat{\mathbf{x}})\mathrm{d}\alpha \, , \tag{5.9}$$

where $\hat{\mathbf{x}}$ is a unit vector in the direction of $\mathbf{x}$, is the radial projection of p onto the unit sphere. The ODF has peaks in the directions in which p has most mass and thus has peaks in the directions of the ridges of p. In DSI, therefore, the peaks of ϕ provide the fibre-orientation estimates. The function ϕ can have multiple pairs of equal and opposite peaks. Each pair provides a separate fibre-orientation estimate, which enables DSI to resolve the orientations of fibres that cross within a single voxel. The ODF also provides anisotropy indices. For example, we can use the standard deviation $(\omega_2[\phi] - 4\pi)^{1/2}$ of ϕ as an analogue of the fractional anisotropy, ν.

Qualitative results from DSI in [33, 34] and subsequent publications show ODF peaks in the expected fibre directions at known crossings in human and animal brain data. However, the results also show ODFs with multiple peaks in grey-matter regions and it is unclear whether these peaks show genuine anatomic structure or simply arise from measurement noise. Diffusion spectrum imaging has clear advantages over DT-MRI and multi-compartment modelling, since it can resolve multiple fibre orientations, it does not require non-linear fitting and it does not involve a model-selection problem. Despite its advantages, DSI is not used as widely as DT-MRI. The main drawback of the technique is that acquisition times are long, since it requires an order of magnitude more measurements than DT-MRI to get sufficient detail in the reconstructed p. Wedeen and Tuch and coworkers [33, 34] use around 500 measurements for DSI. They acquire images with $64 \times 10^{-9}\,\mathrm{m}^3$ voxels, compared with $10 \times 10^{-9}\,\mathrm{m}^3$ voxels typical in DT-MRI, to keep the acquisition time manageable. Furthermore, DSI ignores the effects of non-negligible δ discussed at the end of Sect. 5.2.

5.3.6 A New Generation of Multiple-Fibre Reconstructions

The main drawback of DSI is the long acquisition time. However, in many applications, DSI wastes much of the information in the measurements. The projection of p onto the sphere to obtain the ODF, ϕ, discards the radial component of p to which much of the information in the measurements contributes. In some applications, the radial component of p may be useful. However, the primary interest is often in the angular structure, which provides fibre-orientation estimates and anisotropy indices. An emerging new generation of diffusion MRI reconstruction algorithm reconstructs the angular structure of p directly from the measurements. Rather than acquiring measurements on a grid of wavenumbers, as in DSI, the new methods use sets of wavenumbers chosen to contribute mostly to the angular structure of p. Specifically, methods to date use the spherical acquisition schemes popular in DT-MRI (see Sect. 5.3.1).

Approximations to the ODF

Several methods approximate the ODF from measurements acquired using a spherical acquisition scheme. Tuch's **q**-ball imaging method [34, 35] approximates the ODF by the Funk transform [36] of the measurements. (For brevity in the remainder of the chapter, we shall refer to Tuch's method simply as '**q**-ball'.) The Funk transform is a mapping between functions of the sphere. The value of the Funk transform of a function f at a point $\hat{\mathbf{x}}$ is the integral of f over the great circle perpendicular to $\hat{\mathbf{x}}$. In [34], Tuch shows that, in the absence of noise, the approximation becomes closer as $|\mathbf{q}|$ increases. Qualitative results in [34, 35] show good agreement between **q**-ball and full DSI in a fibre-crossing region in the human brain. Tuch uses high-quality test data with $N = 492$ and with $|\mathbf{q}| = 3.6 \times 10^5 \, \mathrm{m}^{-1}$ ($b = 4.0 \times 10^9 \, \mathrm{s \, m}^{-2}$) and $|\mathbf{q}| = 5.4 \times 10^5 \, \mathrm{m}^{-1}$ ($b = 12.0 \times 10^9 \, \mathrm{s \, m}^{-2}$). Lin et al. [37] propose a similar algorithm independently. They test their algorithm on data acquired from a phantom containing water-filled capillaries in two orientations, which simulates crossing white-matter fibres. The algorithm recovers the orientation of the capillaries consistently.

In Chap. 10 and [38], Ozarslan et al. fit higher-order tensor models (see Sect. 5.3.2) to measurements from a spherical acquisition scheme. They assume that $A(\mathbf{q})$ decays exponentially with increasing $|\mathbf{q}|$ and fixed $\hat{\mathbf{q}}$. This assumption allows them to estimate the measurements on a regular grid of wavenumbers, which they use as input to DSI. The method finds the ridge directions of simple test functions and qualitative results on rat-brain data, with $N = 81$ and $b = 1.5 \times 10^9 \, \mathrm{s \, m}^2$, are promising.

Deconvolution Techniques

Deconvolution methods generalize the fibre-model methods by assuming a distribution of fibre orientations. The diffusion MRI signal is the convolution of the *fibre orientation distribution* (FOD) with the response from a single fibre [30, 39, 40]. Any fibre model can provide the response for a single fibre. References [30, 39] use Gaussian fibre models. Tournier [40] derives a fibre model directly from the data by taking an average signal from the most anisotropic voxels. Deconvolution is linear using a linear set of basis functions, such as the spherical harmonics, for the FOD [39, 40]. The peaks of the FOD provide fibre-orientation estimates. Like the ODF, the FOD can have any number of pairs of equal and opposite peaks and each pair provides a separate fibre-orientation estimate. Thus, deconvolution methods avoid the model-selection problems associated with multi-compartment and fibre models.

Other Methods

Jansons and Alexander's PASMRI algorithm [41] computes another feature of p called the persistent angular structure (PAS). The PAS is the function $\tilde{p}$ of the sphere that, when embedded in three-dimensional space on a sphere of radius r, has Fourier transform that best fits the measurements. Thus

$$\tilde{p} = \arg\min_{\hat{p}} \left[\sum_{i=1}^{N} \left(A(\mathbf{q}_i) - \hat{A}(\mathbf{q}_i; \hat{p}) \right)^2 \right] ,$$

where

$$\hat{A}(\mathbf{q}_i; \hat{p}) = \int \hat{p}(\hat{\mathbf{x}}) \cos(r\mathbf{q}_i \cdot \hat{\mathbf{x}}) d\hat{\mathbf{x}} . \tag{5.10}$$

Jansons and Alexander use a maximum-entropy parametrization of $\tilde{p}$. They fit the $N + 1$ parameters of $\tilde{p}$ using a Levenberg–Marquardt algorithm and numerical approximations of the integrals in (5.10). The function $\tilde{p}$ can have any number of pairs of equal and opposite peaks and each pair provides a fibre-orientation estimate. The parameter r controls the smoothness of $\tilde{p}$.

The iterative optimization required to compute $\tilde{p}$ makes PASMRI a much slower algorithm than the other algorithms discussed in this section. However, Alexander [42] shows that PASMRI reconstructs fibre directions more consistently than **q**-ball. On the human-brain data used for Fig. 5.3, the **q**-ball algorithm fails to resolve the orientations at known fibre-crossings, where PASMRI succeeds. Simulations show that PASMRI is more sensitive than **q**-ball to anisotropy in test functions and recovers ridge directions more reliably, particularly at low b and S. Figures 5.4 and 5.5 show the PAS, computed by PASMRI, and ODF, approximated by **q**-ball, respectively, in the coronal brain slice in Fig. 5.3. The PAS has sharper peaks than the ODF and resolves the crossing fibres in the pons more consistently.

Liu et al. [10] outline a general inversion of their higher-order-tensor series model (see Sect. 5.3.2) of $\log(A)$ to obtain p. They simulate random walks of molecules through restricted media to obtain synthetic MRI measurements. In simulation, the reconstructed p reflects the geometry of several simple media.

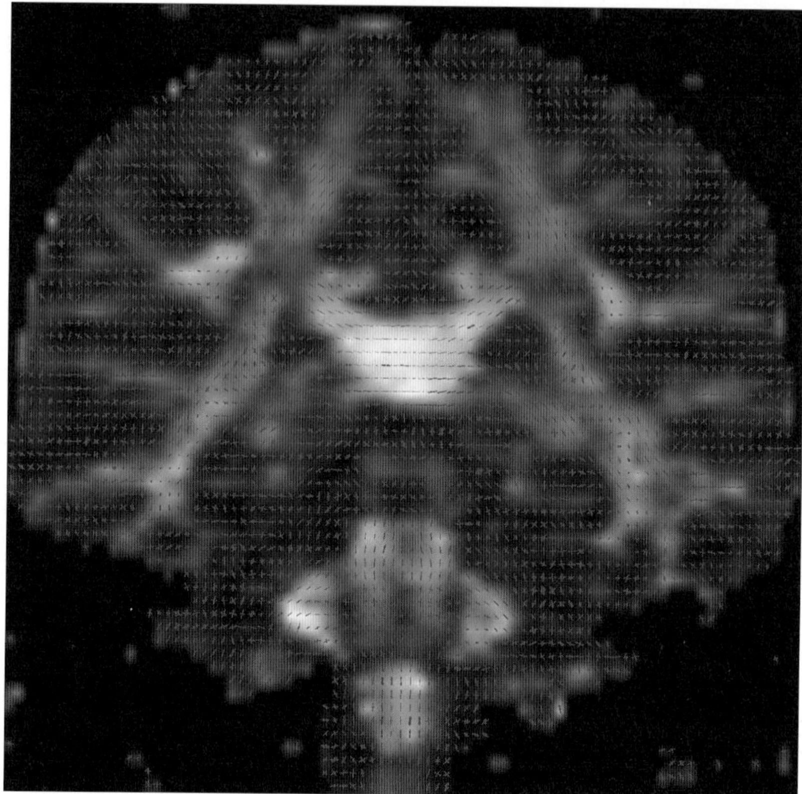

Fig. 5.4. See colour plates. Shows the PAS (in red) in brain voxels of the coronal slice in Fig. 5.3 superimposed on the fractional anisotropy map

Liu et al. use the phase of the MRI measurements and include odd-order tensors in their model, which allows them to determine net motion of particles (advection) as well as symmetric motion.

5.4 Applications

Diffusion-tensor MRI is now a routine clinical technique. Scalar statistics derived from the apparent diffusion tensor, such as $\mathrm{Tr}(D)$ and the fractional anisotropy [16], are used to study a broad range of conditions including stroke, epilepsy, multiple sclerosis, dementia and many other white-matter diseases; see [43] for a recent review. Diffusion MRI is also used to probe the microstructure of a variety of other materials including muscle tissue, e.g. in the heart [44], cartilage [45], plant tissue [46] and porous rock [47].

A major application area of diffusion MRI is fibre-tracking or 'tractography'. References [48, 49] contain reviews of tractography techniques with

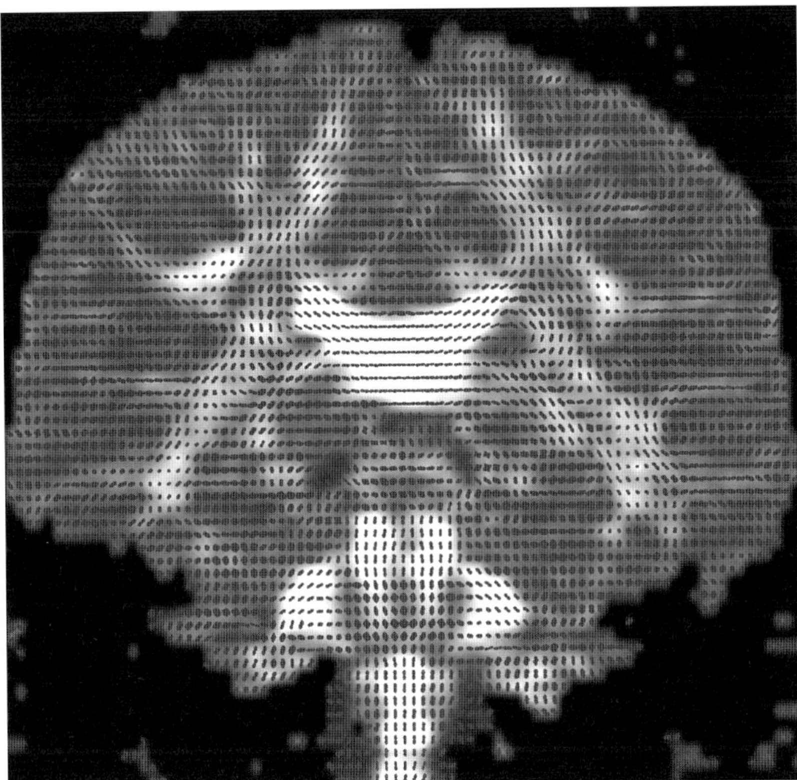

Fig. 5.5. See colour plates. Shows the ODF (in red) approximated using **q**-ball in brain voxels of the coronal slice in Fig. 5.3 superimposed on the fractional anisotropy map

qualitative and quantitative performance comparisons. Chapter 7 by Vilanova et al. also discusses tractography techniques. Simple 'streamline' tractography algorithms trace fibre trajectories by following fibre-orientation estimates from point to point through an image volume. Probabilistic tractography algorithms use a probability density function to model the uncertainty in the fibre-orientation estimate in each voxel. The algorithms run repeated streamline tractography processes with fibre-orientation estimates drawn from the model in each voxel. The fraction of streamlines that pass through a voxel provides an index of the connectivity of that voxel to the starting point. The distributions on the fibre-orientation estimates generally come from modelling the distribution of estimates from repeated trials of adding synthetic noise to the measurements. Some implementations [20, 50] use shape indices, such as the fractional anisotropy, to predict the parameters of the distribution.

Most tractography in the literature uses DT-MRI for fibre-orientation estimates. Several authors [20, 26, 27, 34, 51] use multiple-fibre reconstructions in tractography applications. Tractography algorithms based on multiple-fibre reconstruction use fibre-orientation estimates from multi-compartment models [20, 26, 27] or the peaks of the ODF [34] or PAS [51] together with uncertainty models obtained from simulations. Blyth et al. [27] provide direct evidence that multiple-fibre reconstruction improves tractography results over DT-MRI. One might be tempted to use the PAS, the ODF or the FOD as a direct estimate of the distribution of fibre orientations for probabilistic tractography. However, the physical basis of these functions is a gross simplification of the complex distribution of barriers to diffusion within material such as brain tissue. Any supposed relationship between these features of p and the true distribution of fibre orientations would require a great deal of validation and verification.

Tractography algorithms have undergone intensive development since the introduction of DT-MRI and exciting applications are now beginning to emerge. By mapping fibre pathways in abnormal brains [52, 53], we can monitor disease progression and assist neurosurgical planning. Probabilistic tractography has led to profound insights in human neuroanatomy [26, 54] and highlights region-connectivity differences between normal and patient groups [55]. Behrens et al. [54] use probabilistic tractography to segment the human thalamus into regions that connect to different cortical regions. The segmentation they produce is consistent among individuals and similar to a connectivity-based segmentation of the monkey thalamus performed by histology. Barrick et al. [56] use a similar idea to segment the whole human brain into connected regions. Behrens et al. [57] also propose a method for automatic segmentation based on connectivity information. For the future, tractography and connectivity-mapping hold great promise for studies of brain development [58, 59].

5.5 Discussion

We have reviewed the principles of diffusion MRI measurements and reconstruction. We have seen how the standard diffusion MRI reconstruction algorithms, in particular DT-MRI and DSI, arise from a simple model relating the measurements to the spin-displacement density function p. We have highlighted the drawbacks of these basic approaches: DT-MRI provides only a single fibre-orientation estimate in each voxel and fails at fibre crossings; DSI requires too many measurements for routine use on current hardware. We have reviewed a new generation of multiple-fibre reconstruction algorithms, including multi-compartment and fibre models and all the methods in Sect. 5.3.6, that can resolve the orientations of crossing fibres from sparse sets of measurements, similar to those acquired routinely in DT-MRI.

The new generation of reconstruction algorithms is still in its infancy and requires refinement and validation before routine application in clinical studies. As yet, no single algorithm has emerged as a comprehensive replacement for DT-MRI. The most tested new algorithms, which are multi-compartment models, PASMRI and **q**-ball, all have problems. Multi-compartment models have problems with model selection and model fitting. The **q**-ball algorithm does not resolve crossing fibres reliably on current standard data sets, but does produce acceptable results with a moderate increase in data quality [42]. The PASMRI algorithm works well on current data, but is too computationally heavy in practice. The great interest in fibre tractography continues to expand. Such are the problems caused by fibre crossings that development of the new algorithms will be rapid and we can expect to see them in routine use within the next few years.

We shall conclude with some specific questions for the further development of diffusion MRI reconstruction algorithms:

What New Shape Indices Can We Derive from Multiple-Fibre Reconstructions?

Multiple-fibre reconstructions produce a range of new features of p that can provide new scalar indices of shape beyond the common anisotropy and skewness statistics. We can compute higher-order moments of these functions, which may highlight previously unseen tissue-type boundaries. The number of peaks and relative peak strength of the PAS, ODF or FOD may also provide useful stains for analysis and diagnosis.

How Reliable are Fibre-Orientation Estimates and Shape Indices?

We can determine the accuracy of fibre-orientation estimates in simulation from test functions, as in [41], and also with bootstrap methods from repeated scanner acquisitions, as in [60]. Such experiments on multiple-fibre reconstructions will provide performance comparisons for selecting the best algorithms and uncertainty estimates for probabilistic tractography. We can assess the reliability of shape indices in the same ways. The reliability determines the diagnostic power of shape indices as well as their potential as indicators of fibre-orientation-estimate accuracy in probabilistic tractography. These performance estimates will depend on the imaging parameters, such as $|\mathbf{q}|$, t, N, M and S. We must optimize the trade-off between imaging time and data quality to maximize performance.

Can We Detect and Reject Spurious Structure in Isotropic Areas?

A major concern with multiple-fibre reconstructions is that they often show spurious structure in isotropic regions. Jansons and Alexander [41] and Alexander [61] illustrate this problem on synthetic data for PASMRI and **q**-ball. On scanner data, these methods invariably produce functions with strong peaks in grey-matter and CSF regions. However, the fibre orientation estimates have little or no voxel-to-voxel coherence, which suggests that the peaks come from measurement noise rather than genuine anatomy. The success of the new generation of algorithms will require methods for distinguishing spurious from genuine structure. Voxel classification algorithms, such as Alexander's [22], may help solve the problem, as may methods that analyze voxel-to-voxel consistency.

Can We Do Better than Spherical Acquisition Schemes?

In the literature, multi-compartment models and fibre models, ODF approximations, PASMRI and deconvolution methods mostly use data acquired with a spherical acquisition scheme. However, these methods can work with data acquired with any set of $\mathbf{q}_i$. Other distributions of sample points surely exist that will improve the methods, but the diffusion MRI community is yet to investigate methods for choosing and optimizing these distributions.

What is the Best Model for p in Brain Tissue?

The literature contains a variety of parametric models for p in white-matter fibres; see for example [30, 31, 39, 40]. Multi-compartment, fibre-model and deconvolution methods can use any such model. Quantitative comparisons of these models, again using simulations and bootstrap techniques, will determine which models best fit the data and produce the most reliable fibre-orientation estimates and shape statistics.

Can We Estimate the Fibre-Orientation Distribution Reliably?

Diffusion-weighted MRI [4, 5, 6, 7] and one-dimensional $\mathbf{q}$-space imaging [5] were the first generation of diffusion MRI algorithms. The second generation, diffusion-tensor MRI and DSI, generalizes the first to three-dimensions. The third generation consists of the multiple-fibre reconstructions from data designed to emphasize the angular structure of p. Despite the names of the features of p that these algorithms compute ('orientation-distribution function' and 'fibre-orientation distribution'), only the peaks of these functions are generally considered reliable as fibre-orientation estimates. Perhaps generation four will provide reliable estimates of the true distribution of fibre orientations within each voxel of an image and help distinguish crossing, kissing and diverging patterns of fibres.

The questions above are the tip of an iceberg. The remaining chapters of this book will reveal many other questions that demand answers in this exciting, expanding and fast-moving area of research.

Acknowledgements

The author would like to thank Dr. Claudia Wheeler-Kingshott from the Institute of Neurology, University College London, who provided the MRI data used to generate the images in this chapter. Dr. Dave Tuch, from the Athinoula A. Martinos Imaging Center for Biomedical Imaging, Massachusetts General Hospital, provided the code for the q-ball algorithm. Dr. Alexander's work is supported by the MIAS IRC, EPSRC GR/N14248/01 and MRC D2025/31, and EPSRC GR/T22858/01.

References

1. Pierpaoli C, Jezzard P, Basser P J, Barnett A and Di Chiro G 1996 Diffusion tensor MR imaging of the human brain *Radiology* **201** 637–48
2. Blinkov S and Glezer I 1968 *The human brain in figures and tables* New York, USA: Plenum Press
3. Highley J R, Esiri M M, McDonald B, Cortina-Borja M, Herron B M and Crow T J 1999 The size and fibre composition of the corpus callosum with respect to gender and schizophrenia: a post-mortem study *Brain* **122** 99–110
4. Stejskal E O and Tanner T E 1965 Spin diffusion measurements: spin echoes in the presence of a time-dependent field gradient *The Journal of Chemical Physics* **42** 288–92
5. Callaghan P T 1991 *Principles of Magnetic Resonance Microscopy* Oxford, UK: Oxford Science Publications
6. Merboldt K D, Hanicke W and Frahm J 1985 Self-diffusion NMR imaging using stimulated echoes *Journal of Magnetic Resonance* **64** 479–486
7. LeBihan D and Breton E 1985 Imagerie de diffusion in-vivo par resonance magnetique nucleaire *C. R. Acad. Sci. (Paris)* **301** 1109-1112
8. Lori N F, Conturo T E and Le Bihan D 2003 Definition of displacement probability and diffusion time in q-space magnetic resonance measurements that use finite-duration diffusion-encoding gradients *Journal of Magnetic Resonance* **165** 185–195
9. Mitra P P and Halperin B I 1995 Effects of finite gradient-pulse widths in pulsed-field-gradient diffusion measurements *Journal of Magnetic Resonance* **113** 94–101
10. Liu C, Bammer R, Acar B and Moseley M E 2004 Characterizing Non-Gaussian Diffusion by Using Generalized Diffusion Tensors *Magnetic Resonance in Medicine* **51** 924–937
11. Brihuega-Moreno O, Heese F P, Tejos C and Hall L D 2004 Effects of, and corrections for, cross-term interactions in q-space MRI *Magnetic Resonance in Medicine* **51** 1048–1054
12. Sijbers J, den Dekker A J, Van Audekerke J, Verhoye M, Van Dyck D 1998 Estimation of the noise in magnitude MR images *Magnetic Resonance Imaging* **16** 87–90.
13. Inglis B A, Bossart E L, Buckley D L, Wirth E D, Mareci T H 2001 Visualization of neural tissue water compartments using biexponential diffusion tensor MRI *Magnetic Resonance in Medicine* **45** 580–587.

14. Basser P J, Matiello J and Le Bihan D 1994 MR diffusion tensor spectroscopy and imaging *Biophysical Journal* **66** 259–67

15. Wang Z, Vemuri B C, Chen Y and Mareci T 2003 A constrained variational principle for direct estimation and smoothing of the diffusion tensor field from DWI *Proc. of 18th International Conference on Information Processing in Medical Imaging (Ambleside)* (Springer: LNCS 2732) 660–671

16. Basser P J and Pierpaoli C 1996 Microstructural and physiological features of tissues elucidated by quantitative diffusion tensor MRI *Journal of Magnetic Resonance Series B* **111** 209–19

17. Pajevic S and Pierpaoli C 1999 Color schemes to represent the orientation of anisotropic tissues from diffusion tensor data: application to white matter fibre tract mapping in the human brain *Magnetic Resonance in Medicine* **42** 526–540

18. Jones D K, Horsfield M A and Simmons A 1999 Optimal strategies for measuring diffusion in anisotropic systems by magnetic resonance imaging *Magnetic Resonance in Medicine* **42** 515–525

19. Jones D K 2004 The effect of gradient sampling schemes on measures derived from diffusion tensor MRI: a Monte Carlo study *Magnetic Resonance in Medicine* **51** 807–815

20. Parker G J M and Alexander D C 2003 Probabilistic Monte Carlo Based Mapping of Cerebral Connections Utilising Whole-Brain Crossing Fibre Information *Proc. of 18th International Conference on Information Processing in Medical Imaging (Ambleside)* (Springer: LNCS 2732) 684–695

21. Frank L R 2002 Characterization of anisotropy in high angular resolution diffusion-weighted MRI *Magnetic Resonance in Medicine* **47** 1083–99

22. Alexander D C, Barker G J and Arridge S R 2002 Detection and modeling of non-Gaussian apparent diffusion coefficient profiles in human brain data *Magnetic Resonance in Medicine* **48** 331–40

23. Armitage P and Berry G 1971 *Statistical methods in medical research* Oxford, UK: Blackwell Scientific Publications

24. Ozarslan E and Mareci T H 2003 Generalized diffusion tensor imaging and analytical relationships between diffusion tensor imaging and high angular resolution diffusion imaging *Magnetic Resonance in Medicine* **50** 955–965

25. Press W H, Teukolsky S A, Vettering W T and Flannery B P 1988 *Numerical Recipes in C* New York, USA: Press Syndicate of the University of Cambridge

26. Parker G J M, Luzzi S, Alexander D C, Wheeler-Kingshott C A M, Ciccarelli O and Lambon-Ralph M A 2004 Non-invasive structural mapping of two auditory-language pathways in the human brain *Neuroimage* In press

27. Blyth R, Cook P A and Alexander D C 2003 Tractography with multiple fibre directions *Proc. 11th Annual Meeting of the ISMRM (Toronto)* (Berkeley, USA: ISMRM) 240

28. Tuch D S, Reese T G, Wiegell M R, Makris N, Belliveau J W and Wedeen V J 2002 High angular resolution diffusion imaging reveals intravoxel white matter fiber heterogeneity *Magnetic Resonance in Medicine* **48** 577–582

29. Chen Y, Guo W, Zeng Q, He G, Vemuri B and Liu Y 2004 Recovery of intravoxel structure from HARD DWI *Proc. IEEE International Symposium on Biomedical Imaging (Arlington)* (IEEE)

30. Behrens T E J, Woolrich M W, Jenkinson M, Johansen-Berg H, Nunes R G, Clare S, Matthews P M, Brady J M and Smith S M 2003 Characterization and propagation of uncertainty in diffusion-weighted MR imaging *Magnetic Resonance in Medicine* **50** 1077–1088

31. Assaf Y, Freidlin R Z, Rohde G K and Basser P J 2004 New modelling and experimental framework to characterize hindered and restricted water diffusion in brain white matter *Magnetic Resonance in Medicine* **52** 965–978

32. Neuman C H 1974 Spin echo of spins diffusing in a bounded medium *Journal of Chemical Physics* **60** 4508–4511

33. Wedeen V J, Reese T G, Tuch D S, Dou J-G, Weiskoff R M and Chessler D 1999 Mapping fiber orientation spectra in cerebral white matter with Fourier-transform diffusion MRI *Proc. 7th Annual Meeting of the ISMRM (Philadelphia)* (Berkeley, USA: ISMRM) 321

34. Tuch D S 2002 *Diffusion MRI of Complex Tissue Structure* Doctor of Philosophy in Biomedical Imaging at the Massachusetts Institute of Technology

35. Tuch D S, Reese T G, Wiegell M R and Wedeen V J 2003 Diffusion MRI of complex neural architecture *Neuron* **40** 885–895

36. S Helgason 1999 *The Radon Transform* Birkhäuser

37. Lin C P, Tseng W Y I, Kuo L, Wedeen V J and Chen J H 2003 Mapping orientation distribution function with spherical encoding *Proc. 11th Annual Meeting of the ISMRM (Toronto)* (Berkeley, USA: ISMRM) 2120

38. Ozarslan E, Vemuri B C and Mareci T H 2004 Fiber orientation mapping using generalized diffusion tensor imaging *Proc. IEEE International Symposium on Biomedical Imaging (Arlington)* (IEEE)

39. Anderson A and Ding Z 2002 Sub-voxel measurement of fiber orientation using high angular resolution diffusion tensor imaging *Proc. 10th Annual Meeting of the ISMRM (Honolulu)* (Berkeley, USA: ISMRM) 440

40. Tournier J-D, Calamante F, Gadian D G and Connelly A 2004 Direct estimation of the fiber orientation density function from diffusion-weighted MRI data using spherical deconvolution *NeuroImage* **23** 1176–1185

41. Jansons K M and Alexander D C 2003 Persistent Angular Structure: new insights from diffusion MRI data *Inverse Problems* **19** 1031–1046

42. Alexander D C 2004 A comparison of q-ball and PASMRI on sparse diffusion MRI data *Proc. 12th Annual Meeting of the ISMRM (Kyoto)* (Berkeley, USA: ISMRM) 90

43. Dong Q, Welsh R C, Chenevert T L, Carlos R C, Maly-Sundgren P, Gomez-Hasan D M and Mukherji S K 2004 Clinical applications of diffusion tensor imaging *Journal of Magnetic Resonance Imaging* **19** 6–18

44. Dou J, Reese T G, Tseng W-Y I and Wedeen V J 2002 Cardiac diffusion MRI without motion effects *Magnetic Resonance in Medicine* **48** 105–114

45. Hsu E W and Setton L A 1999 Diffusion tensor microscopy of the intervertebral disc annulus fibrosus *Magnetic Resonance in Medicine* **41** 992–999

46. Li T-Q 1997 Porous structure of cellulose fibers studied by Q-Space NMR Imaging *Langmuir* **13** 3570–3574

47. Mansfield P and Issa B 1994 Studies of fluid transport in porous rocks by echo-planar MRI *Magnetic Resonance Imaging* **12** 275–278

48. Mori S and van Zijl P C M 2002 Fiber tracking: principles and strategies – a technical review *NMR in Biomedicine* **15** 468–480

49. Lori N F, Akbudak E, Shimony J S, Cull T S, Snyder A Z, Guillory R K and Conturo T E 2002 Diffusion tensor fiber tracking of human brain connectivity: acquisition methods, reliability analysis and biological results *NMR in Biomedicine* **15** 494–515

50. Cook P A, Alexander D C and Parker G J M 2004 Modelling noise-induced fibre-orientation error in diffusion-tensor MRI *Proc. IEEE International Symposium on Biomedical Imaging (Arlington)* (IEEE)

51. Parker G J M and Alexander D C 2005 Probabilistic anatomic connectivity derived from the microscopic persistent angular structure of cerebral tissue. *Philosophical Transactions of the Royal Society* In press

52. Clark C A, Barrick T R, Murphy M M, Bell B A 2003 White matter fiber tracking in patients with space-occupying lesions of the brain: a new technique for neurosurgical planning? *NeuroImage* **20** 1601–1608

53. Mori S, Frederiksen K, van Zijl P C M, Steiltjes B, Kraut M A, Solaiyappan M and Pomper M G 2002 Brain white matter anatomy of tumor patients evaluated with diffusion tensor imaging *Annals of Neurology* **51** 377–380

54. Behrens T E J, Johansen-Berg H, Woolrich M W, Smith S M, Wheeler-Kingshott C A M, Boulby P A, Barker G J, Sillery E L, Sheehan K, Ciccarelli O, Thompson A J, Brady J M and Matthews P M 2003 Non-invasive mapping of connections between human thalamus and cortex using diffusion imaging *Nature Neuroscience* **7** 750–757

55. Ciccarelli O, Toosey A T, Parker G J M, Wheeler-Kingshott C A M, Barker G J, Miller D H and Thompson A J 2003 Diffusion tractography based group mapping of major white-matter pathways in the human brain *NeuroImage* **19** 1545–1555

56. Barrick T R, Lawes I N and Clark C A 2004 Automatic segmentation of white matter pathways by application of a region growing algorithm *Proc. 12th Annual Meeting of the ISMRM (Kyoto)* (Berkeley, USA: ISMRM) 619

57. Behrens T E J, Johansen-Berg H, Drobnjak I, Brady J M, Matthews P M, Smith S M and Higham D J 2004 Delineation of functional subunits in the human cortex from diffusion based connectivity matrices *Proc. 12th Annual Meeting of the ISMRM (Kyoto)* (Berkeley, USA: ISMRM) 621

58. Mori S, Itoh R, Zhang J Y, Kaufmann W E, van Zijl P C M, Solaiyappan M and Yarowsky P 2001 Diffusion tensor imaging of the developing mouse brain *Magnetic Resonance in Medicine* **46** 18–23

59. Ulug A M 2002 Monitoring brain development with quantitative diffusion tensor imaging *Developmental Science* **5** 286–292

60. Jones D K 2003 Determining and visualizing uncertainty in estimates of fiber orientation from diffusion tensor MRI *Magnetic Resonance in Medicine* **49** 7–12

61. Alexander D C 2005 Multiple-fibre reconstruction algorithms in diffusion MRI *Annals of the New York Academy of Sciences* In Press

6

Random Noise in Diffusion Tensor Imaging, its Destructive Impact and Some Corrections

Klaus R. Hahn[1], Sergej Prigarin[2], Susanne Heim[3], and Khader Hasan[4]

[1] Institute of Biomathematics and Biometrics, National Research Center for Environment and Health, Ingolstädter Landstr. 1, 85764 Neuherberg, Germany
`hahn@gsf.de`
[2] Institute of Computational Mathematics and Geophysics, pr. Lavrentieva, Novosibirsk, 630090, Russia
`smp@osmf.sscc.ru`
[3] Institute of Statistics, Ludwig-Maximilians-Universität München, Ludwigstr. 33, 80539 Munich, Germany
`susanne.heim@stat.uni-muenchen.de`
[4] Department of Diagnostic and Interventional Imaging, University of Texas Medical School, 6431 Fannin Street, MSB 2.100, Houston, TX 77030, USA
`Khader.M.Hasan@uth.tmc.edu`

Summary. The empirical origin of random noise is described, its influence on DTI variables is illustrated by a review of numerical and in vivo studies supplemented by new simulations investigating high noise levels. A stochastic model of noise propagation is presented to structure noise impact in DTI. Finally, basics of voxelwise and spatial denoising procedures are presented. Recent denoising procedures are reviewed and consequences of the stochastic model for convenient denoising strategies are discussed.

6.1 Introduction

Though the theoretical and experimental basics of Diffusion Tensor Imaging DTI are still in a stage of development, it is well established, that magnetic resonance measurements of diffusing water molecules can reveal unique information about the architecture of normal and diseased brain tissues. See [1] for a recent survey on basic concepts, experimental methods, postprocessing procedures, and potential applications. An enumeration of the limitations of DTI at present would fill a long list. Some of them are caused by the 'artifacts' which comprise effects of subject motion, eddy currents, susceptibility variations, calibration errors, and noise [1, 2].

Random or Johnson noise is essentially white and has its origin in thermal Brownian motion of electrons. Johnson noise is superposed in DTI by two components: noise from the scanner apparatus and noise from the patient's body inside the scanner [3]. The measurement of the magnetization, carrying the anatomical information, results in complex valued data in k-space which give, after Fourier transformation, the signal in configuration or physical space [3]. Johnson noise in the data or signals can be approximated by a complex Gaussian distribution with mean zero, constant standard deviation and independent real and imaginary parts [4].

Consequently, the magnitude of the signal follows the family of Rician distributions [5], which comprises distributions with nearly Gaussian shape for low noise levels. In case of increasing noise however, the distributions become appreciably skewed and have a biased mean value. Hence the expectation value of a noisy signal magnitude is different from its noise-free or true value. Such magnitudes or diffusion weighted images DWI are mapped in the standard model of DTI via the Stejskal-Tanner equations ST to the diffusion tensor [6, 7] and then via several nonlinear transformations to detailed anatomical information of the brain. From a statistical point of view one should realize that in general any nonlinear transformation can transform a Gaussian distribution to a skewed and heavy tailed one with biased mean value. Consequently, a chain of such transformations can create a highly complicated stochastic situation. In fact, nonlinear noise propagation can lead to severe misinterpretations in DTI, which is still one of the central problems.

Several topics are addressed in this chapter. First we present some formal results of stochastics to model noise propagation in DTI. Then, a survey of published results on noise artifacts and denoising methods is presented. The whole range of signal to noise ratios is covered, own results for high noise levels supplement the review. Final aim of this work is to structure the complicated field of noise impact in DTI and to support the application and development of convenient denoising methods.

6.2 Noise Impact

First of all we introduce some fundamental concepts of DTI and of its statistics. In particular, the statistical Delta Method will be introduced. This method describes the large sample convergence to Gaussian distributions for variables which are derived by nonlinear transformations. Second, we present a survey of published results on noise artifacts. These studies comprise results achieved by Monte Carlo simulation and by bootstrap sampling.

6.2.1 Noise Propagation Model

In the following we restrict ourselves to statistical aspects caused by Johnson noise; the influence of non statistical distortions is excluded. In addition, only the standard diffusion tensor with rank=2 is considered, for extensions see Chap. 10 by Özarslan et al. The chain of nonlinear transformations, leading from measured quantities to anatomically relevant observables proceeds as follows: {signals S} $\mapsto$ {magnitudes $|S|$} $\mapsto$ {tensor $\mathbf{d}$} $\mapsto$ {eigenvalues, eigenvectors} $\mapsto$ {anisotropy, tracks} $\mapsto$ {connectivity, etc.} Only for the first transformation, the statistics is completely formalized [5]. We present in the following a closer look at the second map in order to exemplify statistical peculiarities caused by nonlinear mappings. The central concept in standard DTI is the diffusion tensor $\mathbf{d}(\mathbf{x})$ for any voxel $\mathbf{x}$ in e.g. a brain. The three eigenvalues $\lambda_i(\mathbf{x})$ and eigenvectors $|i(\mathbf{x})\rangle$ describe the geometric properties of a diffusion ellipsoid along the fibers. As the tensor is real and symmetric, a convenient braket notation [8] is used, where the ket $|.\rangle$ is a column vector, the bra $\langle.|$ a transposed ket, and $\langle.|.\rangle$ a scalar product. In this notation we get

$$\mathbf{d}(\mathbf{x}) = \begin{pmatrix} d_{11}(\mathbf{x}) & d_{12}(\mathbf{x}) & d_{13}(\mathbf{x}) \\ d_{12}(\mathbf{x}) & d_{22}(\mathbf{x}) & d_{23}(\mathbf{x}) \\ d_{13}(\mathbf{x}) & d_{23}(\mathbf{x}) & d_{33}(\mathbf{x}) \end{pmatrix} = \sum_{i=1}^{3} \lambda_i(\mathbf{x}) |i(\mathbf{x})\rangle \langle i(\mathbf{x})| . \tag{6.1}$$

The ST equations are then

$$|S_j(\mathbf{x})| = |S_0(\mathbf{x})| \exp\left(-b \sum_{i=1}^{3} \lambda_i(\mathbf{x}) \langle i(\mathbf{x})| \mathbf{g}_j\rangle^2 \right), \tag{6.2}$$

incorporating the diffusion weighting b-value which is a function of scanning parameters [7], a normalized diffusion measuring gradient $|\mathbf{g}_j\rangle$, the diffusion weighted image DWI $|S_j(\mathbf{x})|$, $j \geq 1$, and the reference $|S_0(\mathbf{x})|$.

Noise enters the system via the complex signals $S_k(\mathbf{x})$, by $S_{k,noisy}(\mathbf{x}) = \mathbf{Re}[S_k(\mathbf{x})] + \varepsilon_{Re} + i(\mathbf{Im}[S_k(\mathbf{x})] + \varepsilon_{Im})$, for $k \geq 0$, where ε_{Re} and ε_{Im} are independent and normally distributed, $\varepsilon \sim N(0, \sigma)$. The noise level σ is the Rayleigh corrected standard deviation of background noise [4, 5].

To quantify the signal to noise ratio, we define $SNR_k = |S_k(\mathbf{x})|/\sigma$ for $k \geq 0$, where $|S_k(\mathbf{x})|$ is without noise [5]. As SNR_k determines, within the Rician family, the distribution of $|S_{k,noisy}(\mathbf{x})|$, these distributions change in space. In the same way, the statistical properties of derived variables affected by noise, like $\mathbf{d}(\mathbf{x})$, change with $\mathbf{x}$. In short notation, those variables build up random fields.

We introduce now several abbreviations to formulate the least square estimation of the tensor from the measured DWIs for the general case including $n \geq 6$ gradient directions $\langle \mathbf{g}_j| = (g_{1,j}, g_{2,j}, g_{3,j})$. To make the notation more transparent, the dependence on $\mathbf{x}$ and the label $noisy$ is suppressed:

$$\mathbf{D^T} := (D_1, D_2, D_3, D_4, D_5, D_6) = (d_{11}, d_{22}, d_{33}, d_{12}, d_{13}, d_{23})$$
$$(\mathbf{A})_j := (g_{1,j}^2, g_{2,j}^2, g_{3,j}^2, 2g_{1,j}g_{2,j}, 2g_{1,j}g_{3,j}, 2g_{2,j}g_{3,j}) \tag{6.3}$$
$$s_j := -\log(|S_j|/|S_0|)/b,$$

where $(\mathbf{A})_j$ is a row of the $n \times 6$ matrix $\mathbf{A}$. The equation $\mathbf{AD} = \mathbf{s}$ for $\mathbf{D}$ is then solved by $\mathbf{D} = \mathbf{B}^{-1}(\mathbf{A}^T \mathbf{s})$, where $\mathbf{B} = \mathbf{A}^T \mathbf{A}$, see [9]. Introducing the weights $w_{il} = \sum_{k=1}^{6} B_{lk}^{-1} A_{ik}$, we can finally write $D_l = \sum_{i=1}^{n} w_{il} s_i$, and find for the expectation of D_l,

$$\mathbf{E}[D_l] = -\sum_{i=1}^{n} w_{il} \mathbf{E}[\log(|S_i|)]/b + \mathbf{E}[\log(|S_0|)] \sum_{i=1}^{n} w_{il}/b \ . \tag{6.4}$$

This equation shows the origin of a possible bias in D_l, hence in general

$$\mathbf{E}[D_l] \neq -\sum_{i=1}^{n} w_{il} \log(|\mathbf{E}[S_i]|)/b + \log(|\mathbf{E}[S_0]|) \sum_{i=1}^{n} w_{il}/b \ . \tag{6.5}$$

The right hand side of (6.5) describes the tensor components without noise, as the signals S_i are normally distributed. When the DWIs $|S_i|$ are essentially free from bias, $SNR_i > 3$, the function log introduces a (possibly) small bias in D_l, as log is a concave map. This effect is enhanced if the DWIs are biased for $SNR_i \leq 3$. Concave or convex mappings of random variables produce bias effects due to the Jensen inequality [10]. Therefore, any further nonlinear transformation on D_l can, in principle, cause additional bias in the derived variable.

A further important aspect is the shape of the distributions. For high noise level the DWIs, as well as derived variables are not normally distributed. However, as noise is sufficiently reduced, the Delta Method [11] predicts approximate Gaussian statistics for all variables of the DTI chain. This follows from an iterative application of the following Theorem and of its generalizations: If the distributions of a sequence of random variables T_m approach with increasing m the Gaussian distributions $N(\Theta, \tau^2/m)$, where Θ is the expectation value and τ^2/m the variance, then, for any nonlinear transformation $f : T_m \rightarrow f(T_m)$ with $\dot{f}(\Theta) \neq 0$, the distributions of $f(T_m)$ tend to $N(f(\Theta), \dot{f}(\Theta)^2 \tau^2/m))$, see [11] for an exact but less descriptive formulation and for extensions to multivariate cases. Thus, reduction of noise greatly simplifies the structure of the mentioned random fields. However, as Θ depends on the spatial coordinate, variance is still varying in space. The Delta Method does pose only weak restrictions on the distributions of T_m and thus extends the usefulness of the Central Limit Theorems CLT [11] as prerequisites for an application of this method. Appropriate T_m can in DTI experiments be achieved by performing m replications of experiments and consecutive averaging of the m magnitudes $|S_{i,noisy}(\mathbf{x})|$. For low m, due to practical limitations, this is one of the standard procedures in DTI to denoise data.

6.2.2 Noise Artifacts

We review only a selection from the huge number of articles on noise artifacts and emphasize the diversity of artifacts, more technical papers are not considered. The artifacts are investigated by numerical modelling via Monte Carlo simulation MCS [12, 13], perturbation theory [8] and bootstrap sampling [1, 14].

The degree of anisotropy in diffusion is connected to the homogeneitiy of the fiber directions in a measured voxel, as diffusion propagates mainly along the fiber direction, see Chap. 7 by Vilanova et al. for illustrations of anisotropy and nerve fibers in the human brain. In [12] different quantitative indices of anisotropy are investigated. The authors show that rotational variant indices suffer from non random orientational artifacts and can make highly anisotropic white matter structures appear isotropic in vivo. Therefore, rotationally variant indices depending on the eigenvalues are included in their study, like e.g. the fractional anisotropy $FA = (3\sum_{k=1}^{3}(\lambda_k - \lambda)^2/2\sum_{k=1}^{3}\lambda_k^2)^{1/2}$, where $\lambda = \sum_{k=1}^{3}\lambda_k/3$, see [12, 13] for more indices depending on eigenvalues. It is shown by MCS that those indices are biased in the presence of noise. This bias enhances artificially the mean anisotropy and can make isotropic diffusion appear anisotropic. Two sources of this error are detected: a) the mean eigenvalues are biased, where the largest eigenvalue is typically enhanced by noise, the smaller ones are reduced; b) noise introduces sorting bias, i.e. due to overlapping statistical distributions of neighboring eigenvalues, magnitude sorting fails. These bias effects increase with decreasing SNR, the study covers a range of $SNR_0 > 5$. Similar findings are reported in [13], in addition, the eigenvalue distributions are investigated. The dependence of skewness on the angles between main diffusion and laboratory system or diffusion gradients is apparent. This exemplifies that DTI distributions build up random fields. Also negative eigenvalues are detected for higher noise level preventing an interpretation of the tensor as a quantity describing diffusion. Perturbation theory is applied [15] for $SNR_0 > 20$, to calculate power series expansions of the eigenvalues and of eigenvectors of the tensor for different model diffusions. The results for the bias in eigenvalues and in FA of [12, 13] are essentially confirmed. Noise in the eigenvector orientation produces random walk trajectories which should model the nerve fiber pathes. The mean position error of the calculated tracks and the standard deviation are calculated for a total of 256 path steps. Both increased, in different manner, with the step number and the noise level. This may indicate fundamental limits in accuracy for tracking, though only a very simple tracking algorithm is applied [15]. The studies discussed so far deal with $SNR_0 > 5$ for $b \approx 1000\,\mathrm{s\,mm}^{-2}$ and focus more on even higher SNR_0, relevant for clinical investigations. Recently, experiments with higher b-values ($b \gg 1000\,\mathrm{s\,mm}^{-2}$) to measure non-Gaussian diffusion [16] or with high spatial resolution (e.g. $1\,\mathrm{mm}^3$) to reduce partial volume effects are performed. Such data include DWIs with $SNR_k < 3$ (henceforth with $k > 0$), which are strongly influenced by peculiarities of the Rician statistics, and consequently we may find different noise artifacts. The first systematic MCS for higher b-values was published recently [17]. Just one interesting result may be reported. In contrast to the findings of [12, 13, 15], the mean FA can now be essentially unbiased for $b \approx 3000\,\mathrm{s\,mm}^{-2}$, or underestimated for $b > 5000\,\mathrm{s\,mm}^{-2}$.

Non-parametric bootstrap BS analysis offers a more empirical approach to error analysis allowing a better inclusion of non statistical distortions. These

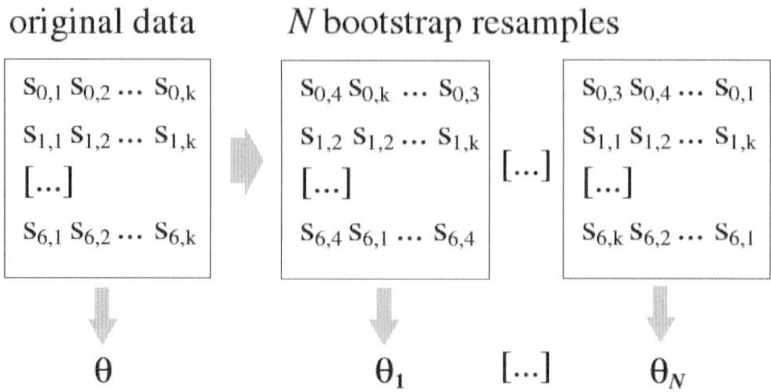

Fig. 6.1. General bootstrap resampling scheme adapted to a typical DTI acquisition of a reference and six diffusion weighted signals, each k times. By random drawing with replacement N bootstrap resamples are obtained. The distribution of a statistic of interest Θ is determined by the $N + 1$ samples

distortions modify the statistical distributions but it is hard to model them in the frame of MCS. The BS draws inferences about some features of unknown distributions by generating multiple replications. The replications are achieved by iterated random drawings with replacement out of a pool of experimental data. See Fig. 6.1 for a BS scheme, applied to a typical DTI acquisition. In this setup k replications of an experiment with 6 diffusion gradients and one reference are performed. A box indicates a complete data set with pool size k, the left box is the purely empirical starting point of the procedure. To the right, artificial resamples created by random drawings are shown. The information in all samples together defines the distribution of interest and allows to study, in an approximate way, the statistical properties of a random variable in a voxel.

By BS in [18] the uncertainty in main diffusion directions is analyzed in vivo. Applying the formalism of dyadic tensors 95% confidence intervals for the angles between the mean and the random directions are calculated. A correlation between this uncertainty and the anisotropy index $C_l = (\lambda_1 - \lambda_2)/(\lambda_1 + \lambda_2 + \lambda_3)$ for $\lambda_1 \geq \lambda_2 \geq \lambda_3$ is found. The uncertainty grows with decreasing C_l qualitatively like C_l^{-1}. Even for high C_l an uncertainty of about 2.5 degrees remains. In [19] BS is applied to distribution specific parameters which can serve as quality measures for DTI data, this could help to detect e.g. data which are corrupted by some machine error in the scanner. For this purpose, the confidence intervals of FA in white matter are determined and submitted to histogram analysis. The mean, modus and height are extracted as quality descriptors. The study particularly investigates the impact of noise and of denoising, as well as motion of the patient on those parameters. In [14] MCS and BS are applied in conjunction. By MCS it is investigated how good a multivariate Gaussian distribution can describe noise in the tensor. Marginal distributions of the tensor and the distributions of the squared rational anisotropy RA, see Chap. 7, are compatible with this assumption. In particular the marginals are well normal distributed already for $SNR_0 > 2$, when only 6 diffusion gradients are applied, and for clinical b-values. The estimation of the covariance matrix is less robust, for a linear regression model the diagonal elements are underestimated by about 20%. In addition, BS for DTI data is introduced in this chapter. Its reliability is shown by MCS on simulated data. BS is also applied to human data under approximate clinical conditions, one result is that in the majority of voxels the statistical properties of the tensor components are compatible with the Gaussian assumption.

6.3 Corrections of Noise Effects

The different denoising methods can be divided into voxelwise and spatial procedures. In the first group, frequently experiments with a small number of gradients close to the minimum number $n_g = 6$ and sometimes with different b-values per experiment are repeated, to average the DWIs or to derive the tensor via regression methods [7]. In multigradient experiments the gradient number is enhanced, $n_g \gg 6$. Different ways to construct the spatial orientation of such gradients were proposed, see [20] for a review and a comparison. Finally, the tensor can be derived from the DWIs by the least squares fit described in Sect. 2.1. Both acquisition schemes reduce noise in the system voxelwise. A complementary technique is offered by spatial denoising, where samples of neighboring voxels are used to estimate the variable of interest. This technique relies on the fact, that anatomical units occupy at least several neighboring voxels in a brain, and that it is possible to detect those regions ROI of 'homogeneity'. Such methods are applied to reduce the sorting bias of tensor eigenvalues [21, 22], or to filter the spatial DWI fields [23, 24], more global assumptions are involved in the denoising methods [25, 26, 27, 28].

6.3.1 Voxelwise Denoising

For $SNR_k > 3$, voxelwise averaging of DWIs derived from repeated measurements introduces, according to the classical CLT [11], unbiased normally distributed mean values with small variance. If, by a high number of replications, the variance is reduced sufficiently one can estimate the derived DTI variables practically without noise influence, due to the Delta Method. In agreement with that it was shown by MCS [15], that for $SNR_0 \approx 20$ bias in the eigenvalues is minimized best by averaging the DWIs before the tensor is derived. For medium $SNR_0 \approx 50$ the results imply an equivalence between DWI and tensor averaging, as the bias in the tensor, see (6.4), is no more relevant. Only at high SNR_0 direct eigenvalue averaging is equivalent to the other methods, as the whole system is now close to the Gaussian limit.

Different orientations in multigradient systems led to the introduction of the condition number $\kappa = \kappa(\mathbf{A})$, which gives an error bound by $\kappa \geq$ (relative error in $\mathbf{D}$)/(relative error in $\mathbf{s}$) [29, 30], for notations see Sect. 6.2.1. In [30] it is shown, that for icosahedral gradients κ is small and independent of rotations of $\mathbf{A}$ in the laboratory system. Within this bound, however, the tensor distributions and the bias effects do depend on SNR_k or on the gradient directions, see (6.2) for an explanation. The number of gradients n_g has also an important influence on bias effects. The MCS in [31] shows, that the fractional anisotropy FA, the mean diffusion $MD = \sum_{k=1}^{3} \lambda_k/3$ and the direction of main diffusion depend on the number n_g of uniformly distributed gradients. Increasing n_g reduces and stabilizes those bias effects, for $SNR_0 = 15$ at least 20 gradients are necessary to achieve reliable anisotropy maps and 30 gradients for reliable directions and MD.

To include $SNR_k \leq 3$ we performed MCS at $SNR_0 \approx 4$. Several three dimensional models of realistic diffusion tensors are explored, with $b = 1000\,\mathrm{s}\,\mathrm{mm}^{-2}$ and $|S_0| = 1000$. The gradients are icosahedral, twelve different gradient sets are used, $n_g \in \{6, 10, 15, 16, 20, 25, 36, 40, 45, 60, 81, 126\}$. In Fig. 6.2 typical results for a 'cigar shaped' diffusion with $d_{11}, d_{22}, d_{33} = .00155, .000354, .000191\,\mathrm{mm}^2\,\mathrm{s}^{-1}$, else *zero* are presented. To minimize SNR_k every gradient set is rotated, such that at least one gradient direction is parallel to the main diffusion direction of the model. This produces maximal Rician bias in the corresponding DWI. The relative bias of the three invariants of the

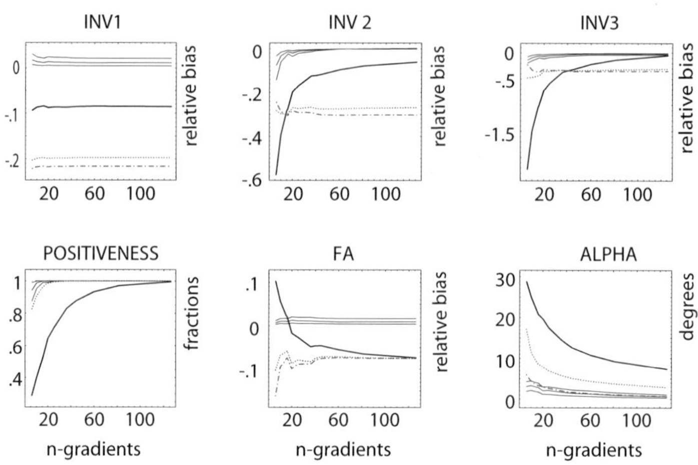

Fig. 6.2. Impact of Rician statistics on DTI variables for $SNR_0 = 4.2$. The model diffusion is 'cigar shaped', $FA = 0.8$ and $MD = 0.0007\,\mathrm{mm}^2\,\mathrm{s}^{-1}$. Relative bias versus number of applied gradients is presented for the invariants $INV1$, $INV2$, $INV3$ and FA, also the fractions of positive definite voxels and the angles between main eigenvector of the model and the averaged main eigenvector of noisy diffusion. Different line styles correspond to different levels of voxelwise averaging: *thick line* (one experiment), *dotted line* (5 replications and DWI averaging DA), *dashed dotted line* (30 replications and DA), *thin lines close together* (30, 50, 100 replications, DA and application of bias correction according to Rician statistics)

tensor $INV1 = \sum_{k=1}^{3} \lambda_k$, $INV2 = \lambda_1\lambda_2 + \lambda_1\lambda_3 + \lambda_2\lambda_3$, $INV3 = \lambda_1\lambda_2\lambda_3$ are shown in the upper panels. Below one finds the fractions of positive definite voxels, the relative bias of *FA* and the angle between the true main diffusion direction and the averaged noisy main diffusion direction. Before averaging, the main directions were calculated by dyadic sorting, see below, and were aligned to the model. In contrast to [31], increasing n_g does not eliminate in all cases the bias effects, see thick lines in panels *INV1*, *INV2*, *FA* and *ALPHA*. This is due to a strong bias in the DWIs, with minimum $SNR_k \approx 1$. When DWI averaging is performed, the bias effects even increase, see dotted and dashed-dotted lines. Due to the classical CLT averaging of DWIs transforms the Rician distributions to nearly normal shape with small variance, centered around the biased Rician mean values. After bias correction [5], the relative bias of the invariants and of *FA* is practically *zero* for 100 replications, the angle bias is below 2 degrees for $n_g \geq 6$. If only 50 or 30 experiments are applied the results deteriorate only slightly (thin lines). Positive definiteness of the tensor is violated drastically before averaging, but denoising by DWI averaging improves the situation considerably, see Fig. 6.2.

6.3.2 Spatial Denoising

In [12] the so called 'lattice' index of anisotropy is proposed, combining eigenvalue and eigenvector information in a ROI. This index shows enhanced robustness in the presence of noise for low anisotropy, compared to intravoxel indices, like *FA*. Also eigenvalue sorting is improved by considering ROIs. In [21] vector sorting is introduced, where the maximum coherence of main eigenvectors in a ROI is involved. By MCS it is shown for isotropic diffusion that this method is superior to magnitude sorting. Dyadic sorting [22] is another improvement. In this method first magnitude sorting is applied to a spatially averaged tensor used as reference, then, by a dyadic overlap measure for tensors, the eigenvalues of the unknown tensor are sorted.

Nonlinear filtering is applied in [23, 24] to DWIs. In those filters the ROIs, or better effective windows, where smoothing is performed, are not only defined by spatial conditions, but also by a distance measure for the DWI to enable edge preservation. Edges are typical features of spatial DTI variables as e.g. anisotropy and fiber directions can change drastically between two voxels. In [23] the diffusion equation by Perona Malik is applied, in [24] a chain of nonlinear Gaussian filters is used. Both methods include only few assumptions about the structure of the signals and seem to be convenient denoising tools for DTI data with $SNR_k > 3$.

Denoising of tensor fields is described in [25, 26], see also Chap. 18 by Pajevic et al., Chap. 19 and 25 by Weickert et al., and Chap. 24 by Westin et al. In [25] B-splines are applied to a discrete set of noisy DT-MRI measurements to obtain a continuous representation of the tensor field, see Chap. 18 for edge preserving representations by NURBS. In such representations differential geometric quantities, like curvature or torsion of fiber tracts, but also the tangent field could be derived directly. In [25] noise affected templates are denoised with good accuracy, except where the field is not homogenous, e.g. in regions where fiber tracts cross. In [26] the Stejskal Tanner Equations ST for complex signals are used; to achieve them formally, replace the DWIs in (6.2) by the corresponding complex signals or complex DWIs. Assuming that sufficiently many complex DWIs are given by the measurements, a smoothed tensor field $\mathbf{d}(\mathbf{x})$ and $S_0(\mathbf{x})$ are derived by a variational principle ensuring positive definiteness of the tensor. The minimization of the variational integral under ST constraints is achieved by an iterative procedure. The method is edge preserving and is tested in model and real data applications.

The main diffusion directions are smoothed in [27, 28]. By a variational regularization, in [27], coherent vector fields are estimated from noisy data. This method conserves discontinuities and reduces the regularization for small anisotropy. In model calculations those properties are verified, for higher noise level an influence of sorting bias leading to orthogonal directional artifacts is observed. The estimated vector field is then used as a prior to estimate, in a second step, also the eigenvalue fields. To this end a diffusion equation including the 'flow' tensor is applied. This 'flow' tensor includes information about the diffusion tensor and controls smoothing and edge preservation. For real data, denoised tensor, eigenvalue and *FA* fields are discussed. In [28] the regularized main directions are estimated by the Bayesian approach. The estimated maximum of the posterior probability for the main direction field relies on a trade-off between DTI data and a priori assumption regarding the low curvature of the nerve fibers. The a priori probability includes information about the behavior of the modelled direction field in the neighborhood or clique around the voxel of interest, leading to a Gibbs random field with interaction, the likelihood includes only voxelwise calculated probabilities. The regularized direction field is finally used to apply a new tracking algorithm to simulated and real data, allowing the treatment of diverging fibers.

Finally we mention a method proposed especially for very high noise levels, $SNR_k < 3$ [32]; DWI averaging is combined with nonlinear DWI filtering [24] and a bias correction, see Fig. 6.2. Human brain data with $1\,\mathrm{mm}^3$ resolution, this is roughly a factor 10 below the clinical voxel volume which produces severe partial volume deficiencies [1], could be denoised successfully.

Both denoising principles discussed in Sect. 6.3 have inherent shortcomings. Voxelwise denoising involves many experiments, therefore patient motion introducing partial volume effects and distortions, as well as temporal instabilities in the scanner are the main limiting factors. Spatial smoothing suffers often from a trade off between blurring and bias caused by the applied method. Blurring occurs when different 'objects' cannot be discriminated by the denoising method and when consequently anatomically separated information is mixed together, like e.g. in the case of two neighbored fiber bundles with different directions. Bias is mainly caused by too strong priors; e.g. edge preserving filters can be tuned for very high quality in edge finding or 'object' discrimination, the price is usually a decreasing flexibility in the linear behavior or a decreasing ability to model curvature.

6.4 Conclusion

What can we learn from our analysis to find convenient strategies for spatial denoising? For very high noise level, $SNR_k < 3$, denoising and bias correction of the DWIs is a suitable procedure [32]. For reduced noise the tensor distributions approach normality [14] and become also reasonable candidates for smoothing. Our own calculations indicate a limit for tensor smoothing well above $SNR_0 \approx 4$ due to the strong bias effects shown in Fig. 6.2. Tensor denoising is particularly important for multigradient designs where DWI averaging of replications, a convenient preprocessing step before spatial denoising, is seldom feasible. For higher SNR_0, when a bias due to the nonlinear DTI chain can be neglected, eigenvector and eigenvalue fields may be convenient variables. In [15] a similar SNR dependent denoising strategy for the reduction of eigenvalue bias is derived by perturbation theory. For $SNR_0 \approx 20$ denoising of the DWIs is recommended, for $SNR_0 \approx 50$ tensor denoising is shown to be equally good, and only for higher SNRs direct eigenvalue denoising is proposed. Additional priors in the denoising method may help to correct effects of minor skewness or kurtosis in the distributions, or may even correct intrinsic partial volume defects, e.g. in the main diffusion directions [28]. But, a spatial dependence in the (co)variance is predicted by the Delta Method already at very low noise levels and may be included in the denoising procedures.

Acknowledgement

We thank the referees and several colleagues from IBB[1] for constructive suggestions. This study is part of the DFG (German research society) project SFB386, 'Statistical analysis of discrete structures'.

References

1. Basser, P. J., Jones, D. K. (2002) Diffusion Tensor MRI: theory, experimental design and data analysis – a technical review. NMR Biomed. **15**, 456–467
2. Conturo, T. E., McKinstry, R. C. et al. (1995) Diffusion MRI: Precision, accuracy and flow effects. NMR Biomed. **8**, 307–332
3. Vlaardingerbroek, M. T., den Boer, L. A. (1996) Magnetic Resonance Imaging. Springer, Berlin Heidelberg
4. Henkelmann, R. M. (1985) Measurement of signal intensities in the presence of noise in MR images. Med. Phys. **12/2**, 232–233

5. Gudbjartsson, H., Patz, S. (1995) The Rican distribution of noisy MRI data. Mag. Res. Phys. **34**, 910–914
6. Basser, P. J., Mattiello, J., LeBihan, D. (1994) MR diffusion tensor spectroscopy and imaging. Biophys. J. **66**, 259–267
7. Basser, P. J., Mattiello, J., LeBihan, D. (1994) Estimation of the effective self-diffusion tensor from the NMR spin echo. Journ. Mag. Res. **B 103**, 247–254
8. Messiah, A. (1972) Quantum Mechanics I. North-Holland Publishing
9. Press, W. P., Vetterling, W. T. et al. (1992) Numerical Recipes. University Press, Cambridge
10. Renyi, A., (1962) Wahrscheinlichkeitsrechnung. VEB Deutscher Verlag der Wissenschaften, Berlin
11. Lehmann, E. L., (1999) Elements of Large-Sample Theory. Springer, New York
12. Pierpaoli, C., Basser, P., (1996) Toward a quantitative assessment of diffusion anisotropy. Mag. Res. Med. **36**, 893–906
13. Skare, S., Tie-Qiang, L. et al. (2000) Noise considerations in the determination of diffusion tensor anisotropy. Mag. Res. Im. **18**, 659–669
14. Pajevic, S., Basser, P., (2003) Parametric and non-parametric statistical analysis of DT-MRI data. Journ. Mag. Res. **161**, 1–14
15. Anderson, A. W. (2001) Theoretical analysis of the effects of noise on diffusion tensor imaging. Mag. Res. Med. **46**, 1174–1188
16. Clark, C. A., Hedehus, M. et al., (2002) In vivo mapping of the fast and slow diffusion tensors in human brain. Mag. Res. Med. **47**, 623–628
17. Jones, D., Basser, P., (2004) 'Squashing peanuts and smashing pumpkins': How noise distorts diffusion-weighted data. Mag. Res. Med. **52**, 979–993
18. Jones, D., (2003) Determining and visualizing uncertainty in estimates of fiber orientation from diffusion tensor MRI. Mag. Res. Med. **49**, 7–12
19. Heim, S., Hahn, K. R. et al. (2004) Assessing DTI data quality using bootstrap analysis. Mag. Res. Med. **52**, 582–589
20. Hasan, K. M, Parker, D. L. et al. (2001) Comparison of gradient encoding schemes for diffusion-tensor MRI. Journ. Mag. Res. Im. **13**, 769–780
21. Martin, K. M., Papadakis, N. G. et al. (1999) The reduction of the sorting bias in the eigenvalues of the diffusion tensor. Mag. Res. Im. **17**, 893–901
22. Basser, P. J., Pajevic, S. (2000) Statistical artifacts in diffusion tensor MRI (DT-MRI) caused by background noise. Mag. Res. Med. **44**, 41–50
23. Parker, G. J.M., Schnabel, J. A. et al. (2000) Nonlinear smoothing for reduction of systematic and random errors in diffusion tensor imaging. Journ. Mag. Res. Im. **11**, 702–710
24. Hahn, K. R., Prigarin, S. et al. (2001) Edge preserving regularization and tracking for diffusion tensor imaging. In: Niessen W.J., Viergever, M.A.(Eds.) Medical image computing and computer-assisted intervention-MICCAI2001, Springer, Berlin, 195–203
25. Pajevic, S., Aldroubi, A. et al. (2002) A continous tensor field approximation of discrete DT-MRI data for extracting microstructural and architectural features of tissue. Journ. Mag. Res. **154**, 85–100
26. Wang, Z., Vemuri, B. C. et al. (2004) A constrained variational principle for direct estimation and smoothing of the diffusion tensor field from complex DWI. IEEE Trans. Med. Im. **23**, 930–939
27. Coulon, O., Alexander, D. C. et al. (2004) Diffusion tensor magnetic resonance image regularization. Med. Im. Anal. **8**, 47–67

28. Poupon, C., Clark, C. A. et al. (2002) Regularization of diffusion-based direction maps for the tracking of brain white matter fascicles. NeuroImage **12**, 184–195
29. Skare, S., Hedehus, M. et al. (2000) Condition number as a measure of noise performance of diffusion tensor data acquisition schemes with MRI. Journ. Mag. Res. **147**, 340–352
30. Batchelor, P. G., Atkinson, D. et al. (2003) Anisotropic noise propagation in diffusion tensor MRI sampling schemes. Mag. Res. Med. **49**, 1143–1151
31. Jones, D., (2004) The effect of gradient sampling schemes on measures derived from diffusion tensor MRI: a Monte Carlo Study. Mag. Res. Med. **51**, 807–815
32. Hahn, K. R., Prigarin, S. et al. (2004) A novel denoising technique for very noisy DTI data. In: Conf. Proc. of 12th Annual Meeting of ISMRM. Kyoto, 1208

7

An Introduction to Visualization of Diffusion Tensor Imaging and Its Applications

A. Vilanova[1], S. Zhang[2], G. Kindlmann[3], and D. Laidlaw[2]

[1] Department of Biomedical Engineering, Eindhoven University of Technology, WH 2.103, 5600 MB Eindhoven, The Netherlands
`a.vilanova@tue.nl`
[2] Department of Computer Science, Brown University, 115 Waterman Street, Box 1910, Providence, RI 02912, USA
`{dhl,sz}@cs.brown.edu`
[3] School of Computing, University of Utah, 50 South Central Campus Drive, Salt Lake City, UT 84112, USA
`gk@cs.utah.edu`

Summary. Water diffusion is anisotropic in organized tissues such as white matter and muscle. Diffusion tensor imaging (DTI), a non-invasive MR technique, measures water self-diffusion rates and thus gives an indication of the underlying tissue microstructure. The diffusion rate is often expressed by a second-order tensor. Insightful DTI visualization is challenging because of the multivariate nature and the complex spatial relationships in a diffusion tensor field. This chapter surveys the different visualization techniques that have been developed for DTI and compares their main characteristics and drawbacks. We also discuss some of the many biomedical applications in which DTI helps extend our understanding or improve clinical procedures. We conclude with an overview of open problems and research directions.

7.1 Introduction

Diffusion tensor imaging (DTI) is a medical imaging modality that can reveal directional information in vivo in fibrous structures such as white matter or muscles. Although barely a decade old, DTI has become an important tool in studying white matter anatomy and pathology. Many hospitals, universities, and research centers have MRI scanners and diffusion imaging capability, allowing widespread DTI applications.

However, DTI data require interpretation before they can be useful. Visualization methods are needed to bridge the gap between the DTI data sets and understanding of the underlying tissue microstructure. A diffusion tensor measures a 3D diffusion process and has six interrelated tensor components. A volumetric DTI data set is a 3D grid of these diffusion tensors that form

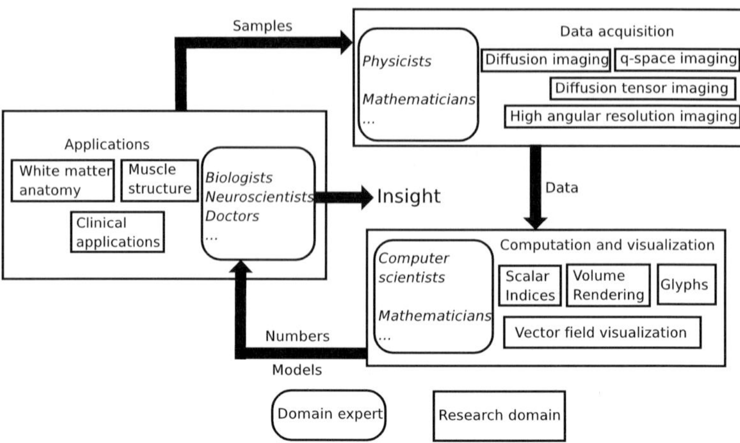

Fig. 7.1. The research context of DTI. Note that all the research domains are interrelated: progress in one domain can easily propagate into the rest of the field

complicated patterns. The multivariate nature of the diffusion tensor and the 3D spatial characteristics of the diffusion tensor field combine to make DTI visualization a challenging task. It is early in the history of visualization of tensor fields and the field is still in an experimental stage. Visualization methods are exploring what users might need to see or evaluate qualitatively on the data. Getting insight on the data allows to identify measures that have statistical and scientific importance to obtain a quantitative evaluation. Applications that involve visualization are beginning to be pursued, but they are even more embryonic than the visualization methods themselves.

This chapter compares current visualization techniques and analyzes their strengths and weaknesses.

DTI research is broadly interdisciplinary. Figure 7.1 gives a simplified illustration of the research domains surrounding DTI. It is worth noting that all of the components in the diagram are interrelated in a loop: new discoveries in one specific area often lead to improvements in the whole DTI field. For example, Pierpaoli et al. found incorrect connections in the neural pathways generated from a DTI data set [1]. Issues like this stimulate research in diffusion imaging and lead to new methods, in this case high angular resolution imaging [2, 3]. In Sect. 7.2, we review techniques for DTI data acquisition In Sect. 7.3, we survey the computation and visualization techniques. We review some applications of DTI in Sect. 7.4, discuss some open issues and problems in Sect. 7.5, and conclude in Sect. 7.6.

7.2 Diffusion Tensor Imaging

As for any visualization method, the merits of DTI visualization methods depend on the quality of the data. Understanding where the data come from, what they measure, and what their limitations are is an important first step in designing and implementing a visualization scheme. We briefly review the diffusion tensor imaging techniques here. Chapter 5 by Alexander presents a more detailed discussion of the subject.

Water molecules in human tissues constantly collide randomly with one another and with other molecules, a phenomenon called Brownian motion. In pure water, this seemingly random movement results in a dynamically expanding Gaussian distribution of water molecules released from one point [4]. In human tissues, however, cell membranes and large protein molecules limit the motion of water molecules. The geometrical and physical properties of the tissue determine the rate and orientation of diffusion. We can thus infer the microstructure of human tissue by measuring the diffusion of the water molecules.

The discovery of the nuclear magnetic resonance (NMR) effect [5, 6] in 1946 was the beginning of work that has led to the current form of diffusion magnetic resonance imaging (MRI). Two important landmarks were the discovery of the spin echo [7], whose signal is perturbed by the water molecule diffusion, and MR imaging [8], which determines exactly where the NMR signal originates within the sample. Diffusion imaging was the first imaging modality to measure the diffusion of water in human tissues in vivo. Although the exact mechanism of the generation of diffusion MRI signals in biological tissues is not fully understood, it is generally believed that the quantity measured by diffusion MRI is a mixture of intracellular diffusion, intercellular diffusion, and the exchange between the two sides of the the cell membrane [9].

Inferring tissue structure from the diffusion process requires exploring the orientation dependence of the diffusion. This dependence can be described by the diffusion propagator $P(r, r', \tau)$, which is the probability of a water molecule traveling from position r' to r in diffusion time τ [10]. In practice, the number of diffusion directions we can measure in a clinical scan is limited by scanning time, making it impossible to reconstruct the diffusion propagator completely. A diffusion tensor [11] describes the orientation dependence of diffusion assuming free diffusion in a uniform anisotropic medium (Gaussian diffusion). For example, a diffusion tensor is a good model for diffusion in uniformly oriented white matter structures such as the corpus callosum, but is insufficient in areas where different tracts cross or merge. The coefficients of the diffusion tensor, $\mathbf{D}$, are related to the diffusion-weighted MRI (DWI) signals by [12] $\tilde{I} = I_0 \exp(\mathbf{b} : \mathbf{D})$, where I_0 is the 0-weighted diffusion image, the tensor $\mathbf{b}$ characterizes the diffusion-encoding gradient pulses used in the MRI sequence, and $\mathbf{b} : \mathbf{D} = \sum_{i=1}^{3} \sum_{j=i}^{3} \mathbf{b}_{ij} \mathbf{D}_{ij}$ is the tensor dot product.

A 3D diffusion tensor is a 3×3 positive symmetric matrix:

$$\mathbf{D} = \begin{bmatrix} \mathbf{D}_{xx} & \mathbf{D}_{xy} & \mathbf{D}_{xz} \\ \mathbf{D}_{xy} & \mathbf{D}_{yy} & \mathbf{D}_{yz} \\ \mathbf{D}_{xz} & \mathbf{D}_{yz} & \mathbf{D}_{zz} \end{bmatrix}$$

Diagonalizing $\mathbf{D}$, we get three positive eigenvalues λ_1, λ_2 and λ_3 (in decreasing order) and their corresponding eigenvectors $\mathbf{e_1}$, $\mathbf{e_2}$ and $\mathbf{e_3}$. Many scalar indices and visualization methods are based on the eigenvalues and eigenvectors of DTI measurements, as discussed in Sect. 7.3.

One geometric representation of Gaussian diffusion is a diffusion ellipsoid. These ellipsoids represent the surface of constant mean-squared displacement of diffusing water molecules at some time τ after they are released from one point. The shape of a diffusion ellipsoid is inherently related to the eigenvalues and eigenvectors of the diffusion tensor: the three principal radii are proportional to the eigenvalues and the axes of the ellipsoid aligned with the three orthogonal eigenvectors of the diffusion tensor. Figure 7.2 shows ellipsoids representing different kinds of diffusion; the difference among the shapes of the ellipsoids are discussed in Sect. 7.3.1.

DTI measurements have been validated within acceptable error on the fibrous muscle tissue of the heart [13, 14]. However, in a voxel containing

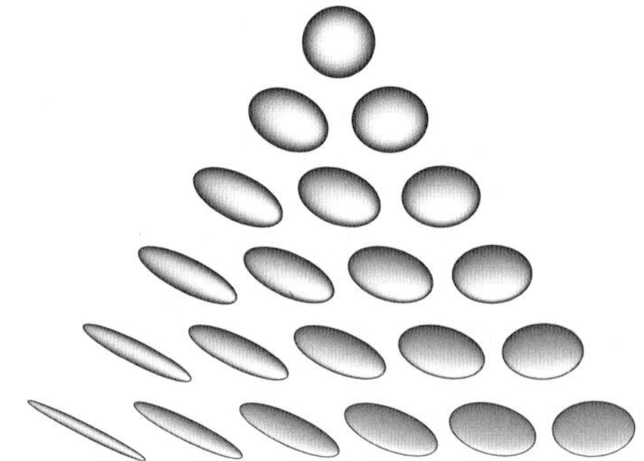

Fig. 7.2. Barycentric space of diffusion tensor ellipsoids

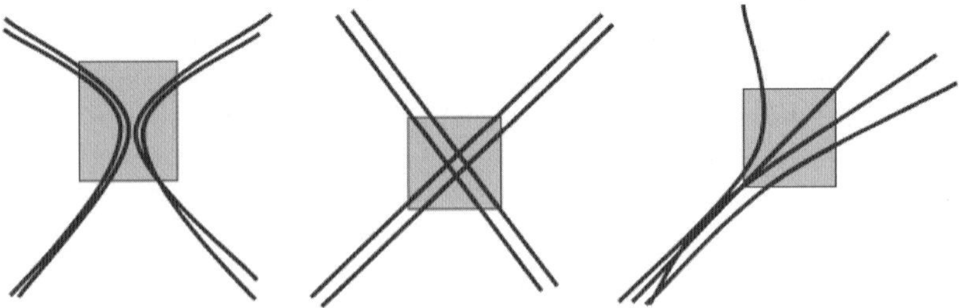

Fig. 7.3. Illustration of regions with planar anisotropy due to the fiber configuration. Gray regions represent voxels with planar anisotropy: (*left*) kissing fibers, (*middle*) two fiber bundles crossing and (*right*) diverging fibers

nonuniformly oriented neural fibers (see Fig. 7.3), DTI measures an average signal from all the fibers within the voxel, which usually results in an apparent reduction of anisotropy and increase in uncertainty [15]. To resolve the uncertainty in these areas, q-space spectral imaging [16] and other high angular resolution diffusion imaging methods [17, 18] have been explored (see Chap. 10 by Özarslan et al.). Beyond these ambiguities introduced in regions where the diffusion is not coherent and cannot be modelled as a tensor, noise in the underlying MR images propagates through the computational pipeline changing the source diffusion weighted images, resulting diffusion tensor images, and visualizations based on them. Understanding the implications of all of these artifacts in visualizations is an active area of current research (see, e.g., Chap. 6 by Hahn et al.).

Image acquisition for DTI is a very active research area. Progress is frequently reported on resolution improvement and reductions in imaging time, noise, and distortion.

7.3 DTI Visualization

Meaningful visualization of diffusion tensor fields is challenging because of its multivariate nature and complex interrelationships. The last decade has seen several approaches to visualizing diffusion tensor data, most of them based on reducing the dimensionality of the data by extracting relevant information from the tensor. One possible classification of the different visualization techniques is by the dimensionality to which the tensor is reduced. Another important characteristic is the ability of these algorithms to show local or global information, where global information means the complex spatial relationships of tensors. Our discussion here groups the visualization methods on the basis of these two criteria. Anisotropy indices reduce the 6D information to a scalar value (1D). *Volume rendering* for DTI uses anisotropy indices to define transfer functions that show the anisotropy and shape of the tensor. *Tensor glyphs* do not reduce the dimensionality of the tensor, instead using primitives that show the 6D tensor as such; however, these techniques cannot show global information. *Vector-field visualization* reduces the tensor field to a vector field, and therefore to 3D information at each point. Several techniques can be used for vector-field visualization that show local as well as global information. Section 7.3.5 describes algorithms in which the vector field is extended with more information from the tensor. This includes techniques where the whole tensor information is taken into account. Finally in Sect. 7.3.6, several interaction schemes in DTI visualization are discussed.

7.3.1 Scalar Indices

The complexity of a DTI data set requires a complicated visualization scheme; however, medical researchers and practitioners alike are trained to read scalar

Table 7.1. Some scalar indices for DTI data. $||\mathbf{D}|| = \sqrt{\mathbf{D} : \mathbf{D}}$ is the tensor norm, $\mathrm{Var}(\lambda)$ and $\mathrm{E}(\lambda)$ are the variance and expectation of the three eigenvalues, a_n is a normalized weighting factor, $\mathbf{A} = \mathbf{D} - \langle\mathbf{D}\rangle\mathbf{I}$

	Scalar Index	Equations
	Mean diffusivity, $\langle\mathbf{D}\rangle$	$\dfrac{\mathbf{D}_{\mathrm{xx}} + \mathbf{D}_{\mathrm{yy}} + \mathbf{D}_{\mathrm{zz}}}{3}, \dfrac{\lambda_1 + \lambda_2 + \lambda_3}{3}, \dfrac{\mathrm{Trace}(\mathbf{D})}{3}$
[19]	Volume ratio, VR	$\dfrac{\lambda_1\lambda_2\lambda_3}{\left(\frac{\lambda_1+\lambda_2+\lambda_3}{3}\right)^3}, 27\dfrac{\mathrm{Determinant}(\mathbf{D})}{\mathrm{Trace}(\mathbf{D})^3}$
[20]	Fractional anisotropy, FA	$\sqrt{\dfrac{3}{2}}\,\dfrac{||\mathbf{D} - \langle\mathbf{D}\rangle\mathbf{I}||}{||\mathbf{D}||}$
[20]	Rational anisotropy, RA	$\dfrac{||\mathbf{D} - \langle\mathbf{D}\rangle\mathbf{I}||}{||\langle\mathbf{D}\rangle\mathbf{I}||}, \dfrac{\sqrt{\mathrm{Var}(\lambda)}}{\mathrm{E}(\lambda)}$
[19]	Lattice index, LI	$\displaystyle\sum_{n=1}^{N} a_n \left(\dfrac{\sqrt{3}}{\sqrt{8}}\dfrac{\sqrt{\mathbf{A} : \mathbf{A}_n}}{\sqrt{\mathbf{D} : \mathbf{D}_n}} + \dfrac{3}{4}\dfrac{\mathbf{A} : \mathbf{A}_n}{\sqrt{\mathbf{D} : \mathbf{D}}\sqrt{\mathbf{D}_n : \mathbf{D}_n}}\right)$
[21]	Linear anisotropy, c_l	$\dfrac{\lambda_1 - \lambda_2}{\lambda_1 + \lambda_2 + \lambda_3}$
	Planar anisotropy, c_p	$\dfrac{2(\lambda_2 - \lambda_3)}{\lambda_1 + \lambda_2 + \lambda_3}$
	Isotropy, c_s	i $\dfrac{3\lambda_3}{\lambda_1 + \lambda_2 + \lambda_3}$

fields on gray-level images slice by slice. Scalar data sets, although limited in the amount of information they can convey, can be visualized with simplicity and clarity and thus interpreted quickly and easily. It can thus be useful to reduce DTI to scalar data sets. Since the advent of diffusion MRI, scalar indices of diffusion MRI data have been designed and visualized successfully alongside multivariate visualization schemes: rather than competing, the two methods complement one another.

The challenges of reducing a tensor-valued diffusion MRI measurement to a scalar index include mapping to a meaningful physical quantity, maintaining invariance with respect to rotation and translation, and reducing the effect of noise. Some scalar indices for DTI data are listed in Table 7.1.

Mean diffusivity (MD), which measures the overall diffusion rate, is the average of the diffusion tensor eigenvalues and is rotationally invariant. Van Gelderen et al. [22] demonstrated that, after a stroke, the trace of the diffusion tensor delineates the affected area much more accurately than the diffusion image in one orientation.

Before the diffusion tensor model was made explicit in 1994 by Basser et al. [11], several different anisotropy indices derived from DWIs were used, such as anisotropic diffusion ratio [23]. Unfortunately, these anisotropy indices depend on the choice of laboratory coordinate system and are rotationally variant: their interpretation varies according to the relative positions of the MR gradient and the biological tissues, usually resulting in an underestimation of the degree of anisotropy [19]. Therefore it is important to use rotationally invariant anisotropy indices such as volume ratio (VR), rational anisotropy (RA) or fractional anisotropy (FA), which are based on the rotationally invariant eigenvalues. Note that both RA and FA can be derived from tensor norms and traces without calculating the eigenvalues.

However, rotationally invariant indices such as RA and FA are still susceptible to noise contamination. Pierpaoli et al. [19] calculated an intervoxel anisotropy index, the *lattice index* (LI), which locally averages inner products between diffusion tensors in neighboring voxels. LI decreases the sensitivity to noise and avoids underestimation of the anisotropy when the neighbor voxels have different fiber orientations.

Because they contract the tensor to one scalar value, FA, RA and LI do not indicate the directional variation of the diffusion anisotropy well. For example, a cigar-shaped and a pancake-shaped ellipsoid can have equal FA while their shapes differ greatly. Geometrical diffusion measures [21] have been developed: linear anisotropy, c_l, planar anisotropy, c_p and spherical anisotropy or isotropy, c_s. By construction, $c_l + c_p + c_s = 1$. Thus, these three metrics parameterize a barycentric space in which the three shape extremes (linear, planar, and spherical) are at the corners of a triangle, as shown in Fig. 7.2. It is worth noting that, unlike FA or RA, geometrical diffusion metrics depend on the order of the eigenvalues and are thus prone to bias in the presence of noise [19].

Figure 7.4 shows one way to compare qualitatively some of the metrics described above by sampling their values on a slice of a DTI data set of a brain. Notice that the mean diffusivity (MD) is effective at distinguishing between cerebrospinal fluid (where MD is high) and brain tissue (lower MD), but fails to differentiate between different kinds of brain tissue. High fractional anisotropy, FA, on the other hand, indicates white matter, because the directionality of the axon bundles permits faster diffusion along the neuron

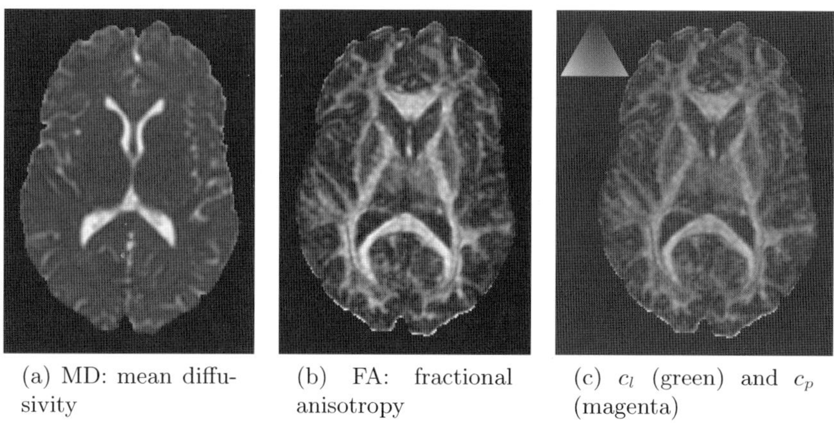

(a) MD: mean diffusivity	(b) FA: fractional anisotropy	(c) c_l (green) and c_p (magenta)

Fig. 7.4. Shape metrics applied to one slice of a brain DTI scan. See color plates

fiber orientation than across it. FA is highest inside thick regions of uniformly anisotropic diffusion, such as inside the corpus callosum. Finally, while both c_l and c_p indicate high anisotropy, their relative values indicate the shape of the diffusion ellipsoid.

7.3.2 Volume Rendering

Volume rendering is a means of visualizing large-scale structure in a tensor field, based on locally measured properties of the tensor data [24]. Volume rendering has the defining property of mapping from the tensor field attributes to a rendered image, without introducing additional geometry. However, volume rendering is inherently flexible in the sense that the volume scene can easily be supplemented with other visualizations (such as glyphs or fiber tracts, described in following sections) to create a more informative image. Compositing all the scene components together creates an integrated visualization in which local and global aspects of the field may be seen in context. The volume of tensor field attributes can either be precomputed and stored as a scalar field, or computed implicitly as part of rendering. In either case, an anisotropy index plays the important role of determining the opacity (thus visibility) of each sample. Each sample is then colored and shaded to indicate local shape characteristics; then samples are composited as the integral of colors and opacities are sampled along each ray.

An essential element of volume rendering is the *transfer function*, which assigns colors and opacities according to locally measured field properties. Traditionally, volume rendering has been applied to visualization of scalar fields, in which the domain of the transfer function is either the scalar value defining the data set or additionally includes derived quantities such as the gradient magnitude [25, 26]. The transfer function is usually implemented as a one-dimensional or two-dimensional lookup table. The transfer function domain variables are quantized to generate indices of table entries that contain the colors and opacity of the transfer function range.

The extension of volume rendering to diffusion tensor fields is thus essentially a matter of determining which quantities should serve as transfer function domain variables. To define opacity, the anisotropy indices in Table 7.1 are used. Fractional anisotropy (FA) is attractive in this respect because it can be expressed in terms of differentiable tensor invariants, so the chain rule can be used to calculate the gradient of FA as a normal for surface shading. Figure 7.5 shows a depiction of basic 3D structure with volume-rendered isosurfaces of fractional anisotropy. Rather than using a polygonal model of the anisotropy isosurface (as with Marching Cubes [27]), these images are computed with an opacity *step function*: opacity is 0.0 or 1.0 depending on whether FA is below or above the indicated threshold.

Color can be assigned in diffusion tensor volume rendering to indicate either the orientation or the shape of the underlying tensor samples. Applying the standard RGB coloring of the principal eigenvector (see Sect. 7.3.4)

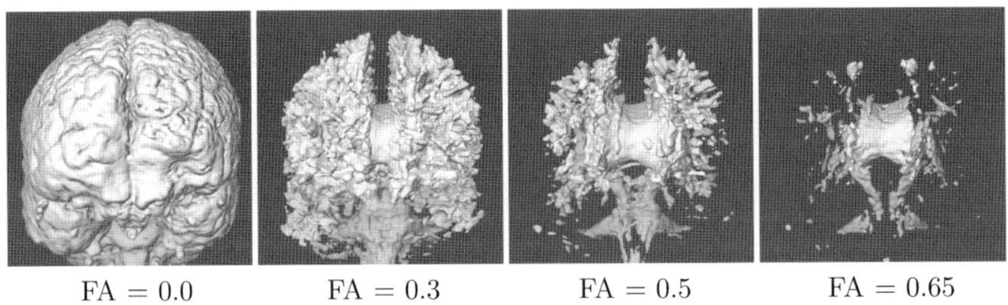

FA = 0.0   FA = 0.3   FA = 0.5   FA = 0.65

Fig. 7.5. Volume-rendered isosurfaces at a range of FA values show basic 3D structure of white matter in a DTI brain scan

allows basic neuroanatomic features to be recognized by their overall color, as in Fig. 6(a). Color can also be used to clarify differences in the shape of anisotropy apart from the anisotropy index used to define opacity. In particular, the difference between linear and planar anisotropy as measured by the c_l and c_p indices (Table 7.1) can be mapped onto the anisotropy isosurface, as in Fig. 6(b) (where the variation from green to magenta for linear to planar anisotropy is the same as in Fig. 4(c)). The rendering indicates how features with orthogonal orientations lead to planar anisotropy at their adjacencies. Locations in the brain characterized by this configuration of white-matter fibers include the right-left transpontine tracts ventral to the inferior-superior corticospinal tracts in the brainstem, and the right-left tracts of the corpus callosum inferior to the anterior-posterior cingulum bundles.

A recent application of volume rendering to diffusion tensor visualization is based on converting the tensor field to scalar fields, as described by Wenger et al. [28]. The approach here is to precompute multiple scalar volumes that can be layered and interactively rendered with 3D texture-mapping graphics hardware [29]. The renderings in Fig. 7.7 show visualizations that combine a volume rendering of the cerebral spinal fluid with a collection of fiber tracts

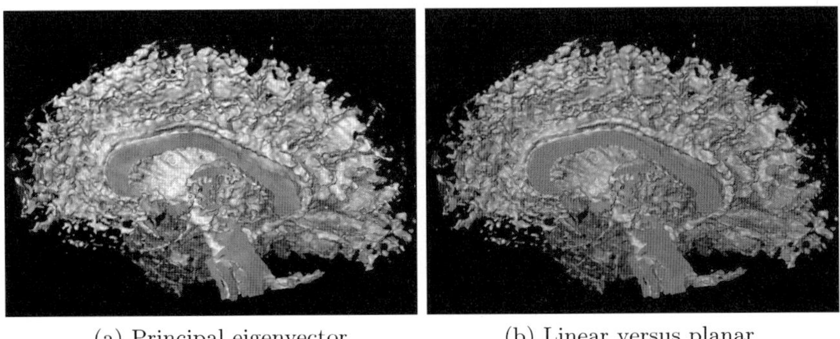

(a) Principal eigenvector   (b) Linear versus planar

Fig. 7.6. Volume renderings of half a brain scan, (**a**) colored according to orientation of principal eigenvector; (**b**) the distribution of linear (*green*) and planar (*magenta*) anisotropy. Surface is defined by FA = 0.4. See color plates

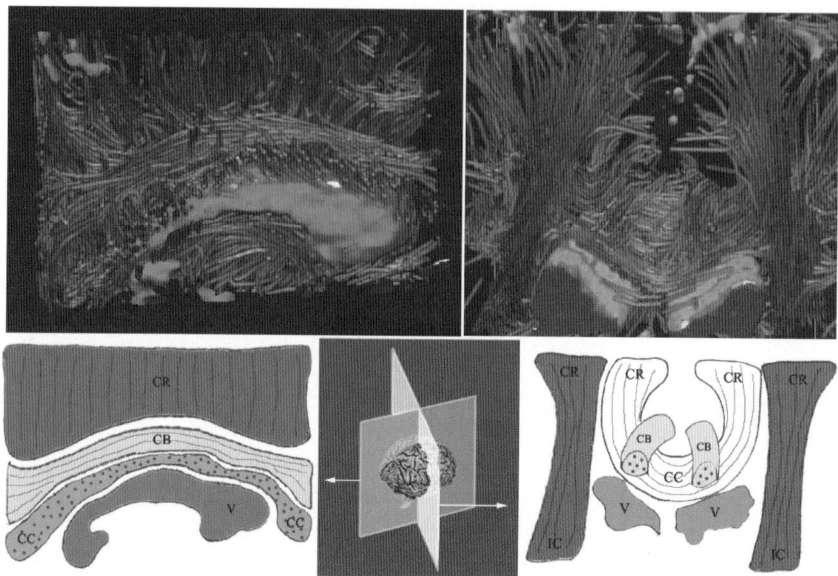

Fig. 7.7. Interactive volume renderings of a human brain data set. The volume renderings (*top*) show collections of threads consistent with major white-matter structures: IC = internal capsule, CR = corona radiata, CB = cingulum bundle, CC = corpus callosum diagrammed on the bottom. Components of the tensor-valued data control thread orientation, color, and density. Direct volume rendering simultaneously shows in blue the cerebral spinal fluid in the ventricles (labeled V) and some sulci for anatomical context. See color plates

rasterized into a color-coded scalar volume to illustrate the relationship between the distribution and orientation of the fiber tracts and the large-scale patterns of anisotropy. The flexible combination of the different scalar volumes into the final rendering permits interactive exploration and generation of visualizations.

There are currently no implementations that can volume render directly from a diffusion tensor volume to an image at interactive rates. The computational speed and flexibility of modern graphics hardware is increasing at such a rate, however, that this should soon be feasible. For example, two-dimensional transfer functions took minutes to render (in software) when introduced in 1988 [26], but can now be rendered at multiple frames per second with commodity graphics hardware [30]. Whether applied to scalar or tensor data, the intrinsically data-parallel nature of volume rendering makes it well suited to the streaming-based processors found on modern graphics hardware [31]. We anticipate that volume-rendering graphics hardware will play an increasing role in the interactive visualization of diffusion tensor data.

7.3.3 Tensor Glyphs

Another avenue of DTI visualization has focused on using tensor glyphs to visualize the complete tensor information at one point. A tensor glyph is a parameterized graphical object that describes a single diffusion tensor with its size, shape, color, texture, location, etc. Most tensor glyphs have six or more degrees of freedom and can represent a diffusion tensor completely. However, tensor glyphs do not expose relationships and features across a diffusion tensor field; rather, they imply these relationships from the visual correlation and features of the individual glyphs. While exploiting many different types of tensor glyphs, from boxes to ellipsoids to superquadrics, tensor glyph designers aim to make the mapping between glyphs and diffusion tensors faithful, meaningful and explicit.

The diffusion ellipsoid described in Sect. 7.2 is the most commonly used representation of a diffusion tensor. Pierpaoli et al. [19], in the first use of ellipsoids as tensor glyphs for DTI, associated ellipsoid size with the mean diffusivity and indicated the preferred diffusion orientation by the orientation of the diffusion ellipsoid. Arrays of ellipsoids were arranged together in the same order as the data points to show a 2D slice of DTI data.

Laidlaw et al. normalized the size of the ellipsoids to fit more of them in a single image [32] (see Fig. 8(a)). While this method forgoes the ability to show mean diffusivity, it creates more uniform glyphs that show anatomy and pathology over regions better than the non-normalized ellipsoids.

Laidlaw et al. [32] also developed a method that uses the concepts of brush strokes and layering from oil painting to emphasize the diffusion patterns. They used 2D brush strokes both individually, to encode specific values, and collectively, to show spatial connections and to generate texture and a sense of speed corresponding to the speed of diffusion. They also used layering and contrast to create depth. This method was applied to sections of spinal cords of

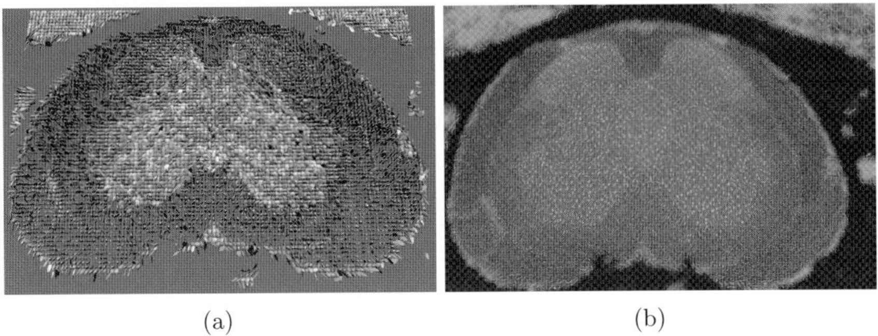

(a)   (b)

Fig. 7.8. (a) Arrays of normalized ellipsoids visualize the diffusion tensors in a single slice. (b) Brush strokes illustrate the orientation and magnitude of the diffusion: background color and texture-map show additional information. See color plates

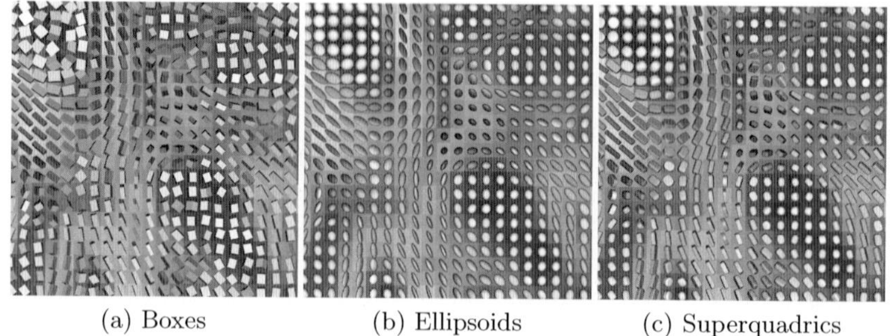

(a) Boxes   (b) Ellipsoids   (c) Superquadrics

Fig. 7.9. A portion of a brain DTI scan as visualized by three different glyph methods (overall glyph sizes have been normalized). See color plates

mice with experimental allergic encephalomyelitis (EAE) and clearly showed anatomy and pathology (see Fig. 8(b)).

Boxes and cylinders have also been used to show the directions and relative lengths of all three eigenvectors. Boxes clearly indicate the orientation of the eigenvectors. They also have fewer polygons and are thus faster to render. But their flat faces usually make it hard to infer the 3D shapes from a 2D image (see Fig. 9(a)).

Kindlmann adapted superquadrics, a traditional surface modeling technique, to generate tensor glyphs [33]. The class of shapes he created includes spheres in the isotropic case, while emphasizing the differences among the eigenvalues in the anisotropic cases. As shown in Fig. 7.10, cylinders are used for linear and planar anisotropy and intermediate forms of anisotropy are represented by approximations to boxes. As with ellipsoid glyphs, a circular cross-section accompanies equal eigenvalues, for which distinct eigenvectors are not defined.

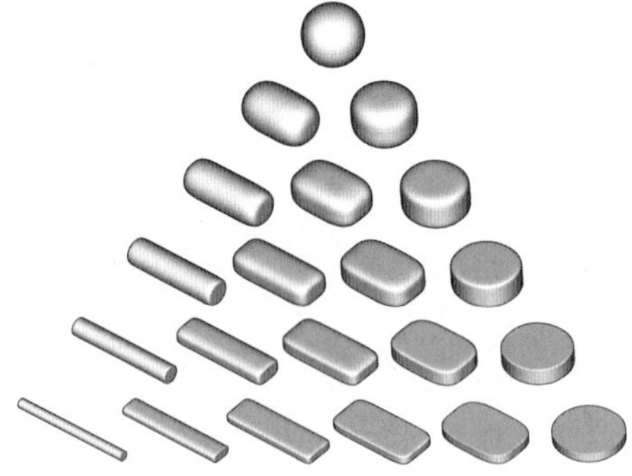

Fig. 7.10. Superquadrics as tensor glyphs, sampling the same barycentric space as in Fig. 7.2

The differences among some of the glyph methods can be appreciated by comparing their results on a portion of a slice of a DTI brain scan, as shown in Fig. 7.9. The individual glyphs have been colored with the principal eigenvector colormap. The directional cue given by the edges of box glyphs 9(a) is effective in linearly anisotropic regions, but can be misleading in regions of planar anisotropy and isotropy, since in these cases the corresponding eigenvectors are not well defined numerically. The rotational symmetry of ellipsoid glyphs 9(b) avoids misleading depictions of orientation, with the drawback that different shapes can be difficult to distinguish. The superquadric glyphs 9(c) aim to combine the best of the box and ellipsoid methods.

7.3.4 Vector Field Visualization

The tensor field can also be simplified to a vector field defined by the main eigenvector, $\mathbf{e_1}$. This simplification is based on the assumption that in the areas of linear anisotropy, $\mathbf{e_1}$ defines the orientation of linear structures. The sign of $\mathbf{e_1}$ has no meaning.

One commonly used method to visualize DTI data is to map $\mathbf{e_1}$ to color, e.g., directly using the absolute value of the $\mathbf{e_1}$ components for the RGB channel: $R = |\mathbf{e_1} \cdot \mathbf{x}|$, $G = |\mathbf{e_1} \cdot \mathbf{y}|$, $B = |\mathbf{e_1} \cdot \mathbf{z}|$. The saturation of this color is weighted by an anisotropy index to de-emphasize isotropic areas (see Fig. 7.11).

Other methods have been proposed to visualize the global information of 2D as well as 3D vector fields [34], and there are well established 2D vector-field visualization methods [35]. Although 2D techniques have been

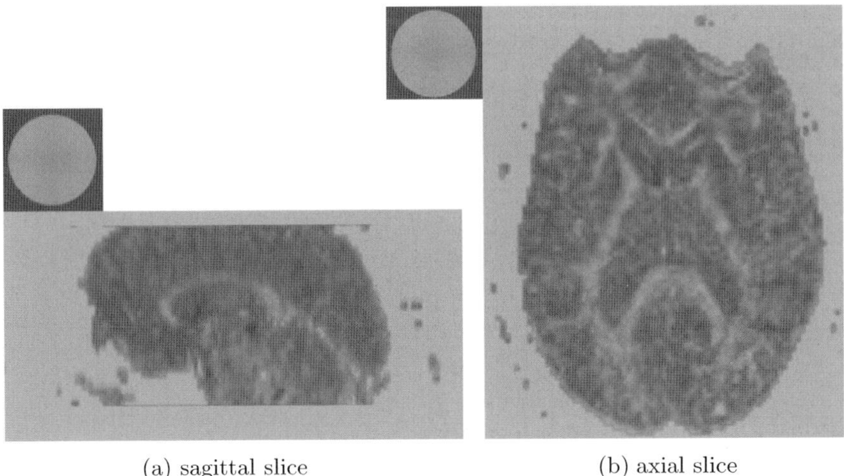

(a) sagittal slice   (b) axial slice

Fig. 7.11. Mapping of $\mathbf{e_1}$ to the RGB channel shown in 2D slices of a healthy volunteer brain. See color plates extended to 3D, the visualization of 3D vector fields is still a challenging problem due to visual cluttering and computational cost.

We concentrate here on 3D DTI data. The most commonly used technique to visualize DTI data is streamline tracing; in DTI-specific literature this is also called fiber tracking [36] or tractography [37]. There is a direct analogy between the streamlines and the linear structures to be visualized (e.g., fibers). Furthermore, streamlines in 3D can easily be visualized by regions in order to avoid cluttering. Streamline tracing is based on solving the following equation:

$$p(t) = \int_0^t \mathbf{v}(p(s))ds \qquad (7.1)$$

where $p(t)$ is the generated streamline and $\mathbf{v}$ corresponds to the vector field generated from $\mathbf{e_1}$. $p(0)$ is set to the initial point of the integral curve.

The streamline technique has three main steps: definition of initial tracking points (i.e., seed points), integration, and the definition of stopping criteria. Seed points are usually user defined: the user specifies one or more regions of interest (ROI). Interior of the ROIs are sampled and the samples are used as seed points (see Fig. 7.12). Equation (7.1) is solved by numerical integration via such schemes as Euler forward and second or fourth-order Runge-Kutta. Stopping criteria avoid calculation of the streamline where the vector field is not robustly defined. In areas of isotropic or planar diffusion, the value of $\mathbf{e_1}$ can be considered random, and thus has no meaning for the underlying structure. The user can usually set a threshold based on the anisotropy indices (e.g., FA, RA or c_l) to describe the areas where the vector field is defined; the value of this threshold depends on the data-acquisition protocol and the nature of the object being scanned. Other criteria can also be used, such as the curvature or length of the streamline.

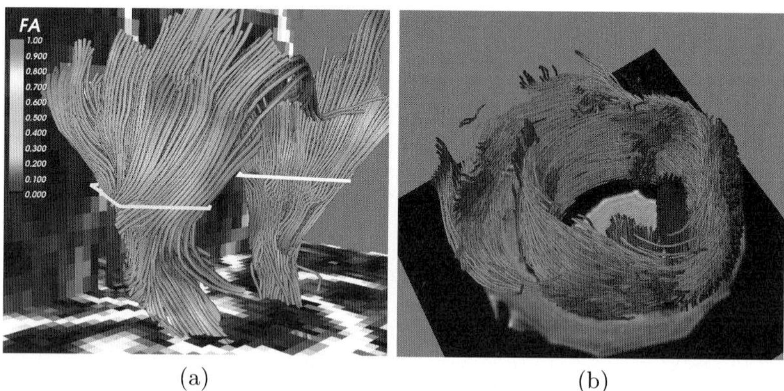

(a)   (b)

Fig. 7.12. (a) Streamline tracing using two ROIs to trace the corona radiata in a data set of a healthy volunteer brain. (b) Streamlines in a data set of a goat heart using the seeding technique of Vilanova et al. [38]. See color plates

Hyperstreamlines are an extension to streamlines for second-order tensor fields [39], first used by Zhang et al. for DTI data [40]. Hyperstreamlines employ all eigenvalues and eigenvectors. A streamline defines the axis of a generalized cylinder whose cross-section perpendicular to the axis is an ellipse defined by e_2 and e_3 and λ_2 and λ_3, respectively.

Streamline-tracing techniques for DTI have several disadvantages that are constantly being addressed. In areas of nonlinear diffusion the main eigenvector is not robustly defined [15]. However, linear structures can be present in areas with nonlinear diffusion, appearing where the linear structure orientation is not coherent within a voxel (see Fig. 7.3) or arising from noise. Most DTI tracing algorithms consider only the areas where the vector field is defined robustly. Several authors have proposed methods to trace within areas of isotropic or planar diffusion following the most probable diffusion orientation based on some heuristics (e.g., [41, 42]). Some of these methods are based on regularization techniques that are commonly used in image processing for noise removal.

Another difficulty in streamlines is seeding. The seed points can be defined by the user. In a healthy person with known anatomy, users can estimate where the interesting bundles are and where to seed. However, in some cases, there are no real clues to the possible underlying structure and user seeding can miss important structures. Defining the seed points to cover the whole volume can be computationally expensive, however, and furthermore, too many seed points clutter the image and make it difficult to extract useful information.

Zhang et al. [40] employed uniform seeding throughout the entire volume and developed a culling algorithm as a postprocessing step to control the streamline density. This allows inside structures to be visible and outside structures still to be adequately represented. The metrics for the culling process include the length of a trajectory, the average linear anisotropy along a trajectory, and the similarity between a trajectory and the group of trajectories already selected.

Vilanova et al. [38] extended Jobard et al.'s seeding algorithm [43] for 3D DTI data (see Fig. 7.12(b)). Here seeding and generation of streamlines depend on a parameter that defines the density of the streamlines (i.e., minimal distance between streamlines). This method allows control of cluttering and less computationally expensive generation of streamlines than seeding the whole volume regularly. However, if the density is set to a low value this method does not guarantee that the important structures are visible, since only the distance between streamline seed points is taken into account.

Generally, the fiber bundles are more interesting than an individual fiber, and several authors have proposed ways to cluster the streamlines to obtain bundles (e.g., [44, 45, 46, 47]). These algorithms differ primarily in the metrics used to define the similarity between streamlines and clusters, which are mainly based on the shape and distance between fiber pairs. Bundles are a compact representation of the data that alleviates cluttering; however, these algorithms have the disadvantage of relying solely on the results of the streamline-tracing algorithm, and therefore are very sensitive to its errors.

7.3.5 Beyond Vector Field Visualization

The previous section presented several visualization methods for which the diffusion tensor data are simplified to the main diffusion orientation to reconstruct the underlying linear structure. In doing this, of course, information is lost. In this section, we present several approaches that try to rectify this loss and use more information than the main eigenvector, e_1.

In DTI, it is assumed that the diffusion tensor gives an indication of the underlying geometrical structure. In the streamline tracing algorithm, the main eigenvector is assumed to represent the tangent vector of an underlying linear structure. However, diffusion does not indicate just linear structures, but also planar structures (e.g., sheet). Similarly to linear anisotropy, it can be assumed that planar anisotropy indicates a planar structure. Therefore, the eigenvectors e_1 and e_2 define the tangent plane of an underlying planar structure, i.e., the streamsurface. Zhang et al. [40] presented an algorithm to generate the streamsurface based on the planar anisotropic characteristics of the data. Figure 7.13(a) shows the results of using their algorithm to trace streamlines and streamsurfaces in the whole volume. In the brain there are no structures which have a planar like shape. However, due to fibers crossing and the partial volume effect planar like structures appear in the DTI data.

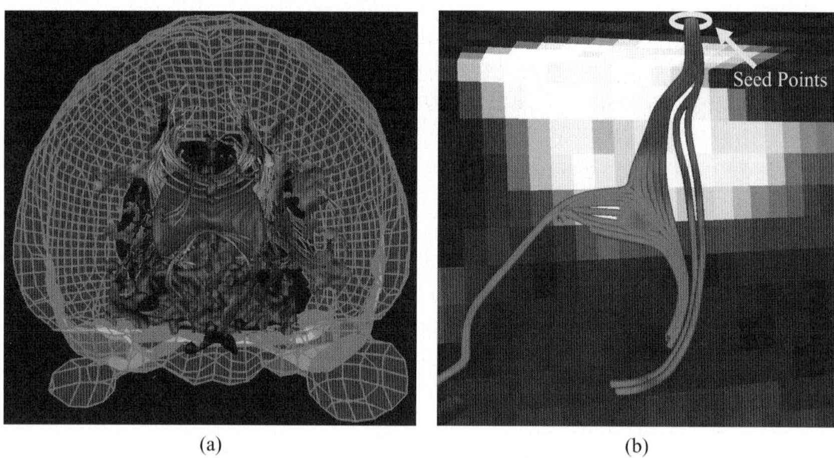

(a)   (b)

Fig. 7.13. Examples of streamsurfaces: (**a**) red streamlines (represented as cylinders) and green streamsurfaces generated using the method of Zhang et al. [40] show linear and planar anisotropy, respectively, together with anatomical landmarks for context; (**b**) Streamlines using seed points (yellow region) trace streamsurfaces and show the possible prolongation of the fiber bundle, generated using the algorithm of Vilanova et al. [38] (see color plates)

Vilanova et al. [38] used a similar algorithm to Zhang et al. in combination with streamline tracing to show the areas where linear structures cross, kiss, converge or diverge (see Fig. 7.3).

Figure 7.13(b) shows streamlines generated by a few seed points (in the yellow circle). Instead of stopping, a streamsurface is traced when a streamline reaches an area of planar anisotropy. In addition, the possible continuations of the initial streamline going through the streamsurface are traced further.

Streamsurfaces are extensions of streamlines, but the tensor information is still simplified and not treated as a whole. Parker et al. [48] and Brun et al. [49] modeled all possible paths from a given starting point. Parker et al. used a front-propagation method with a speed function based on the underlying tensor field. The path between the starting point and any point in the volume is defined by using the time of arrival of the front to each point and a gradient-descent algorithm. A connectivity metric describes the likelihood of connection of each path. Brun et al. [49] modeled the paths as a probability distribution that is discretely represented by weighted samples from it. For each path, a connectivity is also assigned according to the diffusion tensor and the path's shape. Batchelor et al. [50] propose a method based on simulating the diffusion defined by the diffusion tensor, and use a probabilistic interpretation of the time of arrival of the diffusion front to quantify the connectivity of two points. O'Donnell et al. [51] describe a similar idea: a flux vector field based on solving for the steady-state concentration is created. Paths generated in this vector field have a measure of connectivity based on the flow along the paths; the maximum flow indicates the most probable connection. They also present a method based on warping the space locally using a metric defined by the inverse of the diffusion tensor. The minimum-distance path (i.e., geodesic) in this warped space provides a reconstruction of a possible underlying linear structure and a numerical measure of connectivity between two points (i.e., distance).

The advantage of these methods is that they are well defined in the complete space, even in areas with planar or isotropic diffusion. Furthermore, they give a quantitative measure of connectivity. Their drawbacks are that they are computationally expensive and any pair of points in the space is connected. Therefore, it is necessary to define not just a starting point but also end points, or to establish criteria for which points are considered to be connected (e.g., a percentile of the most probable connections).

There have been several efforts to visualize the global information of the second-order tensor field in general [52, 53] (see also Chap. 16 by Hotz et al.). Zheng and Pang [54] presented an extension of the vector-field visualization method LIC (line integral convolution) to tensor data. Similarly, Bhalerao and Westin [55] extended splatting (a scalar volume rendering technique) to tensor data. Cluttering is a problem when these methods are applied to DTI data, since not much more than the outer shell of the anisotropic areas is visible.

Hesselink et al. [56] presented a method to extract topology skeletons of second-order 3D tensor fields. These skeletons are mainly defined by points, lines and surfaces that represent the complex structure of a tensor field in a compact and abstract way. The topology is based on the calculation of degenerate points whose eigenvalues are equal to each other. In Chap. 14, Zheng et al. show that the stable degenerated features in 3D tensor fields form lines. The main drawback of this method is the lack of an intuitive interpretation of the topology skeletons for tensor fields. In real data, the resulting skeletons can be very complex and difficult to analyze.

7.3.6 Interaction

Human-computer interaction (HCI) arises in multiple aspects of DTI visualization: transfer function manipulation, seeding point selection, streamline culling, streamline query, and graphical model exploration, to name a few. We briefly review some of the interaction techniques here.

In volume rendering, transfer functions determine the mapping from the data to color and opacity (see Sect. 7.3.2). The selection of transfer functions often requires expertise; in addition, it is often done by trial and error, so that it is important that the user be able to select the transfer functions intuitively and quickly. Kniss et al. [30] describes a set of widgets that let the user specify multidimensional transfer functions interactively. Wenger et al. [28] applied this idea to DTI volume rendering, employing a set of widgets including a barycentric widget for manipulating the geometrical diffusion measures (see Fig. 7.14).

Interaction permeates the whole process of vector field visualization: both seed points selection and connectivity query involve specifying ROIs. Streamline culling requires selecting certain criteria and setting the corresponding thresholds. Displaying the 3D streamline models often relies on user input

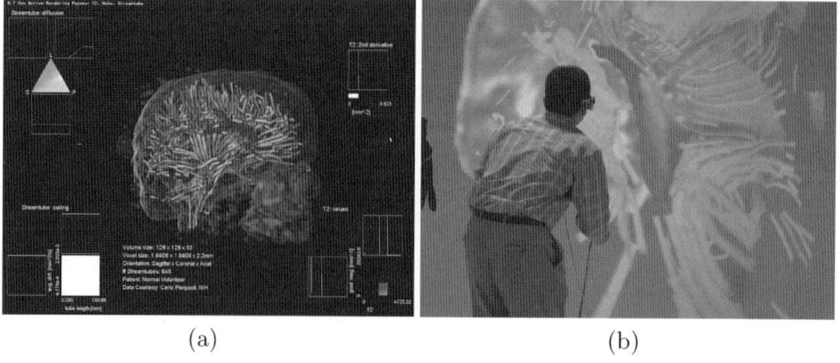

(a)   (b)

Fig. 7.14. (a) An interactive exploration tool for DTI volume rendering. Clockwise from upper left are a 2D barycentric widget, a 1D widget, a 2D Cartesian widget, and a 2D Cartesian culling widget. (b) A user explores a complex 3D model in a virtual reality CAVE. See color plates to show the models at different scales and perspectives. Akers et al. [57] developed a pathway-query prototype to expedite the first two operations, precomputing the pathways and their statistical properties to achieve real-time interaction.

The complexity of the DTI data sets often yields complicated graphical models that are hard to discern in a still picture. Continuing developments in computer graphics constantly change how users interact with these models. Desktop 3D graphics used mouse click and drag to move the models; fishtank virtual reality display systems added stereo and head tracking [58]. The CAVE provided an immersive virtual environment that engaged the user in whole-body interaction [59] (see Fig. 14(b)). However, none of these systems are sufficient alone; each has its strengths and weaknesses depending on certain applications [58].

The interaction schemes can also be combined in hybrid visualization methods. For example, the streamtube-culling widget can be incorporated into the control panel with various other transfer function widgets (see Fig. 14(a)). A traditional 2D structural image slice provides context in a complex 3D scene (see Fig. 14(b)).

Currently, computational power limits our ability to achieve real-time interaction and precomputed models must often be used for sake of speed. In the future, we expect a closer tie between computation and human input for more efficient and effective data exploration.

7.4 Applications

DTI is especially useful in studying fibrous structures such as white matter and muscle: the anisotropy information it provides reveals the fiber orientation in the tissue and can be used to map the white-matter anatomy and muscle structure in vivo [37]. The diffusion coefficient measures a physical property of the tissue and the measurements can be compared across different times, locations, and subjects. Therefore, DTI has frequently been used to identify differences in white matter due to a variety of conditions. Normal conditions such as age and gender have been reported to affect anisotropy and diffusivity; neural developments such as myelination, physical trauma such as brain injury, and neurodegenerative diseases such as multiple sclerosis and HIV have all been indicated by DTI studies to affect white-matter composition, location, or integrity.

The variety of DTI applications provides a valuable testbed for visualization methods. Indeed, without applications to guide the development of computational and visualization tools, these tools are far less likely to be useful. We introduce some of the applications of DTI in this section.

7.4.1 White Matter Normal Conditions

Some normal conditions are reflected in the microstructure of white matter. Significant differences were found in diffusivity and anisotropy of the human corpus callosum with gender and handedness [60]. Age also has significant effect on white matter, usually resulting in reduced FA and increased diffusivity [61, 62]. These factors should be considered when selecting control groups for white-matter pathology studies.

The vector-field visualization methods introduced in Sect. 7.3.4 have been employed to reveal connectivity in a normal brain. A common application is to use neuroanatomy knowledge to select the ROIs and then reconstruct neural pathways running through them. Evidence of occipito-temporal connections within the living human brain was found by tracing neural pathways between two ROIs [63]. Expert-defined ROIs for brainstem fibers and associated fibers have been used to generate corresponding tracts [64]. An exciting trend is to combine functional MRI (fMRI), which measures the changes in blood flow and oxygenation in a brain area, with DTI fiber tracking, so that both activated brain areas and the tract connecting them to other brain areas can be visualized at the same time. For example, foci of fMRI activation have been used as ROIs to reveal axonal connectivity in a cat's visual cortex [65].

7.4.2 White Matter Development

Almost all the neurons that a brain will ever have are present at birth. However, the brain continues to develop for a few years after birth. A significant aspect of brain development is myelinization, the continued growth of myelin around the axons. Myelin acts as an insulating membrane and allows a conduction of nerve impulses from ten to one hundred times faster than along a non-myelinated system and, at birth, few fibers are myelinated. The development of myelin is thus a measure of increasing maturity of the neural system. Previous studies have explored when particular fibers are myelinated; e.g., areas related with primary sensory (vision, touch, hearing, etc.) and motor areas are the first to myelinate [66].

Diffusion tensor imaging has the potential to evaluate brain maturity in newborns. Myelinated fibers have higher anisotropy than non-myelinated ones, i.e., the anisotropy depends on the development phase. The study of newborn brain presents new challenges:

- The anisotropy in the neonatal brain is lower than in the adult brain. Therefore it is more difficult to reconstruct fibers reliably.
- Motion artifacts can play a larger role, since neonates often move more than adults.
- The signal-to-noise ratio is smaller. The neonatal brain is smaller than that of an adult, and hence the voxel size must be smaller, leading to decreased signal.

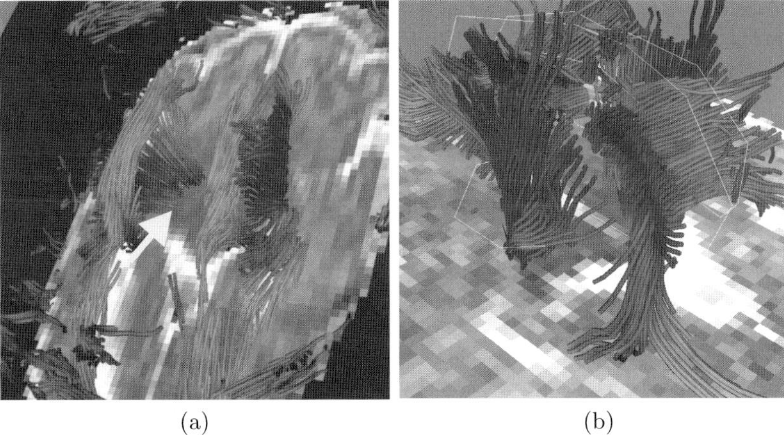

(a)   (b)

Fig. 7.15. Studies of white matter fibers in neonatal brains with different data sets. (a) Premature neonate lacking corpus callosum (see arrow), (b) full-term neonate where no fiber abnormalities were found. Corpus callosum and corona radiata are seen (see color plates)

The first years of life are a critical time for brain development. Early diagnoses of brain lesions can help diminish the consequences of an injury. For example, neonates who suffer hypoxic ischemic brain damage have brain injuries caused by lack of oxygen and nutrients because of blood flow problems. Diffusion weighted imaging has already proved useful in detecting this injury. Diffusion tensor imaging might provide further information about structure and the development of the neonatal brain. Figure 7.15(a) shows the white matter fibers corresponding to a data set of a premature neonate of 26 weeks and scanned at six weeks old. Several fiber structures are visible (e.g., corona radiata in blue). However, the corpus callosum is not visible: the arrow indicates where the fibers are missing. Further investigation of remaining MR images of this neonate confirmed that this patient lacks a corpus callosum. Figure 7.15(b) shows the result of tracing streamlines using ROIs to visualize the corpus callosum and the corona radiata in a full-term neonate scanned at four weeks after birth. The DTI data does not reveal any alteration in the fibers, even though the neonate had meningitis.

7.4.3 White Matter Injury and Disorders

DTI has proven effective in studying a range of white-matter disorders. Some of these disorders are brain injury, brain tumor, focal epilepsy, multiple sclerosis, tuberous sclerosis, Parkinson's disease, Alzheimer's disease, schizophrenia, HIV infection, Krabbe's disease, chronic alcohol dependence, ALS, X-linked ALD, and CADASIL. Reviews of these studies can be found in [67, 68, 69, 70].

We select three application areas in which pathological causes differ greatly, resulting in different patterns and subtleties of the changes in white matter. These cases can be analyzed effectively only by applying processing and visualization methods accordingly.

Brain Tumor

It is estimated that 17,500 people in the U.S. die from primary nervous-system tumors each year [71]. A better understanding of the pathophysiology of brain tumors is essential if we are to find effective treatments. Cortical disconnection syndromes may play a significant role in clinical dysfunction associated with this disorder.

Tractography methods have been applied to study patterns of white-matter tract disruption and displacement adjacent to brain tumors. Wieshmann et al. [72] found evidence of displacement of white-matter fibers of the corona radiata in a patient with low-grade glioma when compared with spatially normalized data collected from 20 healthy volunteers. Mori et al. [73] found evidence of displacement and destruction of the superior longitudinal fasciculus and corona radiata in two patients with anaplastic astrocytoma. Gossl et al. [74] observed distortion of the pyramidal tract in a patient with a high-grade glioma. Witwer et al. [75] found evidence of white-matter tract edema. Zhang et al. [76] observed the pattern of linear and planar diffusion around a tumor and analyzed the asymmetries of white-matter fiber tracts between the tumor and the contralateral hemisphere.

Figure 7.16 shows visual exploration and quantitative analysis of a cancerous brain [76]. The streamtubes and streamsurfaces visualize both linear and planar diffusion. The displacement of fiber tracts around the tumor is accompanied by a cradle of streamsurfaces, indicating a local increase of planar anisotropy. The normalized distribution of anisotropy is calculated on a barycentric space (see Sect. 7.3.1) for both the tumor-bearing side and contralateral side of the brain. The difference in the two distributions (Fig. 16(b)) clearly indicates a decrease in linear anisotropy and an increase in planar anisotropy in the tumor side of the brain.

As Fig. 7.17 indicates, the geometrical alteration of fiber structures surrounding the tumors can have different patterns [38]. In Fig. 17(a), the fibers are pushed to the left by the presence of the tumor; in Fig. 17(b), the fibers seem to be destroyed: the structure around the tumor is not moved, but in the tumor area no fibers are present.

Tumors and their surrounding edema often cause gross changes in the neural fibers around them. DTI can benefit tumor growth study and surgery planning by modeling these changes geometrically. Scalar index analysis complement the geometrical modeling by quantifying these changes.

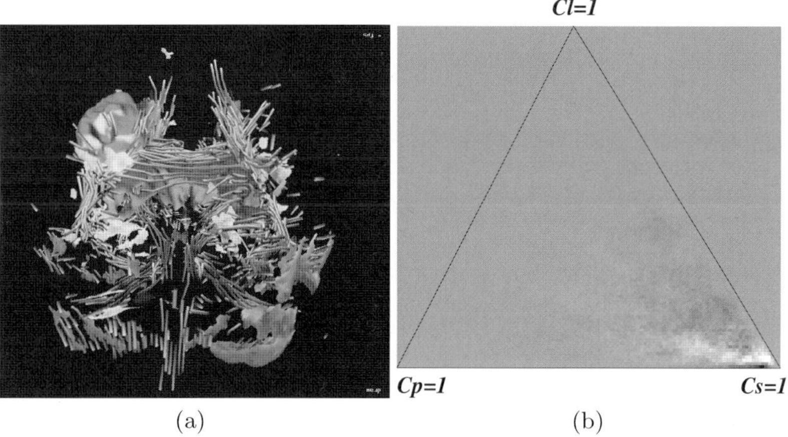

(a) (b)

Fig. 7.16. Visual exploration and quantitative analysis of a cancerous brain. (**a**) A 3D visualization showing streamtubes and streamsurfaces as well as tumor and ventricles. (**b**) The difference histogram obtained by subtracting normalized barycentric histograms calculated from tumor-bearing and contralateral sections. Here zero maps to medium gray because the difference is signed. Note that the most striking difference occurs near the $c_s = 1$ vertex. See color plates

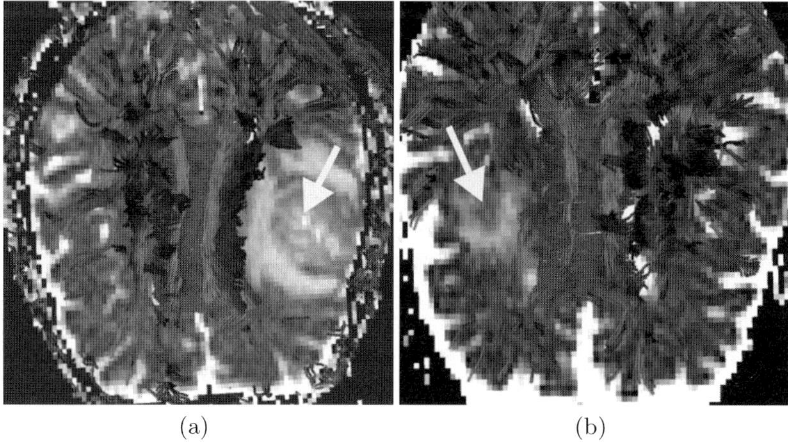

(a) (b)

Fig. 7.17. Two cases of adult tumor brain. (**a**) Fibers are pushed by the tumor. (**b**) No fibers are in the tumor area, indicating the destruction of neural structures there. See color plates

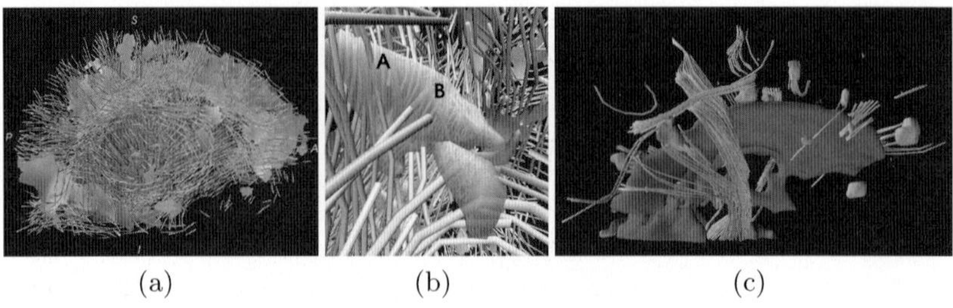

(a)   (b)   (c)

Fig. 7.18. Visualization of coregistered DTI and MS lesion models. (**a**) The whole brain with streamtubes, streamsurfaces, lesion masks and ventricles. (**b**) A closeup view of white matter fibers near the MS lesions. The streamtubes around the lesion area give some clues about white matter structural changes there. (**c**) The same brain and view as (a) but showing only streamtubes that contact the lesions, thus clarifying the white matter structures involved. See color plates

Multiple Sclerosis

Multiple sclerosis (MS) is a chronic disease of the central nervous system that predominantly affects young adults during their most productive years. Pathologically, MS is characterized by the presence of areas of demyelination and T-cell predominant perivascular inflammation in the brain white matter. Recent studies on MS have shown an elevated mean diffusivity and reduced diffusion anisotropy [77] in MS lesion areas. The lesions with more destructive pathology are generally shown to have the highest diffusivity.

Analyzing the interrelationship between the MS lesion and the affected fiber pathways might help in understanding the mechanism of the axonal damage. The visualization of DTI models with coregistered MS lesion masks in Fig. 7.18 can be utilized to determine the relationship between focal lesions and the neuronal tracts that are anatomically related. Figure 18(b) suggests the different effects that the focal lesions might have on the fibers. Note that the streamtubes sometimes continue through the lesions (A) and sometimes break within them (B). Figure 18(c) depicts only the fiber pathways that are confined in the lesion area.

MS lesions are often dispersed and show different levels of severity. Visualizing the affected tracts can clarify the various effects of the lesions. Identifying the gray matter to which these partially damaged tracts connect might help explain the disabling effect of MS. The study of MS remains an active research area. These visualization results might help researchers think about the progression of the pathology and design other experiments which, in turn, might help validate the DTI results.

HIV Neurodegeneration

Human immunodeficiency virus (HIV) is an aggressive disease that affects multiple organ systems and body compartments, including the central nervous system (CNS). Structural imaging studies of HIV patients' brains reveal morphometric changes in the subcortical gray and white matter regions [78]. However, because of the relatively poor sensitivity of structural imaging to white-matter abnormalities in patients with mild HIV [79], the relationship between cognition and white-matter abnormalities in structural MRI has not been fully determined. These limitations can be overcome by DTI. Recent DTI studies have demonstrated white-matter abnormalities among patients with HIV even when fluid-attenuated inversion recovery (FLAIR) structural MRI scans failed to do so [80, 81]. Most recently, Ragin et al. [82] reported strong relationships between whole-brain fractional anisotropy and severity of dementia among a small cohort of HIV patients ($n = 6$).

In cases such as HIV infection, where the white-matter structural changes may be too subtle to detect with structural imaging, DTI can be used to quantify the changes.

7.4.4 Myocardial Structure

Diffusion tensor MRI can also be used to measure directionally constrained diffusion in tissues outside the nervous system. Understanding the complex muscular structure of the mammalian heart is another important application. The efficiency of the heart is due in part to its precise arrangement of myofibers (contractile muscle cells), especially the myocardium (the muscular wall) of the left ventricle, which is responsible for pumping blood to the rest of the body. The pattern of myofiber orientation in the myocardium is *helical*: between the epicardium and endocardium (outer and inner surface) there is roughly a 140-degree rotation of myofiber orientation, from -70 to $+70$ degrees. Computational simulations of heart dynamics require an accurate model of the myofibral orientation in order to model both the contractile mechanics of the myocardium and the pattern of electrical wave propagation within it [83]. The principal eigenvector as measured by DT-MRI has been confirmed to align with the myofiber orientation [13, 14]. Recent work (see Fig. 7.19) has applied superquadric tensor glyphs to visualize the myofiber twisting and to inspect other anatomical features revealed by DT-MRI [84].

As is clear from the descriptions above, the applications of DTI are increasingly diverse. Associated with the breadth of application areas is a need for a wide variety of visualization techniques. Characterizing a tumor's effect on white matter integrity is based on fiber tracking, while the effect of neurodegenerative diseases may be quantified in terms of anisotropy metrics, and myocardial structure is described by a continuous rotation of the principal eigenvector.

7.5 Open Problems

Successfully applying DTI to new research areas and problem domains demands that visualization tools be flexible enough to support experimentation

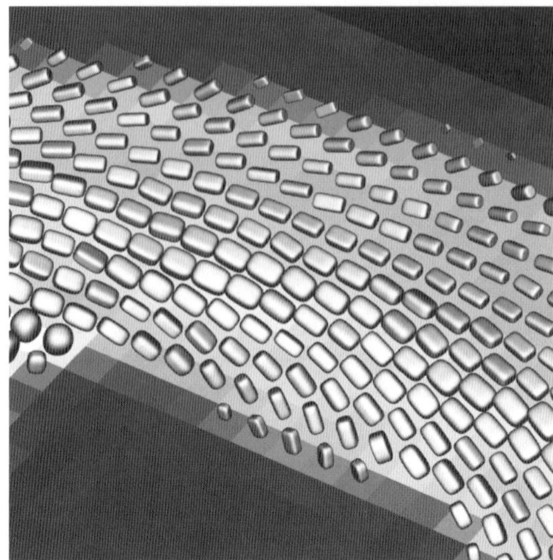

Fig. 7.19. Visualization of transmural twist of myofibers in canine myocardium, seen in a short axis slice. The edges of the superquadric glyphs help show the flat inclination at midwall and the differences among the eigenvalues at various locations

with the range of techniques, so as to evaluate the appropriateness of each. This in turn requires that the modes of interaction efficiently support the exploration and parameter setting needed for creating visualizations, ideally in a manner friendly to application-area experts who may not be visualization experts.

In clinical practice, anisotropy indices, such as FA or trace (see Sect. 7.3.1), are commonly used. Although, they show just a part of the information contained in the tensor, their visualization is similar to what radiologists are used to, and they are easy to understand and quantify. Other visualization techniques based on tractography or fiber tracking are popular probably due to the direct analogy between streamlines and fibers. However, the result of most of these techniques are very sensitive to input parameter values from the user (e.g., seed point). Important information can be missed if the user fails to give the right input when the underlying anatomy is not known. User independence is critical for statistical comparison and evaluation of diseases.

Some methods have tried to achieve more user independence by reconstructing linear structures in the whole volume. The main problems in this case are the computational cost and the huge amount of data to inspect. Therefore, the user should be able to navigate and explore the data interactively and in an intuitive way. For example, meaningful grouping or clustering of data can help navigation. Intuitive interaction for setting of parameters, such as transfer functions or thresholds (e.g., c_l in fiber tracking to define areas with linear structure). Fiber tracking algorithms are prone to error, e.g., due to partial volume effect or numerical integration. Finding and visualizing uncertainty measures for the visualization algorithms could help to reduce the effect of this error.

Visualization techniques are commonly used as exploratory tool to identify measures for quantification. At the moment, measures for quantification only exist for anisotropy indices. Quantification is important to get clinical acceptance. It is necessary to generate statistics and distinguish between diseased and normal, and to build models according to the different demographic and clinical variables that influence the results such as age and sex.

Validation is an important issue for DTI. There have been too few validation studies to be able to conclude that what is measured corresponds to the anatomy [1, 13]. At the moment and to our knowledge, there is no gold standard to validate the results of the techniques developed in this field.

An open problem of a different sort is the communication among different scientific fields. It is important for physicians and technicians to communicate in such a way that the necessary software and tools to advance in the clinical investigations for DTI are developed.

Finally, although not discussed in this chapter, a main research issue is the protocols for DTI data acquisition in order to improve quality and reduce scanning times. Furthermore, much research in image processing has been devoted to scalar but less to vector images, and little work has been done on image processing techniques for tensor data. Filters for noise removal, interpolation, feature extraction, etc. are of importance for the development of DTI (e.g., see the chapters of part V: Image Processing Methods for Tensor Fields). Second order diffusion tensor does not contain enough information to disambiguate areas where a voxel contains non-coherent linear structures. New representations for diffusion that show its more complex behavior are being researched. Visualization and image processing techniques would need to adapt to the complexity of this new data.

7.6 Summary and Conclusions

DTI allows the visualization of tissue microstructure (e.g., white matter or muscle) in vivo. Meaningful visualizations are crucial in analyzing and getting insight into multivariate data such as DTI. We have presented several visualization techniques developed in recent years. All visualization techniques have their advantages and disadvantages. Tensor glyphs are good for giving information at individual points, however, they miss to communicate their relationships. Fiber tracking methods are good for following major coherent fiber structures, but prone to error, e.g., partial volume effects, numerical integration. Fiber tracking methods usually reduce the dimensionality of the tensor from 6D to 3D, based in the assumption that just linear structures are interesting. Other methods were the whole tensor information is used to show the relationships between tensors, suffer from cluttering. A combination of different visualization techniques might be the best solution to provide most insight in the data. However, there are still essential disadvantages, such as robust parameter definition, that must be overcome. These visualization methods ideally should be easy to use to application-area experts who may not be visualization experts.

Some examples of the large variety of DTI applications have been presented. Besides the large amount of research that is devoted to white matter, DTI is not limited to it. Other fields are also gaining from DTI, e.g., heart studies. There is clear evidence that DTI will bring new insights in various fields of research.

DTI is a relative young and exciting new field of research that brings together several disciplines. Research in each of these disciplines is crucial to achieve fruitful results in the application and use of DTI data.

Acknowledgments

We thank the BioMedical NMR group at the Eindhoven University of Technology and Maxima Medical Center in Veldhoven, Drs. Raimond Winslow and Elliot McVeigh of Johns Hopkins University, and Andrew Alexander of the W. M. Keck Laboratory for Functional Brain Imaging and Behavior at the University of Wisconsin-Madison for providing some of the data sets and evaluations used in this chapter. We thank Dr. Mark Bastin of the University of Edinburgh, Dr. Jack Simon of the University of Colorado Health Science Center, and Dr. Robert Paul of the Brown Medical School for providing some of the data sets and for contributing to the section on white matter injury and disorders.

References

1. C. Pierpaoli, A.S. Barnett, S. Pajevic, A. Virta, and P.J. Basser. Validation of DT-MRI tractography in the descending motor pathways of human subjects. In *ISMRM, Conf. Proc.*, p. 501, 2001.
2. D.S. Tuch, R.M. Weisskoff, J.W. Belliveau, and V.J. Wedeen. High angular resolution diffusion imaging of the human brain. In *ISMRM, Conf. Proc.*, p. 321, 1999.
3. L.R. Frank. Anisotropy in high angular resolution diffusion-weighted MRI. *MR in Medicine*, 45(6):935–939, 2001.
4. A. Einstein. Über die von der molekularkinetischen Theorie der Wärme geforderte Bewegung von in ruhenden Flüssigkeiten suspendierten Teilchen. *Annalen der Physik*, 17:549–560, 1905.
5. E.M. Purcell, H.C. Torrey, and R.V. Pound. Resonance absorption by nuclear magnetic moments in a solid. *Physical Review*, 69:37–43, 1946.
6. F. Bloc. Nuclear induction. *Physical Review*, 70:460–474, 1946.
7. E.L. Hahn. Spin echoes. *Physical Review*, 80:580–594, 1950.

8. P.C. Lauterbur. Image formation by induced local interactions: examples employing nuclear magnetic resonance. *Nature*, 242:190–191, 1973.

9. G.J. Stanisz and R.M. Henkelman. Tissue compartments, exchange and diffusion. In *Workshop on Diffusion MRI: Biophysical Issues*, pp. 34–37, 2002.

10. P.T. Callaghan. *Principles of Nuclear Magnetic Resonance Microscopy*. Oxford, 1993.

11. P.J. Basser, J. Mattiello, and D. LeBihan. Estimation of the effective self-diffusion tensor from the NMR spin echo. *MR Journal*, 103(3):247–54, 1994.

12. D. LeBihan. Molecular diffusion nuclear magnetic resonance imaging. *Magn. Reson. Quant.*, 17:1–30, 1991.

13. D.F. Scollan, A. Holmes, R. Winslow, and J. Forder. Histological validation of myocardial microstructure obtained from diffusion tensor magnetic resonance imaging. *Am J Physiol*, 275:2308–2318, 1998.

14. E.W. Hsu, A.L. Muzikant, S.A. Matulevicius, R.C. Penland, and C.S. Henriquez. Magnetic resonance myocardial fiber-orientation mapping with direct histological correlation. *Am J Physiol*, 274:1627–1634, 1998.

15. J.K. Jones. Determining and visualizing uncertainty in estimates of fiber orientation from diffusion tensor MRI. *MR in Medicine*, 49:7–12, 2003.

16. Y. Assaf, A. Mayk, and Y. Cohen. Displacement imaging of spinal cord using q-space diffusion-weighted MRI. *MR in Medicine*, 44:713–722, 2000.

17. D.S. Tuch, T.G. Reese, M.R. Wiegell, N. Makris, J.W. Belliveau, and V.J. Wedeen. High angular resolution diffusion imaging reveals intravoxel white matter fiber heterogeneity. *MR in Medicine*, 48(4):577–582, 2002.

18. L.R. Frank. Characterization of anisotropy in high angular resolution diffusion-weighted MRI. *MR in Medicine*, 47:1083–1099, 2002.

19. C. Pierpaoli and P.J. Basser. Toward a quantitative assessment of diffusion anisotropy. *MR in Medicine*, 36(6):893–906, 1996.

20. P.J. Basser and C. Pierpaoli. Microstructural features measured using diffusion tensor imaging. *MR Journal*, pp. 209–219, 1996.

21. C.F. Westin, S. Peled, H. Gubjartsson, R. Kikinis, and F.A. Jolesz. Geometrical diffusion measures for MRI from tensor basis analysis. In *ISMRM, Conf. Proc.*, p. 1742, April 1997.

22. P. van Gelderen, M.H. de Vleeschouwer, D. Despres, J. Pekar, P.C. van Zijl, and C.T. Moonen. Water diffusion and acute stroke. *MR in Medicine*, 31:154–63, 1994.

23. P. Douek, R. Turner, J. Pekar, N. Patronas, and D. LeBihan. MR color mapping of myelin fiber orientation. *J. Comput. Assist. Tomogr*, 15:923–929, 1991.

24. G. Kindlmann, D. Weinstein, and D.A. Hart. Strategies for direct volume rendering of diffusion tensor fields. *IEEE Trans. on Visualization and Computer Graphics*, 6(2):124–138, 2000.

25. R.A. Drebin, L. Carpenter, and P. Hanrahan. Volume rendering. *Computer Graphics, SIGGRAPH Proc.*, 22(4):65–74, 1988.

26. M. Levoy. Display of surfaces from volume data. *IEEE Computer Graphics & Applications*, 8(5):29–37, 1988.

27. W.E. Lorensen and H.E. Cline. Marching cubes: a high resolution 3D surface reconstruction algorithm. *Computer Graphics, SIGGRAPH Proc.*, 21(4):163–169, 1987.

28. A. Wenger, D. Keefe, S. Zhang, and D.H. Laidlaw. Interactive volume rendering of thin thread structures within multivalued scientific datasets. *IEEE Trans. on Visualization and Computer Graphics*, 2004. In press.

29. B. Cabral, N. Cam, and J. Foran. Accelerated volume rendering and tomographic reconstruction using texture mapping hardware. In *Symposium on Volume Visualization, Conf. Proc.*, pp. 91–98, 1994.

30. J. Kniss, G. Kindlmann, and C. Hansen. Interactive volume rendering using multi-dimensional transfer functions and direct manipulation widgets. In *IEEE Visualization, Conf. Proc.*, pp. 255–262, October 2001.

31. R. Fernando, editor. *GPU Gems: Programming Techniques, Tips, and Tricks for Real-Time Graphics.* Addison-Wesley, 2004.

32. D.H. Laidlaw, E.T. Ahrens, D. Kremers, M.J. Avalos, C. Readhead, and R.E. Jacobs. Visualizing diffusion tensor images of the mouse spinal cord. In *IEEE Visualization, Conf. Proc.*, pp. 127–134, October 1998.

33. G. Kindlmann. Superquadric tensor glyphs. In *Proceedings IEEE TVCG/EG Symposium on Visualization 2004*, pp. 147–154, May 2004.

34. F. Post, B. Vrolijk, H. Hauser, R.S. Laramee, and H. Doleisch. Feature extraction and visualization of flow fields. In *State-of-the-Art EG, Conf. Proc.*, pp. 69–100, 2002.

35. J.J. van Wijk. Image based flow visualization. *Computer Graphics, SIGGRAPH Proc.*, 21(3):745–754, 2002.

36. S. Mori and P.C.M. van Zijl. Fiber tracking: principles and strategies – a technical review. *NMR in Biomedicine*, 15(7-8):468–480, 2002.

37. P.J. Basser, S. Pajevic, C. Pierpaoli, J. Duda, and A. Aldroubi. In vivo fiber tractography using DT-MRI data. *MR in Medicine*, 44:625–632, 2000.

38. A. Vilanova, G. Berenschot, and C. van Pul. DTI visualization with streamsurfaces and evenly-spaced volume seeding. In *VisSym '04 Joint EG – IEEE TCVG Symposium on Visualization, Conf. Proc.*, pp. 173–182, 2004.

39. T. Delmarcelle and L Hesselink. Visualizing second order-tensor fields with hyperstreamlines. *IEEE Computer Graphics & Applications*, 13(4):25–33, 1993.

40. S. Zhang, C. Demiralp, and D.H. Laidlaw. Visualizing diffusion tensor MR images using streamtubes and streamsurfaces. *IEEE Trans. on Visualization and Computer Graphics*, 9(4):454–462, 2003.

41. D. Weinstein, G. Kindlmann, and E.C. Lundberg. Tensorlines: advection-diffusion based propagation through diffusion tensor fields. In *IEEE Visualization, Conf. Proc.*, pp. 249–253, 1999.

42. L. Zhukov and A.H. Barr. Oriented tensor reconstruction: tracing neural pathways from diffusion tensor MRI. In *IEEE Visualization, Conf. Proc.*, pp. 387–394, 2002.

43. B. Jobard and W. Lefer. Creating evenly-spaced streamlines of arbitrary density. In *Visualization in Scientific Computing. Proc. of the EG Workshop*, pp. 43–56. Springer Verlag, 1997.

44. Z. Ding, J.C. Gore, and A.A. Anderson. Classification and quantification of neuronal fiber pathways using diffusion tensor MRI. *MR in Medicine*, 49(4):716–721, 2003.

45. A. Brun, H-J. Park, H. Knutsson, and C.-F. Westin. Coloring of DT-MRI fiber traces using Laplacian eigenmaps. In *EUROCAST, Conf. Proc.*, volume 2809 of *LNCS*, February 2003.

46. S. Zhang and D.H. Laidlaw. Hierarchical clustering of streamtubes. Technical Report CS-02-18, Brown University Computer Science Dep., August 2002.

47. I. Corouge, G. Gerig, and S. Gouttard. Towards a shape model of white matter fiber bundles using diffusion tensor MRI. In *IEEE International Symposium on Biomedical Imaging, Conf. Proc.*, pp. 344–347, 2004.

48. G.J.M. Parker, C.A. Wheeker-Kingshott, and G.J. Barker. Distributed anatomical connectivity derived from diffusion tensor imaging. *IPMI, LNCS*, 2082:106–120, 2001.

49. A. Brun, M. Björnemo, R. Kikinis, and C.-F. Westin. White matter tractography using sequential importance sampling. In *ISMRM, Conf. Proc.*, May 2002.

50. P.G. Batchelor, D.L.G. Hill, F. Calamante, and D. Atkinson. Study of connectivity in the brain using the full diffusion tensor from MRI. In *IPMI, Conf. Proc.*, pp. 121–133, 2001.

51. L. O'Donnell, S. Haker, and C.F. Westing. New approaches to estimation of white matter connectivity in diffusion tensor MRI: elliptic PDE's and geodesics in tensor-warped space. In *MICCAI, Conf. Proc.*, pp. 459–466, 2002.

52. X. Zheng and A. Pang. Volume deformation for tensor visualization. In *IEEE Visualization, Conf. Proc.*, pp. 379–386, 2002.

53. A. Sigfridsson, T. Ebbers, E. Heiberg, and L. Wigström. Tensor field visualisation using adaptive filtering of noise fields combined with glyph rendering. In *IEEE Visualization, Conf. Proc.*, pp. 371–378, 2002.

54. X. Zheng and A. Pang. Hyperlic. In *IEEE Visualization, Conf. Proc.*, pp. 249–256, 2003.

55. A. Bhalerao and C.-F. Westin. Tensor splats: Visualising tensor fields by texture mapped volume rendering. In *MICCAI, Conf. Proc.*, pp. 294–901, 2003.

56. L. Hesselink, Y. Levy, and Y. Lavin. The topology of symmetric, second-order 3D tensor fields:. *IEEE Trans. on Visualization and Computer Graphics*, 3(1):1–11, 1997.

57. D. Akers, A. Sherbondy, R. Mackenzie, R. Dougherty, and B. Wandell. Exploration of the brain's white matter pathways with dynamic queries. In *IEEE Visualization, Conf. Proc.*, October 2004.

58. Ç. Demiralp, D.H. Laidlaw, C. Jackson, D. Keefe, and S. Zhang. Subjective usefulness of CAVE and fishtank VR display systems for a scientific visualization application. In *IEEE Visualization Poster Compendium*, 2003.

59. S. Zhang, Ç. Demiralp, D. Keefe, M. DaSilva, B.D. Greenberg, P.J. Basser, C. Pierpaoli, E.A. Chiocca, T.S. Deisboeck, and D.H. Laidlaw. An immersive virtual environment for DT-MRI volume visualization applications: a case study. In *IEEE Visualization, Conf. Proc.*, pp. 437–440, October 2001.

60. R. Westerhausen, C. Walter, F. Kreuder, R.A. Wittling, E. Schweiger, and W. Wittling. The influence of handedness and gender on the microstructure of the human corpus callosum: a diffusion-tensor magnetic resonance imaging study. *Neuroscience Letters*, 351:99–102, 2003.

61. A. Pfefferbaum, E.V. Sullivan, M. Hedehus, K.O. Lim, E. Adalsteinsson, and M. Moseley. Age-related decline in brain white matter anisotropy measured with spatially corrected echo-planar diffusion tensor imaging. *MR in Medicine*, 44(2):259–268, 2000.

62. M. O'Sullivan, D.K. Jones, P.E. Summers, R.G. Morris, S.C.R. Williams, and H.S. Markus. Evidence for cortical disconnection as a mechanism of age-related cognitive decline. *Neurology*, 57:632–638, 2001.

63. M. Catani, D.K. Jones, R. Donato, and D.H. Ffytche. Occipito-temporal connections in the human brain. *Brain*, 126:2093–2107, 2003.

64. S. Wakana, H. Jiang, L.M. Nagae-Poetscher, P.C.M. van Zijl, and S. Mori. Fiber tract based atlas of human white matter anatomy. *Radiology*, 230:77–87, 2004.

65. D.-S. Kim, M. Kima, I. Ronena, E. Formisano, K.-H. Kima, K. Ugurbila, S. Moric, and R. Goebel. In vivo mapping of functional domains and axonal connectivity in cat visual cortex using magnetic resonance imaging. *MRI Journal*, 21(10):1131–1140, 2003.

66. J.J. Volpe. *Neurology of the Newborn*. W.B. Saunders Company, 1995.

67. K.O. Lim and J.A. Helpern. Neuropsychiatric applications of DTI – a review. *NMR in Biomedicine*, 15(7-8):587–593, 2002.

68. M.A. Horsfield and D.K. Jones. Applications of diffusion-weighted and diffusion tensor MRI to white matter diseases – a review. *NMR in Biomedicine*, 15(7-8):570–577, 2002.

69. M. Kubicki, C.-F. Westin, S.E. Maier, H. Mamata, M. Frumin, H. Ersner-Hershfield, R. Kikinis, F.A. Jolesz, R. McCarley, and M.E. Shenton. Diffusion tensor imaging and its application to neuropsychiatric disorders. *Harvard Rev. of Psychiatry*, 10:234–336, 2002.

70. P.C. Sundgren, Q. Dong, D. Gomez-Hassan, S.K. Mukherji, P. Maly, and R. Welsh. Diffusion tensor imaging of the brain: review of clinical applications. *Neuroradiology*, 46(5):339–350, 2004.

71. N.I. Bohnen, K. Radharkrishnan, B.P. O'Neil, and L.T. Kurland. *Descriptive and Analytic Epidemiology of Brain Tumours. Cancer of the Nervous System.* Blackwell Publishing, 2001.

72. U.C. Wieshmann, M.R. Symms, G.J. Parker, C.A. Clark, L. Lemieux, G.J. Barker, and S.D. Shorvon. Diffusion tensor imaging demonstrates deviation of fibres in normal appearing white matter adjacent to a brain tumour. *J. Neurol. Neurosurg. Psychiatry*, 68(4):501–3, 2000.

73. S. Mori, K. Frederiksen, P.C. van Zijl, B. Stieltjes, M.A. Kraut, M. Solaiyappa, and M.G. Pomper. Brain white matter anatomy of tumor patients evaluated with diffusion tensor imaging. *Ann. Neurol.*, 51(3):337–8, 2002.

74. C. Gossl, L. Fahrmeir, B. Putz, L.M. Auer, and D.P. Auer. Fiber tracking from DTI using linear state space models: detectability of the pyramidal tract. *Neuroimage*, 16(2):378–88, 2002.

75. B.P. Witwer, R. Moftakhar, K.M. Hasan, P. Deshmukh, V. Haughton, A. Field, K. Arfanakis, J. Noyes, C.H. Moritz, M.E. Meyerand, H.A. Rowley, A.L. Alexander, and B. Badie. Diffusion-tensor imaging of white matter tracts in patients with cerebral neoplasm. *J. Neurosurg.*, 97(3):568–75, 2002.

76. S. Zhang, M.E. Bastin, D.H. Laidlaw, S. Sinha, P.A. Armitage, and T.S. Deisboeck. Visualization and analysis of white matter structural asymmetry in diffusion tensor MR imaging data. *MR in Medicine*, 51(1):140–147, 2004.

77. D.J. Werring, C.A. Clark, G.J. Barker, A.J. Thompson, and D.H. Miller. Diffusion tensor imaging of lesions and normal-appearing white matter in multiple sclerosis. *Neurology*, 52:1626–1632, 1999.

78. R.H. Paul, R. Cohen, and R. Stern. Neurocognitive manifestations of HIV. *CNS Spectrums*, 7(12):860–866, 2003.

79. R.H. Paul, R. Cohen, B. Navia, and K. Tashima. Relationships between cognition and structural neuroimaging findings in adults with human immunodeficiency virus type-1. *Neurosci. Biobehav. Rev.*, 26(3):353–9, 2002.

80. N. Pomara, D.T. Crandall, S.J. Choi, G. Johnson, and K.O. Lim. White matter abnormalities in HIV-1 infection: a diffusion tensor imaging study. *Psychiatry Res.*, 106(1):15–24, 2001.

81. C.G. Filippi, A.M. Ulug, E. Ryan, S.J. Ferrando, and W. van Gorp. Diffusion tensor imaging of patients with HIV and normal-appearing white matter on MR images of the brain. *American Journal of Neuroradiology*, 22:277–283, 2001.

82. A. B. Ragin, P. Storey, B. A. Cohen, L. G. Epstein, and R. R. Edelman. Whole brain diffusion tensor imaging in HIV-associated cognitive impairment. *American Journal of Neuroradiology*, 25(2):195–200, 2004.

83. F.B. Sachse. *Computational Cardiology: Modeling of Anatomy, Electrophysiology, and Mechanics*. LNCS Vol. 2966. Springer Verlag, 2004.

84. D.B. Ennis, G. Kindlmann, P.A. Helm, I. Rodriguez, H. Wen, and E.R. McVeigh. Visualization of high-resolution myocardial strain and diffusion tensors using superquadric glyphs. In *ISMRM, Conf. Proc.*, May 2004.

8

Anatomy-Based Visualizations of Diffusion Tensor Images of Brain White Matter

James C. Gee, Hui Zhang, Abraham Dubb, Brian B. Avants, Paul A. Yushkevich, and Jeffrey T. Duda

Departments of Bioengineering, Computer and Information Science, and Radiology University of Pennsylvania, 3600 Market Street, Philadelphia, PA 19104, USA
`gee@rad.upenn.edu`

Summary. In this chapter, we consider the task of anatomically labeling diffusion tensor images of cerebral white matter to facilitate visualization as well as quantitative comparison of these data. The analogous labeling problem for structural magnetic resonance images of the brain has been extensively studied and we propose that advances in atlas-based techniques may be leveraged to anatomically segment the fiber-tractographic maps derived from diffusion tensor data. The feasibility of the approach is demonstrated with data acquired of the corpus callosum, and implications of the results for callosal morphometry are discussed.

8.1 Introduction

Diffusion tensor (DT) imaging is a recent innovation in magnetic resonance imaging (MRI) [1]. The measurement made at each voxel in a DT-MR image is a symmetric second order tensor, which describes the local diffusive behavior of water at the corresponding point in the imaged material. The DT may be represented by an ellipsoid describing the root mean squared displacement in each direction from the center of the voxel. DT imaging has proved useful, because of the added insight it provides into the structure of fibrous tissue, such as white matter in the brain, which contains bundles of fibrous axons. In this type of tissue, although water is relatively free to diffuse along the axis of the fibers, diffusion is hindered in perpendicular directions by cell membranes that bound the fibers. Measurements acquired from these regions thus tend to be anisotropic, i.e., the rate of diffusion is dependent on direction [2]. Furthermore, the major axis of the DT points along the axis of the bundled fibers, which allows these fibers to be traced in vivo through DT images. In the brain, this affords the possibility of connectivity maps being constructed [3, 4], since the fibers are axons which form connections in the brain.

DT-MRI and its visualization are discussed in detail in various chapters of this volume. Here, we consider the problem of anatomically labeling fiber

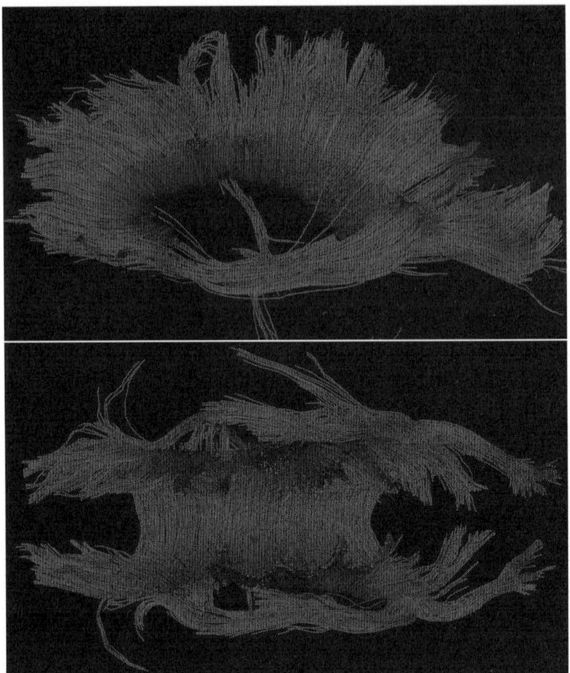

Fig. 8.1. Visualization of the corpus callosum as extracted via fiber tractography [5] from the diffusion tensor MR image of a female human brain (see color plates). Views are from the side (*top*) and top (*bottom*) of the brain, with the head facing toward the left. The corpus callosum is the connecting band of white matter fibers that provide the primary means of communication between the two cerebral hemispheres

tracts that have been extracted from diffusion tensor images of brain white matter using any of the available fiber tracking methods in the literature. The proposed approach is especially useful for visualizations of the corpus callosum, the connecting band of fibers that provide the primary means of communication between the two cerebral hemispheres. Typical tracings of this tract originate from a region of interest corresponding to the corpus callosum on the midsagittal plane. The fiber tracings are then extended toward the cortical regions in both hemispheres that the fibers interconnect. As exemplified in Fig. 8.1, the result provides a vivid depiction of the anatomy of the callosum in much the same way that structural MRI is able to produce exquisite pictures of soft tissue such as the human brain. However, just as anatomical localization is a difficult task with brain images, so is the analogous problem of identifying the particular gray matter regions interconnected by different sets of fiber bundles within the corpus callosum. This anatomic labeling of white matter is prerequisite for the conduct of cross-sectional or longitudinal DT-MRI studies of health and disease. We thus foresee the development of algorithmic solutions to the white matter labeling problem emerging as a major focus in research and clinical applications of diffusion tensor imaging.

In this chapter, we sketch out an approach for labeling diffusion tensor images of cerebral white matter that leverages advancements in both fiber tractography and atlas-based techniques for brain image segmentation. The proposed method is demonstrated on DT-MRI data acquired of the corpus callosum, and implications of the results for callosal morphometry are discussed.

8.2 Methods

The goal of the proposed tract labeling and visualization algorithm is to take as input tractographic maps of brain white matter and to differentiate the fiber bundles in these maps according to the gray matter regions that they interconnect. Figure 8.5 depicts such a cortex-based anatomic parcellation, in this case of the corpus callosum shown in Fig. 8.1. A prerequisite for implementation of the algorithm is a labeled atlas of the brain and a method for warping the atlas into detailed alignment with the corresponding structural MR images of the diffusion tensor data. In the examples to follow, high resolution T1-weighted images are used because of the anatomic detail that they can contain. Lower quality structural images may be used but these will limit the anatomic fidelity of subsequent atlas-based segmentations. Because the brain labels are determined over the structural scan for an individual and then superimposed on the diffusion tensor image of the individual, another factor that will affect the reliability of the tract labeling results is the degree to which the structural and DT images are co-registered.

Once the different gray matter regions of interest in the diffusion tensor images are identified via atlas-based registration, the previously extracted white matter fiber tracts can in principle be associated with the regions at which the tracts terminate, and their labels determined accordingly. In practice, routine clinical DT-MRI studies, such as those used in the experiments here, are too noisy for existing tractography methods to reliably trace fibers all the way to the gray-white interface. One way to proceed in this situation is to propagate the gray matter labels into the white matter until they intersect the fiber tracts. This can be accomplished in a principled way by computing a Voronoi tessellation of the image volume, where the cells correspond to different labels. To help ensure the veracity of the final results depicted in the figures below, an additional constraint is imposed that precludes labeling of fiber bundles which do not terminate within a certain distance – 15 mm in the examples – from the cortex.

In the remainder of this section, the steps above are illustrated through their application to the task of labeling the callosal tract in Fig. 8.1. Figure 8.2 depicts the brain atlas and its warped version after registration to the T1-weighted structural image of the female subject whose corpus callosum is

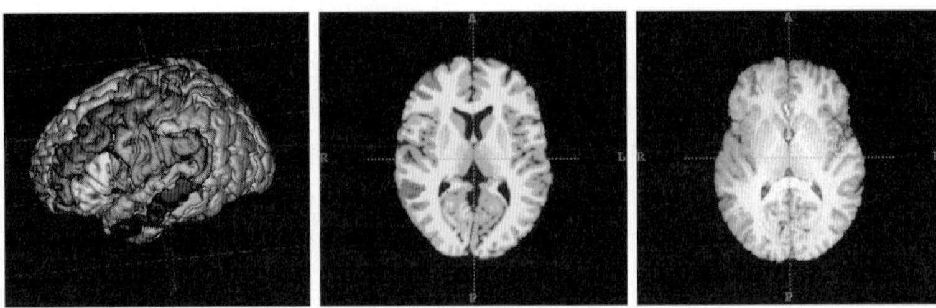

Fig. 8.2. Atlas-based brain image segmentation (see color plates). (*Left*) A surface rendering of the labeled atlas used in this work. (*Middle*) The gray matter labels for one hemisphere are shown superimposed on the underlying structural image of the brain atlas. (*Right*) The atlas is registered to the corresponding T1-weighted structural image of the female subject whose corpus callosum is depicted in Fig. 8.1, and the warped gray matter labels for one hemisphere are shown superimposed on the subject's structural image. The following brain regions are delineated in the atlas, further details of which can be found in [6]: precentral gyrus; superior temporal gyrus; middle temporal gyrus; inferior temporal gyrus; superior frontal gyrus; middle frontal gyrus; inferior frontal gyrus; supramarginal gyrus; postcentral gyrus; parahippocampal gyrus; occipitotemporal gyrus; superior parietal lobule; inferior parietal lobule; occipital lobe

shown in Fig. 8.1. The registration result was obtained with the method detailed in [7], but a variety of other techniques are potentially applicable [7, 8].

The degree of anatomic correspondence between the atlas and structural images after registration can be appreciated in Fig. 8.4. The superimposed gray matter labels seen in Fig. 8.2 are used to obtain the three-dimensional Voronoi partition – shown in Fig. 8.3 – of the structural image volume. Given this partition, callosal fibers can be associated with the gray matter region at which they terminate. Figures 8.5 and 8.6 depict this anatomic parcellation for the corpus callosum of our original female subject and a second, male subject, respectively.

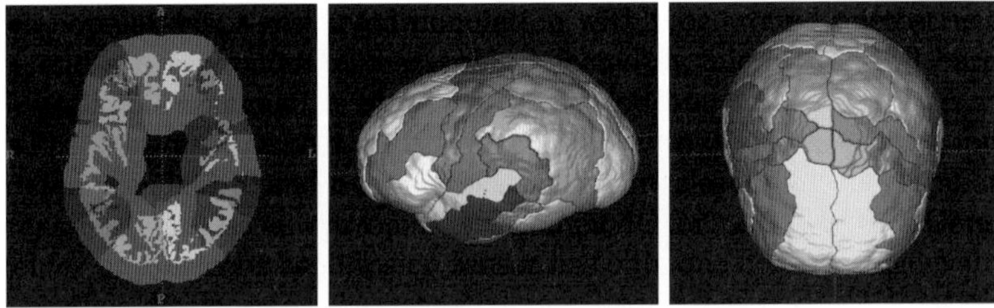

Fig. 8.3. Voronoi partition derived from the individualized atlas (see color plates). (*Left*) The distance-constrained Voronoi tessellation superimposed on the individualized gray matter labels on which the tessellation is based. (*Middle* and *Right*) Surface renderings of the same three-dimensional Voronoi partition

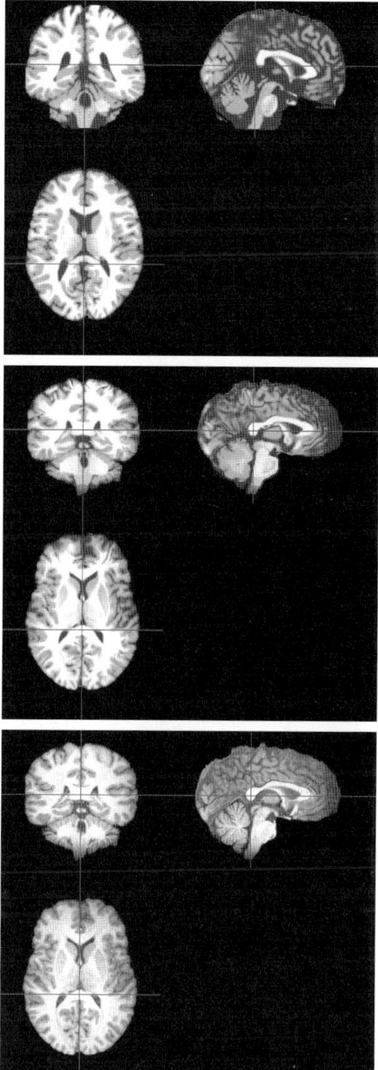

Fig. 8.4. Highly detailed correspondence obtained between the registered atlas and subject images. The atlas (*top*) is non-rigidly registered (*middle*) to the female subject (*bottom*) by optimizing in multiresolution fashion a robust mean squares metric under the constraints of a viscous fluid transformation model [7, 7]. The cursor is positioned at the same location in the three volumes

8.3 Discussion

The advent of diffusion tensor imaging has provoked considerable interest in part because of the new and unique information it provides into the structure

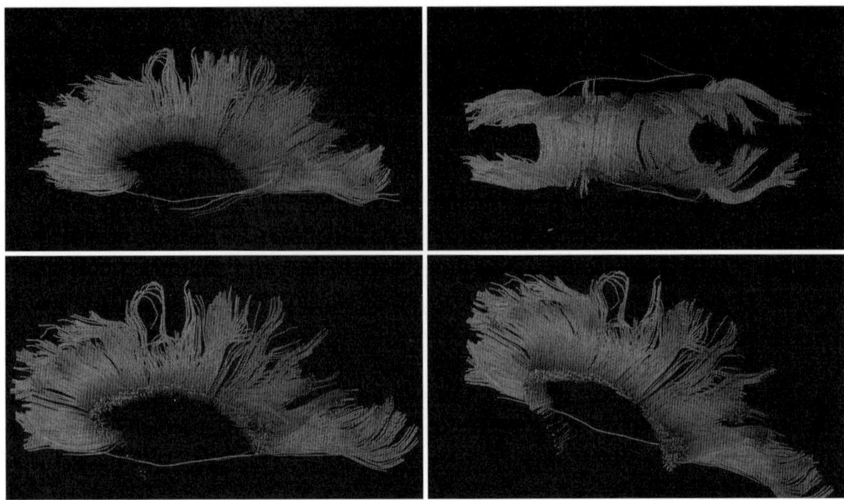

Fig. 8.5. Visualization of the anatomically labeled version of the callosal tract depicted in Fig. 8.1 (see color plates). The color legend is the same as that for the atlas in Fig. 8.2. The *bottom* row shows the tract within one hemisphere (*oblique view*) and its appearance at the midsagittal plane (*bottom left*)

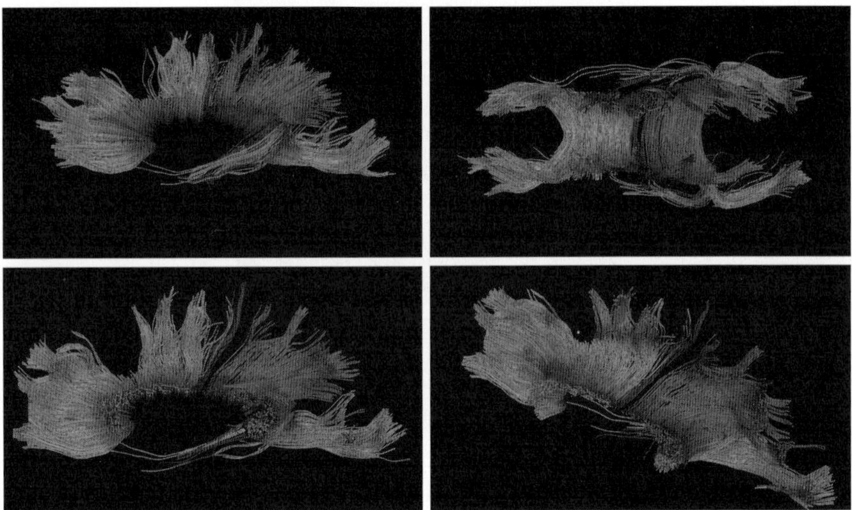

Fig. 8.6. Visualization of the anatomically labeled version of the callosal tract from a male subject (see color plates). The color legend is the same as that for the atlas in Fig. 8.2. The *bottom* row shows the tract within one hemisphere (oblique view) and its appearance at the midsagittal plane (*bottom left*)

of white matter regions in the brain. However, in order to be able to use this information reliably in clinical interpretation or cross-sectional studies, the measurements must be characterized with respect to the underlying anatomy, which would make possible their reference on a common anatomical basis. The development of methods for anatomic labeling of brain white matter is therefore expected to become a major avenue for research in diffusion tensor visualization and analysis.

In this chapter, we have proposed a scheme for identifying white matter tracts extracted from DT-MRI brain studies of an individual using cortical labels transferred from an atlas that has been warped into alignment with the individual's corresponding structural image. Individualization of the atlas is obtained via very high dimensional registration. The warped cortical labels are resampled into the space of the diffusion tensor data, which is co-registered with the structural image, and used to generate a Voronoi partitioning of the image volume, where the cells correspond to different labels. By determining the cell at which a fiber bundle terminates, subject to distance constraints from the cortex, we automatically obtain the label of the fiber bundle and color it accordingly. Feasibility of the approach was demonstrated using tractographic maps of the corpus callosum, producing a refined anatomic parcellation of this white matter tract according to the gray matter regions it interconnects.

Callosal morphology as a potential clinical diagnostic criterion has attracted much attention in the research community [10]. Recently, many investigators have focused on shape and size variations of the corpus callosum between distinct populations. There appears to be evidence confirming possible morphological differences between normal subjects and those subjects afflicted with schizophrenia [11, 12, 13], prenatal alcohol exposure [14], dyslexia [15], Alzheimer disease [16], Williams syndrome [17] or chromosome 22q11 deletion syndrome [18]. If these effects are found to be distinctive enough, we can hope to be able to use these differences in a diagnostic manner. Even barring such a diagnostic success, understanding the pathologies of a disease, in this case morphometric differences, may aid in uncovering the cause.

Most studies of the corpus callosum (CC) searching for group differences have used the Witelson partition or similar partitions [19, 20]. The Witelson partition consists of subdividing the CC using cuts perpendicular to the longest line segment that can be formed by connecting two points on the midsagittal plane of the structure. The first third is called the anterior third; the next sixth, the anterior midbody; the following sixth, the posterior midbody; the next two-fifteenths the isthmus; and the remaining fifth the splenium. Studies typically report statistical differences in the overall or relative size of the whole CC or one of these parts of the CC. Because this approach may fail to reveal statistically relevant differences which either bridge boundaries between partitions or perhaps occur on scales smaller than the partition and are cancelled out by other competing effects within the same partition, some studies have instead applied deformation-based morphometry [21, 22, 23], where a CC template is registered to subject callosa, and the resulting set of transformations are used to search for differences in any subregion of the CC, potentially even distributed effects which are not confined to a single contiguous region.

A more important shortcoming of existing partitioning schemes, however, is their dependence on heuristic albeit systematic specifications of the CC partitions. The availability of DT-MRI enables an alternative, more principled approach, in which the CC is partitioned according to rigorous anatomic definitions as advanced in this work. Current applications of deformation-based callosal morphometry also have limitations; specifically, they use only the two-dimensional boundary information of the CC as it appears on the midsagittal plane, and morphological variations within the body of the CC must be inferred from the boundary correspondences.

In related work [24], Huang et al. provide proof-of-concept of the use of diffusion tensor imaging as a rigorous basis for anatomically partitioning the CC. Moreover, they leverage the partition boundaries as additional landmarks with which to guide deformation-based morphometry within the callosum. In this work, we extend the heuristically obtained parcellations of Huang et al., and present a principled approach to the tract labeling problem and its automatic implementation via atlas registration. These developments when combined with the fully volumetric tractographic maps derived from DT-MRI brain studies open an exciting new realm for research in cerebral connectivity.

References

1. Basser, P.J., Matiello, J., Le Bihan, D.: MR diffusion tensor spectroscopy and imaging. Biophysical Journal, **66**, 259–267 (1994)
2. Pierpaoli, C., Jezzard, P., Basser, P.J., Barnett, A., Di Chiro, G.: Diffusion tensor imaging of the human brain. Radiology, **201**, 637–648 (1996)
3. Mori, S., van Zijl, P.C.M.: Fiber tracking: principles and strategies – a technical review. NMR in Biomedicine, **15**, 468–480 (2002)
4. Lori, N.F., Akbudak, E., Shimony, J.S., Cull, T.S., Snyder, A.Z., Guillory, R.K., Conturo, T.E.: Diffusion tensor fiber tracking of human brain connectivity: acquisition methods, reliability analysis and biological results. NMR in Biomedicine, **15**, 493–515 (2002)
5. Fillard, P., Gerig, G.: Analysis tool for diffusion tensor MRI. In: Peters, T.M., Ellis, R.E. (ed) Medical Image Computing and Computer-Assisted Intervention. Springer-Verlag, Berlin (2003)
6. Dubb, A., Yushkevich, P.A., Xie, Z., Gur, R.C., Gur, R.E., Gee, J.C.: Regional structural characterization of the brain of schizophrenia patients. In: Barillot, C., Haynor, D.R., Hellier, P. (ed) Medical Image Computing and Computer-Assisted Intervention. Springer-Verlag, Berlin (2004)
7. Avants, B.B., Schoenemann, P.T., Gee, J.C.: Landmark and intensity driven Lagrangian frame diffeomorphic image registration: Application to functionally and structurally-based inter-species comparison. Medical Image Analysis, to appear.

8. Toga, A.W.: Brain Warping. Academic Press, San Diego (1999)
9. Avants, B., Sundaram, T., Duda, J., Ng, L., Gee, J.: Non-rigid image registration. In: Yoo, T.S. (ed) Insight into Images: Principles and Practice for Segmentation, Registration, and Image Analysis. A.K. Peters, Wellesey (2004)
10. Zaidel, E., Iacoboni, M.: The Parallel Brain: The Cognitive Neuroscience of the Corpus Callosum. MIT Press, Cambridge (2003)
11. David, A.S.: Schizophrenia and the corpus callosum: Developmental, structural and functional relationships. Behav. Brain Res., **64**, 203–211 (1992)
12. Delisi, L.E., Tew, W., Xie, S., Hoff, A.L.: A prospective follow-up study of brain morphology and cognition in first-episode schizophrenic patients: Preliminary findings. Biol. Psychiatry, **39**, 349–360 (1995)
13. Lewine, R., Flashman, L., Gulley, L., Beardsley, S.: Sexual dimorphism in the corpus callosum and schizophrenia. Schizophren. Res., **4**, 63–64 (1991)
14. Sowell, E.R., Mattson, S.N., Thompson, P.M., Jernigan, T.L., Riley, E.P., Toga, A.W.: Mapping callosal morphology and cognitive correlates: Effects of heavy prenatal alcohol exposure. Neurology, **57**, 235–244 (2001)
15. Hynd, G.W., Hall, J., Novey, E.S., Eliopulos, D.: Dyslexia and corpus callosum morphology. Arch. Neurol., **52**, 32–38 (1995)
16. Hampel, H., Teipel, S.J., Alexander, G.E., Horowitz, B., Teichberg, D., Shapiro, M.B., Rapoport, S.I.: Corpus callosum atrophy is a possible indicator of region and cell type specific neuronal degneration in Alzheimer disease. Arch. Neurol., **55**, 193–198 (1998)
17. Tomaiuolo, F., Di Paolo, M., Caravale, B., Vicari, S., Petrides, M., Caltagirone, C.: Morphology and morphometry of the corpus callosum in Williams syndrome: A T1-weighted MRI study. NeuroReport, **13**, 2281–2284 (2002)
18. Shashi, V., Muddasani, S., Santos, C.C., Berry, M.N., Kwapil, T.R., Lewandowski, E., Keshavan, M.S.: Abnormalities of the corpus callosum in nonpsychotic children with chromosome 22q11 deletion syndrome. NeuroImage, **21**, 1399–1406 (2004)
19. Thompson, P.M., Narr, K.L., Blanton, R.E., Toga, A.W.: Mapping structural alterations of the corpus callosum during brain development and degeneration. In: Zaidel, E., Iacoboni, M. (ed) The Parallel Brain: The Cognitive Neuroscience of the Corpus Callosum. MIT Press, Cambridge (2003)
20. Bermudez, P., Zatorre, R.J.: Sexual dimorphism in the corpus callosum: Methodological considerations in MRI morphometry. NeuroImage, **13**, 1121–1130 (2001)
21. Davatzikos, C., Vaillant, M., Resnick, S.M., Prince, J.L., Letovsky, S., Bryan, R.N.: A computerized approach for morphological analysis of the corpus callosum. J. Comput. Assist. Tomogr., **20**, 88–97 (1996)
22. Pettey, D.J., Gee, J.C.: Sexual dimorphism in the corpus callosum: A characterization of local size variations and a classification driven approach to morphometry. NeuroImage, **17**, 1504–1511 (2002)
23. Dubb, A., Gur, R., Avants, B., Gee, J.: Characterization of sexual dimorphism in the human corpus callosum. Neuroimage, **20**, 512–519 (2003)
24. Huang, H., Jiang, H., Wakana, S., Poetscher, L., Zhang, J., Miller, M.I., van Zijl, P.C., Mori, S.: DTI-based parcellation of white matter: Application to the corpus callosum. In: Proc. Intl. Soc. Mag. Reson. Med., ISMRM, Berkeley (2004)

Variational Regularization
of Multiple Diffusion Tensor Fields

Ofer Pasternak[1], Nir Sochen[2], and Yaniv Assaf[3,4]

[1] Tel-Aviv University, School of Computer Science, Ramat-Aviv, 69978 Tel-Aviv, Israel
`oferpas@post.tau.ac.il`
[2] Tel-Aviv University, Department of Applied Mathematics, Ramat-Aviv, 69978 Tel-Aviv, Israel
`sochen@post.tau.ac.il`
[3] Tel-Aviv University, Department of Neurobiochemistry, Faculty of Life Sciences, 69978 Tel-Aviv, Israel
[4] Wohl Institute for Advanced Imaging, Functional Brain Imaging unit Sourasky Medical Center, 6 Weizmann st., 64239 Tel-Aviv, Israel
`asafyan@zahav.net.il`

Summary. Diffusion Tensor Imaging (DTI) became a popular tool for white matter tract visualization in the brain. It provides quantitative measures of water molecule diffusion anisotropy and the ability to delineate major white matter bundles. The diffusion model of DTI was found to be inappropriate in cases of partial volume effect, such as Multiple Fiber Orientations (MFO) ambiguity. Recently, a variety of image processing methods were proposed to enhance DTI results by reducing noise and correcting artifacts, but most techniques were not designed to resolve MFO ambiguity. In this Chapter we describe variational based DTI processing techniques, and show how such techniques can be adapted to the Multiple Tensor (MT) diffusion model via the Multiple Tensor Variational (MTV) framework. We show how the MTV framework can be used in separating differently oriented white matter fiber bundles.

9.1 Introduction

Diffusion Weighted Magnetic Resonance Imaging (DW-MRI) enables the measurement of the apparent water self-diffusion along a specified direction [1, 2, 3, 4]. Diffusion Tensor Imaging (DTI) uses multiple Diffusion Weighted Images (DWIs) to extract anisotropic diffusion effects [1]. DTI is based on the assumptions that each voxel can be represented by a single diffusion compartment and that the diffusion within this compartment has a Gaussian distribution. Under those assumptions DTI states the relation between the signal attenuation, E, and the diffusion tensor, D, as follows [2, 3]:

$$E(q_k) = \frac{A(q_k)}{A(0)} = \exp(-bq_k^T D q_k) \, , \tag{9.1}$$

where $A(q_k)$ is the DWI for the kth applied diffusion gradient direction, $A(0)$ is a non weighted image and b is a constant reflecting the experimental diffusion weighting [1]. D is a second order tensor, i.e., a 3×3 positive semidefinite symmetric matrix, and therefore at least 6 DWIs from different non-collinear applied gradient directions are required to uniquely calculate it [2]. One of the promising applications based on DTI is fiber tracking (See Chap. 7 by Vilanova et al.), producing $3D$ visualization of white matter tracts in the brain, by integrating over the field of principle eigenvectors [5, 6, 7]. Principle eigenvectors are found using the tensor spectral decomposition

$$D = \sum_{a=1}^{3} \lambda^a U^a (U^a)^T \, , \tag{9.2}$$

for three eigenvectors U^a and three positive eigenvalues λ^a. The ratio between the eigenvalues determines the diffusion anisotropy, with measures such as Fractional Anisotropy (FA)[3]. Fiber tracking techniques have provided visualization of white matter tracts, resembling known anatomical structures in the brain [6, 7], but at the same time they also reveal DTI's limitations. DTI was found to produce erroneous orientations in voxels with partial volume, i.e., exhibiting more than one compartment [4], where the assumption of a single diffusion compartment no longer holds. A specific type of partial volume occurs in voxels containing Multiple Fiber Orientations (MFO), where diffusion is not restricted to a Single Fiber Orientation (SFO) and therefore is not accurately described by a Gaussian distribution. In addition to the MFO modeling limitation, DTI has to deal with machine noise and with various artifacts accompanying the DWI acquisition process. The effect of noise and artifacts on DWIs is hard to model, much yet to remove [8]. The errors propagate and accumulate through the tracking process and can create large diversions from initially small signal changes. Since the DTI algorithm does not contain any inherent mechanism to eliminate artifacts or to reduce noise effects it requires either pre or post processing. In this chapter we focus on the variational approach for DTI denoising, and show how this approach could be applied on the multiple tensor diffusion model, aiming to reduce the errors resulting from partial volume effects while reducing noise effects.

9.2 Variational Approach for DTI Denoising

Variational frameworks for denoising images usually consists of a functional which minima is considered to be provided by a regularized image [9]. Considering an initial image $I_0(x, y, z)$ in the image domain Ω then an appropriate functional with a denoised image $I(x, y, z)$ as minimizer will have the following form:

$$F(I) = \int_{\Omega} (\alpha K(I, I_0) + R(\nabla I)) \, d\Omega \, . \tag{9.3}$$

The first term of the functional, the fidelity term, is used to constrain the solution to the original image with the function K. The second part of the functional, the regularization term, adds neighborhood alignment constraints to the desired solution with the function R. The regularization term aims to reduce overall edges in the image, which are measured with the gradient, ∇I, values. The relative influence of both terms is determined by the parameter α. Small variations in gradients assumed to be caused by noise, whereas large variations are attributed to edges or contour lines. Adapting variational framework to the processing of diffusion data would be by concerning different diffusion measures as scalar, vector or matrix valued images.

9.2.1 Scalar Diffusion Images

Raw diffusion data is usually in the form of DWIs, which are scalar images. DWIs are then further analyzed to fit diffusion models such as DTI. Applying the variational framework on the set of DWIs is one possible way to achieve smoother DTI results, such as FA values and principle eigenvectors [10, 11]. An example for such functional is [10]

$$F(I) = \int_{\Omega} \left(\alpha(I - I_0)^2 + \phi(|\nabla I|) \right) d\Omega \, . \tag{9.4}$$

Minimization by gradient descent of (9.4) gives the diffusion flow

$$\frac{\partial I}{\partial t} = \alpha(I_0 - I) + div \left(\frac{\phi'(|\nabla I|)}{|\nabla I|} \nabla I \right) \, . \tag{9.5}$$

The function ϕ should smooth insignificant edges while preserve the significant ones. Example of different functions are Perona-Malik's $\phi(|\nabla I|) = e^{-(|\nabla I|/K)^2}$ [12], Total Variation $\phi(|\nabla I|) = |\nabla I|$ [13] or Charbonnier et al. $\phi(|\nabla I|) = \sqrt{1 + \frac{|\nabla I|^2}{k^2}}$ [14]. Since DWIs have a scalar value for each pixel, they are dealt as regular gray valued images, and do not require additional constraints (For scalar images regularization see [15]).

9.2.2 Multi-Valued Diffusion Images

Diffusion data can also be regularized at the diffusion tensor level, after fitting the DWIs to the DTI model [16, 17]. The reasoning is that achieving smooth variation of tensors will supply smoothed FA maps and fiber tracts. In general the functional to minimize has a similar shape to (9.4) only now the scalar images, I, are replaced with tensor valued images, $D(x, y, z) = (d_{kl}(x, y, z))$ as follows:

$$F(D) = \int_{\Omega} \left(\alpha \|D - D_0\|^2 + \phi(|\nabla D|) \right) d\Omega \, . \tag{9.6}$$

The Frobenius norm is usually used for matrix norm as $\|D\| = \sqrt{\sum_{k,l} d_{kl}^2}$. The matrix gradient can be calculated as $|\nabla D| = \sum_{k,l} |\nabla d_{kl}|$ for isotropic flow or could be calculated with other schemes (For vector and matrix valued image regularization see [18]). When handling tensors it is important that the solution will preserve the diffusion tensor properties, i.e., D has to be symmetric positive semidefinite. Some methods monitor the tensor properties explicitly by decomposing the tensor to formats which promise to maintain symmetric positive semidefiniteness, such as the Cholesky decomposition ($D(x) = LL^T(x)$, with L being a lower triangular matrix) [17], or by decomposing D to $D = R^T R$ where $R \in GL(n, \mathbb{R})$, the Lie group of invertible $n \times n$ real matrices [16]. The necessity of explicitly monitoring the positive semidefinite nature of the tensor is brought to question by Weickert and Brox [18] where they prove that there exits a finite different scheme for diffusion filtering that implicitly preserves positive semidefiniteness of the initial matrix field for all iteration levels, providing that the filtering method applies the same diffusivities on all tensor channels. For some DTI applications such as fiber tracking, it is enough to regularize only the tensor orientations. Therefore, regularization of all tensor channels is not needed. The minimization in this case is done by changing the orientations of the eigenvectors [19] computed by the spectral decomposition (9.2):

$$F(U) = \int_\Omega \left(\alpha |U - U_0|^2 + \phi_1(|\nabla U|) \right) d\Omega \, , \qquad (9.7)$$

where U is a vector consisting all the components of the eigenvectors. With this kind of regularization the orthonormal ratio between the eigenvectors has to be preserved, and it is done by simultaneously rotating all 3 of them with the same angle, determined by a momentum vector comprising the different flows of $\frac{\partial U_i^a}{\partial t}$ for each element U_i of U [19]. The results are smoothed eigenvector maps, which can directly be used for fiber tracking, or could be used for reconstruction of the reoriented diffusion tensor.

9.2.3 Simultaneous Fitting and Regularization

The variational framework could also be used for estimating a regularized tensor field. The estimation is done by fitting the DWIs to the diffusion model [20, 21] and does not require an initial tensor field. Simultaneous fitting and smoothing is achieved by finding the tensor field, D, minimizing the following:

$$F(D) = \int_\Omega \left(\alpha (M(D) - I_0)^2 + \phi(|\nabla D|) \right) d\Omega \, . \qquad (9.8)$$

Both (9.8) and (9.6) share the same regularization term, whereas (9.8) is restricted by a different fidelity term, consisted of M, a diffusion model dependent function, and I_0, the normalized DWIs. In the DTI case, M estimates the DWIs which would fit D by (9.1). The fitting term measures how far are the predicted DWIs for the currently estimated diffusion tensor from the measured DWIs. Minimization by gradient descent of (9.8) leads to the flow

$$\frac{\partial D}{\partial t} = \alpha M'(D)(I_0 - M(D)) + div\left(\frac{\phi'(|\nabla D|)}{|\nabla D|}\nabla D\right)$$
(9.9)

The simultaneous fitting and smoothing should provide better results than smoothing a prior fitted tensor field, since the fitting procedure itself in a noisy situation is ill-posed, and adding the regularization stabilizes it [9].

9.3 Multiple Tensor Variational Framework for Fitting and Regularizing Diffusion Weighted Images

Chapter 5 by Alexander explains that the DTI model shows some inaccuracies in areas of complex architecture where the assumptions of DTI do not hold. A specific case is fiber orientation ambiguity, where fiber bundles with different orientations reside in the same voxel. Trying to fit the attenuation signal from Multiple Fiber Orientations (MFO) voxels to the DTI model (9.1) usually results with low FA tensors with an oblate form ($\lambda^1 \simeq \lambda^2 \gg \lambda^3$), or sometimes even spherical form ($\lambda^1 \simeq \lambda^2 \simeq \lambda^3$) with no significant diffusion orientation [22]. The principle eigenvector in those cases will not necessarily be aligned with any of the fiber orientations [4], causing either a deviation of the delineated tract, or a premature termination of the tracing procedure when arriving to MFO voxels. In the recent years advanced diffusion models and acquisition techniques were introduced aiming to overcome limitations of the DTI model [23, 24, 25, 26, 27]. One of those methods is presented in Chap. 10 by Özarslan et al. In the previous section variational framework for DTI fitting and denoising were described, but those are confined within the limitation of DTI diffusion model. In this section we will describe application of the variational framework on a Multiple Tensor (MT) diffusion model [23], which we call the Multiple Tensor Variational (MTV) framework.

9.3.1 Multiple Tensor Model

The MTV framework [28] is based on the MT water molecules diffusion model [23]. The model is based on the assumption that each voxel is consisted of discrete number of homogeneous regions, which are in slow exchange, i.e., separated by a distance much greater than the diffusion mixing length. It is further assumed that the diffusion within each region is Gaussian, i.e., fully described by a tensor. Under those assumptions the attenuation signal is described as a finite mixture of Gaussians,

$$E(q_k) = \sum_{i=1}^{n} f_i E_i(q_k) \, ,$$
(9.10)

for n components, with each component described as

$$E_i(q_k) = \exp(-bq_k^T D_i q_k) \tag{9.11}$$

and f_i as the weight of the i'th component in the mixture of Gaussian diffusion densities E_i. To ensure that the volume fractions are properly bounded ($f_i \in [0,1]$) and normalized ($\sum_i f_i = 1$) the weights are calculated through the soft-max transform

$$f_i = \frac{\exp \eta_i}{\sum_{j=1}^n \exp \eta_j} \, , \tag{9.12}$$

where $\eta_i \in \mathbb{R}$. Using (9.2) and (9.12), the modelled signal takes the form

$$E(q_k) = \sum_{i=1}^n \frac{e^{\eta_i}}{\sum_{j=1}^n e^{\eta_j}} e^{-bq_k^T (\Sigma_{a=1}^3 \lambda_i^a U_i^a (U_i^a)^T) q_k} \, , \tag{9.13}$$

where λ_i^a (U_i^a) are the a'th eigenvalue (eigenvector) of the i'th diffusion tensor.

9.3.2 Variational Framework for the Multi-Tensor Model

The MTV framework estimates the MT vector field while smoothing it by the minimization of the following functional:

$$S_1(\eta, D) = \int_\Omega \left[\alpha_0 H + \sum_i (\alpha_1 \phi_1(|\nabla \eta_i|) + \alpha_2 \phi_2(|\nabla D_i|)) \right] d\Omega \, , \tag{9.14}$$

where $H = \sum_{k=1}^d (E(q_k) - \hat{E}(q_k))^2$, for d different acquisition directions. $\hat{E}$ is the measured diffusion signal attenuation and E is calculated using (9.13). During the regularization the tensors have to maintain their symmetric positive semidefinite attributes and in addition should remain anisotropic. Anisotropy is enforced in order to resemble neuronal fibers cylindrical shape and in this way to avoid fitting of MFO voxels to a single isotropic tensor as would happen with DTI fitting. In order to allow addition of anisotropy constraints and in order to delimit the regularization to the principle eigenvector orientations the tensor components were spectral decomposed using (9.2). Consequently a regularization scheme based on (9.7) was separately preformed on the eigenvalues and eigenvectors:

$$S_2(\eta, \lambda, U) = \int_\Omega \left[\alpha_0 H + \sum_{i=1}^n (\alpha_1 \phi_1(|\nabla \eta_i|) + \alpha_2 \phi_2(|\nabla U_i^1|) \right.$$
$$\left. + \sum_{a=1}^3 \alpha_3 \phi_3(|\nabla \lambda_i^a|)) \right] d\Omega \, . \tag{9.15}$$

The eigenvectors are regularized using the rotation scheme [19]. The rotation momentum was determined solely by the flow of the principle eigenvector for each tensor, $\frac{\partial U_i^1}{\partial t}$. This momentum vector is then used to build a rotation matrix with the Rodrigues' formula [29], applied on all three eigenvectors, resulting with preservation of orthonormality. The eigenvalues are regularized channel by channel as independent scalar images. The regularization is constrained to positive eigenvalues and to anisotropic ratio by projection to the allowed range ($\lambda > \lambda_{min} > 0, \frac{\lambda_i^1}{\lambda_i^2} > minRate > 1$). Furthermore the second and the third eigenvectors were set to remain equal during the regularization ($\lambda_i^2 = \lambda_i^3$). The minimum of S_2 solves the Euler-Lagrange equations found by the gradient descent scheme. The resulting is a system of coupled diffusion-like equations:

$$\frac{\partial X_i}{\partial t} = \alpha_X \mathrm{div}\left(\frac{\phi_X'(|\nabla X_i|)}{|\nabla X_i|} \nabla X_i \right) - \alpha_0 \frac{\partial H}{\partial X_i} \qquad (9.16)$$

where X is replaced by the parameters λ_a^i, U_i^1 and η_i. The gradient descent scheme used the Neumann boundary condition and the initial conditions $X_i(t = 0) = (X_i)_0$. The functional (9.15) is based on the calculation of gradients, which is straightforward for scalar parameters, but requires a specialized gradient scheme for eigenvectors. This is since two tensors with oppositely oriented eigenvectors are in fact equal, due to the symmetric nature of the diffusion measured in DWIs, whereas in contrast the angular difference or metric difference between the opposite eigenvectors is large. Therefore, to calculate the gradients of the principle eigenvectors a modified gradient calculation scheme [19] is used: eigenvector orientations in a neighborhood are flipped to create sharp angles, following with channel by channel difference computation. The computation difficulties related to the tensor fields can be avoided by confining the diffusion model to a fixed sets of tensors [30]. The fitting is done by finding the relative weights of the different tensors in each voxel, thus reducing the problem to scalar valued data. The cost of this simplification is lower angular resolution and requires a choice of tensor bases which takes in account the various eigenvalues relations which are found in brain tissue.

9.3.3 MTV as a General Framework

DTI fitting, DTI regularization and MT fitting are all special cases of the more general MTV model. DTI results can be achieved with MTV by using only the fitting term ($\alpha_1 > 0, \alpha_i = 0 | i \neq 1$) with single component fitting ($n = 1$). Adding the fitting term to the single component fitting ($\alpha_i > 0, n = 1$) and using DTI output as an initial state, reduces MTV to DTI regularization. The advantage of MTV is clearly the addition of more than one orientation per voxel. Using only the fitting term without restriction to a single component ($\alpha_1 > 0, \alpha_i = 0 | i \neq 1$) reduces MTV to MT. Fitting the MT model in MFO voxels is known to be ill-posed, especially in noisy setups, since the diffusion shape becomes planar or spherical and could be equally fitted to more than one set of orientations. The addition of the regularization terms should stabilize the fitting process [9], since additional constraints provide better specification to the desired solution. However, MTV can not promise to prevent from local minima entrapment, which is a problem shared by all variational methods when the functional is not convex. The regularization term should have the most effect in MFO voxels, where ambiguity causes lower fidelity term penalties. The desired outcome are smoother tracts in MFO voxels which continue the denoised orientations of tracts found at neighboring SFO voxels.

9.4 Simulations

Comparing simulations of DTI, DTI based variational regularization and MTV regularization, demonstrates the effect of the variational regularization. The simulations also show how fiber ambiguity can be resolved by MTV. The algorithms were implemented as MATLAB code, and were tested on both synthetic and experimental DWIs.

Observing a noise free simulation of perpendicular fibers, crossing each other, shows that DTI does not correctly identify the orientations of either fibers in the crossing area (Fig. 9.1a). The fitting was done with 99 simulated DWIs corresponding to 99 applied gradient directions distributed equally over a unit sphere, simulated using (9.10) ($b = 1,000$ s/mm^2, $\lambda_1 = 1.5 \times 10^{-3}$ mm^2/s, $\lambda_2 = \lambda_3 = 0.4 \times 10^{-3}$ mm^2/s). MFO voxels appear where both fibers reside in the same voxels, and in those voxels the principle eigenvectors found are aligned between the two simulated fiber orientations. Addition of the regularization term creates smooth tract continuity inside the MFO voxels areas, but correct orientation can not be recovered since the model is limited to single component per voxel (Fig. 9.1b). Removing this limitation using the MTV framework (Fig. 9.1c) allows the successful fitting of both fiber orientations.

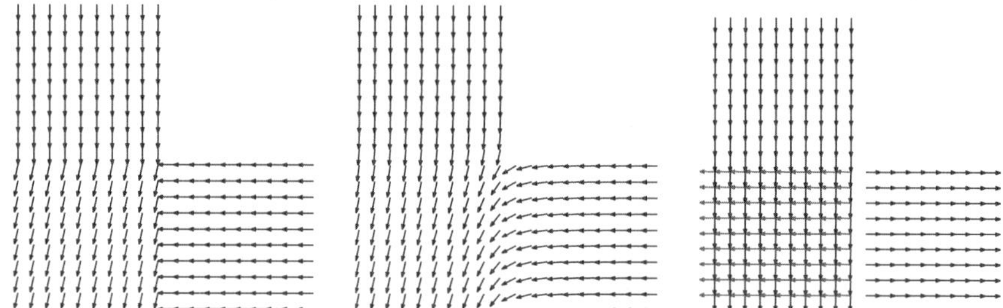

Fig. 9.1. (See colour plates) Synthetic data. Computer simulation of crossing fibers. (**a**) *Left*: DTI results. *Middle*: (**b**) DTI variational regularization (VR) results. (**c**) *Right*: MTV results.Each arrow represents a voxel. Voxels represented by more than one arrow have multiple components. Only components with a considerable volume fraction are shown ($f_i > 0.3$)

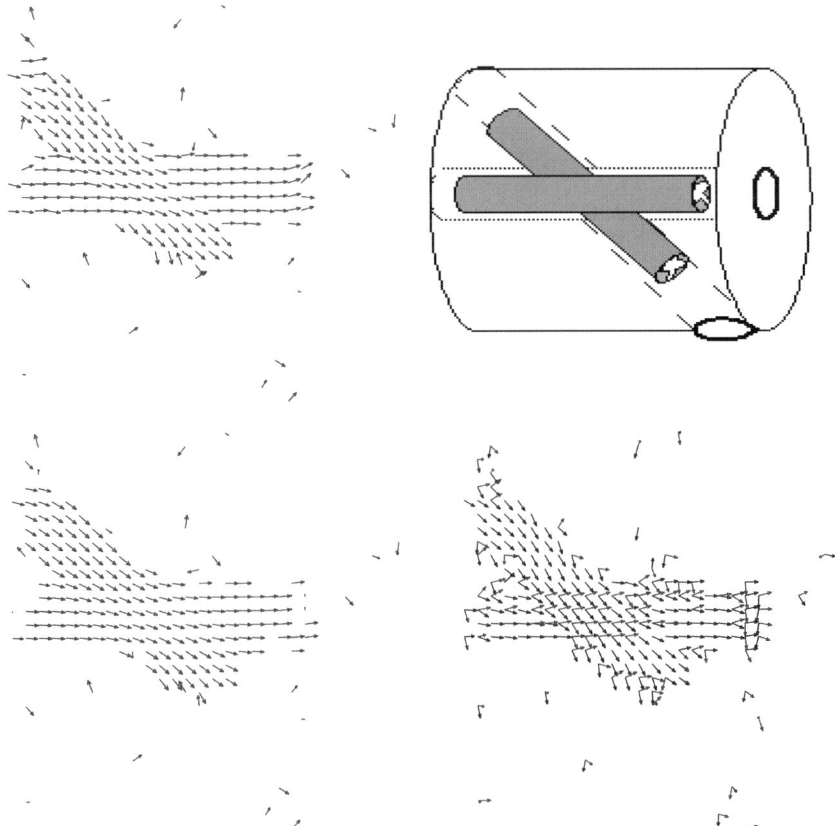

Fig. 9.2. (See colour plates) Phantom. (**a**) *Top Right*: Excised spinal cords placed crossing at 45 degrees (illustration). (**b**) *Top Left*: DTI results. (**c**) *Bottom Left*: Regularization results. (**d**) *Bottom Right* MTV results. Only components with a considerable volume fraction are shown ($f_i > 0.3$) The directions supplied by MTV are parallel to the original fiber orientations

Observing the fitting of DW-MRI acquired from a phantom reinforces the synthethic results in conditions similar to regular MRI acquisitions. The phantom used consisted of two sections of a freshly excised cervical pig spinal cord which were placed crossing at 45 degrees (Fig. 9.2a), and was scanned on a $7T$ spectrometer (PGSE, $TR/TE = 2000/200\,\mathrm{ms}$, $\Delta/\delta = 150/40\,\mathrm{ms}$, $FOV = 5\,\mathrm{cm}$, $32{\times}32$ pixels, $15\,\mathrm{mm}$ slice thickness, $0.14G/\,\mathrm{mm}$ gradient strength, $b = 1725\,\mathrm{s/mm}^2$) providing 31 DWIs corresponding to 31 non-collinear gradient directions. Similar to the synthetic case, MTV was able to provide correct fiber directions in the MFO voxels area (Fig. 9.2d), where both DTI and variational regularization of DTI fails (Fig. 9.2b,c). Noise reduction achieved with the variational framework is more noticeable observing fiber tracking images (Fig. 9.3). Fiber tracking was generated from the tensor field outcome

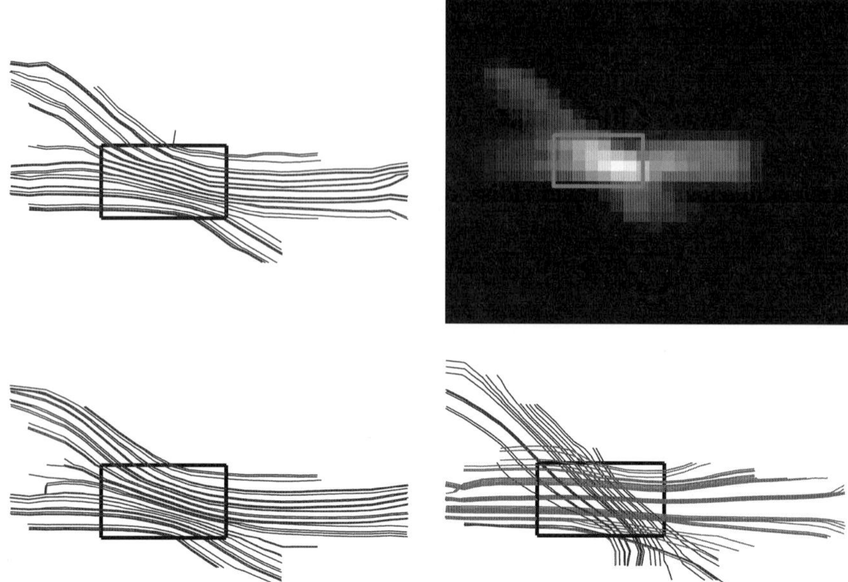

Fig. 9.3. (See colour plates) Fiber Tracking. (**a**) *Top Right*: T_2 non diffusion weighted reference image. (**b**) *Top Left*: DTI resulted fiber tracking. (**c**) *Bottom Left*: Fiber tracking of a regularized tensor field. (**d**) *Bottom Right*: MTV resulted fiber tracking. The tracking originated from the ROI, marked with a rectangle

of the three algorithms. The tracts provided by DTI (Fig. 9.3b) show many fluctuations and sharp edges, most of those are eliminated using the variational frameworks (Fig. 9.3c,d).

9.5 Concluding Remarks

The variational framework is a powerful tool for the modelling and regularization of various mappings. It is applied, with great success, to scalar and vector fields in image processing and computer vision. Recently It has been generalized to deal with tensor fields which are of great interest to brain research via the analysis of DWIs and DTI. We review in this chapter few approaches to the determination of neuronal fiber bundles from DTI, with emphasis on variational methods. We show that the more realistic model of multi-fiber voxels conjugated with the variational framework provides much improved results and better accuracy of the fiber tracking algorithms. Based on the success of our model to perform intra-voxel separation between different bundles of neuronal fibers we currently study cases of partial volume between different type of tissues, such as at the endings of fiber bundles in cortical areas.

Acknowledgments

The authors thank Prof. Peter Basser for letting us use data collected in his lab (spinal cord images). We acknowledge the support of the Edersheim-Leve-Gitter Functional Human Brain Mapping Unit of Tel-Aviv University, the Adams super-center for brain research, The Israel Academy of Sciences, Israel Ministry of Science and technology, and the Tel-Aviv University research fund.

References

1. D. Le Bihan, J.-F. Mangin, C. Poupon, C.A. Clark, S. Pappata, N. Molko, and H. Chabriat. Diffusion tensor imaging: concepts and applications. *Journal of Magnetic Resonance Imaging*, 13:534–546, 2001.
2. P.J. Basser and C. Pierpaoli. A simplified method to measure the diffusion tensor from seven MR images. *Magnetic Resonance in Medicine*, 39:928–934, 1998.
3. P.J. Basser and C. Pierpaoli. Microstructural and physiological features of tissues elucidated by quantitative-diffusion-tensor MRI. *Journal of Magnetic Resonance*, 111(3):209–219, June 1996.
4. C. Pierpaoli and P.J. Basser. Toward a quantitative assessment of diffusion anisotropy. *Magnetic Resonance in Medicine*, 36(6):893–906, 1996.
5. S. Mori and P.C. van Zijl. Fiber tracking: principles and strategies – a technical review. *NMR Biomed.*, 15:468–480, 2002.
6. M. Catani, R.J. Howard, S. Pajevic, and D.K. Jones. Virtual in vivo interactive dissection of white matter fasciculi in the human brain. *NeuroImage*, 17:77–94, 2002.
7. P.J. Basser, S. Pajevic, C. Pierpaoli, J. Duda, and A. Aldroubi. In vivo fiber tractography using DT-MRI data. *Magnetic Resonance in Medicine*, 44:625–632, 2000.
8. A.W. Anderson. Theoretical analysis of the effects of noise on diffusion tensor imaging. *Magnetic Resonance in Medicine*, 46:1174–1188, 2001.
9. G. Aubert and P. Kornprobst. *Mathematical Problems in Image Processing: Partial Differential Equations and the Calculus of Variations*, volume 147 of *Applied Mathematical Sciences*. Springer-Verlag, 2002.
10. G.J.M. Parker, J.A. Schnabel, M.R. Symms, D.J. Werring, and G.J. Garker. Nonlinear smoothing for reduction of systematic and random errors in diffusion tensor imaging. *Journal of Magnetic Resonance Imaging*, 11(6):702–710, 2000.
11. B.C. Vemuri, Y. Chen, M. Rao, T. McGraw, Z. Wang, and T. Mareci. Fiber tract mapping from diffusion tensor MRI. In *Proceedings of the IEEE Workshop on Variational and Level Set Methods (VLSM'01)*. IEEE, 2001.
12. P. Perona and J. Malik. Scale-space and edge detection using anisotropic diffusion. *IEEE Trans. Pattern Anal. Mach. Intell.*, 12(7):629–639, 1990.
13. L.I. Rudin, S. Osher, and E. Fatemi. Nonlinear total variation based noise removal algorithms. In *Proceedings of the eleventh annual international conference of the Center for Nonlinear Studies on Experimental mathematics : computational issues in nonlinear science*, pp. 259–268. Elsevier North-Holland, 1992.

14. P. Charbonnier, L. Blanc-Féraud, G. Aubert, and M. Barlaud. Two deterministic half-quadratic regularization algorithms for computed imaging. In *ICIP (2)*, pp. 168–172, 1994.

15. J. Weickert. *Anisotropic Diffusion in Image Processing*. Teubner-Verlag, 1998.

16. C. Chefd'hotel, D. Tschumperlé, R. Deriche, and O.D. Faugeras. Constrained flows of matrix-valued functions: Application to diffusion tensor regularization. In *Proceedings of the 7th European Conference on Computer Vision-Part I*, pp. 251–265. Springer-Verlag, 2002.

17. T. McGraw, B.C. Vemuri, Y. Chen, M. Rao, and T.H. Mareci. DT-MRI denoising and neuronal fiber tracking. *Med. Imag, Analysis*, 8:95–111, 2004.

18. J. Weickert and T. Brox. Diffusion and regularization of vector- and matrix-valued images. *Inverse Problems, Image Analysis and Medical Imaging. Contemporary Mathematics*, 313:251–268, 2002.

19. D. Tschumperlé and R. Deriche. Orthonormal vector sets regularization with PDE's and applications. *Int. J. Comput. Vision*, 50(3):237–252, 2002.

20. Z. Wang, B.C. Vemuri, Y. Chen, and T. Mareci. A constrained variational principle for direct estimation and smoothing of the diffusion tensor field from DWI. In Christopher J. Taylor and J. Alison Noble, editors, *IPMI*, volume 2732 of *Lecture Notes in Computer Science*, pp. 660–671. Springer, 2003.

21. D. Tschumperlé and R. Deriche. Variational frameworks for DT-MRI estimation, regularization and visualization. In *2nd IEEE Workshop on Variational, Geometric and Level Set Methods in Computer Vision (VLSM'03)*, 2003.

22. D.C. Alexander, G.J. Barker, and S.R. Arridge. Detection and modeling of non-gaussian apparent diffusion coefficient profiles in human brain data. *Magnetic Resonance in Medicine*, 48:331–340, 2002.

23. D.S. Tuch, T.G. Reese, M.R. Wiegell, N.G. Makris, J.W. Belliveau, and V.J. Wedeen. High angular resolution diffusion imaging reveals intravoxel white matter fiber heterogeneity. *Magnetic Resonance in Medicine*, 48:577–582, 2002.

24. Y. Assaf, R.Z. Freidlin, G.K. Rohde, and P.J. Basser. A new modeling and experimental framework to characterize hindered and restricted water diffusion in brain white matter. In *Proceedings of 12th Annual Meeting of the ISMRM*, page 251, 2004.

25. E. Ozarslan and T.H. Mareci. Generalized diffusion tensor imaging and analytical relationships between diffusion tensor imaging and high angular resolution diffusion imaging. *Magnetic Resonance in Medicine*, 50(5):955–965, 2003.

26. D.S. Tuch. *Diffusion MRI of complex tissue structure*. PhD thesis, Division of Health Sciences and Technology, Massachusetts Institute of Technoloy, 2002.

27. K.M. Jansons and D.C. Alexander. Persistent angular structure: new insights from diffusion MRI data. *Inverse Problems*, 19:1031–1046, 2003.

28. O. Pasternak, N. Sochen, and Y. Assaf. Separation of white matter fascicles from diffusion MRI using ϕ-functional regularization. In *Proceedings of 12th Annual Meeting of the ISMRM*, page 1227, 2004.

29. O. Faugeras. *Three-dimensional computer vision: a geometric viewpoint*. MIT Press, 1993.

30. A.R. Manzanares and M. Rivera. Brain nerve bundles estimation by restoring and filtering intra-voxel information in diffusion tensor MRI. In *2nd IEEE Workshop on Variational, Geometric and Level Set Methods in Computer Vision (VLSM'03)*, pp. 71–80. IEEE, 2003.

10

Higher Rank Tensors in Diffusion MRI

Evren Özarslan[1,2], Baba C. Vemuri[2,3], and Thomas H. Mareci[1,2,4]

[1] Department of Physics, University of Florida, Gainesville, FL32611, USA
[2] McKnight Brain Institute, University of Florida, Gainesville, FL32610, USA
[3] Department of Computer and Information Science and Engineering, University of Florida, Gainesville, FL32611, USA
[4] Department of Biochemistry and Molecular Biology, University of Florida, Gainesville, FL32610, USA
`evren@mbi.ufl.edu, vemuri@cise.ufl.edu`

Summary. In this work we review how the diffusivity profiles obtained from diffusion MRI can be expressed in terms of Cartesian tensors of ranks higher than 2. When the rank of the tensor being used is 2, one recovers traditional diffusion tensor imaging (DTI). Therefore our approach can be seen as a generalization of DTI. The properties of generalized diffusion tensors are discussed. The shortcomings of DTI experienced in the presence of orientational heterogeneity may cause inaccurate anisotropy values and incorrect fiber orientations. Employment of higher rank tensors is helpful in overcoming these difficulties.

10.1 Introduction

The dependence of the magnetic resonance signal intensity on the direction of the applied diffusion sensitizing gradients has been exploited to calculate the local orientations in fibrous tissues, which may eventually lead to the construction of anatomical connections within different regions of the brain. The most common approach used to model orientational dependence of the diffusivities, called diffusion tensor MRI or diffusion tensor imaging (DTI) [1, 2], has employed a Cartesian tensor of rank-2 that has yielded a simple scheme to calculate anisotropy values as well as local orientations of the fibers from multidirectional diffusion measurements. However, the underlying assumption of DTI, i.e. the orientational homogeneity within the voxels, may be too restrictive for the imaging of neural tissue. The incapability of DTI to resolve more than one fiber orientation has prompted recent interest in the development of more sophisticated techniques. A review of DTI along with some of the techniques developed to overcome the failure of DTI in regions of tissue with complex microstructure by Alexander can be found in Chap. 5. Also note that a recent method by Pasternak et al. based on modeling the signal in a variational framework using multiple rank-2 tensors is detailed in the preceding chapter. In this chapter, we present a technique that we have recently introduced called generalized diffusion tensor imaging that uses tensors of rank possibly higher than 2.

10.1.1 Background

The dynamics of magnetization within the tissue is governed by the Bloch-Torrey equation [3], which, upon simplification to keep its diffusion related parts, takes the form

$$\frac{\partial \psi}{\partial t} = -i\gamma \mathbf{r} \cdot \mathbf{G}\psi + D\nabla^2\psi \, , \tag{10.1}$$

where $\mathbf{r}$ is the position vector, γ is the gyromagnetic ratio, D is the apparent diffusion coefficient and $\mathbf{G}$ is the linear magnetic field gradient, whose direction $\mathbf{g}$ is assumed to be time independent. In the above expression $\psi := M_+ \exp(iw_0 t + t/T_2)$, where w_0 is the Larmor frequency, T_2 is the spin-spin relaxation constant and M_+ is the complex representation for local transverse magnetization. Integral of M_+ over the voxel yields the signal S received from that voxel. The components of $\mathbf{g}$ can be written in terms of the spherical coordinates as

$$\mathbf{g} := \frac{\mathbf{G}}{||\mathbf{G}||} = \begin{pmatrix} g_1 \\ g_2 \\ g_3 \end{pmatrix} = \begin{pmatrix} \sin\theta \cos\phi \\ \sin\theta \sin\phi \\ \cos\theta \end{pmatrix} \, , \tag{10.2}$$

where θ is the polar and ϕ is the azimuthal angle.

The solution to (10.1) yields the well known Stejskal-Tanner equation [4], that relates the applied diffusion gradient to the MR signal, given by

$$S(\mathbf{g}) = S_0 \exp(-\gamma^2\delta^2||\mathbf{G}||^2(\Delta - \delta/3)D(\mathbf{g})) = S_0 \exp(-b\,D(\mathbf{g})) \, , \tag{10.3}$$

where δ is the duration of the gradient pulses and Δ is the time difference between the leading edges of these pulses.

In DTI, one replaces the diffusivity in (10.1) with a rank-2 symmetric positive definite tensor, which results in an approximate signal attenuation expression given by

$$S(\mathbf{g}) = S_0 \exp(-b\,\mathbf{g}^{\mathrm{T}}\mathbf{D}\mathbf{g}) \, . \tag{10.4}$$

Comparison of the last two equations indicates that DTI assumes a diffusivity profile that is specified by the quadratic forms of the rank-2 tensor, i.e.,

$$D(\mathbf{g}) = \mathbf{g}^{\mathrm{T}}\mathbf{D}\mathbf{g} \, . \tag{10.5}$$

10.1.2 Generalized Diffusion Tensor Imaging

As an extension of the transition from a diffusion coefficient (a rank-0 tensor) to the rank-2 diffusion tensor, we have proposed to use Cartesian tensors of rank higher than 2 to model the orientational dependence of diffusivities [5]. In this scheme, generalization of (10.4) is given by

$$S = S_0 \exp\left(-b \sum_{i_1=1}^{3} \sum_{i_2=1}^{3} \cdots \sum_{i_l=1}^{3} D_{i_1 i_2 \ldots i_l} g_{i_1} g_{i_2} \cdots g_{i_l}\right), \qquad (10.6)$$

where $D_{i_1 i_2 \ldots i_l}$ represents the components of the rank-l tensor. In this case, the diffusivity profile implied by the rank-l tensor can be expressed as

$$D(\mathbf{g}) = \sum_{i_1=1}^{3} \sum_{i_2=1}^{3} \cdots \sum_{i_l=1}^{3} D_{i_1 i_2 \ldots i_l} g_{i_1} g_{i_2} \cdots g_{i_l}. \qquad (10.7)$$

Note that (10.7) implies that

$$D(-\mathbf{g}) = \begin{cases} D(\mathbf{g}), & \text{if } l \text{ is even} \\ -D(\mathbf{g}), & \text{if } l \text{ is odd} \end{cases}. \qquad (10.8)$$

However, the latter case would yield negative diffusivities which are nonphysical. Therefore, the rank of the tensor model has te be even in which case antipodal symmetry of the diffusivities is also ensured. Furthermore, (10.7) also implies that the rank-l tensor is a totally symmetric tensor, i.e.,

$$D_{i_1 i_2 \ldots i_l} = D_{(i_1 i_2 \ldots i_l)}, \qquad (10.9)$$

where $(i_1 i_2 \ldots i_l)$ stands for all permutations of the indices. This is because the rank-l tensor links the components of the same l vectors to a scalar, therefore the order of these vectors do not affect the result. A totally symmetric tensor in three dimensional space has

$$N_l := \binom{l+2}{2} = \frac{(l+1)(l+2)}{2} \qquad (10.10)$$

distinct components [6], where each of these distinct elements is repeated

$$\mu := \binom{l}{n_x} \binom{l - n_x}{n_y} = \frac{l!}{n_x! \, n_y! \, n_z!} \qquad (10.11)$$

times[1], where n_x, n_y and n_z are respectively the number of x, y and z indices included in the full sequence of subscripts defining the component of

---

[1] Note that the properties of the higher order diffusion tensor as described in the text follows from the expression given in (10.7). A similar expression is found in the linear theory of elasticity where the elastic energy U (a scalar) is obtained

the tensor. For example, for D_{xxxz}, i.e., xxxz component of the rank-4 tensor, $n_x = 3$, $n_y = 0$ and $n_z = 1$. Therefore, using (10.11), it is easy to see that the multiplicity, μ, of this component is 4.

These findings can be incorporated into (10.6) to yield a simplified expression for the generalized Stejskal-Tanner equation:

$$S = S_0 \exp\left(-b \sum_{k=1}^{N_1} \mu_k D_k \prod_{p=1}^{1} g_{k(p)}\right) , \qquad (10.12)$$

where D_k is the k-th distinct element of the tensor, and $g_{k(p)}$ is the component of the gradient direction specified by the p-th index of D_k.

A rank-l tensor contains the information stored in tensors of rank smaller than l. Therefore, once a rank-l tensor is calculated, the components of the lower rank tensors can be derived from this rank-l tensor. For example the rank-0 tensor has only 1 component and is given in terms of the components of the rank-2 tensor by $D = 1/3(D_{xx} + D_{yy} + D_{zz})$. The derivations of these relations involve using the irreducible representation of the tensor and are given in [5].

10.2 Quantification of Anisotropy from Higher Rank Tensors

One of the most widely utilized achievements of DTI has been the parametrization of anisotropy, which produces a new contrast mechanism between highly structured tissue and others[2]. It has been found in numerous studies that changes in the neural tissue integrity due to many pathologies are reflected on the values obtained from anisotropy maps [7]. Many indices have been proposed to date that relate the observed signal intensities to an anisotropy value. Most of these formulations are based upon the rank-2 tensor model of DTI. In Chap. 17, Moakher and Batchelor present a new approach to the quantification of anisotropy from rank-2 diffusion tensors. However, the failure of DTI in the presence of orientational heterogeneity introduces a major problem in the anisotropy values calculated. This is because when there is more than one orientation within the voxel of interest, using the rank-2 tensor model gives rise

---

from the elasticity tensor E (a rank-4 tensor) through the relationship

$$U = \frac{1}{2} E_{ijkl}\, \zeta_{ij}\, \zeta_{kl} .$$

The differences in the properties of the elasticity tensor when compared to the rank-4 diffusion tensor stem from the fact that the former links the components of the strain tensor ζ (a rank-2 tensor) to a scalar whereas the diffusion tensor links the components of a vector (a rank-1 tensor) to a scalar.

[2] In Chap. 12, Kindlmann presents a comprehensive work on tensor invariants including anisotropy indices as well as other invariants.

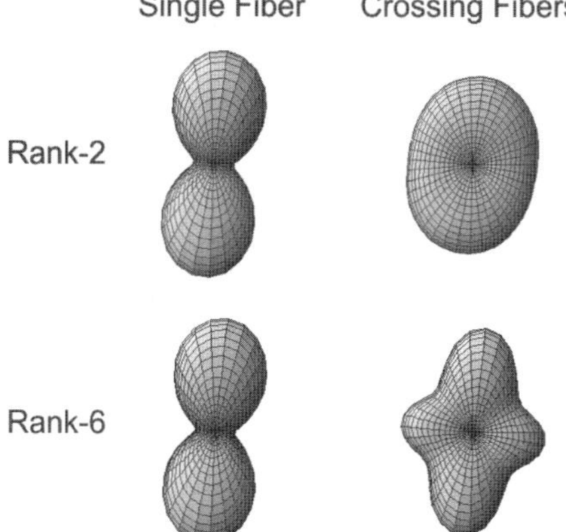

Fig. 10.1. Simulations of the diffusivity profiles from rank-2 (*top*) and rank-6 (*bottom*) tensors from a unidirectional voxel (*left*) and a voxel with two different fiber orientations (*right*). See colour plates

to an excessive smoothing of the diffusivity profile, hence a reduction in the anisotropy value [8]. In Fig. 10.1, we show the diffusivity profiles as implied by rank-2 and rank-6 tensors for simulated unidirectional and directionally heterogeneous voxels. It is clear that employment of a rank-2 tensor gives rise to a significant change in the diffusivity profiles in the presence of multiple orientations. As a result, one may expect inaccurate anisotropy values in such voxels if a rank-2 tensor model is used.

10.2.1 Generalization of Trace

The most widely used indices such as Fractional Anisotropy (FA) and Relative Anisotropy (RA) [9] are not readily generalizable to accomodate diffusivity profiles that are more general than those that can be generated by rank-2 tensors. Therefore, we attempt to express these indices in a way that may make it feasible to generalize them to higher rank tensors as well as to arbitrary functions defined on the surface of a unit sphere. We note that FA and RA can be expressed in terms of the trace of the square of a matrix $\mathsf{R} := \mathsf{D}/\mathrm{trace}(\mathsf{D})$ as

$$\mathrm{FA} = \sqrt{\frac{1}{2}\left(3 - \frac{1}{\mathrm{trace}(\mathsf{R}^2)}\right)}, \text{ and } \mathrm{RA} = \sqrt{3\,\mathrm{trace}(\mathsf{R}^2) - 1} \ . \tag{10.13}$$

The trace of a rank-2 tensor can be expressed as the integral of the quadratic forms of the tensor given by

$$\mathrm{trace}(\mathsf{D}) = \frac{3}{2\pi}\int_{\Omega} \mathbf{g}^{\mathrm{T}}\mathsf{D}\mathbf{g}\,\mathrm{d}\mathbf{g}\ , \tag{10.14}$$

where Ω is the unit hemisphere. Note that this expression can be generalized to functions whose domains are the unit hemisphere because $\mathbf{g}^{\mathrm{T}}\mathbf{D}\mathbf{g}$ is a function on Ω. We will denote this generalized trace operation with 'gentr'. For functions $f(\mathbf{g})$, with antipodal symmetry on the unit sphere, this operation is given by

$$\mathrm{gentr}(f(\mathbf{g})) = \frac{3}{2\pi} \int_{\Omega} f(\mathbf{g})\,\mathrm{d}\mathbf{g} \ . \tag{10.15}$$

Insertion of (10.7) into the above expression enables one to calculate the generalized trace of a rank-l tensor. We have shown that the generalized trace of a rank-l diffusion tensor is independent of the tensor rank and is just 3 times the mean diffusivity value [8].

10.2.2 Anisotropy in Terms of Variance

In this work, we formulate anisotropy in terms of the variance of the normalized diffusivity profile where normalization is achieved (in analogy with the definition of R above) via the expression

$$D_{\mathrm{N}}(\mathbf{g}) = \frac{D(\mathbf{g})}{\mathrm{gentr}(D(\mathbf{g}))} \ . \tag{10.16}$$

Next, instead of trace($\mathbf{R}^2$), we propose to use the quantity $\mathrm{gentr}(D_{\mathrm{N}}(\mathbf{g})^2)$. When a rank-$l$ tensor model is used, this quantity can be shown to be given by

$$\mathrm{gentr}(D_{\mathrm{N}}(\mathbf{g})^2) = \frac{1}{6\pi\langle D\rangle^2} \sum_{k_1=1}^{N_l} \sum_{k_2=1}^{N_l} \mu_{k_1} \mu_{k_2} D_{k_1} D_{k_2} \tag{10.17}$$

$$\times \left(\int_{\Omega} \mathrm{d}\mathbf{g} \prod_{p_1=1}^{l} \prod_{p_2=1}^{l} g_{k_1(p_1)} g_{k_2(p_2)} \right) ,$$

where mean diffusivity, $\langle D\rangle$, is just

$$\langle D\rangle = \frac{1}{2\pi} \sum_{i_1=1}^{3} \sum_{i_2=1}^{3} \cdots \sum_{i_l=1}^{3} D_{i_1 i_2 \ldots i_l} \int_{\Omega} g_{i_1} g_{i_2} \cdots g_{i_l}\,\mathrm{d}\mathbf{g} \ . \tag{10.18}$$

Note that the integrals in (10.17 and 10.18) can be evaluated analytically.

It is straightforward to show that the variance of the normalized diffusivities is related to $\mathrm{gentr}(D_N(\mathbf{g})^2)$ through the relationship

$$V := \mathrm{variance}(D_{\mathrm{N}}(\mathbf{g})) = \frac{1}{3}\left(\mathrm{gentr}(D_{\mathrm{N}}(\mathbf{g})^2) - \frac{1}{3} \right) \ . \tag{10.19}$$

This variance value takes its minimum value of 0 only when diffusivities along all directions are equal. This value is independent of l, i.e., the minimum value is the same for all tensor models. This is in contrast with the supremum value, which is achieved when the diffusivity profile is expressed as proportional to the outer product of same l vectors given by

$$D_{i_1 i_2 \ldots i_l} = D\, g'_{i_1} g'_{i_2} \cdots g'_{i_l} \ . \tag{10.20}$$

The variance value associated with this tensor is

$$\operatorname{sup\ variance}(D_{\mathrm{N}}(\mathbf{g})) = \frac{l^2}{9(2l+1)} \ . \tag{10.21}$$

In (10.20), $\mathbf{g}'$ is the unit vector specifying the direction of greatest diffusion coefficient and D is this maximal diffusivity. The form of the supremum value in (10.21) implies that

- the supremum value depends on the rank of the model
- there is a limit to the anisotropy of the profiles that can be characterized by lower rank tensor models
- when an arbitrary function is given[3] this supremum value is ∞.

As a result of the last of these findings, a general anisotropy index can be defined as a monotonic function that maps the interval $[0, \infty)$ to $[0, 1)$. Based on this, we define the generalized anisotropy index as

$$\mathrm{GA} := 1 - \frac{1}{1 + (250V)^{\varepsilon(V)}} \ , \tag{10.22}$$

where

$$\varepsilon(V) := 1 + \frac{1}{1 + 5000V} \ . \tag{10.23}$$

The particular form of this index differs from those of FA and RA in that FA and RA emphasize the variations among pixels with very low anisotropy values. However, the sensitivity of the GA images to changes in variance values is suppressed when those variance values are very small. As a result, the formulation of GA index as given in (10.22–10.23) ensure that the emphasized variations in the variance values are within a window that is more consistent with the variance values observed in the real datasets, increasing the contrast of the anisotropy images.

In Fig. 10.2, we show the GA images implied by rank-2 and rank-6 tensors where the sample is an excised rat brain acquired at 17.6T. Also included are the difference maps demonstrating how much the variance and GA values calculated from rank-6 tensors differ from those calculated from rank-2 tensors. Complicated architecture of the brain stem is distinguished as the bright pixels in the difference maps.

---

[3] Note that in this case the required tensor model is ∞.

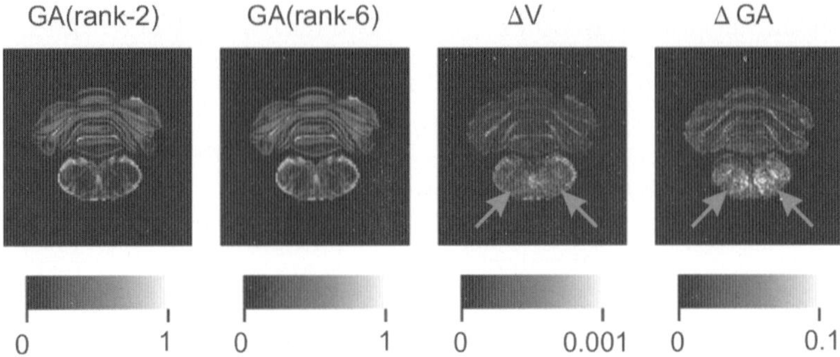

Fig. 10.2. GA values from rank-2 (left column) and rank-6 (second column) tensors from a coronal slice of an excised rat brain image. The right two columns show the difference between the variance and GA values when these two tensor models were used (see colour plates)

10.3 Fiber Orientations Implied by Higher Rank Tensors

The underlying hypothesis in the utilization of diffusion weighted imaging to map fiber orientations in tissue is that the major orientations along which diffusion occurs coincide with the fiber orientations. Therefore, in order for one to have a correct orientation map, he needs to accurately estimate a function $\overline{P}(\mathbf{x}, t_{\mathrm{d}})$ that is just the probability of water molecules to move a distance $\mathbf{x}$ during a time t_{d}. It is known from q-space imaging [10] that the average of this function over the voxel is just the Fourier transform of the signal attenuations (assuming $\delta << \Delta$), where the signal is envisioned to be on the reciprocal space of $\mathbf{x}$ defined by the gradient directions:

$$\overline{P}(\mathbf{x}, t_{\mathrm{d}}) = \int \mathrm{d}\mathbf{q} \, \frac{S(\mathbf{q})}{S_0} \, \exp(-i2\pi\mathbf{q} \cdot \mathbf{x}) \,, \qquad (10.24)$$

where $\mathbf{q} := (2\pi)^{-1}\gamma\delta G\mathbf{g}$.

Note that in the rank-2 tensor model of traditional DTI, making the substitution (from (10.4))

$$\frac{S(\mathbf{q})}{S_0} = \exp\left(-4\pi^2 q^2 t_{\mathrm{d}} \mathbf{g}^{\mathrm{T}} \mathbf{D}\mathbf{g})\right) \qquad (10.25)$$

into (10.24) results in the well-known oriented Gaussian displacement profile for water molecules

$$\overline{P}(\mathbf{x}, t_{\mathrm{d}}) = \frac{1}{\sqrt{(4\pi t_{\mathrm{d}})^3 \det(\mathbf{D})}} \, \exp\left(\frac{-\mathbf{x}^{\mathrm{T}} \mathbf{D}^{-1} \mathbf{x}}{4 t_{\mathrm{d}}}\right) \,. \qquad (10.26)$$

Although (10.25) is known to be incorrect for large values of $\mathbf{q}$, DTI has been found to be quite successful in the determination of fiber directions when the voxel of interest is unidirectional.

In the case of rank-2 DTI, in order to find the fiber direction, it is sufficient to diagonalize the diffusion tensor because the peak of the displacement and diffusivity profiles coincide and are given by the principal eigenvector of the diffusion tensor.

In this work, we generalize these ideas to the case when diffusion is characterized by a tensor of rank possibly higher than 2. Following the same lines with the above formulation, we make the same monoexponentiality assumption as in (10.25), and write

$$\frac{S(\mathbf{q})}{S_0} = \exp\left(-4\pi^2 q^2 t_\mathrm{d} D(\mathbf{g})\right) , \tag{10.27}$$

where in the case of a rank-l tensor model, $D(\mathbf{g})$ will be given by (10.7). It is a formidable task to analytically calculate the $\overline{P}(\mathbf{x}, t_\mathrm{d})$ function corresponding to a rank-l tensor model. Therefore, we adopt a numerical scheme in which we sample the q-space on a rectangular regular lattice using (10.27). We use a $64 \times 64 \times 64$ grid such that the largest q-value corresponds to a b-value of $60000 \, \mathrm{s/mm}^2$. Then we apply the FFT algorithm to estimate the displacement probabilities [11].

In Fig. 10.3, we show the simulations of 1, 2 and 3 fiber systems. Clearly rank-2 DTI fails to give meaningful results when there are more than one fiber directions. As seen in the third column, the peaks of the diffusivity profiles do not correspond to the fiber orientations when there are more than one fiber orientation. Increasing the rank of the tensor model however, enables the visualization of the different fiber bundles. In the last column, we apply a sharpening transformation to the isosurfaces of the displacement probability

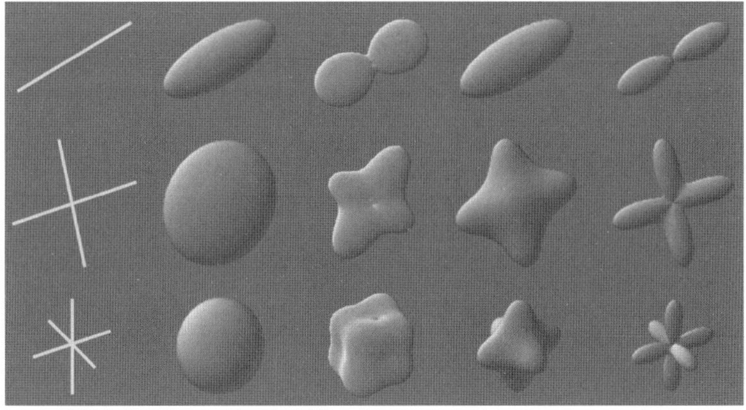

Fig. 10.3. The simulation results (see colour plates). The three rows show the 1, 2 and 3 fiber systems from top to bottom. The different columns show the orientations of the cylinders, probability isosurfaces obtained using rank-2 DTI, diffusivity profiles, equiprobability surfaces from rank-6 DTI, and these probability surfaces after a sharpening transformation (from *left* to *right*)

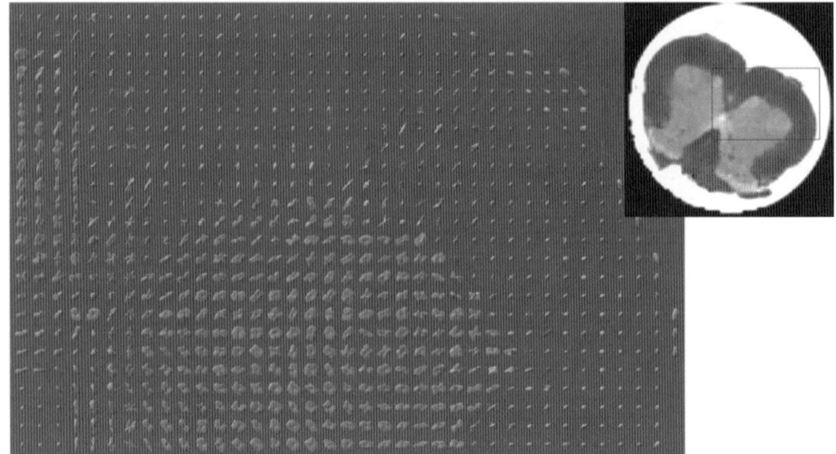

Fig. 10.4. Isosurfaces of displacement probability functions implied by a rank-6 tensor model from a selected region of interest (ROI) in an excised rat spinal cord image. The top right image is from a non-diffusion weighted dataset showing the ROI where the probability isosurfaces were calculated (see colour plates)

profile that involves the removal of the largest sphere that fits into the surface. This step can be thought of as an operation analogous to disregarding of the smaller eigenvalues of the diffusion tensor in traditional DTI.

Figure 10.4 shows the sharpened isosurfaces of the displacement profiles calculated on a slice of excised rat spinal cord imaged at 14.1 T. The rank of the tensor model employed was 6. Fiber crossings are visible in many areas in the spinal cord, particularly in the ventral nerve roots that travel among white-matter fiber bundles in a direction perpendicular to them and causing partial volume effects. Also note the complicated structure in gray-matter where most fibers are oriented in the plane of the image.

Acknowledgments

We would like to acknowledge Dr. Tim M. Shepherd of Neuroscience department for useful discussions. This work was supported by National Institutes of Health grant numbers P41-RR16105 and R01-NS42075. The magnetic resonance images were acquired in the Advanced Magnetic Resonance Imaging and Spectroscopy Facility of the McKnight Brain Institute. The experiments on animal tissue were performed with the approval of the University of Florida Institutional Animal Care and Use Committee.

References

1. Basser P. J., Mattiello J., et al. (1994) MR diffusion tensor spectroscopy and imaging. Biophys. J. **66** (1), 259–267.
2. Basser P. J., Mattiello J., et al. (1994) Estimation of the effective self-diffusion tensor from the NMR spin echo. J. Magn. Reson. B **103**(3), 247–254.
3. Torrey H. C. (1956) Bloch equations with diffusion terms. Phys. Rev. **104**(3), 563–565.
4. Stejskal E. O., Tanner J. E. (1965) Spin diffusion measurements: Spin echoes in the presence of a time-dependent field gradient. J. Chem. Phys. **42**(1), 288–292.
5. Özarslan E., Mareci T. H. (2003) Generalized diffusion tensor imaging and analytical relationships between diffusion tensor imaging and high angular resolution diffusion imaging. Magn. Reson. Med. **50**, 955–965.
6. Schouten J. A. (1989) Tensor Analysis for Physicists. New York Dover Publications.
7. Dong Q., Welsh R. C., et al. (2004) Clinical applications of diffusion tensor imaging. J. Magn. Reson. Imaging **19**(1), 6–18.
8. Özarslan E., Vemuri B. C., et al. (2004) Generalized scalar measures for diffusion MRI using trace, variance and entropy. Magn. Reson. Med., *accepted.*
9. Basser P. J. (1995) Inferring microstructural features and the physiological state of tissues from diffusion–weighted images. NMR Biomed. **8**, 333–344.
10. Callaghan P. T. (1991) Principles of Nuclear Magnetic Resonance Microscopy. Oxford Clarendon Press.
11. Özarslan E., Vemuri B. C., et al. (2004) Multiple fiber orientations resolved by generalized diffusion tensor imaging. Proc. Intl. Soc. Mag. Reson. Med. 89.

Visualization of Tensor Fields

11

Strategies for Direct Visualization of Second-Rank Tensor Fields

Werner Benger[1,2] and Hans-Christian Hege[1]

[1] Zuse-Institute Berlin, Takustrasse 7, D-14195 Berlin-Dahlem, Germany
[2] Max-Planck Institute for Gravitational Physics (Albert-Einstein Institute), Am Mühlenberg 1, D-14476 Golm/Potsdam, Germany
{benger,hege}@zib.de

Summary. Tensor field visualization aims either at depiction of the full information contained in the field or at extraction and display of specific features. Here, we focus on the first task and evaluate integral and glyph based methods with regard to their power of providing an intuitive visual representation. Tensor fields are considered in a differential geometric context, using a coordinate-free notation when possible. An overview and classification of glyph-based methods is given and selected innovative visualization techniques are presented in more detail. The techniques are demonstrated for applications from medicine and relativity theory.

11.1 Introduction

We consider tensor fields which are given either analytically or numerically on a discrete mesh. For the last kind of data we assume that the we are able to reconstruct the underlying continuous field approximately employing some interpolation method (as described in Chap. 17 by Moakher and Batchelor, Chap. 18 by Pajevic et al., and Chap. 19 by Weickert and Welk).

Depicting tensor fields, two major problems arise: first, the large number of degrees of freedom to be displayed at each point and, second, for data in more than two dimensions, the view occlusion to be minimized. The tensor degrees of freedom have to be mapped to graphical degrees of freedom like color, transparency, reflectivity, texture patterns and shape. Encoding all degrees of freedom of a tensor field into the parameter space of just one of these categories is difficult, if not impossible.

Ideally one would like to map all degrees of freedom to graphical encodings at each point in space. However, texture patterns and shaped objects are spatially extended, and color plus transparency encompass essentially only four degrees of freedom. The occlusion problem is usually tackled by employing transparency and depicting sparsely distributed thin objects like, e.g., lines. Direct tensor field visualization techniques can thus be differentiated

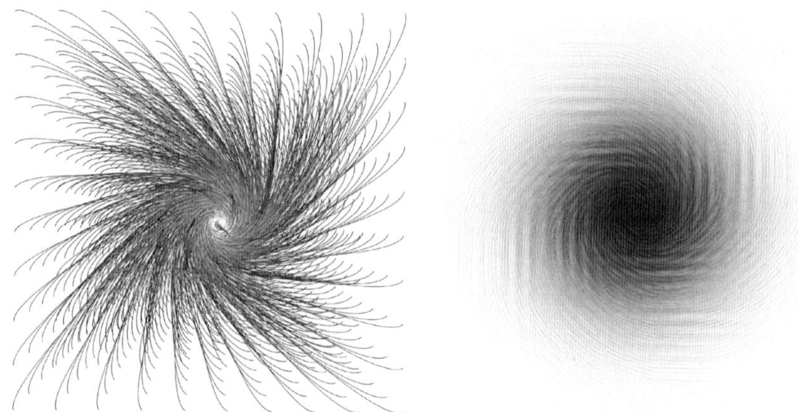

Fig. 11.1. Maelstrom of spacetime around a rotating black hole, visualized via integral lines (*left*) and vertex-based glyphs (*right*) See also color plates

in those computing integral lines or surfaces, and others displaying the field per vertex in the entire volume by drawing tiny objects, so-called 'glyphs', cf. Fig. 11.1. We will discuss the benefits of both approaches, concentrating on the mathematical aspects of integral manifolds in the first part, and focusing on rendering glyphs in the second part of the chapter.

We do not delve into feature based (indirect) visualization methods that aim at extraction and graphical representation of specific structural features of the tensor field, like e.g. topological ones. For further information about this class of visualization techniques, see Chap. 13 by Tricoche et al., Chap. 14 by Zheng et al., and Chap. 15 by Wischgoll and Meyer.

11.1.1 Basic Notation

In computer graphics, one usually considers vector operations in Euclidean space E^n with dimension n. A more general concept is a *differentiable manifold*[1]. A *curve* γ within a manifold is a continuous map $\gamma : \mathbb{R} \to M : s \mapsto \gamma(s)$,

---

[1] A *manifold* is a topological Hausdorff space that looks locally like the ordinary Euclidean space E^n, i.e. every point has an open neighbourhood homeomorphic to an open subset of E^n. To work with these objects one uses *coordinate charts* which are homeomorphisms between open sets of M and open sets of E^n. A collection of charts which cover M is called an *atlas* of M. The homeomorphisms of two overlapping charts provide a transition map from a subset of E^n to some other subset of E^n. If all these maps are k times continuously differentiable, then the atlas is an C^k *atlas*. C^k atlases are called equivalent if their union is a C^k atlas (this is an equivalence relation). A C^k *manifold* is defined to be a manifold together with an equivalence class of C^k atlases. If all the connecting maps are infinitely often differentiable, then one speaks of a C^∞ *manifold* or *differentiable manifold*

where s is called the *curve parameter*. The set of all points of a curve within a manifold is a *line*; it can be thought of as an equivalence class of infinitely many curves with different parameterizations.

In contrast to Euclidean space, a manifold is not necessarily a vector space. However, associated with a manifold M is a *tangential space* $T_p(M)$ at each point $p \in M$. Tangential spaces[2] are vector spaces, their elements are *tangential vectors* which can be thought of as the vectors which are tangent to lines through point p. A *covariant tensor* of rank n is a multilinear map $T_p(M)^n \to \mathbb{R}$ that maps n tangential vectors to a real number. Its co-ordinates with respect to a specific basis are given by applying it to combinations of n basis vectors of the n vector spaces.

The set of all tangential spaces on all points of a manifold[3] is called the *tangential bundle* $\mathcal{T}(M)$. This is an example of a vector bundle, i.e. a vector space depending on parameters – the parameters being in a manifold. Choosing a specific vector v_p at each point $p \in M$ gives a *vector field* (also called 'section of a bundle'). Since the tensor product is independent of any choice of the basis, tensor products of tangential bundles on M can be taken. The component-free treatment of tensors carries over – again independently of co-ordinates. In this geometric setting, a *tensor field* is a section of a tensor field bundle, which assigns a tensor to each point $p \in M$.

A covariant tensor of rank 1 thus is a linear functional on $T_p(M)$ and is also called *co-vector*. In Euclidean space, there is an isomorphism between tangential vectors and co-vectors, and there is no need to distinguish them. In curved space, such as the surface of sphere, this not anymore true.

All these terms are defined without any coordinates. Expressing mathematical statements in a co-ordinate free fashion guarantees that the statements are valid not only in certain coordinates but in any chart. But for numerical compuations, one needs to deal with representations of these objects in coordinate systems. For a n-dimensional manifold, a tensor g of rank two is represented by a $n \times n$ matrix (g) in a coordinate system. Such a tensor may also be used to map a tangential vector to a co-vector. Tangential vectors which are mapped to their isomorphic representation as co-vectors (same numerical representation in Euclidean space) are called *eigenvectors*. In Euclidean space, this corresponds to the matrix multiplication $gv_i = \lambda_i v_i$

---

[2] Suppose M is a C^k manifold ($k \geq 1$) and p is a point in M. Select a chart $\phi : U \to R^n$ where U is an open subset of M containing p. Suppose two curves $\gamma_1 : (-1, 1) \to M$ and $\gamma_2 : (-1, 1) \to M$ with $\gamma_1(0) = \gamma_2(0) = p$ are given such that $\phi \circ \gamma_1$ and $\phi \circ \gamma_2$ are both differentiable at 0. Then γ_1 and γ_2 are called *tangent at* 0, if the ordinary derivatives of $\phi \circ \gamma_1$ and $\phi \circ \gamma_2$ coincide. This is an equivalence relation and the equivalence classes are the *tangent vectors* of M at p. The equivalence class of the curve γ is written as $\gamma'(0)$. The tangent space of M at p, denoted by $T_p(M)$, is defined as the set of all tangent vectors; it does not depend on the choice of the chart.

[3] The elements of the tangential bundle $\mathcal{T}(M)$ are pairs (p, v) with $p \in M$ and $v \in T_p(M)$. $\mathcal{T}(M)$ itself is is a manifold of dimension $2n$.

with g the tensor, v_i the ith eigenvector and λ_i the ith eigenvalue. There may be at most n independent eigenvalues and eigenvectors. The eigenvector which corresponds to the largest eigenvalue is called the *principal eigenvector*. A visualization scheme for eigenvalues is presented in Chap. 12 by Kindlmann.

If only m out of n eigenvectors are linearly independent with $m < n$, then the matrix (g) is singular, i.e. not invertible. In this case, at most m eigenvalues will differ. However, the reverse is not true: linearly independent eigenvectors may still share the same eigenvalues. In this case, the eigenvalues are said to be *degenerated* and the points in a manifold where the tensor's eigenvalues degenerate are called *degenerated points* of the tensor field[4]. If all eigenvalues are identical, then the tensor is *isotropic*. However, the term 'degenerate' is also used for bi-linear forms and metric tensor fields: here it denotes a tensor field which is not invertible on specific points, subregions or the whole domain. Both notions of 'degenerate' do not neccessarily coincide.

11.1.2 Classification and Properties of Tensor Fields

At first, we need to determine the *symmetry properties* with respect to permutations of indices of a rank two tensor field: is it *symmetric*, like the diffusion tensor field in magneto-resonance imaging (DT-MRI) or like the metric tensor field in general relativity; is it *antisymmetric*, or does it contain *no symmetries* at all, like the Jacobi matrix of a general vector field? Any general tensor field can be decomposed into a symmetric and an antisymmetric part, so one can defer the visualization of a generic tensor field into two sub-tasks. In three dimensions, an antisymmetric tensor field of rank 2 consists of three independent components and is thus equivalent (homeomorphic) to a vector field. For an n-dimensional manifold, the number of independent quantities for general tensors of rank 2 is n^2, whereby the symmetric part contributes $n(n+1)/2$ components and the antisymmetric part $n(n-1)/2$. The homeomorphism between the antisymmetric part and a vector field thus only exists in three dimensions.

An important property of a tensor field that needs to be known before selecting an appropriate visualization method is its *definiteness:* A multilinear map $g : V \times V \rightarrow \mathbb{R} : (\mathbf{x}, \mathbf{y}) \mapsto g(\mathbf{x}, \mathbf{y})$, with V a vector space, is *positive definite* if $\forall \mathbf{v} \in V$ with $\mathbf{v} \neq \mathbf{0} : g(\mathbf{v}, \mathbf{v}) > 0$. If $g(\mathbf{v}, \mathbf{v}) \geq 0$, then g is called positive semi-definite. This property is equivalent to requiring all eigenvalues of the tensor field to be positive at each point $p \in M$.

For positive-definite symmetric three-dimensional tensors of rank two we may compute linear, planar and spherical shape factors [WPG$^+$97] from its eigenvalues: $c_l = (\lambda_{max} - \lambda_{med})/tr(g)$, $c_p = 2(\lambda_{med} - \lambda_{min})/tr(g)$ and $c_s = 3\lambda_{min}/tr(g)$, where $tr(g) = \lambda_{max} + \lambda_{med} + \lambda_{min}$ is the trace of the tensor. The three shape factors obey the relationship $c_l + c_p + c_s = 1$ and can thus be interpreted as barycentric coordinates within a triangle.

---

[4] See also Chap. 14 by Zheng, Tricoche and Pang as well as Chap. 16 by Hotz et al.

11.2 Visualization via Integral Manifolds

Because powerful vector field visualization techniques already exist, we want to try these first. A straightforward approach is to employ vector field visualization methods to the eigenvectors of a tensor field. Since field lines are very useful for vector field visualization, we review vector field integral methods first and discuss their applicability to eigenvector fields. Dealing also with time-dependent fields, we take a spacetime point of view (see also [TWHS05]). However, tensor fields are richer in information and thus can only partially be represented by eigenvector integral lines. A more appropriate approach is visualization of geodesics.

11.2.1 Integral Lines in Vector Fields

An *integral line* $q \subset M$ on a vector field $v \in \mathcal{T}(M)$ within a manifold M with starting point $q_0 \in M^5$ is defined via

$$\dot{q} \equiv \frac{d}{ds} q(s) = v(q(s)) \quad \text{with} \quad q(0) = q_0 \,. \tag{11.1}$$

Integral lines are also called *trajectories* or *tangent curves*. They describe the path of a point-like particle in the flow of a vector field. In coordinates, q describes spatial and temporal information; usually only three-dimensional, but possibly time-dependent (non-stationary) vector fields are considered. Then we may use the time coordinate as the curve parameter and equation (11.1) reduces to three equations

$$\dot{q}^a(s) = v^a(q^t(s), q^1(s), q^2(s), q^3(s)), \quad q^t(s) = s \tag{11.2}$$

whereby $a = 1, 2, 3$ describes spatial coordinates.

In the case of a stationary vector field or when investigating a vector field at some instance of time, we may drop the time dependency and by solving

$$\dot{q}^a(s) = v^a(q^t(s), q^1(s), q^2(s), q^3(s)), \quad q^t(s) = q^t(0) \tag{11.3}$$

we get lines known as *field lines* or *stream lines*. They correspond to the flow direction of many particles which are spread around in the volume of the vector field. Path lines and stream lines are both one-dimensional manifolds; they can't cross each other, since at each point their direction is uniquely determined by the given vector field. A stream line is a static object, all of its points belong to the same time slice, whereas a path line is constructed by points from different time instances. A path line can be considered as the projection of a stream line within an time-dependent n-dimensional manifold

---

[5] If M is a spacetime manifold, we call a point, i.e. a spatial location together with a specific point in time, an 'event'.

onto an $n-1$ dimensional spatial submanifold. This projection *may* intersect itself.

Beside the inspection of lines that start from a single event q_0, we can also study the behavior of a bundle of lines that start from a set of events, e.g. some 'initial seed' line $q_0(\tau) : I \to M$ with $I \subset \mathbb{R}$. The *integral surface* $S \subset M$ within a vector field $v \in \mathcal{T}(M)$ with initial seed line q_0 is then constructed from all integral lines that pass through an event on this initial seed line:

$$S = \{q : \mathbb{R} \to M, \ \dot{q}(s) = v(q(s)), \ q(0) = q_0(\tau)\} \ . \tag{11.4}$$

It contains a natural parametrization $S(s, \tau)$ by the initial seed parameter τ and the integration length s. The intersection of an 2-dimensional surface within a n-dimensional manifold with a $n-1$ sub-manifold does not necessarily yield a one-dimensional manifold and thus may lead to lines that can self-intersect.

A commonly used choice is to use a timelike initial seed line $q_0(\tau) = (\tau, q^1, q^2, q^3)$ with fixed spatial coordinates q^1, q^2, q^3 (we can call such a seed line a 'location', since it describes a point in space independent of time). The resulting integral surface will then be spanned by a timelike tangential vector ∂_t and a spacelike tangential vector ∂_s. For a fixed time coordinate t the projection of the integral surface into a time slice $dt = 0$ yields a line, called a '*streak line*'. It is formed by the location of all particles that have passed (or will pass) through a specific point $q_0(t)$ at some time t. For stationary vector fields, integral lines will be independent of time, and so streak lines will coincide with stream lines.

Another choice is to use a spacelike initial seed line $q_0(\tau) = (q^0, q^1(\tau), q^2(\tau), q^3(\tau))$. The image of the seed line under evolution, the line $S(s, \tau)|_{s=const}$ is called a '*material line*' or '*time line*'. The surface S is called a *stream surface*. Improved algorithms for computing a stream surface, based on the original one by Hultquist [Hul92], are given in [Sta98] and [GTS$^+$04].

Sometimes higher dimensional initial seed data are used, revealing surfaces or volumes evolving under the flow map of the underlying vector field. For instance, evolving a timelike two-dimensional initial seed surface (spatially a line) yields *streak surfaces* in the spatial projection of the resulting timelike volume. In general, these spatial projections are not manifolds and may penetrate themselves like streak lines.

11.2.2 Eigenvector Stream Lines

It is a straightforward approach to employ vector field visualization methods to the principal eigenvectors of a tensor field g. However, treatment of eigenvectors needs to consider the following two aspects:

- The principal eigenvector is undefined in isotropic regions. Its direction is ambiguous and may vary due to slight numerical instabilities.

- The sign of eigenvectors is undefined, since $-\mathbf{v}$ is a solution of the eigenvalue equation $g \cdot \mathbf{v} = \lambda \mathbf{v}$ as well. We may call a vector whose sign is left open a '*pre-vector*' (as a not yet fully determined vector).

The difference among pre-vector and vector fields is important. For instance, it is possible to find a pre-vector field representing the tangential vectors of a non-orientable manifold. Consider, e.g., a three-dimensional pre-vector field that is tangential to a Moebius strip in a volume, and getting smoothly zero farther away from the Moebius strip. Since the Moebius strip is a non-orientable manifold, also its associated tangential pre-vector field cannot be oriented globally to yield a vector field. Thus in general it is not possible to apply unmodified vector field visualization methods to eigenvectors. Furthermore, due to the eigenvector ambiguity within isotropic regions, unmodified vector field visualizations find and display features which are not a property of the data field, but stem from the numerical eigenvalue extraction algorithm (isotropy artifacts). Modified interpolation and/or integration methods are required for eigenvector fields:

- When interpolating eigenvectors within a cell, all vectors contributing to the interpolation must be oriented such that they point into the same half-space, i.e. $\mathbf{v}_i \cdot \mathbf{v}_j \geq 0$ ('*local alignment*').
- Interpolating eigenvectors yields different results than interpolating the tensor field and computing the eigenvector at each interpolation point. The choice of the most appropriate interpolation method for tensor fields is an open issue by itself (see Chaps. 17–19).
- Stream line integration advances a point $q(s)$ of the stream line q to the next point $q(s + ds)$ by a small step size ds via

$$q(s + ds) = q(s) + ds\ \dot{\mathbf{q}}(s) , \tag{11.5}$$

whereby the new tangential direction is the direction of the vector field $\mathbf{v}$ at the point of interest $q(s)$

$$\dot{\mathbf{q}}(s) = \mathbf{v}\big|_{q(s)} . \tag{11.6}$$

Here, $\mathbf{v}$ is the solution of the eigenvalue equation $G\mathbf{v} = \lambda\mathbf{v}$ at the point $q(s)$ such that $\mathbf{v} \cdot q(s) \geq 0$. This last condition of local alignment during integration is essential and needs to be added to a usual stream line integration algorithm.
- Local alignment does not cure the problems arising from isotropy artifacts. Stream lines of the principal eigenvector only lead to reasonable results in regions with one dominant eigenvalue. An alternative, less vulnerable integration algorithm is to start stream lines in regions with high linearity and to advance it according to the deviation vector[6] $g \cdot \dot{\mathbf{q}}$:

---

[6] The operation $g \cdot \dot{\mathbf{q}}$ actually yields a co-vector, such that the deviation vector is the isomorphic correspondence, which is no longer numerically identical in the case of a non-flat base manifold.

$$\mathbf{v} = g \cdot \dot{\mathbf{q}} \quad \rightarrow \quad q(s + ds) = q(s) + ds\,\mathbf{v}\,. \qquad (11.7)$$

Integral lines of deviation vector fields are e.g. used in [ZP03b]. The method of 'tensor lines' [WKL99] combines this method by blending the oriented principal eigenvector $\mathbf{v}_{max}$ and the deviation vector with the linearity shape factor c_l at the point $q(s + 1)$:

$$\mathbf{v} = c_l\,\mathbf{v}_{max} + (1 - c_l)\left[(1 - w)\,\dot{\mathbf{q}}(s) + w\,g \cdot \dot{\mathbf{q}}\right]\,. \qquad (11.8)$$

Hereby w is a user-controlled 'stiffness' parameter in the range $[0, 1]$ which is said to be selected depending on the type of data.

- Both integral lines as solution of (11.7) and tensor lines don't provide a unique direction at each point in space, thus intersections of lines may occur – in contrast to non-intersecting stream lines.

11.2.3 Visualization of Eigenvector Stream Lines

Hyperstreamlines [DH93] are a widely known technique for visualizing eigenvector streamlines. They encode the median and minimal eigenvectors as elliptical cross-section and the eigenvalue maximum as color along the streamline. However, they severely suffer from isotropy artifacts and, while they are good for inspecting single lines, they are afflicted with view occlusion problems when depicting a large data volume. An alternative approach is to use the technique of illuminated stream lines [ZSH96] upon eigenvector fields. As the cross-section is infinitely small here, we may encode the additional tensor field quantities as transparency and line distribution density. To reduce or even avoid anisotropy artifacts, the transparency is set proportional to the isotropy, using the spherical shape factor c_s. Consequently, lines in isotropic regions of undefined principal eigenvector become invisible, although a stream line of the principal eigenvector field continues there technically. The seed points for the stream line integration, which determines the density and number of stream lines, are set dominantly in regions where one eigenvector is dominant (density chosen to be proportional to the linear shape factor c_l), because only then there is a unique direction. As a result, stream lines start in highly linear regions, may traverse through planar regions but are less dense there and vanish in isotropic parts of the volume data set.

This approach is very suitable for full three-dimensional visualization of a data set as in Fig. 11.2 and is able to display most of the tensor field features, including isotropic and linear regions in a comprehensible way (see Fig. 11.3). However, due to the three-dimensional nature of stream lines, it is not applicable to two-dimensional slices or for point-wise detailed inspection of a data set. Also, planar regions are not visualized correctly, since eigenvector stream lines visually suggest only one direction there.

An alternative approach on visualizing vector fields is line integral convolution (LIC). Its extension to tensor fields leads to methods such as HyperLIC, see [ZP03a] or Chap. 16 by Hotz et al.

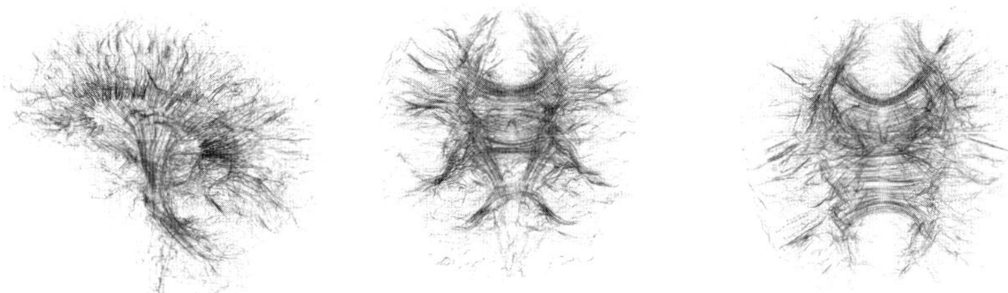

Fig. 11.2. Front, side and top view of stream lines along the maximum eigenvector in linear regions of a human brain data set. See also color plates

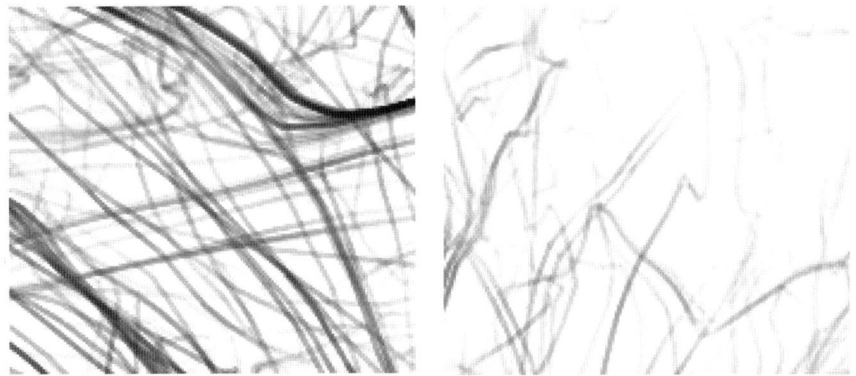

Fig. 11.3. Magnification of two regions showing stream lines along the principal eigenvector. *Left*: stable lines in linear regions, depicted pronouncedly. *Right*: unstable lines in more isotropic regions, depicted more transparently

11.2.4 Geodesics

A positive definite tensor field of rank two can be interpreted as a metric tensor field and used to measure distances among points in space and time. This interpretation can be used to compute embedding diagrams as in [Hot02, BAS02].

[OHW02] interpreted a diffusion tensor field as a metric tensor field and computed geodesics there. They employed Dijkstra's algorithm and a level set method to compute all possible geodesics originating from a single point. Here, we review the computation of a single geodesic as a corresponding extension of stream lines within a vector field to tensor fields.

An *extremal line* is the shortest or longest (i.e. most extreme) connection between two points. It is determined by the metric tensor field. A curve $q(s)$ is the most extreme connection between two points $A = q(s_1)$ and $B = q(s_2)$ if and only if

$$\int_{s_1}^{s_2} \sqrt{|g(\dot{q}(s), \dot{q}(s))|}\, ds = \text{minimum} . \tag{11.9}$$

We may employ the Lagrange formalism to derive a differential equation for the curve $q(s)$. If we take the *square* of the length of the tangential vectors as Lagrange function,

$$\mathcal{L}(q^k(s), \dot{q}^k(s)) = g(\dot{q}(s), \dot{q}(s)) = \dot{q}^\mu \dot{q}^\nu g_{\mu\nu} \tag{11.10}$$

then the parameterization of the curve becomes fixed and the solutions are extremal lines parameterized by their affine parameters. These curves are called *geodesics*. By inserting (11.10) into the Euler-Lagrange-equations and a little algebra we arrive at the coordinate expression for the geodesic equation

$$\ddot{q}^\lambda + \Gamma^\lambda_{\mu\nu} \dot{q}^\mu \dot{q}^\nu = 0 \, , \tag{11.11}$$

whereby $\Gamma^\lambda_{\mu\nu}$ are the so-called *Christoffel symbols* and $\ddot{q}^\lambda$ denotes the second derivative of the coordinate expression $q^\lambda(s)$ by the curve parameter. They abbreviate an expression involving only the metric and its first partial derivatives:

$$\Gamma^\lambda_{\mu\nu} := \frac{1}{2} g^{\lambda\alpha} \left(g_{\mu\alpha,\nu} + g_{\nu\alpha,\mu} - g_{\mu\nu,\alpha} \right) \, . \tag{11.12}$$

Here, the comma denotes the partial derivative by a coordinate function, i.e. $g_{\mu\alpha,\nu} \equiv \partial g_{\mu\alpha}/\partial x^\nu$. The partial derivative of a tensor $g_{\mu\alpha,\nu}$ (or even of a vector $v^\mu{}_{,\nu}$) does not yield a tensor again; it may be zero in all components in one coordinate system while non-zero in another ones. Consequently, the Christoffel symbols $\Gamma^\lambda_{\mu\nu}$ do not form a tensor, too. The Christoffel symbols can be used to define the *covariant derivative* of a tensor field that does not depend on the choice of coordinates. This covariant derivative is denoted by a semicolon, e.g. $v^\mu{}_{;\nu}$. Its coordinate expression for a vector field is given by

$$v^\mu{}_{;\nu} = v^\mu{}_{,\nu} + \Gamma^\mu_{\lambda\nu} v^\lambda \, . \tag{11.13}$$

The *directional derivative* of a vector field is just the linear combination of covariant derivatives and the components of the direction of interest. This operation is written as $\nabla_u v := v^\mu{}_{;\nu} u^\nu \partial_\mu$. Differently from partial derivatives, covariant derivatives in general do not commute: $v^\mu{}_{,\nu,\lambda} = v^\mu{}_{,\lambda,\nu}$, but $v^\mu{}_{;\nu;\lambda} \neq v^\mu{}_{;\lambda;\nu}$. As the covariant derivative yields a tensor, so does the difference of two covariant derivatives. This tensor is the Riemannian curvature tensor:

$$K^\mu_{\nu\lambda\sigma} v^\sigma = v^\mu{}_{;\nu;\lambda} - v^\mu{}_{;\lambda;\nu} \, . \tag{11.14}$$

It is used in general relativity to form the left-hand side of the Einstein field equations of the gravitational field (via contraction). The Riemann tensor is a map $K : V \times V \times V \to V$ and is defined in coordinate free notation with $u, v, w \in V$ based on the directional derivative ∇ and the commutator $[u, v] = u(v) - v(u)$:

$$K(u, v)w := \nabla_u \nabla_v w - \nabla_v \nabla_u w - \nabla_{[u,v]} w \, . \tag{11.15}$$

The Riemann tensor only depends on the metric, its first and second partial derivatives. The first partial derivatives may vanish in a certain coordinate system, but the second ones do not. Thus, the Riemann tensor allows a coordinate-independent classification of the underlying metric tensor fields. If all of its components vanish in one coordinate system, then the metric space associated with the tensor field is said to be *flat*.

11.2.5 Geodesic Deviation

The difference among close geodesics as depicted by the cross-section of a geodesic bundle depends on differences of the Christoffel symbols and thus directly visualizes the Riemann tensor. Let $\Phi(s,t) : \mathbb{R}^2 \to M$ denote a two-dimensional family of geodesics such that for fixed parameter t the curves $\gamma(s) := \Phi(s, t = const.)$ are geodesics. Let $\delta := \frac{d}{dt}\Phi(s,t) \in \mathcal{T}(M)$ denote the deviation vector of points on the geodesics with same parameter $s \in \mathbb{R}$, also known as the *Jacobi field* of the geodesics [O'N83]. Here the dot denotes the derivative by the geodesic parameter s, which is given by the directional derivative along the geodesic:

$$\dot{\delta} := \frac{d}{ds}\delta \equiv \nabla_{\dot{\gamma}}\delta \tag{11.16}$$

We may also describe the deviation by an vector field $\delta \in \mathcal{T}(M)$ that is transported along the geodesic bundle, i.e. its evolution is described by the flow map along the geodesics. This requires its Lie derivative $\mathcal{L}_{\dot{\gamma}}\delta$ to vanish (see [Ben04] for illustration):

$$0 = \mathcal{L}_{\dot{\gamma}}\delta \equiv [\dot{\gamma}, \delta] = \dot{\gamma}\delta - \delta\dot{\gamma} = \nabla_{\dot{\gamma}}\delta - \nabla_{\delta}\dot{\gamma} \tag{11.17}$$

and we see that

$$\nabla_{\dot{\gamma}}\delta = -\nabla_{\delta}\dot{\gamma} \ . \tag{11.18}$$

If we compute the second derivative by the affine parameter we get

$$\ddot{\delta} := \frac{d^2}{ds^2}\delta \equiv \nabla_{\dot{\gamma}}\nabla_{\dot{\gamma}}\delta = -\nabla_{\dot{\gamma}}\nabla_{\delta}\dot{\gamma} \ . \tag{11.19}$$

Recalling definition (11.15) of the Riemann tensor $K(u,v)w$ and inserting $u = \delta$, $w = v = \dot{\gamma}$ yields:

$$K(\delta, \dot{\gamma})\dot{\gamma} = \nabla_{\delta}\nabla_{\dot{\gamma}}\dot{\gamma} - \nabla_{\dot{\gamma}}\nabla_{\delta}\dot{\gamma} - \nabla_{[\delta,\dot{\gamma}]}\dot{\gamma} \ . \tag{11.20}$$

$\nabla_{\dot{\gamma}}\dot{\gamma} = 0$ is just the geodesic equation and from (11.17) we know that $[\delta, \dot{\gamma}] = 0$. Thus we see that the second derivative of the deviation vector is linearly related to the Riemann curvature tensor:

$$\ddot{\delta} = K(\delta, \dot{\gamma})\dot{\gamma} \ . \tag{11.21}$$

The evolution of the deviation vector in a chart is given by the coordinate expression

$$\ddot{\delta}^{\mu}\partial_{\mu} = K^{\mu}{}_{\alpha\beta\nu}\delta^{\alpha}\dot{\gamma}^{\beta}\dot{\gamma}^{\nu}\,\partial_{\mu}\;. \tag{11.22}$$

In flat space $K = 0$ in any coordinate system and no focusing happens. The deviation vector then describes just a linear expansion of a geodesic bundle like a cone, depending on its initial cross-section δ and opening angle $\dot{\delta}$. The influence of curved space on a geodesic bundle, e.g. as depicted in Fig. 11.4, is also known as 'Ricci focusing' and plays a central role in gravitational lens theory. See also Fig. 11.12. An extensive discussion of theory and application can be found in [SSE94, SEF99].

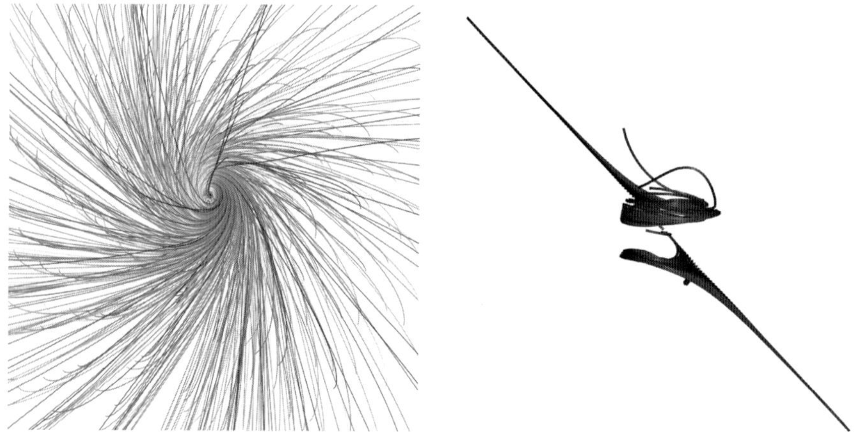

Fig. 11.4. Particle geodesics in the vicinity of a rotating black hole. The congruence of the geodesics is a direct visualization of the Riemann tensor, which is a central component of the Einstein equations describing the gravitational field in general relativity. The change of proper distances among geodesic paths thus indicates that the spacetime is non-Euclidean, i.e. it has a non-vanishing Riemann tensor due to some mass distribution. See also color plates

11.3 Vertex-Based Visualization Methods

A symmetric tensor of rank two at a point p may be represented graphically by the set of all vectors $\mathbf{v}$ which are mapped to the same length ℓ, i.e. $g(\mathbf{v}, \mathbf{v}) = \ell$. This set of vectors corresponds to a set of points which have distance ℓ from the point p as measured with a metric tensor g. The coordinate expression is quadratic, so these points form a quadric surface, i.e. an ellipsoid (a hyperboloid in general) for a positive definite tensor field on a three dimensional base manifold. If g is a metric tensor, this surface can be interpreted physically as the shape of a light sphere emitted from a certain point.

11.3.1 Rendering Metric Ellipsoids

The quadric surface is defined by all vectors with the same length ℓ when measured with the tensor field g as a metric, i.e. $g(\mathbf{v}, \mathbf{v}) = \ell$. Any unit vector $\mathbf{e}$ has a corresponding 'metric' unit vector $\mathbf{v} = \mathbf{e}/\sqrt{g(\mathbf{e}, \mathbf{e})}$ which fulfills $g(\mathbf{v}, \mathbf{v}) = 1$:

$$g(\mathbf{v}, \mathbf{v}) = g\left(\frac{\mathbf{e}}{\sqrt{g(\mathbf{e}, \mathbf{e})}}, \frac{\mathbf{e}}{\sqrt{g(\mathbf{e}, \mathbf{e})}}\right) = \frac{g(\mathbf{e}, \mathbf{e})}{\sqrt{g(\mathbf{e}, \mathbf{e})}\sqrt{g(\mathbf{e}, \mathbf{e})}} = 1 \ . \tag{11.23}$$

Thus, each vertex of an arbitrarily triangulated sphere may be radially scaled by $1/\sqrt{g(\mathbf{e}, \mathbf{e})}$, where $\mathbf{e}$ is the unit radial direction of the vertex relative to the sphere's center, to yield a metric ellipsoid. However, due to the discrete representation of the sphere as a graphical primitive, the vertex with the maximal or minimal extent of the metric ellipsoid might be missed. A more precise alternative is to use tensor's eigendecomposition to set up a projection matrix while drawing a unit sphere; the maximal extent is then ensured to correspond to the sphere's pole. Due to the numerical overhead of the eigenvector computation this variant is slower, but allows using any graphical primitive instead of a sphere (e.g. a hedgehog).

11.3.2 Projection of Metric Ellipsoids

For rendering the quadric surface of a tensor, it is sufficient to just draw a two-dimensional ellipse instead of a truly three-dimensional object that is projected by the 3D graphics engine. For depicting such an ellipsoid, we can draw a rectangle with an arbitrary texture on it. This rectangle needs to be oriented perpendicular to the view direction and transformed by a transformation matrix according to the projection of the tensor field in the view plane.

Let $\mathbf{z}$ be the view direction and $\mathbf{x}, \mathbf{y}$ be two orthonormal vectors describing the view plane. A point $\mathbf{q}$ on the view plane can be computed from two parameters (a, b) via $\mathbf{q} = a\mathbf{x} + b\mathbf{y}$. We get the projected ellipsoid by considering a ray $\mathbf{p} = \mathbf{q} + \lambda\mathbf{z}$ that is orthogonal to the view plane (we could model rays for perspective projection as well). Points on the ellipsoid obey $g(\mathbf{p}, \mathbf{p}) = 1$, which yields a quadratic equation in the ray parameter λ

$$1 = g(\mathbf{q} + \lambda\mathbf{z}, \mathbf{q} + \lambda\mathbf{z}) \equiv g(\mathbf{q}, \mathbf{q}) + 2\lambda g(\mathbf{q}, \mathbf{z}) + \lambda^2 g(\mathbf{z}, \mathbf{z}) \ . \tag{11.24}$$

For the projection of the ellipsoid on the view plane we are interested in the set of parameters (a, b) where the ray is tangential to the ellipsoid, i.e. where the discriminant of (11.24) vanishes:

$$\frac{g(\mathbf{q}, \mathbf{z})^2}{g(\mathbf{z}, \mathbf{z})^2} - \frac{g(\mathbf{q}, \mathbf{q}) - 1}{g(\mathbf{z}, \mathbf{z})} = 0 \equiv g(\mathbf{q}, \mathbf{z})^2 - g(\mathbf{q}, \mathbf{q})g(\mathbf{z}, \mathbf{z}) + g(\mathbf{z}, \mathbf{z}) \ . \tag{11.25}$$

Substituting $\mathbf{q} = a\mathbf{x} + b\mathbf{y}$ into ((11.25)) yields a quadratic expression in (a, b):

$$a^2\big[g(\mathbf{x}, \mathbf{z})^2 - g(\mathbf{x}, \mathbf{x})g(\mathbf{z}, \mathbf{z})\big] + 2ab\big[g(\mathbf{x}, \mathbf{z})g(\mathbf{y}, \mathbf{z}) - g(\mathbf{x}, \mathbf{y})g(\mathbf{z}, \mathbf{z})\big]$$
$$+ b^2\big[g(\mathbf{y}, \mathbf{z})^2 - g(\mathbf{y}, \mathbf{y})g(\mathbf{z}, \mathbf{z})\big] + g(\mathbf{z}, \mathbf{z}) = 0 \ . \quad (11.26)$$

The coefficients in (11.26) for a^2, $2ab$ and b^2 are the components of a bilinear form describing the *shadow* of the metric ellipsoid in the coordinates (a, b). Note that in this derivation we never used coordinates on the 3-vectors, i.e. this derivation was completely coordinate-free. We may also write (11.26) as

$$(a\ b)\left[g(\mathbf{z}, \mathbf{z}) \overbrace{\begin{pmatrix} g(\mathbf{x}, \mathbf{x}) & g(\mathbf{x}, \mathbf{y}) \\ & g(\mathbf{y}, \mathbf{y}) \end{pmatrix}}^{=:\pi(g)} - \begin{pmatrix} g(\mathbf{x}, \mathbf{z})^2 & g(\mathbf{x}, \mathbf{z})g(\mathbf{y}, \mathbf{z}) \\ & g(\mathbf{y}, \mathbf{z})^2 \end{pmatrix} \right] \begin{pmatrix} a \\ b \end{pmatrix} = g(\mathbf{z}, \mathbf{z})$$

$$\underbrace{\qquad\qquad\qquad\qquad\qquad\qquad\qquad}_{=:\sigma(g)}$$

$$(11.27)$$

whereby $\pi(g)$ is the intersection of the ellipsoid with the view plane $g(\mathbf{q}, \mathbf{q})$ and $\sigma(g)$ is the 'shadow ellipsoid'. With (v, w) the eigenvectors of this 2×2 metric and (λ, μ) the corresponding eigenvalues, i.e.

$$\sigma g \cdot v = \lambda v \qquad \sigma g \cdot w = \mu w \ , \qquad (11.28)$$

the orientation of the resulting projected ellipsoid in 3D is given by evaluating the eigenvectors as linear combination of the basis $\{\mathbf{x}, \mathbf{y}\}$:

$$\mathbf{p}_1 = (v_x/\sqrt{\lambda})\mathbf{x} + (v_x/\sqrt{\lambda})\mathbf{y} \qquad (11.29)$$
$$\mathbf{p}_2 = (w_x/\sqrt{\mu})\mathbf{x} + (w_x/\sqrt{\mu})\mathbf{y} \ . \qquad (11.30)$$

The two three-dimensional vectors $\mathbf{p}_1, \mathbf{p}_2$ are orthonormal with respect to the metric tensor g (i.e. $g(\mathbf{p}_i, \mathbf{p}_j) = \delta_{ij}$) and are completely contained in the view plane $\mathbf{x}, \mathbf{y}$. Since the eigenvalue equation of $\sigma(g)$ is just quadratic, it can be solved faster and more precisely than the eigenvalue equation of the full 3×3 tensor matrix. From the visualization side, the advantage of this method is that we can use an arbitrary image as texture on the distorted rectangle.

11.3.3 Selected Glyph-Based Visualization Methods

Many alternatives to the quadric surfaces have been proposed that are superior in enhancing certain features of the tensor field and that are more sensitive to deviations. Here, we review some glyph-based methods that provide alternatives to quadric surfaces ('metric ellipsoids').

Superquadrics. [Kin04] uses superquadrics, i.e. surfaces of the form $ax^n + by^n + cz^n = 1$ with $n > 2$, to reduce ambiguities on the appearance of view-projected quadric surfaces. See also Chap. 12 by Kindlmann.

Reynold Glyphs. Reynold glyphs [MSM95] are an inverse mapping of the metric ellipsoid, mapping each unit vector $\mathbf{e}$ to $\mathbf{e} \cdot \sqrt{g(\mathbf{e},\mathbf{e})}$ instead of $\mathbf{e}/\sqrt{g(\mathbf{e},\mathbf{e})}$ as with the quadric surface.

Haber Glyphs. Haber [Hab90] used a disc and a rod instead of an ellipsoid to encode the eigenvalues of a tensor at each point. This glyph is useful for depicting anisotropy more easily than ellipsoids, but is also vulnerable to isotropy artifacts.

Shape Icons. To allow reading off directly the relationships of the shape factors, [WMM$^+$02] used a combination of a sphere, a disc and a needle at each vertex. Each component is scaled accordingly to the spherical, planar and linear shape factor. The method is robust against isotropy artifacts, but suffers under visual clutter like any opaque tensor glyph.

Van Gogh Keystrokes. [LAK$^+$98] were inspired by the key strokes in the oil paintings of Van Gogh for their tensor field visualization. At each vertex of a planar slice, the projected ellipsoid is drawn with an elliptical shape, whereby an additional texture indicates the tensor components orthogonal to the slice. The method provides a pattern-like qualitative overview when viewed from a large scale, but still allows a quantitative inspection when viewed closely.

Tensor Glow. Here, the idea is to avoid rendering three-dimensional objects as a tensor glyph, but instead to only compute the projection of the tensor ellipsoid on the view plane on the fly, depending on the view direction [Ben04]. The actual graphics primitive is just a rectangle which is stretched and oriented according to the visible projection as derived in (11.29) and (11.30). This rectangle can be rendered very fast and equipped with an arbitrary, even animated texture. It is thus very suitable to provide the impression of a glowing flash of light dissipating into space, which is an intuitive rendering of a metric tensor field.

Tensor Cones. Inspired by the frequently used light cones in general relativity, tensor cones [Ben04] are constructed from little cones with elliptical cross-sections. An arbitrary input vector field has to be provided which forms the original axis of these cones. Their extruded cross-section is computed from the 2×2 tensor in the projection orthogonal to the original axis. Finally, the three left over components of the tensor field along the vector field are used to tilt the cones according to the deviation vector. The tensor cones incorporate the full tensor information content, but depend on a certain input vector field. This allows to display simultaneously a vector field and a tensor field.

Tensor Schlieren. This is an experimental technique [Ben04], inspired by the visual appearance of Schlieren photography [Set01]. Here the deviation of the view direction by the tensor field is visualized by decreased transparency at locations of large deviations. The visual appearance is like a fuzzy geometry that changes with view position or rotation of the data volume. This technique is not limited to positive definite tensor fields.

Tensor Splats. This technique has been described in detail in [BH04] and [BH]. The basic idea is to replace the complex geometries of glyphs by transparent splats equipped with a texture-like pattern that incorporates the same information content. As a result, tensor splats are able to visualize entire three-dimensional volumes of a tensor field and intuitively provide a notion of the tensor field's important properties.

11.3.4 Comparison of Visualization Techniques using DT MRI Data

Diffusion weighted magnetic resonance imaging (DW MRI) is a technique that measures the diffusion properties of water molecules in tissues. With the availability of such measured tensor field data for medical purposes, the interest of visualizing such data has grown rapidly in the last years (see Part B). We will compare selected visualization methods upon an example data set using exactly the same view parameters.

Metric Ellipsoids. As first approach, we may employ metric ellipsoids with colors indicating the trace of the tensor. We find that this representation clearly depicts the properties of the tensors at each point, Fig. 11.5, but we need to enlarge the image such that each ellipsoids becomes visible on their own. When inspecting the entire image as an overview, hardly anything can be seen at all because the structures of the ellipsoids fall below the image resolution, cf. also Fig. 11.11 (top). Equivalently we could use volume rendering of the trace as a scalar field. But even when zoomed onto an interesting regions, the ellipsoids are hard to interpret because we only see their projected shape.

Tensor Glow. Employing the method of tensor glow in Fig. 11.6 reduces the visual clutter. In the variant used here, the projected glow pattern is not normalized, but its transparency is proportional to the trace of the tensor

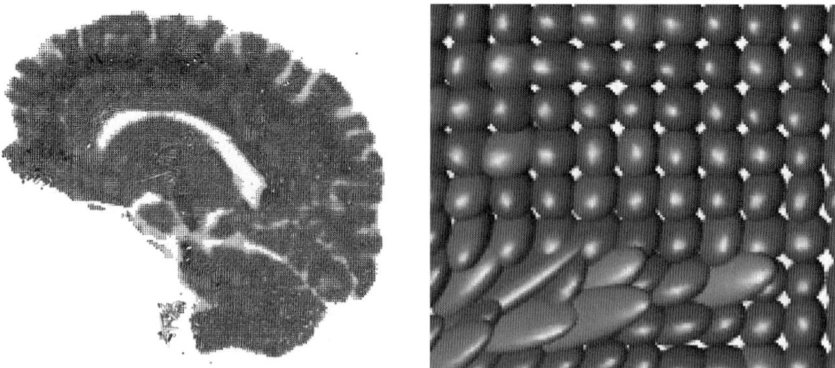

Fig. 11.5. Metric ellipsoids applied to a slice of the human brain: overview (*left*) and enlargement (*right*). See also color plates

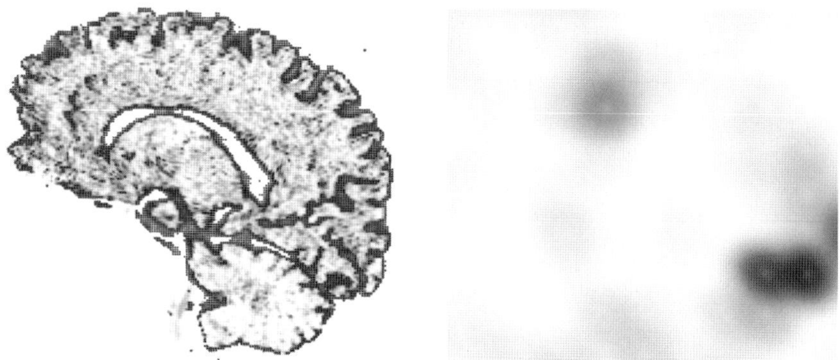

Fig. 11.6. Tensor glow technique applied to a slice of the human brain: overview (*left*) and enlargement (*right*). See also color plates

field. Other variants are possible, too. Using e.g. an isotropy indicator were a reasonable approach. Employing these settings upon the human brain tensor field enhances regions of high trace. This is the region where water may flow rapidly. Such areas are depicted clearly, in an overview as well as in an enlargement. We also get an glimpse of the orientation of the flow, but it is not too prominent as the anisotropy is not overwhelmingly large. The tensor glow method is thus applicable and helps to enhance certain features, but one gets the impression that it should be possible to do better.

Tensor Cones. Although specifically developed for relativistic data, using tensor cones for brain data Fig. 11.7 resulted in a pleasant surprise: it displays some global structure information more clearly than both metric ellipsoids and tensor glow. This is due to the larger sensitivity of the appearance of tensor cones to variations of the tensor field. As a consequence, we get a good

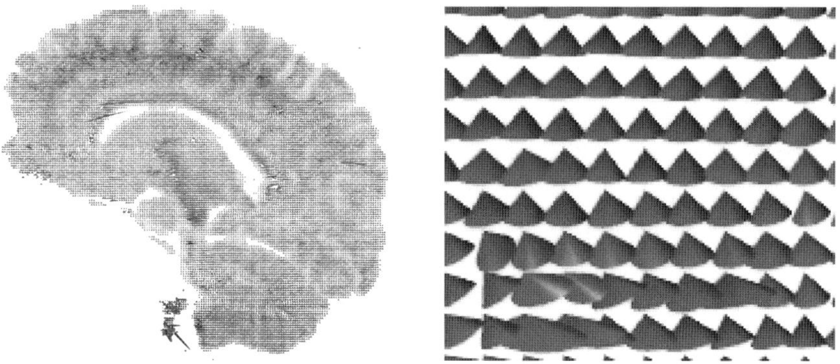

Fig. 11.7. Tensor cones applied to a slice of the human brain: overview (*left*) and enlargement (*right*). See also color plates

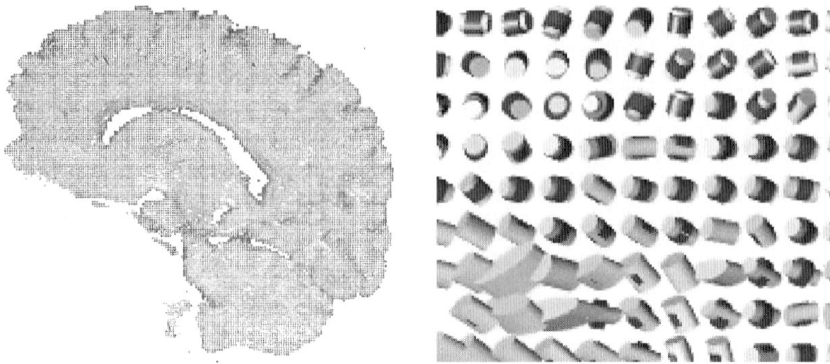

Fig. 11.8. Haber glyphs applied to a slice of a human brain: overview (*left*) and enlargement (*right*). See also color plates

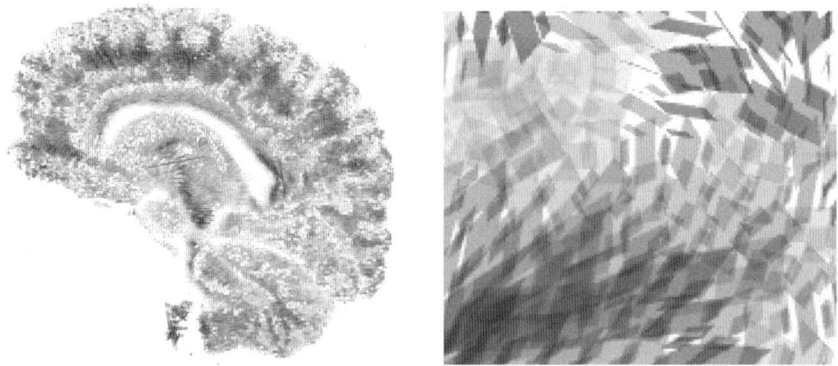

Fig. 11.9. Tensor schlieren applied to a slice of a human brain: overview (*left*) and enlargement (*right*). See also color plates

overview of all structures contained in the data set. However, the interpretation is difficult since the user-chosen vector field probe is an arbitrary input parameter. So we can study the tensor field properties by visual inspection, but it still requires some mental effort.

Haber Glyphs. Haber glyphs have some history in computational fluid dynamics. They are very sensitive to anisotropy and are thus able to enhance global structures in an overview similar to the tensor cones, but without dependence on an user-chosen input vector field. The enlarged view as in Fig. 11.8 also gives a hint of some large structures that incorporate a flow. However, to really recognize the details, we require an extreme enlargement such that all glyphs become resolved. A drawback of Haber glyphs are their anisotropy artifacts, as the glyphs are randomly oriented in isotropic areas.

Tensor Schlieren. In contrast to tensor cones and Haber glyphs, the technique of tensor schlieren uses transparency as a fundamental part of the visualization technique. Thus, it is more suitable for large-scale overviews. However, transparency is not an invariant quantity here, but depends on the view direction, as the purpose of tensor schlieren is to enhance regions where the principal eigenvector is perpendicular to the view direction. Tensor schlieren are thus especially suitable for an interactive environment rather than for static, two-dimensional images. However, even for static images it yields the best overview, Fig. 11.9, of the brain visualizations discussed so far: it reduces visual clutter by rendering large regions transparent (those where the principal eigenvector is parallel to the view direction), while strongly displaying the orientation of the minor eigenvector in other regions. We thus get a good structural overview plus directional information in each area.

Tensor Splats. While tensor schlieren produces view-dependent images encoding the orientation of the tensor field's eigenvectors by intensity, the technique of tensor splats [BH04] employs view-independent graphical primitives oriented according to the eigenvectors and uses colors for depicting the relationships of the eigenvalues. Transparency is used to encode the isotropy, i.e. isotropic regions are visually removed from the image. The result Fig. 11.10 is a strong enhancement for all anisotropic features, cf. also Fig. 11.11 (bottom), with clear depiction of difference among minor and median eigenvectors as well. The tensor splat technique intentionally displays various features redundantly in different manners to compensate the reduction of visual information by projection of the glyph geometry onto the two-dimensional view plane. Green, e.g., indicates a linear region independent from its orientation and is thus clearly distinguishable from a red disk seen from aside. Tensor splats thus appear to provide the best view of the discussed methods and are also appropriate for full three-dimensional volume visualization.

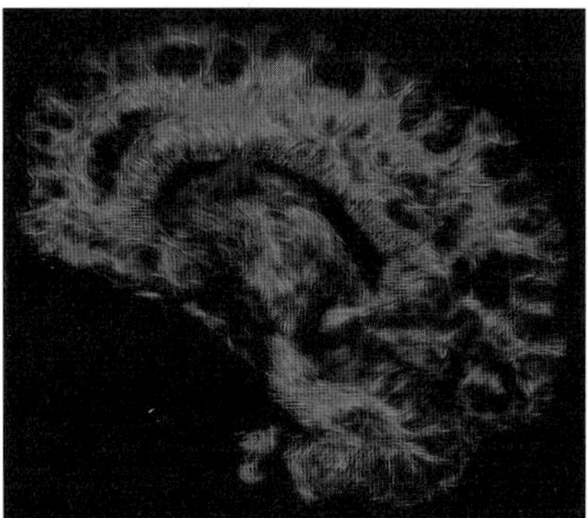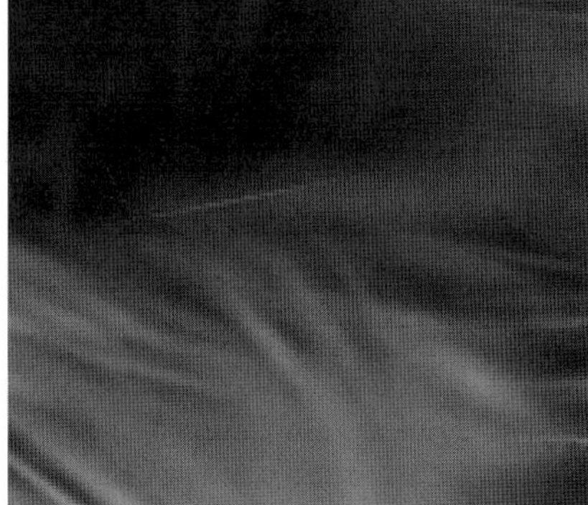

Fig. 11.10. Tensor splats applied to a slice of a human brain: overview (*left*) and enlargement (*right*). See also color plates

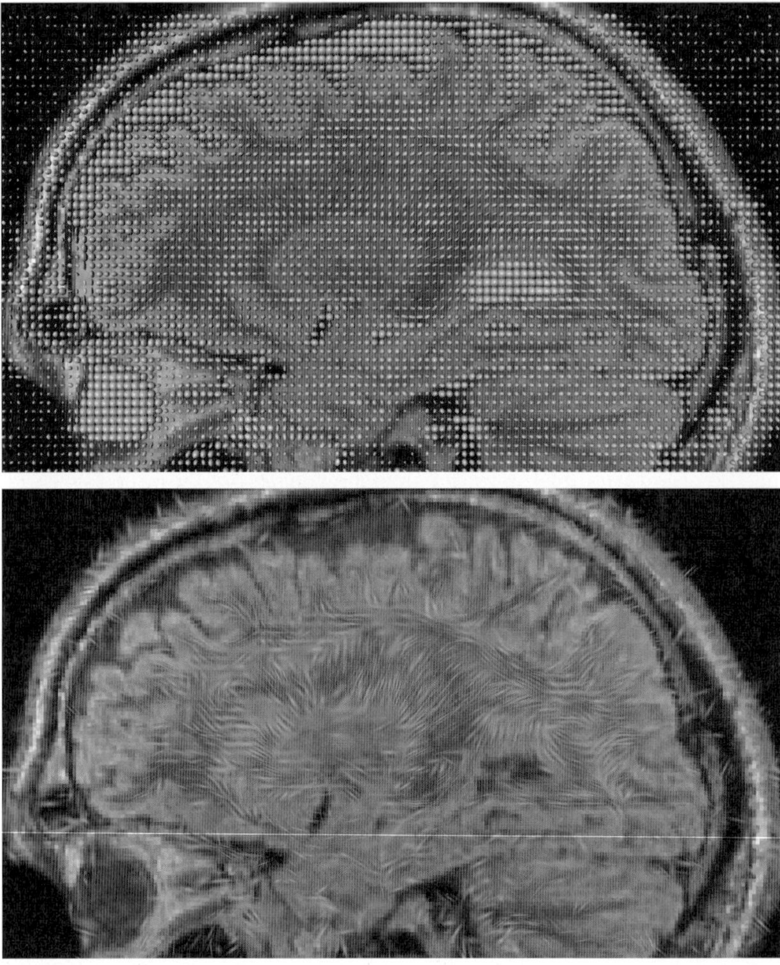

Fig. 11.11. Comparison of metric ellipsoids with tensor splats technique applied to a slice through a diffusion tensor field acquired from a human brain (see color plates)

11.4 Summary

Table 11.1 compares various tensor field visualization methods. The table is ordered according to the tensor field quantities which are used for the visualization. It is not possible to provide a general scoring of these methods and to determine the 'best' visualization method – each method has advantages that might cause it to be superior to others in specific applications. For instance, tensor ellipsoids are straightforward to understand, but suffer from the problem of visual clutter. Tensor splats clearly display relevant features of a tensor

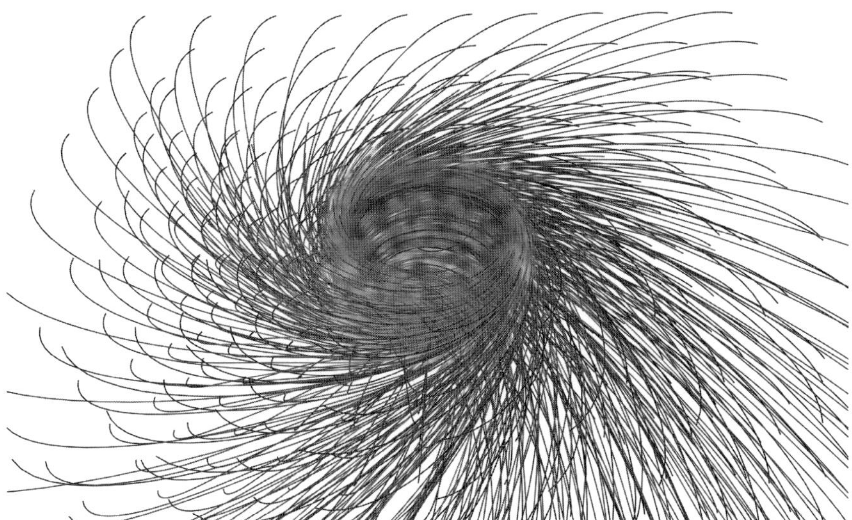

Fig. 11.12. Geodesics in the spacetime of a rotating black hole, indicating the 'event horizon' of the black hole at the location of their congruence (see color plates)

field even in 3D volume, but require some experience for understanding the visual effects – as with most tensor field visualization methods.

Nevertheless some criteria might help to select an appropriate method for a particular application:

- *Number of quantities:* Does the method make use of the full information content of the tensor field or does it work by reduction to fewer quantities? Some methods display a reduced set and include parameters that allow to browse other quantities as well, such that multiple images are required to get a complete impression of the tensor field. These parameter-dependent tensor quantities are denoted by numerical indices such as 'g_{00}', whereas parameter-independent quantities are denoted by coordinate components such as 'g_{xx}'.
- *Robustness against visual clutter:* Is a method suitable for three-dimensional data volumes or is it limited to two-dimensional slices only?
- *Isotropy artifacts:* Visualization methods based on eigenvectors have to address/handle ambiguities in isotropic regions.
- *Limitation to positive definite tensors:* Can the method handle tensor fields with negative or zero eigenvalues? Tensor fields like in DT-MRI or Riemannian metric tensors are always positive definite, such that the corresponding quadric surface is an ellipsoid. The stress tensor in CFD or the extrinsic curvature tensor in general relativity may contain negative eigenvalues as well.
- *Limitation to symmetric tensors:* Can the method display asymmetric tensor fields?

Table 11.1. Comparison and assessment of selected tensor field visualization methods. The entries in column 'Q' tells the number of quantities depicted by the method, '$\smile$' stand for the robustness against visual clutter, $tr(g)$ indicates how far the methods suffer under eigenvector ambiguities in isotropic regions, the '+'/'sym' columns shows the methods requires the tensor field to be positive definite or symmetric. Although geodesics incorporate the derivatives of the tensor field, too, they are only able to display a subset of the full parameter space depending on their initial conditions, so the number of depictable quantities is quoted. See text for further details

Tensor Encoding	Q	Viz Method	$\smile$	$tr(G)$	'+'	sym
$g_{xx}, g_{xy}, g_{yy},$ g_{yz}, g_{zz}, g_{zx}	6	Quadric surface	bad	good	no	yes
		Metric ellipsoids	bad	good	yes	yes
		Reynold Glyph	bad	good	yes	yes
$\mathbf{v}_{max}, \lambda_{max}, \lambda_{med}, \lambda_{min}$	6	Haber Glyph	bad	bad	yes	yes
		Tensor Schlieren	good	bad	yes	yes
$g_{00}, g_{01}, g_{11},$ g_{12}, g_{22}, g_{20}	6+3	Tensor Cones	bad	bad	yes	yes
g_{00}, g_{01}, g_{11}	3	Deformation Surfaces	bad	good	no	no
$g_{00}, g_{01}, g_{11},$ $tr(g)$	4	Color Coding	good	good	no	no
$\mathbf{v}_{max}, tr(g), c_p, c_l$	6	Tensor Splats	good	good	yes	yes
$g(\mathbf{x}, \mathbf{x}), g(\mathbf{x}, \mathbf{y}), g(\mathbf{x}, \mathbf{y})$ $\mathbf{x}(\vartheta, \varphi), \mathbf{y}(\vartheta, \varphi)$	3-6	Tensor Glow	good	medium	yes	yes
$g_{xx}, g_{xy}, g_{yy},$ $tr(g), \lambda_{max}$	5	Van Gogh keystrokes	bad	good	yes	yes
$\mathbf{v}_{max}, \lambda_{max}, \lambda_{med},$ $\lambda_{min}, \partial \mathbf{v}_{max}$	9	Hyperstreamlines	good	bad	yes	no
	9	Tensor Lines	good	good	yes	no
$g_{mn}, \partial g_{mn}$	'24"	Geodesic	good	good	yes	yes
$g_{mn}, \partial g_{mn}, \partial\partial g_{mn}$	'78"	Geodesics Bundle	good	good	yes	yes

Which method is best suited for a specific application therefore depends on both, the characteristics of the tensor field and the features to be emphasized.

Acknowledgments

The DT-MRI brain dataset used for comparison was provided generously by Gordon Kindlmann and Andrew L. Alexander. The data set used in Fig. 11.11 was provided by Hagen Kitzler. We thank Konrad Polthier and Peter Deuflhard for fruitful discussions.

References

[BAS02]   M. Bondarescu, M. Alcubierre, and E. Seidel, *Isometric embeddings of black hole horizons in three-dimensional flat space*, Class. Quant. Grav. **19** (2002).

[Ben04]   W. Benger, *Visualization of general relativistic tensor fields via a fiber bundle data model*, Ph.D. thesis, Free University Berlin, August 2004, published by Lehmanns Media, Berlin, 2005.

[BH]   W. Benger and H.-C. Hege, *Analysing curved spacetimes with tensor splats*, Proc. 10th Marcel Grossmann Meeting on General Relativity, Rio de Janeiro, July 20-26, 2003, to appear.

[BH04]   ______, *Tensor splats*, Conference on Visualization and Data Analysis 2004 (R. Erbacher et al., ed.), Proc. of SPIE, Vol. 5295, 2004, IS&T/SPIE Electronic Imaging Symposium, San Jose, CA.

[DH93]   T. Delmarcelle and L. Hesselink, *Visualizing second order tensor fields with hyperstream lines*, IEEE Computer Graphics and Applications **13** (1993), 25–33.

[GTS$^+$04] C. Garth, X. Tricoche, T. Salzbrunn, T. Bobach, and G. Scheuermann, *Surface techniques for vortex visualization*, VisSym 2004, Symposium on Visualization, Konstanz, Germany, May 19-21, 2004, Eurographics Association, 2004, pp. 155–164, 346.

[Hab90]   R.B. Haber, *Visualization techniques for engineering mechanics*, Comp. Sys. in Engineering **1** (1990), no. 1, 37–50.

[Hot02]   I. Hotz, *Isometric embedding by surface reconstruction from distances*, IEEE Visualization 2002, 2002, pp. 251–257.

[Hul92]   J.P.M. Hultquist, *Constructing stream surfaces in steady 3d vector fields*, Visualization, IEEE Computer Society, 1992, pp. 171–178.

[Kin04]   G.L. Kindlmann, *Superquadric tensor glyphs.*, VisSym 2004, Symposium on Visualization, Konstanz, Germany, May 19-21, 2004, Eurographics Association, 2004, pp. 147–154.

[LAK$^+$98] D.H. Laidlaw, E.T. Ahrens, D. Kremers, M.J. Avalos, R.E. Jacobs, and C. Readhead, *Visualizing diffusion tensor images of the mouse spinal cord.*, IEEE Visualization, 1998, pp. 127–134.

[MSM95]   J.G. Moore, S.A. Schorn, and J. Moore, *Methods of classical mechanics applied to turbulence stresses in a tip leakage vortex*, Proc. ASME Gas Turbine Conf., Houston, Texas, no. 95-GT-220, 1995.

[OHW02]   L. O'Donnell, S. Haker, and C.-F. Westin, *New approaches to estimation of white matter connectivity in diffusion tensor MRI: Elliptic PDEs and geodesics in a tensor-warped space*, Fifth Int. Conf. Medical Image Computing and Computer-Assisted Intervention (MICCAI'02) (Tokyo, Japan), 2002, pp. 459–466.

[O'N83]   B. O'Neill, *Semi-riemannian geometry, with applications to relativity*, Academic Press, Inc., 1983.

[SEF99]   P. Schneider, J. Ehlers, and E.E. Falco, *Gravitational lenses*, Springer Verlag Berlin Heidelberg, 1999.

[Set01]   G.S. Settles, *Schlieren and shadowgraph techniques: Visualizing phenomena in transparent media*, Springer Verlag, 2001.

[SSE94]   S. Seitz, P. Schneider, and J. Ehlers, *Light propagation in arbitrary spacetimes and the gravitational lens approximation*, Class. Quant. Grav (1994).

[Sta98]   D. Stalling, *Fast texture-based algorithms for vector field visualization*, Ph.D. thesis, Free University Berlin, 1998.

[TWHS05]   H. Theisel, T. Weinkauf, H.-C. Hege, and H.-P. Seidel, *Topological methods for 2d time-dependent vector fields based on stream lines and path lines*, IEEE Trans. Visual. Comp. Graph. (TVCG) **11** (2005), no. 4.

[WKL99]   D. Weinstein, G. Kindlmann, and E. Lundberg, *Tensorlines: Advection-diffusion based propagation through diffusion tensor fields*, IEEE Visualization 1999, IEEE Computer Society Press, 1999, pp. 249–253.

[WMM$^+$02]   C.F. Westin, S.E. Maier, H. Mamata, A. Nabavi, F.A. Jolesz, and R. Kikinis, *Processing and visualization for diffusion tensor MRI*, Medical Image Analysis **2** (2002), no. 6, 93–108.

[WPG$^+$97]   C.F. Westin, S. Peled, H. Gudbjartsson, R. Kikinis, and FA. Jolesz, *Geometrical diffusion measures for MRI from tensor basis analysis*, Proceedings of ISMRM, Fifth Meeting, Vancouver, Canada, April 1997, p. 1742.

[ZP03a]   X. Zheng and A. Pang, *HyperLIC*, IEEE Visualization 2003, 2003, pp. 249–256.

[ZP03b]   ———, *Interaction of light and tensor fields*, VisSym '03, 2003, pp. 157–166.

[ZSH96]   M. Zöckler, D. Stalling, and H.-C. Hege, *Interactive visualization of 3d-vector fields using illuminated streamlines*, IEEE Visualization '96, Oct./Nov. 1996, pp. 107–113.

Tensor Invariants and their Gradients

Gordon Kindlmann

School of Computing, University of Utah, 50 South Central Campus Drive, Salt
Lake City, UT 84112, USA
gk@cs.utah.edu

Summary. Second-order tensors may be described in terms of *shape* and *orientation*. Shape is quantified by tensor *invariants*, which are fixed with respect to coordinate system changes. This chapter describes an anatomically-motivated method of detecting edges in diffusion tensor fields based on the *gradients* of invariants. Three particular invariants (the mean, variance, and skewness of the tensor eigenvalues) are described in two ways: first, as the geometric parameters of an intuitive graphical device for representing tensor shape (the *eigenvalue wheel*), and second, in terms of their physical and anatomical significance in diffusion tensor MRI. Tensor-valued gradients of these invariants lead to an orthonormal basis for describing changes in tensor shape. The spatial gradient of the diffusion tensor field may be projected onto this basis, producing three different measures of edge strength, selective for different kinds of anatomical boundaries. The gradient measures are grounded in standard tensor analysis, and are demonstrated on synthetic data.

12.1 Background and Notation

As described in Chap. 5 by Alexander, fields of water diffusion tensors may be measured *in vivo* with magnetic resonance imaging (MRI), providing a valuable tool for assessing the organization of tissue microstructure. A diffusion tensor $\mathbf{D}$ is numerically estimated by its matrix representation in the orthonormal *laboratory frame* $\mathcal{L} = \{\mathbf{b}_1, \mathbf{b}_2, \mathbf{b}_3\}$ associated with the MRI scanner [1]:

$$[\mathbf{D}]_{\mathcal{L}} = \begin{bmatrix} D_{11} & D_{12} & D_{13} \\ D_{12} & D_{22} & D_{23} \\ D_{13} & D_{23} & D_{33} \end{bmatrix} .$$

Unit-length eigenvectors $\mathbf{e}_i$ can be found to form an orthonormal *principal frame* $\mathcal{E} = \{\mathbf{e}_1, \mathbf{e}_2, \mathbf{e}_3\}$, in which the matrix representation of $\mathbf{D}$ has the eigenvalues λ_i along the diagonal:

$$[\mathbf{D}]_{\mathcal{E}} = \begin{bmatrix} \lambda_1 & 0 & 0 \\ 0 & \lambda_2 & 0 \\ 0 & 0 & \lambda_3 \end{bmatrix} \Rightarrow [\mathbf{D}]_{\mathcal{L}} = R \begin{bmatrix} \lambda_1 & 0 & 0 \\ 0 & \lambda_2 & 0 \\ 0 & 0 & \lambda_3 \end{bmatrix} R^{\mathrm{t}} .$$

Column i of rotation matrix R is unit-length eigenvector representation $[\mathbf{e}_i]_{\mathcal{L}}$. Diagonalizing a matrix representation of $\mathbf{D}$ into eigenvalues and eigenvectors separates the tensor into shape and orientation information, respectively. Herein, tensor 'shape' refers to the unordered set of three eigenvalues.

12.2 From Principal Invariants to Eigenvalues

The eigenvalues of a symmetric tensor $\mathbf{D}$ are computed by solving its cubic characteristic polynomial:

$$\det(\lambda \mathbf{I} - \mathbf{D}) = 0$$

The determinant of $\lambda \mathbf{I} - \mathbf{D}$ may be computed in the laboratory frame:

$$\det(\lambda I - [\mathbf{D}]_{\mathcal{L}}) = \begin{vmatrix} \lambda - D_{11} & -D_{12} & -D_{13} \\ -D_{12} & \lambda - D_{22} & -D_{23} \\ -D_{13} & -D_{23} & \lambda - D_{33} \end{vmatrix} = \lambda^3 - J_1\lambda^2 + J_2\lambda - J_3 \;;$$

$$\begin{aligned} J_1 &= D_{11} + D_{22} + D_{33} \\ J_2 &= D_{11}D_{22} + D_{11}D_{33} + D_{22}D_{33} - D_{12}^2 - D_{13}^2 - D_{23}^2 \\ J_3 &= 2D_{12}D_{13}D_{23} + D_{11}D_{22}D_{33} - D_{13}^2 D_{22} - D_{11}D_{23}^2 - D_{12}^2 D_{33} \end{aligned} \tag{12.1}$$

On the other hand, evaluating $\det(\lambda \mathbf{I} - \mathbf{D})$ in the principal frame $\mathcal{E}$ gives:

$$J_1 = \lambda_1 + \lambda_2 + \lambda_3 \;; \quad J_2 = \lambda_1\lambda_2 + \lambda_1\lambda_3 + \lambda_2\lambda_3 \;; \quad J_3 = \lambda_1\lambda_2\lambda_3 \tag{12.2}$$

J_1, J_2, J_3 are the *principal invariants* [2], with coordinate free expression:

$$J_1 = \text{tr}(\mathbf{D}) \;; \quad J_2 = \frac{\text{tr}(\mathbf{D})^2 - \text{tr}(\mathbf{D}^2)}{2} \;; \quad J_3 = \det(\mathbf{D}) \tag{12.3}$$

Equation (12.1) is how the principal invariants are computed in practice, based on the matrix components of the tensor represented in the laboratory frame. Equation (12.2) shows how J_i are functions of λ_i alone.

Another useful invariant J_4 is computed from the principal invariants:

$$\begin{aligned} J_4 = \text{tr}(\mathbf{D}^{\text{t}}\mathbf{D}) &= J_1^2 - 2J_2 \\ &= D_{11}^2 + 2D_{12}^2 + 2D_{13}^2 + D_{22}^2 + 2D_{23}^2 + D_{33}^2 \\ &= \lambda_1^2 + \lambda_2^2 + \lambda_3^2 \end{aligned}$$

J_1 and J_4 both describe tensor *size*, either by the sum of the eigenvalues, or their squares, respectively. Much of the DT-MRI literature has noted the utility of the J_i invariants as measures of tensor shape that do not require diagonalization [1, 3, 4]. Computing eigenvalues, however, is simply arithmetic combination of principal invariants to create new invariants. The standard formulas for solving cubic polynomials define [5, 6]:

$$Q = \frac{J_1^2 - 3J_2}{9} \; ; \; R = \frac{-9J_1J_2 + 27J_3 + 2J_1^3}{54} \; ; \; \Theta = \frac{1}{3}\cos^{-1}\left(\frac{R}{\sqrt{Q^3}}\right) \quad (12.4)$$

With these, the three eigenvalues (themselves invariants) are:

$$\begin{aligned}
\lambda_1 &= J_1/3 + 2\sqrt{Q}\cos(\Theta) \\
\lambda_2 &= J_1/3 + 2\sqrt{Q}\cos(\Theta - 2\pi/3) \\
\lambda_3 &= J_1/3 + 2\sqrt{Q}\cos(\Theta + 2\pi/3)
\end{aligned} \quad (12.5)$$

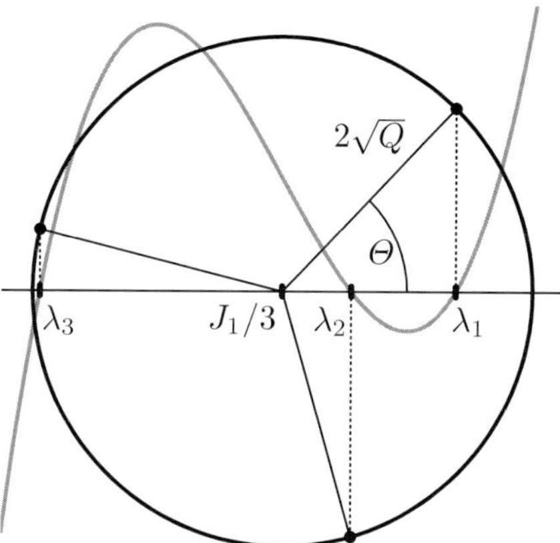

Fig. 12.1. Characteristic polynomial in gray, eigenvalues λ_i, and wheel parameters J_1, Q, Θ

12.3 Eigenvalue Wheel

The structure of (12.5) suggests a geometric analogy, shown in Fig. 12.1 [7]. A wheel with three equally placed spokes is centered on the real number line at $J_1/3$. The radius of the wheel is $2\sqrt{Q}$, and Θ measures the orientation. The eigenvalues are the projection of the spoke ends onto the horizontal axis. The wheel geometry can be expressed in terms of statistics of the unsorted eigenvalues, starting with their *central moments* μ_1, μ_2, μ_3:

$$\begin{aligned}
\mu_1 &= \langle \lambda_i \rangle = J_1/3 \\
\mu_2 &= \langle (\lambda_i - \mu_1)^2 \rangle = 2Q \\
\mu_3 &= \langle (\lambda_i - \mu_1)^3 \rangle = 2R
\end{aligned} \quad (12.6)$$

The eigenvalue mean, variance and standard deviation are μ_1, μ_2, and $\sigma = \sqrt{\mu_2}$, respectively. The skewness of the eigenvalues α_3 is defined as [5][1]:

---

[1] 'Skewness' can also refer to μ_3, as in Chap. 5.

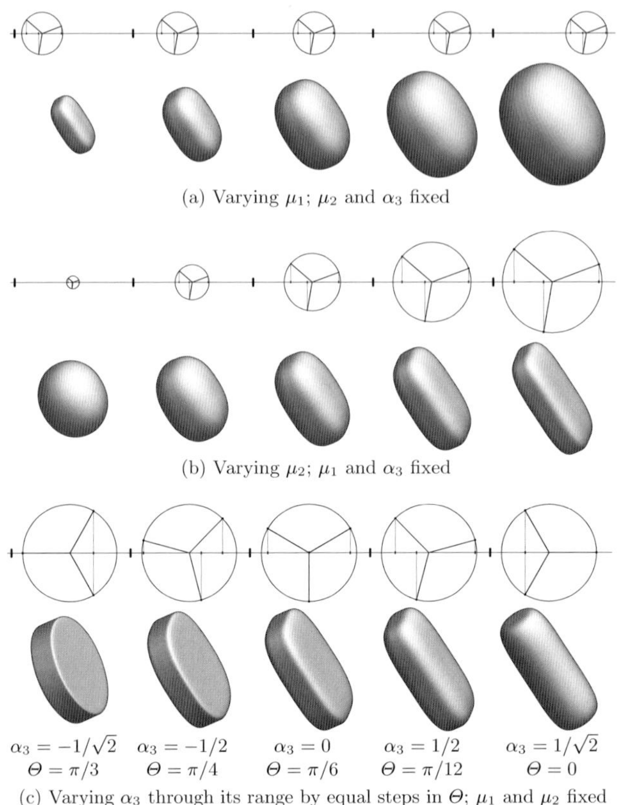

(a) Varying μ_1; μ_2 and α_3 fixed

(b) Varying μ_2; μ_1 and α_3 fixed

| $\alpha_3 = -1/\sqrt{2}$ | $\alpha_3 = -1/2$ | $\alpha_3 = 0$ | $\alpha_3 = 1/2$ | $\alpha_3 = 1/\sqrt{2}$ |
| $\Theta = \pi/3$ | $\Theta = \pi/4$ | $\Theta = \pi/6$ | $\Theta = \pi/12$ | $\Theta = 0$ |

(c) Varying α_3 through its range by equal steps in Θ; μ_1 and μ_2 fixed

Fig. 12.2. Visualizations of shape variations associated with changing eigenvalue mean μ_1 (wheel location), variance μ_2 (wheel radius) and skewness α_3 (spoke angle)

$$\alpha_3 = \frac{\mu_3}{\sigma^3} = \frac{R}{\sqrt{2Q^3}} = \frac{\cos(3\Theta)}{\sqrt{2}} \Rightarrow \Theta = \frac{1}{3}\cos^{-1}(\sqrt{2}\,\alpha_3) \qquad (12.7)$$

Note that the eigenvalue statistics determine the wheel parameters. The *geometric* intuition that the wheel's location, radius, and orientation may be varied in isolation is grounded in the *statistical* property that mean, variance, and skewness are orthogonal. That is, viewing μ_1, μ_2, and α_3 as scalar functions over the space of unsorted eigenvalue triples $(\lambda_1, \lambda_2, \lambda_3)$, and letting $\nabla_\lambda J$ be the gradient of scalar invariant J over $(\lambda_1, \lambda_2, \lambda_3)$, one finds:

$$\nabla_\lambda \mu_1 \cdot \nabla_\lambda \mu_2 = 0 \; ; \; \nabla_\lambda \mu_1 \cdot \nabla_\lambda \alpha_3 = 0 \; ; \; \nabla_\lambda \mu_2 \cdot \nabla_\lambda \alpha_3 = 0 \; . \qquad (12.8)$$

The orthogonality of μ_1, μ_2, α_3 was described by Bahn [8] with cylindrical coordinates for $(\lambda_1, \lambda_2, \lambda_3)$ space. Previous work in continuum mechanics defined related orthogonal measures with the mean, variance, and skewness of the logarithms of the strain tensor eigenvalues [9]. Figure 12.2 illustrates the orthogonal invariants with eigenvalue wheels and superquadric glyphs [10].

12.4 Anatomical Significance of Eigenvalue Statistics

The measures described in the previous sections take on physical meaning when interpreted in the context of a particular application domain, such as diffusion tensor imaging. The diffusion tensor eigenvalues are the apparent diffusion coefficients (ADCs) along the eigenvectors [1]. Eigenvalue mean μ_1 is the *bulk mean diffusivity* [11], the average of ADC over all possible directions. This readily distinguishes the cerebral spinal fluid (CSF) of the ventricles (high μ_1) from the white and gray matter (lower μ_1). An important empirical fact is that μ_1 is essentially constant across white and gray matter [11, 12, 13]. Isolating this degree of freedom permits μ_2 and α_3 to better characterize the brain tissue features that DT-MRI is uniquely capable of detecting.

The variance of the eigenvalues μ_2 measures the directional dependence of the ADC, which indicates anisotropic microstructure. As described in Chap. 5, anisotropy is generally low in gray matter, and high in white matter, due in part to myelinated axon sheaths [14]. Basser and Pierpaoli defined the *fractional* and *relative* anisotropy measures with μ_2 [15]:

$$\mathrm{FA} = \sqrt{\frac{3}{2}}\frac{\|\mathbf{D}-\mu_1\mathbf{I}\|}{\|\mathbf{D}\|} = 3\sqrt{\frac{\mu_2}{2J_4}} \; ; \; \mathrm{RA} = \frac{\|\mathbf{D}-\mu_1\mathbf{I}\|}{\|\mu_1\mathbf{I}\|} = \sqrt{\frac{\mu_2}{\mu_1^2}} \, . \qquad (12.9)$$

The empirical constancy of μ_1 in brain tissue helps compensate for the unfortunate property (visible in Fig. 12.2(a)) that varying μ_1 separately from μ_2 and α_3 effectively changes the anisotropy defined by FA or RA. This assumes, however, that CSF can be masked out with μ_1, which can be somewhat challenging given the limited spatial resolution of DT-MRI.

Eigenvalue skewness α_3 isolates the variation between anisotropic tensors which are 'planar' (large in two axes and small in the other) versus 'linear' (large along one axis, small in the others). This shape variation is not measured by the usual anisotropy metrics: from (12.8) and (12.9), skewness is in fact *orthogonal* to FA and RA. There are two related aspects to the anatomical significance of eigenvalue skewness. The phenomenon of *partial voluming* is a basic characteristics of discretely sampled medical images, in which the sample value records a measurement over some spatial extent related to the spacing between samples. Previous analysis of partial voluming in DT-MRI demonstrated a bias towards planar anisotropy caused by measurement mixing of adjacent regions of linear anisotropy along orthogonal orientations [16, 17]. Planar anisotropy can also arise in more complex configurations. For example, previous work in visualizing regions of significant planar anisotropy characterized locations where populations of differently-oriented fibers apparently mix at a fine scale, far below that of the image resolution [18]. A location with this configuration is the intersection of the medial-lateral tracts of the corpus callosum and inferior-superior tracts of the corona radiata, as confirmed by high-angular resolution diffusion imaging in [19].

12.5 Edge Detection with Invariant Gradients

One strategy for image processing on diffusion tensor data is to locally decompose the space of tensor values (at each tensor sample) into shape changes and orientation changes, enabling a more anatomically driven approach to edge and feature detection. Measuring spatial changes in eigenvalue mean μ_1 could isolate the boundary of the cerebral spinal fluid. Rapid changes in μ_2 might indicate the transition from gray matter to white matter, as well as structural variations within white matter. Changes in α_3 might signal the partial voluming between regions of orthogonally oriented white matter structures. In all cases, disregarding changes in tensor *orientation* may reduce the chance of falsely identifying structural boundaries. Implementing this strategy involves the *gradients* of eigenvalue statistics. This generalizes previous work decomposing tensor changes into changes in the isotropic component, and changes in anisotropy and orientation (the deviator) [20].

Some elements of tensor analysis are reviewed herein [2]. Though a diffusion tensor $\mathbf{D}$ is often identified with its matrix components in the laboratory frame, $\mathbf{D}$ is in fact an element of $L(\mathbb{R}^3, \mathbb{R}^3)$, the set of linear transforms from $\mathbb{R}^3$ to $\mathbb{R}^3$ (see Chap. 1 by Hagen and Garth). $L(\mathbb{R}^3, \mathbb{R}^3)$ is a vector space [21], so every tensor *is* also a vector. Though potentially confusing, recognizing $L(\mathbb{R}^3, \mathbb{R}^3)$ as a vector space grounds the tensor analysis below on our geometric intuition about bases, projections, and gradients from vector calculus. The double contraction $\mathbf{C}:\mathbf{D} = \mathrm{tr}(\mathbf{C}^{\mathrm{t}}\mathbf{D})$ endows $L(\mathbb{R}^3, \mathbb{R}^3)$ with an inner (or dot) product. The tensor norm is defined as $\|\mathbf{D}\| = \sqrt{\mathbf{D}:\mathbf{D}}$. The tensor product of vectors $\mathbf{u} \otimes \mathbf{v}$ is defined by $(\mathbf{u} \otimes \mathbf{v})\mathbf{x} = \mathbf{u}(\mathbf{v} \cdot \mathbf{x})$ for all vectors $\mathbf{x}$. The Kronecker delta δ_{ij} is 1 if $i = j$ and 0 otherwise. The coordinate-free *spectral decomposition* of a symmetric tensor $\mathbf{D}$ into eigenvalues and unit-length eigenvectors is:

$$\mathbf{D} = \sum_i \lambda_i \mathbf{e}_i \otimes \mathbf{e}_i \qquad (12.10)$$

Just as invariants characterize tensor shape, gradients of invariants characterize changes in tensor shape. Herein, 'invariant gradient' denotes differentiation with respect to the tensor value (in $L(\mathbb{R}^3, \mathbb{R}^3)$), rather than differentiation with respect to the spatial domain of the image ($\mathbb{R}^3$). The tensor-valued gradient of a scalar invariant J is notated here with $\boldsymbol{\nabla} J$ (rather than ∇J):

$$\boldsymbol{\nabla} J : L(\mathbb{R}^3, \mathbb{R}^3) \mapsto L(\mathbb{R}^3, \mathbb{R}^3) \; ; \; \boldsymbol{\nabla} J = \frac{\partial J}{\partial \mathbf{D}} \; ; \; ([\boldsymbol{\nabla} J]_{\mathcal{L}})_{ij} = \frac{\partial J}{\partial D_{ij}}$$

By differentiating the spectral decomposition (12.10), one finds $\boldsymbol{\nabla} \lambda_i = \mathbf{e}_i \otimes \mathbf{e}_i$, and thus $\boldsymbol{\nabla} \lambda_i : \boldsymbol{\nabla} \lambda_j = \delta_{ij}$. That is, $\{\boldsymbol{\nabla} \lambda_1, \boldsymbol{\nabla} \lambda_2, \boldsymbol{\nabla} \lambda_3\}$ is an orthonormal basis for shape change around a given tensor value. However, this basis lacks the immediate anatomical significance associated with the eigenvalue statistics (described in the previous section), and the gradients of sorted eigenvalues are not defined when two or more eigenvalues are equal.

To address this, an alternative orthonormal basis for shape change is proposed, based on the (tensor-valued) gradients of μ_1, μ_2, and α_3. From the first-order Taylor expansion of J around $\mathbf{D}$, $J(\mathbf{D}+\boldsymbol{\epsilon}) = J(\mathbf{D})+\boldsymbol{\epsilon}:\boldsymbol{\nabla}J+O(\boldsymbol{\epsilon}^2)$, the gradients of the J_i invariants can be computed as [2]:

$$\begin{array}{ll} \boldsymbol{\nabla}J_1(\mathbf{D}) = \mathbf{I} & \boldsymbol{\nabla}J_2(\mathbf{D}) = \mathrm{tr}(\mathbf{D})\mathbf{I} - \mathbf{D} \\ \boldsymbol{\nabla}J_3(\mathbf{D}) = \det(\mathbf{D})\mathbf{D}^{-1} & \boldsymbol{\nabla}J_4(\mathbf{D}) = 2\mathbf{D} \end{array} \qquad (12.11)$$

Expressions for $\boldsymbol{\nabla}\mu_1$, $\boldsymbol{\nabla}\mu_2$, and $\boldsymbol{\nabla}\alpha_3$ may then be built up from (12.4), (12.6), (12.7), and (12.11), using the standard rules of vector calculus. The spectral decomposition (12.10) allows the double contraction of the gradients of invariants J and K to be reduced to a simple three-dimensional vector dot product:

$$\begin{aligned} \boldsymbol{\nabla}J : \boldsymbol{\nabla}K &= \left(\textstyle\sum_i \partial J/\partial\lambda_i \,\mathbf{e}_i \otimes \mathbf{e}_i\right) : \left(\textstyle\sum_j \partial K/\partial\lambda_j \,\mathbf{e}_j \otimes \mathbf{e}_j\right) \\ &= \textstyle\sum_{i,j}(\partial J/\partial\lambda_i)(\partial K/\partial\lambda_j)\delta_{ij} \\ &= \textstyle\sum_i(\partial J/\partial\lambda_i)(\partial K/\partial\lambda_i) \\ &= \nabla_\lambda J \cdot \nabla_\lambda K \end{aligned}$$

Then, (12.8) establishes the mutual orthogonality of $\boldsymbol{\nabla}\mu_1$, $\boldsymbol{\nabla}\mu_2$, and $\boldsymbol{\nabla}\alpha_3$.

Where defined, the eigenvalue gradients $\boldsymbol{\nabla}\lambda_i$ have constant unit magnitude. $\|\widehat{\boldsymbol{\nabla}}\mu_1\| = 1/3$ is also constant, but the gradients of μ_2 and α_3 have varying magnitude, because their ranges are bounded. $\boldsymbol{\nabla}\mu_2$ vanishes when all eigenvalues are equal (μ_2 at minimum), and $\boldsymbol{\nabla}\alpha_3$ vanishes when two eigenvalues are equal (α_3 at extremum). Still, the space of shape changes is always three-dimensional, so some scheme is required to 'fix' the $\{\boldsymbol{\nabla}\mu_1, \boldsymbol{\nabla}\mu_2, \boldsymbol{\nabla}\alpha_3\}$ basis to consistently span the space of shape variation. Developing this scheme is a focus of ongoing work. One inelegant approach is to, at each tensor sample in an image being processed, slightly perturb the tensor values if there is equality between eigenvalues, so that $\boldsymbol{\nabla}\mu_2$ and $\boldsymbol{\nabla}\alpha_3$ become non-zero.

Normalized invariant gradients are then defined by:

$$\widehat{\boldsymbol{\nabla}}J = \boldsymbol{\nabla}J/\|\boldsymbol{\nabla}J\| \; ; \; J = \mu_1, \mu_2, \alpha_3$$

12.6 Application to Diffusion Tensor Images

The tensor field is assumed to be a continuous and differentiable function $\mathbf{D} : \mathbb{R}^3 \mapsto Sym_3$, as is ensured by the band-limited nature of MRI measurements. The gradient of $\mathbf{D}$ is a *third-order* tensor, described by Pajevic et al. [20]:

$$\nabla\mathbf{D} : \mathbb{R}^3 \mapsto Sym_3^3 \; ; \; \nabla\mathbf{D} = \frac{\partial\mathbf{D}}{\partial\mathbf{x}} \; ; \; ([\nabla\mathbf{D}]_\mathcal{L})_{ijk} = \frac{\partial D_{ij}}{\partial x_k}$$

The double contraction of a second-order tensor with a third-order tensor is a first-order tensor – a vector. Double contracting invariant gradient $\boldsymbol{\nabla}J$ with field gradient $\nabla\mathbf{D}$ creates a vector ∇J, measuring spatial changes of J in the tensor field $\mathbf{D}$. This is simply the chain rule applied to $J(\mathbf{D}(\mathbf{x}))$:

$$\nabla J : \mathbb{R}^3 \mapsto \mathbb{R}^3 \; ; \; \nabla J(\mathbf{x}) = \boldsymbol{\nabla}J(\mathbf{D}(\mathbf{x})):\nabla\mathbf{D}(\mathbf{x}) \; ; \; ([\nabla J(\mathbf{x})]_\mathcal{L})_k = \sum_{i,j}\frac{\partial J}{\partial D_{ij}}\frac{\partial D_{ij}}{\partial x_k}$$

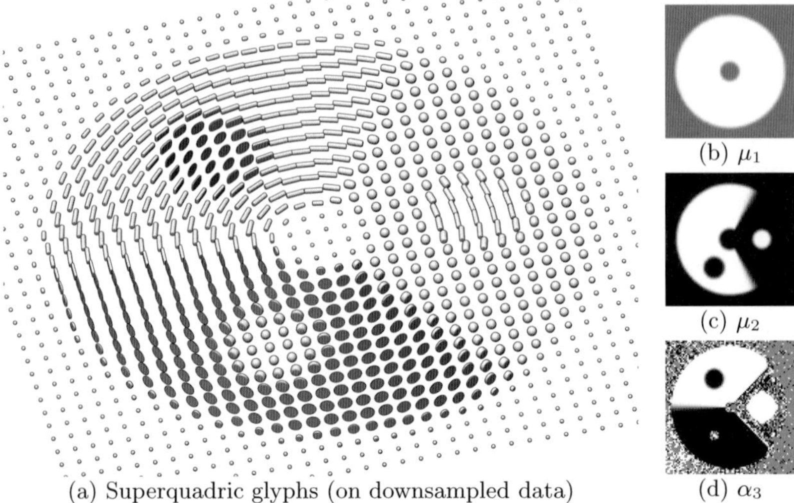

(a) Superquadric glyphs (on downsampled data)   (b) μ_1 (c) μ_2 (d) α_3

Fig. 12.3. Synthetic tensor image for testing gradient measures. Superquadric glyphs are shown in (**a**). Eigenvalue statistics are shown in grayscale in (**b**), (**c**), and (**d**)

Note that $|\nabla J|$ is effectively scaled by $\|\boldsymbol{\nabla}J\|$. This has implications for how spatial changes (edges) in shape are detected. Because $\|\boldsymbol{\nabla}\lambda_i\| = 1$, the spatial eigenvalue gradients $\nabla\lambda_i$ will collectively indicate any and all shape changes in a tensor field, while $\nabla\mu_2$ and $\nabla\alpha_3$ fail in this respect. For example, $\nabla\mu_2$ does not detect changes in anisotropy around a field location with an isotropic tensor. This motivated the definition of $\{\widehat{\boldsymbol{\nabla}}\mu_1, \widehat{\boldsymbol{\nabla}}\mu_2, \widehat{\boldsymbol{\nabla}}\alpha_3\}$ – an *anatomically relevant* orthonormal basis for tensor shape change. With this in mind, a novel 'equi-sensitive' spatial gradient of invariant J is defined as:

$$\nabla J : \mathbb{R}^3 \mapsto \mathbb{R}^3 \; ; \; \nabla J(\mathbf{x}) = \widehat{\boldsymbol{\nabla}}J(\mathbf{D}(\mathbf{x})) : \nabla\mathbf{D}(\mathbf{x})$$

Note that $\nabla J \neq \nabla J/|\nabla J|$. Rather, $\nabla J = \nabla J/\|\boldsymbol{\nabla}J\|$, assuming $\|\boldsymbol{\nabla}J\| > 0$.

The spatial gradients are demonstrated with a two-dimensional synthetic dataset shown in Fig. 12.3. There are four types of materials (isotropic low diffusivity, isotropic high diffusivity, planar anisotropic, and linear anisotropic), with boundaries between every material pair. Eigenvalue statistics are evaluated at each tensor sample and shown in Figs. 12.3(b), 12.3(c), and 12.3(d). The gradient measurement results are shown in Fig. 12.4. Figure 12.4(a) shows a measure of both shape and orientation gradients, $\|\nabla\mathbf{D}\| = \sqrt{\sum_{ijk}(\partial D_{ij}/\partial x_k)^2}$ [20]. However, note that Figs. 12.4(b) and 12.4(c) indicate shape changes only, and with equal sensitivity, as intended. Finally, Figs. 12.4(d), 12.4(e), and 12.4(f) show how the edges in the three degrees of freedom in shape can be detected in isolation.

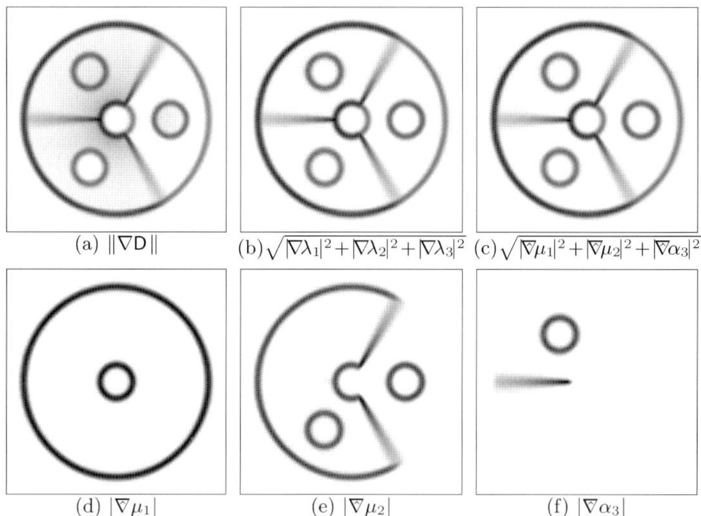

(a) $\|\nabla \mathbf{D}\|$ (b) $\sqrt{|\nabla\lambda_1|^2+|\nabla\lambda_2|^2+|\nabla\lambda_3|^2}$ (c) $\sqrt{|\nabla\mu_1|^2+|\nabla\mu_2|^2+|\nabla\alpha_3|^2}$

(d) $|\nabla\mu_1|$ (e) $|\nabla\mu_2|$ (f) $|\nabla\alpha_3|$

Fig. 12.4. Gradient magnitudes of synthetic data, shown with inverted grayscale

12.7 Discussion

This chapter describes a method for detecting changes (edges) in tensor shape within diffusion tensor fields. A particular set of three tensor invariants (the eigenvalue statistics μ_1, μ_2, α_3) was leveraged for both its orthogonality and its relevance to anatomical feature detection. Tensor analysis was used to create a tensor-valued orthonormal basis for shape change, against which the spatial gradient of the tensor field is measured. Various aspects of this work require further development, most importantly the robust and efficient computation of the invariant-based orthonormal basis for shape change, since this must be calculated anew at every tensor value. Ongoing work is validating the utility of this approach on real data, as well as assessing the impact of noise in the MRI measurements. In the interests of space, the practical details of efficiently measuring the derivatives of the tensor components (for $\nabla \mathbf{D}$) have not been explored here, though continuous tensor field models from convolution or splines (see Chap. 18) provide a natural basis for this.

References

1. PJ Basser, J Mattiello, and D Le Bihan. Estimation of the effective self-diffusion tensor from the NMR spin-echo. *Journal of Magnetic Resonance, B*, 103(3):247–254, 1994.
2. GA Holzapfel. *Nonlinear Solid Mechanics*, Chap. 1. John Wiley and Sons, Ltd, England, 2000.

3. AM Uluğ and PCM van Zijl. Orientation-independent diffusion imaging without tensor diagonalization: Anisotropy definitions based on physical attributes of the diffusion ellipsoid. *Journal of Magnetic Resonance Imaging*, 9:804–813, 1999.

4. KM Hasan, PJ Basser, DL Parker, and AL Alexander. Analytical computation of the eigenvalues and eigenvectors in DT-MRI. *Journal of Magnetic Resonance*, 152:41–47, 2001.

5. EW Weisstein. *CRC Concise Encyclopedia of Mathematics*, pp. 362–365, 1652. CRC Press, Florida, 1999.

6. WH Press, BP Flannery, SA Teukolsky, and WT Vetterling. *Numerical Recipes: The Art of Scientific Computing*. Cambridge University Press, Cambridge (UK) and New York, 2nd edition, 1992.

7. RWD Nickalls. A new approach to solving the cubic: Cardan's solution revealed. *The Mathematical Gazette*, 77:354–359, November 1993.

8. MM Bahn. Invariant and orthonormal scalar measures derived from magnetic resonance diffusion tensor imaging. *Journal of Magnetic Resonance*, 141:68–77, 1999.

9. JC Criscione, JD Humphrey, AS Douglas, and WC Hunter. An invariant basis for natural strain which yields orthogonal stress response terms in isotropic hyperelasticity. *Journal of Mechanics and Physics of Solids*, 48:2445–2465, 2000.

10. G Kindlmann. Superquadric tensor glyphs. In *Proceedings IEEE TVCG/EG Symposium on Visualization 2004*, pp. 147–154, May 2004.

11. PJ Basser and DK Jones. Diffusion-tensor MRI: theory, experimental design and data analysis – a technical review. *Nuclear Magnetic Resonance in Biomedicine*, 15:456–467, 2002.

12. C Pierpaoli, P Jezzard, PJ Basser, A Barnett, and G DiChiro. Diffusion tensor MR imaging of the human brain. *Radiology*, 201(3):637–648, 1996.

13. AM Uluğ, N Beauchamp, RN Bryan, and PCM van Zijl. Absolute quantitation of diffusion constants in human stroke. *Stroke*, 28(3):483–490, 1997.

14. C Beaulieu. The basis of anisotropic water diffusion in the nervous system – a technical review. *Nuclear Magnetic Resonance in Biomedicine*, 15:435–455, 2002.

15. C Pierpaoli and PJ Basser. Toward a quantitative assessment of diffusion anisotropy. *Magnetic Resonance in Medecine*, 33:893–906, 1996.

16. DC Alexander, GJ Barker, and SR Arridge. Detection and modeling of non-gaussian apparent diffusion coefficients profiles in human brain data. *Magnetic Resonance in Medecine*, 48:331–340, 2002.

17. AL Alexander, KM Hasan, M Lazar, JS Tsuruda, and DL Parker. Analysis of partial volume effects in diffusion-tensor MRI. *Magnetic Resonance in Medicine*, 45:770–780, 2001.

18. MR Wiegell, HBW Larsson, and VJ Wedeen. Fiber crossing in human brain depicted with diffusion tensor MR imaging. *Radiology*, 217(3):897–903, Dec 2000.

19. DS Tuch, RM Weisskoff, JW Belliveau, and VJ Wedeen. High angular resolution diffusion imaging of the human brain. In *Proceedings 7th Annual Meeting of ISMRM*, page 321, 1999.

20. S Pajevic, A Aldroubi, and PJ Basser. A continuous tensor field approximation of discrete DT-MRI data for extracting microstructural and architectural features of tissue. *Journal of Magnetic Resonance*, 154:85–100, 2002.

21. K Hoffman and R Kunze. *Linear Algebra*. Prentice-Hall, Inc., Englewood Cliffs, NJ, 1971.

13

Visualizing the Topology of Symmetric, Second-Order, Time-Varying Two-Dimensional Tensor Fields

Xavier Tricoche[1], Xiaoqiang Zheng[2], and Alex Pang[2]

[1] University of Utah, Salt Lake City, UT 84112, USA
   tricoche@sci.utah.edu
[2] University of California, Santa Cruz, CA 95064, USA
   {zhengxq,pang}@cse.ucsc.edu

Summary. We introduce the underlying theory behind degenerate points in 2D tensor fields to study the local field properties in the vicinity of linear and nonlinear singularities. The structural stability of these features and their corresponding separatrices are also analyzed. From here, we highlight the main techniques for visualizing and simplifying the topology of both static and time-varying 2D tensor fields.

13.1 Fundamental Notions of Two-Dimensional Tensor Field Topology

13.1.1 Basic Definitions

Eigenvector Fields

We consider symmetric, second-order two-dimensional, real tensor fields that we call *tensor fields* hereafter. The tensor values of such fields correspond to symmetric, linear transformations that map vectors to vectors in the plane. When considered in a Cartesian coordinate system, tensor fields can be represented by matrix-valued functions mapping points to 2×2 symmetric matrices. Tensor fields are fully characterized by their real eigenvalues and orthogonal eigenvectors. Hence the basic idea behind tensor field topology is to analyze the qualitative properties of a tensor field through the structure of its associated fields of eigenvectors. To formalize the notion of tensor topology, one needs a systematic way to associate a tensor field with the classified pair of corresponding eigenvector fields. This is done by sorting the eigenvectors according to the real eigenvalues.

Definition 1. *Let $\lambda_1 \geq \lambda_2$ be the two real eigenvalues of the tensor field $\mathbf{T}$, i.e. λ_1 and λ_2 are both scalar fields as functions of the coordinate vector $\mathbf{x}$.*

The corresponding eigenvector fields $\mathbf{e}_1$ *and* $\mathbf{e}_2$ *are called* major *and* minor *eigenvector field, respectively. Positions at which* $\lambda_1 = \lambda_2$ *are associated with isotropic tensor values and constitute singularities.*

Line Fields and Covering Spaces

Similar to streamlines integrated over vector fields, tensor field lines [5] are defined as follows.

Definition 2. *A tensor field line* computed in a smooth continuous eigenvector field, *is a curve that is everywhere tangent to the direction of the field. By analogy with vector fields, we associate the set of all tensor field lines in a particular eigenvector field with a mathematical* flow.

Because of the very nature of eigenvectors, the tangency is expressed at each position in the domain in terms of lines. For this reason, an eigenvector field is essentially a *line field*. This implies that classical theorems ensuring existence and uniqueness of streamlines cannot be directly applied here.

However, there exists a fundamental relationship between vector and eigenvector fields that can be formally characterized in terms of covering space. A rigorous introduction to this notion of algebraic topology is beyond the scope of this presentation and we restrict ourselves to an illustration of the basic idea. More details can be found in [6]. Consider the configuration illustrated in Fig. 13.1(a). An eigenvector field is defined over the bottom layer. This layer is covered by two similar layers over which two normalized vector fields are defined that point in opposite directions. A projection operator associates every pair of opposite vectors with a single eigenvector (line) direction in the bottom layer. Using this construct, an eigenvector field can be interpreted as the projection of two opposite vector fields. Moreover, the *path lifting property* ensures that streamlines integrated over the vector fields defined in the covering space project onto tensor field lines in the eigenvector field. This eventually provides the theoretical framework for tensor field line integration. We mentioned previously that eigenvector fields become degenerate at positions where the tensor field is isotropic, that is, has two equal eigenvalues.

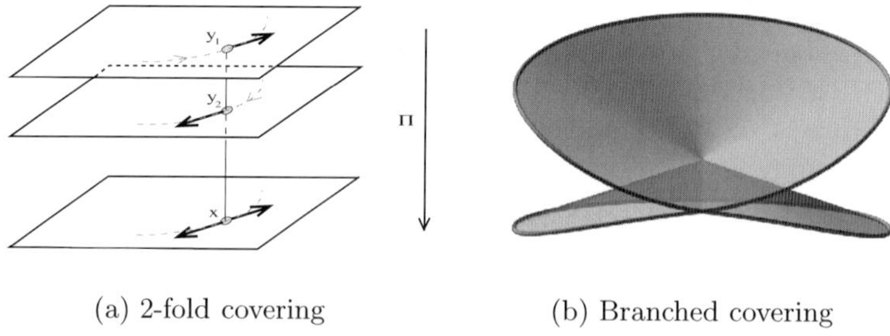

(a) 2-fold covering   (b) Branched covering

Fig. 13.1. Covering spaces

This degeneracy corresponds to a so-called branch of the covering space. In the case of a 2-fold covering of a two-dimensional space, this configuration is equivalent to the complex map $z \mapsto z^2$ defined over the unit ball around zero, as shown in Fig. 13.1(b). In other words, a degenerate point is associated with a single critical point at the branch point in the covering space through the projection operator.

Tensor Index

The relationship between vector and tensor fields can also be used to extend the notion of Poincaré index to the tensor setting. Analogous to the vector case, one defines the index of a closed curve as the number of rotations of the eigenvector fields along this curve. Since these fields are orthogonal, the tensor index has the same value for both of them. By continuity of the eigenvector fields, the index of any closed curve will take values that are multiples of $\frac{1}{2}$. As a matter of fact, the eigenvector direction reached after full rotation along the curve must be the same as the one we started from. Because of the orientation indeterminacy of eigenvectors, this direction might in fact correspond to a rotation by π of the starting eigenvector. An example is shown in Fig. 13.2.

The tensor index is independent of the coordinate frame. Moreover, it remains invariant under local continuous transformations of the eigenvector field since it takes discrete values. Additionally a curve enclosing a region exhibiting uniform flow has index 0 and the index of a curve enclosing a set of curves is the sum of their individual indices.

13.1.2 Degenerate Points

The map associating a tensor value with the corresponding pair of eigenvectors is singular at locations where the tensor value is isotropic.

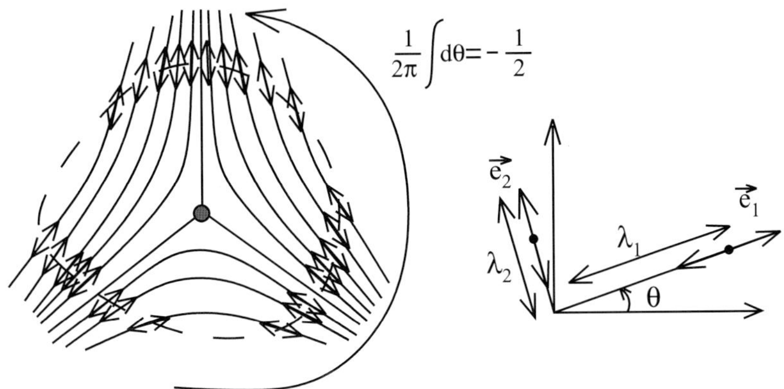

Fig. 13.2. Tensor index of a trisector

Definition 3. *A degenerate point of a two-dimensional tensor field is a location where the field is isotropic. At this position, every non-zero vector is an eigenvector.*

Because of the indeterminacy of the eigenvectors at degenerate points, tensor lines can intersect there. In the following, we successively consider the linear and nonlinear cases.

Degenerate Points in Planar Linear Fields

A tensor field is called linear if its scalar components are linear functions of the space variable $\mathbf{p} = (x, y)^T$. In this case, the linear system providing the position of a degenerate point has a unique solution in general. For the sake of simplicity, we assume that the degenerate point is located at the origin of the coordinate system and rewrite the tensor field as follows.

$$\mathbf{T}(\mathbf{p}) = \begin{pmatrix} \alpha(\mathbf{p}) & \beta(\mathbf{p}) \\ \beta(\mathbf{p}) & -\alpha(\mathbf{p}) \end{pmatrix} + \gamma(\mathbf{p})\mathbf{I_2} \ , \tag{13.1}$$

where γ is the mean value of the real eigenvalues, $\alpha(\mathbf{p}) = \alpha_1 x + \alpha_2 y$ and $\beta(\mathbf{p}) = \beta_1 x + \beta_2 y$ are linear functions of (x, y), and $\mathbf{I_2}$ is the identity matrix. By definition, the right term is isotropic and has no influence on the eigenvectors of $\mathbf{T}$. The remaining matrix is called the *deviator part* of the symmetric tensor, denoted $\mathbf{D}$. Observe that it is zero by construction at a degenerate point.

To characterize the flow pattern around a linear degenerate point, we extract directions of radial convergence, i.e. tensor lines reaching the degenerate point along straight lines. For convenience, we reformulate the eigensystem in polar coordinates, using the fact that it is independent of the distance to the origin in the linear case. We obtain

$$\mathbf{D}_\theta \, \mathbf{e}_\theta \times \mathbf{e}_\theta = \left(\begin{pmatrix} \alpha_\theta & \beta_\theta \\ \beta_\theta & -\alpha_\theta \end{pmatrix} \begin{pmatrix} \cos\theta \\ \sin\theta \end{pmatrix} \right) \times \begin{pmatrix} \cos\theta \\ \sin\theta \end{pmatrix} = 0 \ , \tag{13.2}$$

where $\alpha_\theta = \alpha(\cos\theta, \sin\theta) = \alpha_1 \cos\theta + \alpha_2 \sin\theta$ and $\beta_\theta = \beta(\cos\theta, \sin\theta) = \beta_1 \cos\theta + \beta_2 \sin\theta$, by linearity. Straightforward calculus yields

$$\tan 2\theta = \frac{\beta_1 \cos\theta + \beta_2 \sin\theta}{\alpha_1 \cos\theta + \alpha_2 \sin\theta} \ . \tag{13.3}$$

Setting $u = \tan\theta$ finally leads to the following cubic polynomial equation:

$$\beta_2 u^3 + (\beta_1 + 2\alpha_2)u^2 + (2\alpha_1 - \beta_2)u - \beta_1 = 0 \ . \tag{13.4}$$

Equation (13.4) has either 1 or 3 real roots that correspond to angles along which the tensor lines radially reach the origin. These angles are defined modulo π and one obtains 6 possible angle solutions for radial eigenvectors. For a given minor or major eigenvector field, one finally gets up to 3 radial eigenvectors. Consequently the linear case exhibits two major types of degenerate

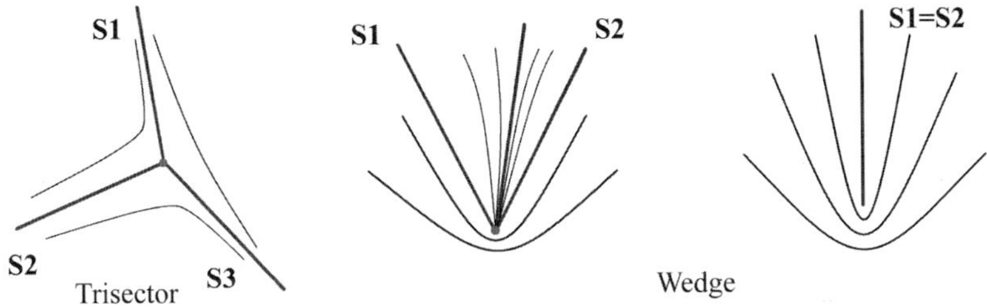

Fig. 13.3. Linear degenerate points

points as shown in Fig. 13.3. In the case of a *trisector*, the 3 directions computed previously bound so-called hyperbolic sectors, as defined in the next section. In the case of a *wedge point*, 3 radial directions correspond to the pattern shown in the middle of Fig. 13.3, while a single radial direction leads to the type depicted on the right. The analysis of the general, nonlinear case will clarify the special role of radial directions as *separatrices* of the linear topology. Considering the tensor index, it can be seen that trisectors have index $-\frac{1}{2}$ while both types of wedge points have index $\frac{1}{2}$. Again, refer to Fig. 13.2.

Nonlinear Degenerate Points

The configurations seen previously are in fact the simplest types of degenerate points. Using the notations of (13.1) it can be shown that a degenerate point is linear if and only if the following condition holds:

$$\delta := \begin{vmatrix} \dfrac{\partial\alpha}{\partial x} & \dfrac{\partial\alpha}{\partial y} \\[2mm] \dfrac{\partial\beta}{\partial x} & \dfrac{\partial\beta}{\partial y} \end{vmatrix} \neq 0 \; . \tag{13.5}$$

Observe that the determinant δ can also be used to distinguish wedge points from trisectors [3]. To study the geometric properties of tensor lines in the vicinity of a nonlinear degenerate point, we return to previous considerations about branched covering spaces (see Sect. 13.1.1). It follows from the local structure of the covering space that the vector field defined over it is wrapped by the projection operator around the degenerate point. Refer to Fig. 13.1(b). For example, Fig. 13.4 shows the vector field corresponding to a trisector point. Standard results from the qualitative theory of dynamical systems [1] tell us that the local flow structure in the vicinity of nonlinear vector field singularities always consists of a set of curvilinear sectors that exhibit one of three possible patterns:

- *parabolic*: streamlines reach the singularity in one direction but leave the neighborhood in the other.
- *hyperbolic*: streamlines leave the neighborhood in both directions.

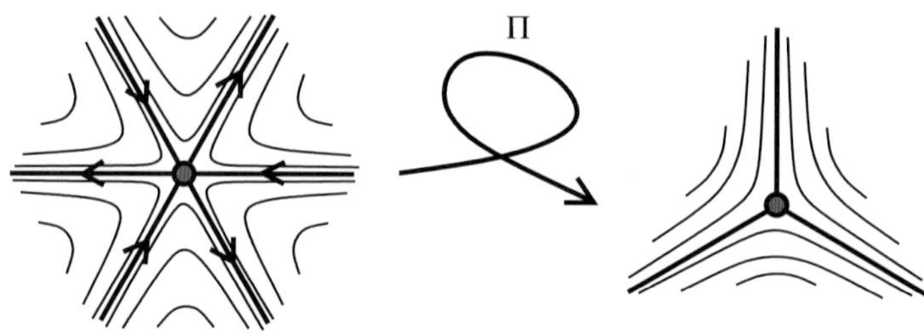

Fig. 13.4. Wrapping of monkey saddle onto trisector point

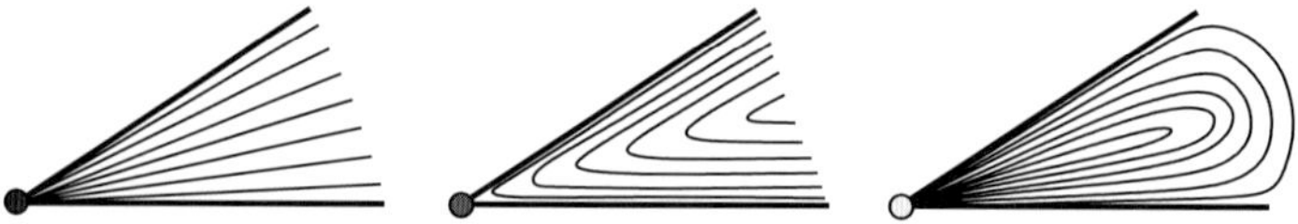

Fig. 13.5. Parabolic, hyperbolic, and elliptic sector types

- *elliptic*: streamlines reach the singularity in both directions.

From the preceding discussions, we conclude that the same sector decomposition characterizes nonlinear degenerate points. These sectors are shown in Fig. 13.5. This relationship leads to the following definition of separatrices and topological graph of a tensor field.

Definition 4. *The boundary curve of a hyperbolic sector in the vicinity of a degenerate point is called the* separatrix. *The set of all degenerate points and associated separatrices is called the* topology *of the tensor field.*

Back in the linear case, the definition above implies that the radial directions computed previously, correspond to the separatrices of linear degenerate points. Observe that in the case of a wedge point with two separatrices, two radial directions are actual separatrices whereas the third one is simply included in the parabolic sector and has no topological significance.

Eigenvalues Near Degenerate Points

Although extracting 2D singularities is simple (see Sect. 13.2), finding 3D degenerate tensors is non trivial, as explained in Chap. 14 by Zheng et al. A 3D degenerate tensor is similarly defined as one with at least two equal eigenvalues. Since 3D degenerate tensors are defined solely on eigenvalues, one might be tempted to calculate the eigenvalues at each point and try to find those that are equal. Although the issue is raised in 3D, we explain the difficulty in a 2D context. The approach above is not viable because the eigenvalues are sorted on each grid point. Unless the singularity coincides with the data point, the majors are always larger than the minors at the data points. There is no way to find the points where the major equals the minor

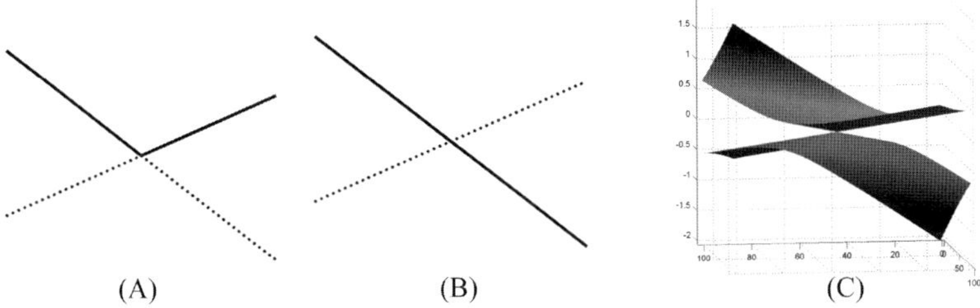

Fig. 13.6. Eigenvalues around a degenerate tensor

just from the interpolated eigenvalues. Of course, one may blame the sorting step. For example, in Fig. 13.6(A), we plot the eigenvalues on a line passing through a degenerate tensor. The solid line represents the major eigenvalues and the dotted line the minor. If we know the major and minor at discrete points, we cannot recover the degenerate points; but if we switch the order of the major and the minor after the degenerate tensor as in Fig. 13.6(B), and have the two groups of eigenvalues on discrete points, we can recover the singularities through interpolation on each group. The question becomes: can we consistently group the eigenvalues into two groups on a 2D domain, where each of them is differentiable? If this could be done, we could use bilinear or bicubic interpolation on each group to get the eigenvalue fields easily, and then recover the singularities.

However, from Fig. 13.6(C), we see that this is impossible. The figure plots the eigenvalues around a degenerate tensor on a 2D domain. Separating the eigenvalues into two differentiable groups, corresponds to separating the structure into two differentiable surfaces. But from Fig. 13.6(C), we see that the eigenvalues around a degenerate point form two conical structures. It is easy to see that there is no way to separate this structure into two differentiable surfaces. This conclusion in 2D is easily extended to 3D.

13.1.3 Structural Stability and Bifurcations

In cases where the tensor field depends on an additional parameter (e.g. time), the stability of the topological features described previously becomes an essential notion. In fact, the structures considered previously only correspond to instantaneous states of an evolving topology. Both the position and nature of degenerate points may change as the parameter is modified. They can be created or annihilated, which affects the connectivity of the topological graph. In particular, an important question is the persistence of degenerate points under small perturbations of the underlying parameter. This property is called *local stability*. Structural transformations are called *bifurcations* by analogy with the terminology used for vector fields. In this section, we restrict our considerations to simple cases of local and global bifurcations.

Structural Stability

The observations proposed next follow the line of reasoning used in the qualitative study of vector fields [7]. In the following, we provide a set of criteria that determine the stability of degenerate points and separatrices.

Degenerate Points

Similar to critical points in vector fields, degenerate points obtained in the linear, non-singular case (i.e. trisectors and wedges) are the only stable ones. As a matter of fact, it can be easily shown that arbitrarily small perturbations can transform nonlinear degenerate points into a set of linear degenerate points. The stability of trisectors and wedges is explained by the invariance of the tensor index. The stability of each type of wedge points is due to the fact that they correspond to different sets of solutions of the cubic polynomial in (13.4), which are both stable.

Separatrices

Following our analogy with the vector case, we may see that separatrices corresponding to the boundary curves of hyperbolic sectors at both ends are unstable. Examples are shown in Fig. 13.7.

The intuitive justification of this assertion is geometric in nature: adding an arbitrarily small angular perturbation to the line field around any point along such a separatrix suffices to break the connection.

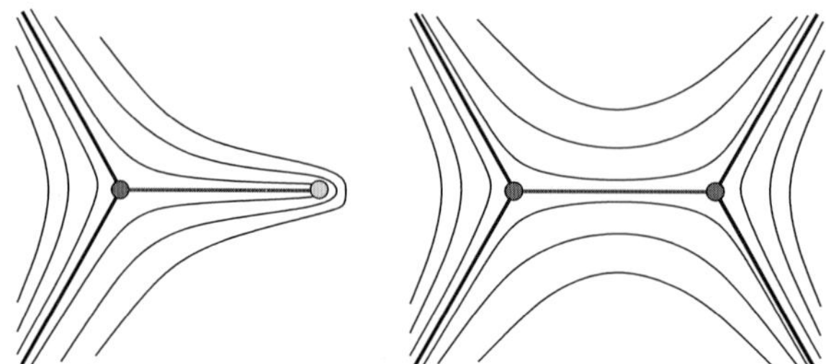

Fig. 13.7. Unstable separatrices

Local Bifurcations

Previous considerations now allow us to describe typical bifurcations associated with the instability of degenerate points. Note that we do not consider homogeneous merging, as described by Delmarcelle in [3] since it creates unstable structures.

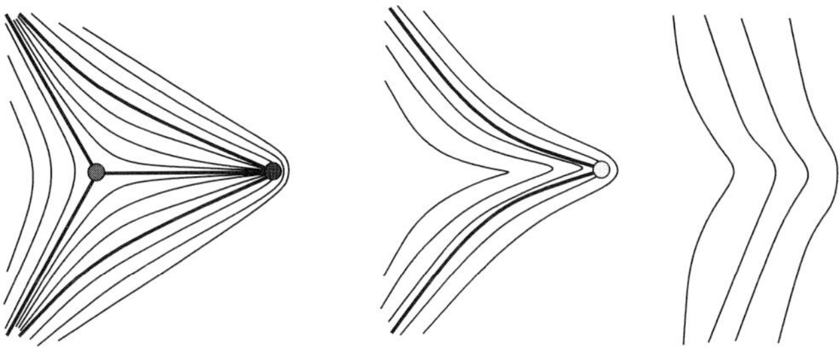

Fig. 13.8. Pairwise annihilation

Pairwise Creation and Annihilation

A wedge and a trisector have opposite indices. Therefore a closed curve enclosing a trisector and a wedge has index 0 which suggests that the combination of both degenerate points is structurally equivalent to a uniform flow. The local transition from a uniform flow to a wedge and a trisector is a *pairwise creation*. The reverse bifurcation is called *pairwise annihilation*. An example is shown in Fig. 13.8.

Wedge Bifurcation

This type of bifurcation was suggested by the remarks on the structural stability of wedge points. Each type of wedge corresponds to a specific number of real roots of the cubic polynomial in (13.4), either 1 or 3. The transition from one type to another implies the appearance or disappearance of a parabolic sector.

Global Bifurcations

In contrast to local bifurcations, global bifurcations induce changes in the connectivity of the topological graph and typically involve large regions in the domain of definition. The bifurcations mentioned here are related to previous considerations about unstable separatrices. They occur when two separatrices emanating from two degenerate points become closer, merge and then split. At the instant of merging, an unstable connection exists. As it breaks, it forces the swapping of both separatrices. This modifies the behavior of most curves in the concerned region. An example is proposed in Fig. 13.9, involving 2 trisectors.

13.2 Basic Topology Visualization

The topological approach was first introduced for the visualization of planar vector fields. Helman and Hesselink pioneered this field in 1989 [8]. They proposed a scheme for the extraction, characterization and depiction of linear

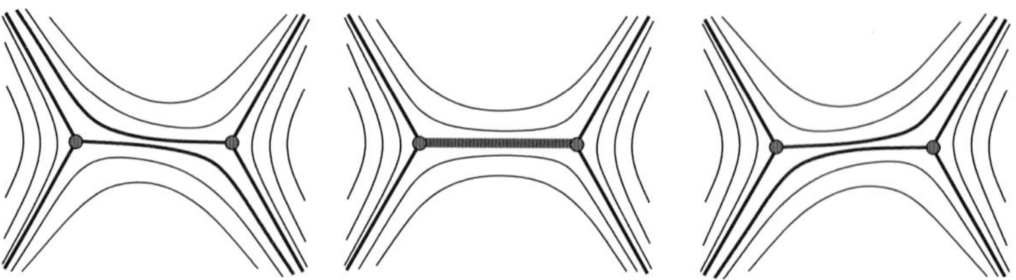

Fig. 13.9. Global bifurcation with trisector-trisector connection

critical points. This early work inspired Delmarcelle who extended the original scheme to symmetric, second-order planar tensor fields [4] as part of his work on general techniques for tensor field visualization [3]. The method can be applied to either the minor or major eigenvector field. Basically, degenerate points are searched in the data set on a cell-wise basis, where the interpolation scheme is typically linear or bilinear. The corresponding equations to solve are then either linear or quadratic. To distinguish between wedge points and trisectors, Delmarcelle used the determinant δ. Refer to (13.5). He showed that a negative value of δ characterizes a trisector, while a positive one corresponds to a wedge point. The cubic polynomial (13.4) yields the angle coordinates of the separatrices. Since angular solutions are defined modulo π, for each of them a test must be carried out to determine which one of both possible orientations actually corresponds to a radial direction in a particular eigenvector field. In the case of a wedge point, special care must be taken if the polynomial has three real roots. Indeed, one of the solutions must be discarded since it lies within the parabolic sector. This is done by retaining the two angles spanning the largest interval smaller than π, since Delmarcelle showed that parabolic sectors are always smaller than π in the linear case [3]. The edges of the topological graph are finally obtained by numerical integration of the separatrices, as tensor lines of the line field under consideration. Classical schemes for the integration of differential equations like Runge-Kutta [9] can be adapted to ensure consistency of two consecutive directions along the curve. In that way, the problem induced by the direction indeterminacy of eigenvectors can be avoided. Observe however that a small step size is required in the vicinity of degenerate points because of fast changing flow directions. This can be done by assigning the Frobenius norm of the deviator as an artificial norm to the tensor field since it provides a measure for the anisotropy. Delmarcelle also suggested a way to embed the missing information conveyed by the eigenvalues by means of a color-coding scheme applied over a LIC-like texture [2] representing the eigenvector flow as shown in Fig. 13.10(a). A possible extension of the original topology extraction technique consists in detecting half-singularities located on the boundary of the considered domain. The purpose of topology analysis is namely to characterize the flow behavior in terms of limit sets of the tensor lines, which leads to a partition of the domain in regions where all contained tensor lines connect the same limit set(s). We saw previously that degenerate

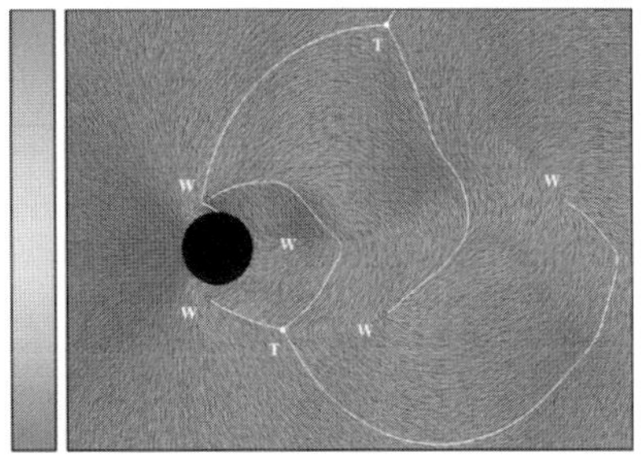 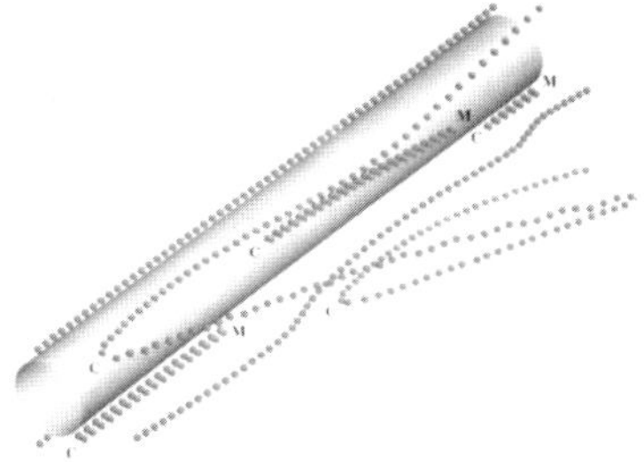

(a) Steady 2D tensor field   (b) Discrete Tracking

Fig. 13.10. Original tensor topology visualization by Delmarcelle (from [4])

points are such limit sets. Yet, dealing with bounded domains implies that
the boundary itself must be part of this classification. This line of reasoning
has already been considered by Scheuermann et al. for vector fields [10]. The
same idea applies to the tensor setting: points where the flow is tangential to
the boundary correspond to additional limit sets of the topology. They are
associated with new separatrices if the tensor line touching the boundary is
bent inward. Simple computation leads to the following equation for deter-
mining the exact position of a touching point: $\alpha\beta \sin 2\theta - \beta^2 \cos 2\theta = 0$, where
α, β and θ are functions of the edge parameterization, and $(\cos\theta, \sin\theta)^T$ is the
normalized direction of the considered boundary edge. The notations corre-
spond to (13.1). Usually, the restriction of the tensor field along the boundary
is linear over each edge. In that case, α and β are linear, too. Solving this
quadratic equation while checking if the positions obtained actually lie on the
edge (i.e. $0 \leq t \leq 1$) yields positions of tangential contact.

13.3 Topology Simplification

Topology-based visualization of symmetric tensor fields usually provides synthetic graph depictions of large and complex data sets while conveying the essential structural information of the considered phenomenon. Unfortunately,
in certain cases, the intricacy of the flow results in a cluttered representation that exhibits a large number of degenerate points and separatrices. This
problem typically arises in the analysis of turbulent data sets where numerous structures of various scales are present. In that case, it becomes tedious
to distinguish between important properties of the data and insignificant details. Observe that this problem is worsened in practice by typical low-order
interpolation schemes (like linear or bilinear interpolation) that cause artifacts. Moreover, noise is frequently present in numerical simulations which
introduces additional confusing features. An example is given in Fig. 13.11.

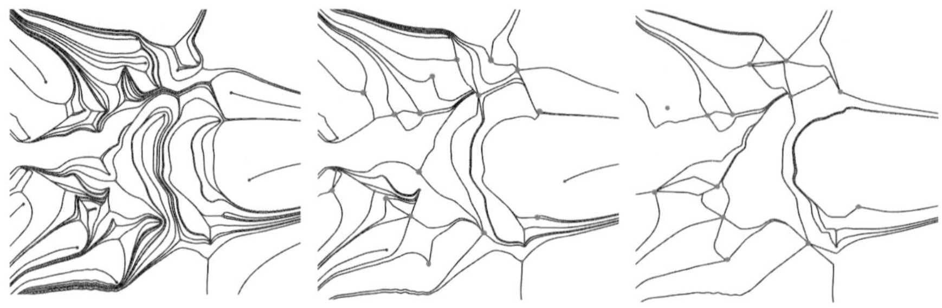

Fig. 13.11. Original and scaled topology (see color plates)

To solve this problem, simplification methods are required that discard insignificant features according to criteria specific to the considered application. The corresponding transformation of the topology must ensure consistency with the original to permit reliable analysis of the final results. Two different methods have been designed to tackle this problem, based on two different assumptions about the cause of the topological complexity.

13.3.1 Topology Scaling

The first approach is of geometric nature. Assuming that the topological complexity is inherent to the data (e.g. we have a turbulent flow) the task consists in clarifying the depiction by highlighting large scale structures while neglecting small scale details. Practically, the method is based on the observation that close degenerate points, when seen from afar, cannot be distinguished from one another and seem to be merged into a more complex, locally equivalent singularity. From the theoretical point of view, the merging of an arbitrary number of linear degenerate points creates a nonlinear singularity, as discussed in Sect. 13.1.2. These facts are the basic ingredients of the scheme proposed by Tricoche et al. [12] to scale the topology.

The first step of the method provides a segmentation of the domain into regions in which all degenerate points are sufficiently close to another, according to a prescribed proximity threshold. A bottom-up clustering scheme is therefore applied on the positions of the original singularities. The second step replaces, in each region, the contained singularities by a single one, mimicking their merging. To this end, the grid structure is locally deformed and a degenerate tensor value is assigned to a grid vertex. The interpolation scheme in the new cells ensures that this degenerate point is the only one present in the region. Further, by preserving the original field values on the region boundary, global consistency is maintained. The final step consists in extracting the structure of these nonlinear singularities. This is done by looking for radial flow directions on a cell-wise basis and characterizing the types of the various sectors surrounding the degenerate point (refer to Fig. 13.5). The separatrices are extracted as bounding curves of hyperbolic sectors and integrated over the whole domain to obtain the simplified topological graph. Results are shown in Fig. 13.11.

13.3.2 Continuous Topology Simplification

As opposed to the previous method, the second technique proposed by Tricoche et al. [13] is specifically designed to remove insignificant degenerate points from the topological graph. In other words, the topological complexity is treated as an artifact and must therefore be removed while keeping important properties unchanged. We saw previously how *bifurcations* locally modify the topology while preserving consistency with the surrounding eigenvector flow. More specifically, a *pairwise annihilation* consists of the simultaneous cancellation of a trisector and a wedge point. Therefore, imposing such bifurcations on the original data permits us to prune undesired features.

Practically, the method assumes that the tensor field is defined over a piecewise linear triangulation. First, the topological graph is computed and degenerate points are assigned to pairs of trisectors and wedges. Next, each pair of singularities is associated with a scalar value that evaluates its importance in the overall topology. Any user-prescribed criterion can be used for this purpose. A natural idea is to penalize very close degenerate points since they cause visual clutter. However, application specific knowledge can be applied to weigh individual degenerate points and, by extension, the pairs they belong to. The pairs are then sorted according to their importance and processed sequentially. For each of them, a connected cell-wise region is determined that contains the pair and no other degenerate point. In terms of tensor index, the boundary of the region has index 0 and the enclosed eigenvector flow is uniform. Finally the tensor values at the internal vertices are slightly modified in a way that guarantees that both degenerate points disappear. This deformation is controlled by angular constraints on the new eigenvector values and is based on specific properties of piecewise linear tensor fields. As a result, a pairwise annihilation has been enforced while the surrounding structure is unchanged. The corresponding results for the same data set are shown in Fig. 13.12. Looking at an enlargement, we can see that preserved features are not affected by the removals taking place in the same area, see Fig. 13.13.

13.4 Topology Tracking

Theoretical results show that bifurcations are the key to understanding and properly visualizing parameter-dependent tensor fields: they transform the topology and explain how stable structures arise. Typical examples in practice are time-dependent datasets. This basic observation motivates the design of techniques that permit us to accurately visualize the continuous evolution of topology.

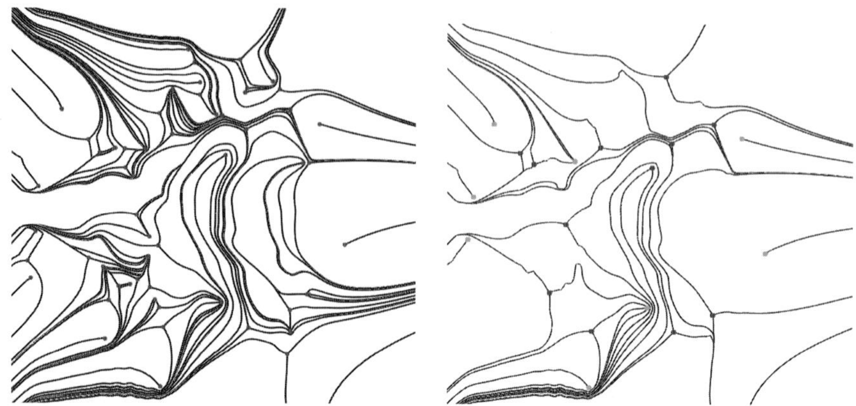

Fig. 13.12. Progressive topology simplification by enforced bifurcations (see color plates)

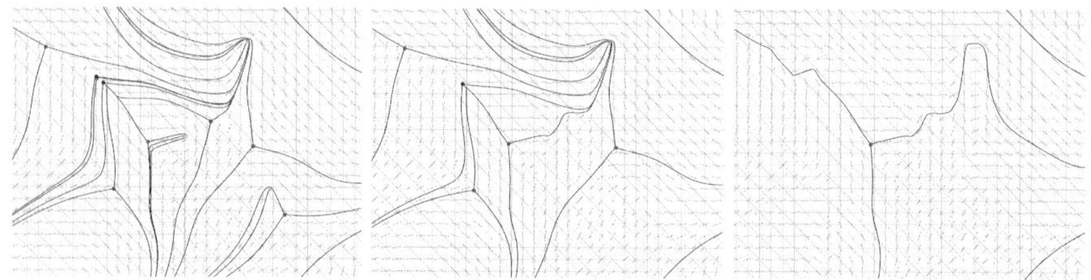

Fig. 13.13. Local topology simplification (see color plates)

An early method was proposed by Delmarcelle and Hesselink [4]. They extended their original scheme for tensor topology visualization to the time-dependent case. The method is restricted to a graphical connection between the successive positions of degenerate points and associated separatrices, leading to a connection if consistency was preserved. However no connection is made if a structural transition has occurred and bifurcations are not visualized. Instead, the comparison between successive time steps is used to infer the nature of the corresponding transitions: either creation or annihilation.

Tricoche et al. proposed a different approach in [11]. The central idea of their technique is to handle the three-dimensional space made of the Euclidean space on one hand and the parameter space on the other hand as a continuum. The time-dependent tensor data is assumed to lie on a fixed triangulation. A 'space-time' grid is constructed by linking corresponding triangles through prisms over the parameter space as shown in Fig. 13.14(a). The choice of a suitable interpolation scheme permits an accurate and efficient tracking of degenerate points through the grid along with the detection of local bifurcations. More precisely, linear space interpolation ensures that each triangle contains at most a single degenerate point at any position in time. Therefore, pairwise creations and annihilations are constrained to take place on the

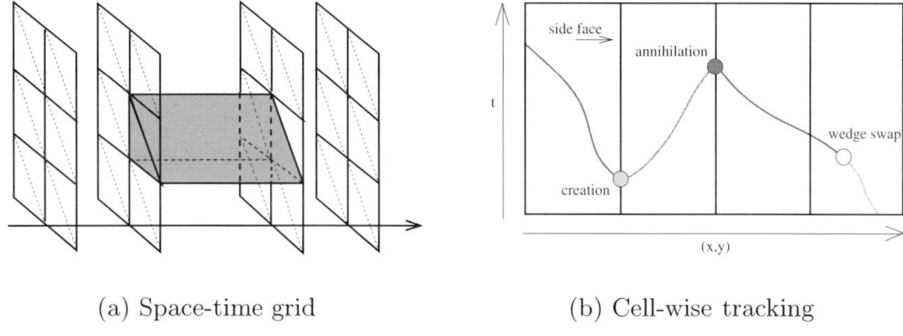

(a) Space-time grid   (b) Cell-wise tracking

Fig. 13.14. Data structure for topology tracking

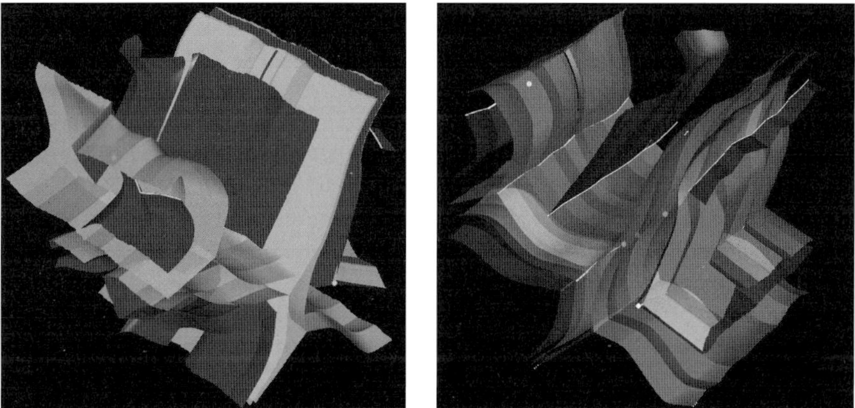

Fig. 13.15. Visualization of the complete topology evolution (see color plates)

side faces of the prisms which simplifies their detection. The principle is illustrated in Fig. 13.14(b). Individual degenerate points are tracked over prisms and potential wedge bifurcations are detected in their interior. The corresponding segments are then reconnected and pairwise creations/annihilations are found. The paths followed by degenerate points yield curves over the 3D grid. Separatrices integrated from them span separating surfaces that are obtained by embedding corresponding curves in a single surface. These surfaces are used further to detect modifications in the global topological connectivity: consistency breaks correspond to global bifurcations. See Fig. 13.15.

13.5 Conclusion

The topological approach provides a powerful framework for the visualization of planar, symmetric, second-order tensor fields. Essential properties of tensor data sets can be efficiently depicted by extracting the singularities of the associated eigenvector fields and integrating the set of separatrices that forms their connectivity. This yields synthetic, graph-type representations that capture the structural characteristics of tensor fields.

In this chapter we have introduced the essential theoretical notions that found the concept of topology in the tensor setting. By clarifying the relationship between vector and tensor topology, the vast mathematical tradition of dynamical systems can be leveraged to analyze eigenvector fields. From the visualization viewpoint, we have discussed the implementation of the basic topology-based technique, and described extensions that address the visual clutter induced by turbulent or noisy fields, as well as their transient nature.

References

1. A. Andronov, E. Leontovich, I. Gordon, and A. Maier. *Qualitative Theory of Second-Order Dynamic Systems*. Israel Program for Scientific Translations, 1973.
2. B. Cabral and L. Leedom. Imaging vector fields using line integral convolution. *Computer Graphics (SIGGRAPH Proceedings)*, 27(4):263–272, 1993.
3. T. Delmarcelle. *The Visualization of Second Order Tensor Fields*. PhD Thesis. Stanford University, 1994.
4. T. Delmarcelle and L. Hesselink. The topology of symmetric, second-order tensor fields. In *IEEE Visualization*, pp. 140–147, 1994.
5. R. Dickinson. A unified approach to the design of visualization software for the analysis of field problems. *Three-Dimensional Visualization and Display Techniques*, 1083:173–180, 1989.
6. B. Gray. *Homotopy Theory. An Introduction to Algebraic Topology*. Pure and Applied Mathematics. Academic Press, 1975.
7. J. Guckenheimer and P. Holmes. *Nonlinear Oscillations, Dynamical Systems and Linear Algebra*. Springer, 1983.
8. J. Helman and L. Hesselink. Representation and display of vector field topology in fluid flow flow data sets. *IEEE Computer*, 22(8):144–152, 1989.
9. W. Press, S. Teukolsky, W. Vetterling, and B. Flannery. *Numerical Recipes in C, Second Edition*. Cambridge University Press, 1992.
10. G. Scheuermann, B. Hamann, K. Joy, and W. Kollmann. Visualizing local topology. *Journal of Electronic Imaging*, 9(4):356–367, 2000.
11. X. Tricoche, G. Scheuermann, and H. Hagen. Tensor topology tracking: A visualization method for time-dependent 2D symmetric tensor fields, 2001.
12. X. Tricoche, G. Scheuermann, and H. Hagen. Scaling the topology of symmetric second order tensor fields. pp. 171–184, 2003.
13. X. Tricoche, G. Scheuermannn, and H. Hagen. Topology simplification of symmetric, second order 2D tensor fields. pp. 275–292, 2003.

Degenerate 3D Tensors

Xiaoqiang Zheng[1], Xavier Tricoche[2], and Alex Pang[1]

[1] University of California, Santa Cruz, CA 95064, USA
   {zhengxq,pang}@cse.ucsc.edu
[2] University of Utah, Salt Lake City, UT 84112, USA
   tricoche@sci.utah.edu

Summary. Topological analysis of 3D tensor fields starts with the identification of degeneracies in the tensor field. In this chapter, we present a new, intuitive and numerically stable method for finding degenerate tensors in symmetric second order 3D tensor fields. This method is based on a description of a tensor having an isotropic spherical component and a linear or planar component. As such, we refer to this formulation as the *geometric approach*. In this chapter, we also show that the stable degenerate features in 3D tensor fields form lines. On the other hand, degenerate features that form points, surfaces or volumes are not stable and either disappear or turn into lines when noise is introduced into the system. These topological feature lines provide a compact representation of the 3D tensor field and are useful in helping scientists and engineers understand their complex nature.

14.1 Introduction

Tensor fields, especially second-order tensor fields, are useful in many medical, mechanical and physical applications such as: fluid dynamics, meteorology, molecular dynamics, biology, astrophysics, mechanics, material science and earth science. Effective tensor visualization methods can enhance research in a wide variety of fields. However, developing an effective algorithm can be difficult because of the large amount of information contained in 3D tensor fields: there are nine independent components in each tensor and six for a symmetric tensor. Users in many research fields are especially interested in real symmetric tensors. In some applications, the data themselves are inherently symmetric. In other cases, symmetric tensor data can be obtained through various decomposition techniques.

The main motivation and goal of this chapter is to develop a simple yet powerful representation of 3D real symmetric tensor fields. Topology-based methods can yield simplified and effective depictions in many visualization fields. These methods consist of two parts: identifying the critical features, and their separatrices. Together, they divide the data space into regions with locally similar characteristics. Different types of topology can be extracted from a data field depending on how the critical features are defined. In this chapter, we are interested in features defined by the relative magnitudes of the eigenvalues. That is, when some of the eigenvalues are equal, the resulting degeneracy is a critical feature. We assume that the tensor fields are continuous and differentiable. A typical tensor field is one where the tensors are 'randomly' distributed in the tensor space, and does not have any inherent constraints such as having two equal eigenvalues at all times. On the other hand, a degenerate tensor field may have, by definition, two repeated eigenvalues everywhere – such as in momentum flux tensor fields defined as: $\Pi = V \cdot V^T$ for a flow field V. In this case, the tensor field is degenerate everywhere. The degenerate features are important in that they are the backbone from which the separatrices are anchored, and they provide a launching point for further analyses into the tensor field. For example, these features may form the basis for seeding hyperstreamlines [7].

Early work on using topology-based method to visualize tensor fields by [1, 2] lays an important background for this research project. It defines the tensor topology based on degenerate features and discusses its nature for the 2D case in great detail, and provides useful knowledge for the 3D case. But we find this early work insufficient in studying 3D tensor topology. Not only is the dimensionality of the features unknown, but how to numerically extract the topological structures is also obscure. In their previous work, Hesselink et al. mentioned that the dimension of the degenerate features can be points, lines, surfaces or subvolumes. This claim itself is essentially true, but it does not point out the dimension of features in a typical 3D tensor field. By analogy, although the critical features (defined by locations where the velocity is zero) in 3D vector fields can be lines, surfaces or even subvolumes, we know they are mostly isolated points in a typical vector field. This knowledge is the foundation for the study of topological structure in vector visualization. All the subsequent study on separatrices are based on the extraction of the critical *points*. On the other hand, no topological results on 3D real symmetric tensor fields have been published to date indicating that critical features in tensor fields form *lines*.

Our recent research [8], we found that the degenerate features in 3D tensor fields form feature lines that are stable even in the presence of noise. In the next section, we discuss the dimensionality of features in 3D tensor fields. Then, we quickly review the traditional method of finding degenerate features in 3D tensors fields based on *discriminants*, followed by the *constraint function* approach presented in [8]. Both of these methods are considered implicit functional approaches. This is followed by a presentation of our new method based on the geometric interpretation of a tensor.

14.2 Dimensionality of Degenerate Features

Similar to the 2D case described by Tricoche et al. in Chap. 13, a 3D real symmetric tensor can be decomposed into three orthogonal eigenvectors, each of which has a real eigenvalue associated with it. They are labeled as major, medium and minor eigenvectors according to the relative order of their eigenvalues. A tensor is degenerate when two or more of the eigenvalues are equal. The corresponding position in the tensor field is called a degenerate point. It follows that degenerate points are the only places where hyperstreamlines can cross each other, and therefore they are critical features in the tensor fields. The collection of these degenerate points constitutes the topological features of interest. Although the experience in flow visualization shows that a visualization restricted to topology alone may be incomplete and ignore essential features like vortex core lines, this analysis remains an important step towards better understanding of the complicated nature of 3D tensor data.

Before we can extract these topological features from 3D tensor fields, we need to know their dimension. Algorithms to locate points, lines, surfaces and volumes employ very different strategies. During our earlier work [8], we discovered that for most typical 3D tensor fields, the dimension of the topological feature is *one*, i.e. the collection of degenerate points form lines. This conclusion can be shown using an early theorem by von Neumann and Wigner which states that the real symmetric degenerate matrices form a variety of codimension two [5]. Codimension is defined as the difference between the dimension of a space and the dimension of a subspace contained in it. Read symmetric tensors in 3D have six independent components. Therefore they form a tensor space of dimension six. A double degenerate tensor where two eigenvalues are equal can be uniquely specified using four parameters. In other words, double degenerate tensors form a subspace A of dimension four in 6D tensor space. In a typical setting, tensor fields defined in 3D space usually form a subspace B of dimension three in the same 6D tensor space. The degenerate tensors are then the intersection of these two subspaces. It can be shown by transversality that these dimensions satisfy the following formula: $\text{codim}(A \cap B) = \text{codim}(A) + \text{codim}(B)$, which yields $\text{codim}(A \cap B) = 2 + 3 = 5$, that is this intersection usually has a dimension one, i.e. forms lines. From the same line of reasoning, we know that degenerate tensors are isolated points in most cases if the data is specified in a 2D space. Since most numerical algorithms are designed to capture points, the basic block of our feature extraction algorithm is to locate 3D degenerate tensors on a 2D patch and then to connect them into lines afterwards.

While the main features are lines, it is still possible to obtain features that are points, surfaces or subvolumes. Features that form points, surfaces or subvolumes are less common in most 3D tensor fields and are usually induced by symmetry constraints. Such features are considered unstable and do not persist under perturbation. For example, a triple degenerate point where three eigenvalues are equal can be uniquely specified using one parameter (scaling of an identity matrix). In this case, previous computation yields a codimension $5 + 3 = 8 > 6$, which results in an unstable feature. Hence we focus our tensor feature extraction on lines rather than surfaces or subvolumes. Having said that, our extraction algorithm still needs to extract points first as these form the basis for finding the lines. Because of this design criterion, features that are surfaces (e.g. in the single point load data) or subvolumes may not be detected as readily as feature lines. This limitation is not insurmountable, but is rather based on the effective use of limited resources in finding features that are not as common nor as stable.

14.3 Implicit Function Approach

The first family of methods to analyze degenerate tensors is through implicit functions. In this family, a tensor is degenerate if and only if its value makes an implicit function equal zero. Here we introduce two formulations: *discriminant* and *constraint function*. Note that since degenerate tensors form a variety of codimension two, an ideal formulation of the implicit constraint defining degenerate tensors should have two implicit functions. But neither of the two formula shown below has this property.

14.3.1 Discriminants

Hesselink et al. [2] define degenerate points as those tensors having at least two equal eigenvalues. Fortunately, we do not need to conduct the eigen-decomposition to find the degenerate points. A tensor has two (or three) equal eigenvalues if and only if its discriminant equals zero. The discriminant D_3 of a tensor T with eigenvalues λ_1, λ_2 and λ_3 is defined as,

$$T = \begin{pmatrix} T_{00} & T_{01} & T_{02} \\ T_{01} & T_{11} & T_{12} \\ T_{02} & T_{12} & T_{22} \end{pmatrix} \tag{14.1}$$

$$D_3(T) = (\lambda_1 - \lambda_2)^2 (\lambda_2 - \lambda_3)^2 (\lambda_3 - \lambda_1)^2 \tag{14.2}$$

This can be reformulated into a form that does not require eigen-decomposition to determine eigenvalues as follows:

$$P = T_{00} + T_{11} + T_{22} \tag{14.3}$$

$$Q = \begin{vmatrix} T_{00} & T_{01} \\ T_{01} & T_{11} \end{vmatrix} + \begin{vmatrix} T_{11} & T_{12} \\ T_{12} & T_{22} \end{vmatrix} + \begin{vmatrix} T_{22} & T_{02} \\ T_{02} & T_{00} \end{vmatrix} \tag{14.4}$$

$$R = \begin{vmatrix} T_{00} & T_{01} & T_{02} \\ T_{01} & T_{11} & T_{12} \\ T_{02} & T_{12} & T_{22} \end{vmatrix} \tag{14.5}$$

$$D_3(T) = Q^2 P^2 - 4RP^3 - 4Q^3 + 18PQR - 27R^2 \qquad (14.6)$$

From (14.2), we can easily find that a discriminant is (a) always non-negative; (b) equal to zero if and only if at least two of the eigenvalues are equal. And it is ideal for computation and numerical purposes because although it is defined on eigenvalues, we do not really need to carry out an expensive eigen-decomposition. Instead, we only need to compute (14.6) which is a polynomial of order six to get the discriminant.

An interesting geometric mapping of the three real eigenvalues is the Cardano circle or the eigenwheel (see Chap. 12 by Kindlmann). This is illustrated in Fig. 14.1 where the three roots are the x-intercepts of the three axes that are 120 degrees apart. Note that the roots λ_1, λ_2 and λ_3 are increasing from left to right. The angle of the axes associated with the largest eigenvalue and the positive X axis is labeled as α. It is obvious that a double degeneracy occurs when $\alpha = 0$ resulting in $\lambda_1 = \lambda_2$, and $\alpha = 180$ resulting in $\lambda_2 = \lambda_3$. We refer to the first type of double degeneracy as Type L for linear, and the second type of double degeneracy as Type P for planar. A triple degenerate point occurs when all three eigenvalues are equal, and the radius of the circle reduces to zero. A very rare event indeed.

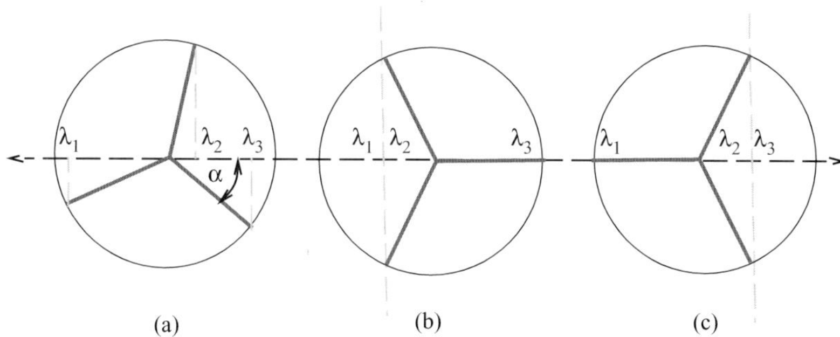

Fig. 14.1. Cardano's circle. The center of the circle is the mean of the three eigenvalues, and the eigenvalues are the x-coordinates of the line segments. (**a**) Relative positions of eigenvalues along the x-axis, (**b**) type L double degenerate point where the minor and medium eigenvalues are equal, and (**c**) type P double degenerate point where the medium and the major eigenvalues are equal

14.3.2 Constraint Functions

In [8], an alternative formulation of degenerate points leading to a more stable numerical solution was presented. We briefly highlight the results here.

Although Equation 14.6 provides an elegant representation for evaluating the discriminant without having to perform eigen-decomposition, it is difficult to solve. In (14.6), the discriminant of a real symmetric tensor is a polynomial of order six. Since it is always non-negative, the degenerate tensor also happens to be its minimum. Rather than using a minimization approach to find the degenerate tensors, the numerical analysis community recommends a root-finding strategy such as conjugate gradient for better numerical stability. A good method widely used to find the root of an equation is to detect the change of signs and then to recursively bisect the domain of interest. But because the degenerate feature is itself a minimum, there is no change of sign at all. Relying on the gradients is also dangerous, because the gradients are notoriously unstable unless they are very close to the feature. Due to this high-orderedness and singularity, directly finding the root of a cubic discriminant stably is very difficult. Instead, we look for another representation of the discriminant.

In our previous investigation, we found that while Hilbert [3] pointed out that not all non-negative polynomials can be broken down into the sum of squares of polynomials, the cubic discriminant can be written as the sum of the squares of *seven* polynomials. We also learned that not only can the discriminant of a second-order tensor of any dimension be expressed as the sum of squares [4], but our solution to the 3D case of *seven* equations is optimal [6] in the number of equations. Therefore, the definition of degenerate tensors can also be expressed as the tensors where the seven *constraint functions* are all zero at the same time. We use these seven cubic equations to extract the feature lines from 3D tensor fields. The seven discriminant constraints are:

$$
\begin{aligned}
f_x(T) &= T_{00}(T_{11}^2 - T_{22}^2) + T_{00}(T_{01}^2 - T_{02}^2) + T_{11}(T_{22}^2 - T_{00}^2) \\
&\quad + T_{11}(T_{12}^2 - T_{01}^2) + T_{22}(T_{00}^2 - T_{11}^2) + T_{22}(T_{02}^2 - T_{12}^2) \\
f_{y1}(T) &= T_{12}(2(T_{12}^2 - T_{00}^2) - (T_{02}^2 + T_{01}^2) + 2(T_{11}T_{00} + T_{22}T_{00} \\
&\quad - T_{11}T_{22})) + T_{01}T_{02}(2T_{00} - T_{22} - T_{11}) \\
f_{y2}(T) &= T_{02}(2(T_{02}^2 - T_{11}^2) - (T_{01}^2 + T_{12}^2) + 2(T_{22}T_{11} + T_{00}T_{11} \\
&\quad - T_{22}T_{00})) + T_{12}T_{01}(2T_{11} - T_{00} - T_{22}) \\
f_{y3}(T) &= T_{01}(2(T_{01}^2 - T_{22}^2) - (T_{12}^2 + T_{02}^2) + 2(T_{00}T_{22} + T_{11}T_{22} \\
&\quad - T_{00}T_{11})) + T_{02}T_{12}(2T_{22} - T_{11} - T_{00}) \\
f_{z1}(T) &= T_{12}(T_{02}^2 - T_{01}^2) + T_{01}T_{02}(T_{11} - T_{22}) \\
f_{z2}(T) &= T_{02}(T_{01}^2 - T_{12}^2) + T_{12}T_{01}(T_{22} - T_{00}) \\
f_{z3}(T) &= T_{01}(T_{12}^2 - T_{02}^2) + T_{02}T_{12}(T_{00} - T_{11}) \\
D_3(T) &= f_x(T)^2 + f_{y1}(T)^2 + f_{y2}(T)^2 + f_{y3}(T)^2 \\
&\quad + 15f_{z1}(T)^2 + 15f_{z2}(T)^2 + 15f_{z3}(T)^2
\end{aligned}
\tag{14.7}
$$

A tensor is degenerate if and only if all of its seven constraint functions are zero. This is the condition that we employ to extract the degenerate 3D tensors. Its first advantage is that the constraint functions are only cubic polynomials, instead of a polynomial of order of six which tend to oscillate more. This property leads to a more stable and accurate numerical algorithm. In addition, the requirement that all seven constraint functions be zero at

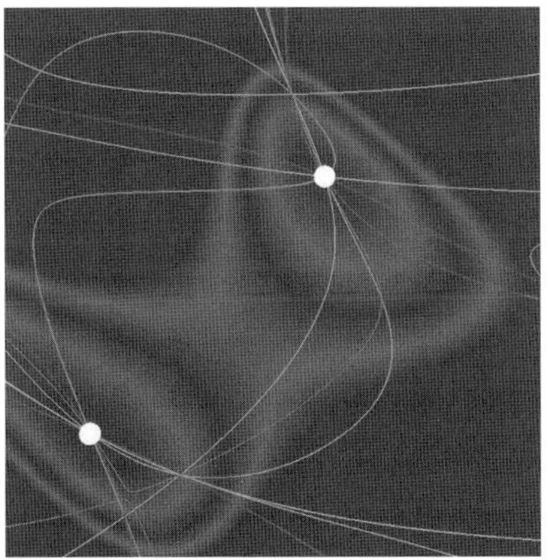

(a) Two degenerate points

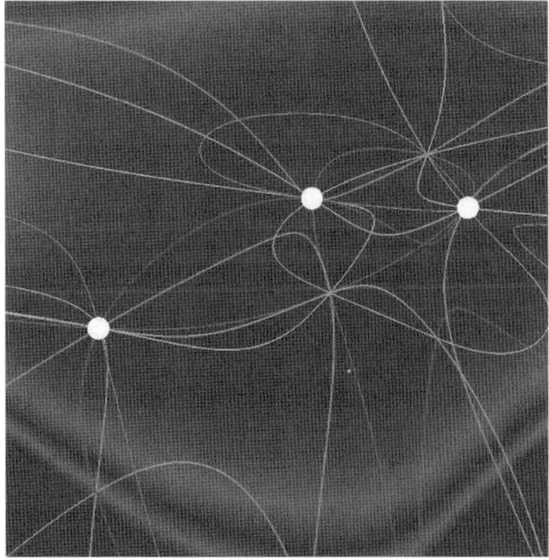

(b) Three degenerate points

Fig. 14.2. White dots are degenerate points indicating places where all seven constraint functions are zero. Each colored curve corresponds to a constraint function being equal to zero. Places where multiple curves intersect are where multiple constraint functions are satisfied simultaneously. The background is pseudo-colored by the discriminant functions. The data is a 2D slice of a randomly generated 3D tensor field. See color plates

the same time depends on the tensor value only and not on the gradient calculated from adjacent tensors. Hence, the algorithm yields a more accurate result than the algorithms that rely on finding degenerate points where the gradients of the discriminants are zeros. Its second advantage is that the constraint functions can be both positive or negative, as opposed to always being non-negative. This property allows us to perform a fast and inexpensive check for the existence of features. And finally, the reformulation also does not require eigen-decomposition.

To find the degenerate lines, we visit all the cells in the data. For each cell, we first examine all the faces and find their intersections with the feature lines, if any. After all the degenerate points are extracted, we revisit the cells and connect them to form lines. Note that in our current implementation, we only consider regular hexahedral cells.

To find the degenerate points on a 2D face, we employ an iterative root finding method that satisfies all the seven constraint functions simultaneously. Note that although we are looking at a 2D face, the tensors are still 3D. Assume the tensor at location X is denoted by $T(X)$. For the feature points X^*, we have $\overrightarrow{CF}(X^*) = CF_i(X^*) = 0$, for $i = 1, \ldots, 7$, where $\overrightarrow{CF}(X)$ is an assembly of the seven constraint functions into one vector function. Using the Newton-Raphson method and an initial guess of X_n, we have the following conceptual algorithm,

$$X_{n+1} = X_n - \left(\frac{\partial \overrightarrow{CF}}{\partial X}\right)^{-1} \cdot \overrightarrow{CF}\Bigg|_{X=X_n}$$
$$= X_n - \left(\frac{\partial \overrightarrow{CF}}{\partial T} \cdot \frac{\partial T}{\partial X}\right)^{-1} \cdot \overrightarrow{CF}\Bigg|_{X=X_n} \tag{14.8}$$

Note that we calculate the $\frac{\partial \overrightarrow{CF}}{\partial X}$ from the chain rule using $\frac{\partial \overrightarrow{CF}}{\partial T}$ and $\frac{\partial T}{\partial X}$ rather than from the interpolated values of $\overrightarrow{CF}$ on the grid using finite difference methods for higher precision. $\frac{\partial \overrightarrow{CF}}{\partial T}$ is calculated from the formula of the tensor constraints, and $\frac{\partial T}{\partial X}$ is from the interpolated tensor values. We used both the bilinear and bicubic natural spline interpolations.

However, (14.8) does not work because on a cell face, X is only 2D while $\overrightarrow{CF}$ is 7D. Thus, $\frac{\partial \overrightarrow{CF}}{\partial X}$ is a 7×2 matrix. There are a number of ways to deal with such a system. In our case, we find that the least square estimator involving the transpose of the matrix works quite well.

$$X_{n+1} = X_n - \left(\frac{\partial \overrightarrow{CF}}{\partial X}^T \cdot \frac{\partial \overrightarrow{CF}}{\partial X}\right)^{-1} \left(\frac{\partial \overrightarrow{CF}}{\partial X}^T \cdot \overrightarrow{CF}\right)\Bigg|_{X=X_n} \tag{14.9}$$

This new hybrid algorithm minimizes the square error terms among the seven constraints. Using the center of each cell as the initial guess for an intersection point, we find that this method converges to the actual intersection point within five iterations in most non-degenerate cases with precisions up to 10^{-9}, and it almost never misses a feature point if it exists. Even if it happens, as evidenced by disconnected feature lines, the missing points can be recovered by subdividing the cell face or tracing the tangents of the feature lines [9]. This Newton-Raphson based method on constraint functions is superior in speed, accuracy and precision compared to other methods developed directly based on the cubic discriminants. For example, we also implemented a comparison algorithm based on cubic discriminant that searched for its minimum using conjugate gradient methods. Not only is it about 50 times slower, using any precision less than 10^{-6} will yield a false negative rate of over 50%.

14.4 Geometric Approach

Since we want to extract the degenerate tensors in a root-finding framework, it is desirable to have a system of equations with an equal number of equations as there are unknowns. However, neither the discriminant nor the constraint functions satisfy this condition. An equation based on discriminant is under-specified since there is only one equation but with two unknowns. An equation based on constraint functions is over-specified because there are seven equations with two unknowns. The formulation on constraint functions is better than its discriminant counterpart numerically because an over-specified

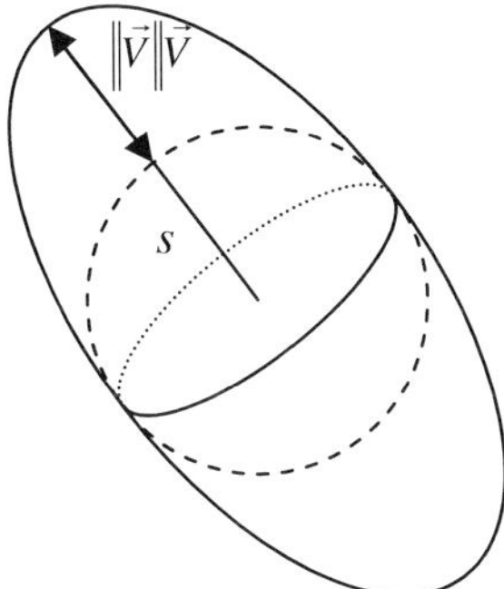

Fig. 14.3. Relationship between s and V and the degenerate tensor glyph

system is easier to solve using the modified Newton-Raphson algorithm and achieves high convergence rates and precision. In this section, we present another extraction algorithm based on the geometric properties of 3D tensors that meets the desired criterion of a well defined system.

Theorem 1. *A tensor T is degenerate if and only if it can be written as the sum of a spherical tensor and a linear tensor* (see Fig. 14.3).

A linear tensor transforms all vectors onto a line. The sufficiency of this theorem is easy to prove. To show its necessity, we simply subtract the duplicate eigenvalues from the diagonal components of the tensor. It is easy to show that the remaining tensor has two duplicate zero eigenvalues. In other words, the rank of the remaining tensor is at most rank one, i.e., linear. Depending on the sign of the other eigenvalue, a linear real symmetric tensor can always be written as the product of a vector, its transpose and an extra sign. This gives us a simple way to write a degenerate tensor,

$$T = sI \pm V \cdot V^T \tag{14.10}$$

where s is a scalar, I is a 3×3 identity matrix and V is a 3×1 vector. An advantage of this formula is that it can distinguish between type P and type L double degenerate points: T is type P with equal major and medium eigenvalues if the minus sign holds; and T is type L with equal minor and medium eigenvalues if the plus sign holds. In applications where the users are only interested in the major hyperstreamline topology, they only need to keep the minus sign, since the major hyperstreamlines are only degenerate at type P features. The three eigenvalues are: $\lambda_1 = \lambda_2 = s$, and $\lambda_3 = s \pm \|V\|^2$. One of the eigenvectors is $e_3 = V/\|V\|$ and the other two eigenvectors are any two orthogonal vectors that are also perpendicular to e_3. Besides its simplicity, this equation also clearly states that all 3D degenerate tensors form a four-parameter family. A degenerate tensor on a 2D patch of a typical 3D real symmetric tensor field can be found by solving:

$$T(x,y) = sI \pm V \cdot V^T \tag{14.11}$$

Finding the location (x,y) of a four-parameter degenerate tensor on a 2D patch means we will have six unknowns. Since there are six independent components in real symmetric tensors, we can write a system of six equations with six unknowns. Such well-defined systems can be solved using any standard numerical method such as Newton-Raphson or one of its variants. And since the problem is well-defined, we also expect it to have stable and isolated solutions.

For the initial guess in the Newton-Raphson method, we use the center of the patch, (x_0, y_0), in place of the position parameters (x, y). Suppose the tensor at (x_0, y_0) is T_0 and suppose that its eigenvalues are $(\lambda_1 \leq \lambda_2 \leq \lambda_3)$ and its normalized eigenvectors are (e_1, e_2, e_3), respectively. Without loss of generality, we also assume that we are extracting type P degenerate features. The algorithm for extracting type L degenerate features is similar in form. To obtain the initial estimates of the four parameters (s, V), we use the following heuristic,

$$s_0 = \frac{\lambda_2 + \lambda_3}{2} \tag{14.12}$$

$$V_0 = \sqrt{s_0 - \lambda_1} \cdot e_1 \tag{14.13}$$

Using s_0 and V_0 for the initial guess, we iteratively update the six parameters using the Newton-Raphson method until convergence to a solution. Since each equation is a simple quadratic equation, taking derivatives is trivial. When the algorithm converges, not only do we have the location of the degenerate feature, but we also get the eigenvalues and eigenvectors of the tensor values at that point from s and V. Besides its simplicity, the disadvantage of this algorithm is also obvious – we need to invert a 6×6 matrix during each iteration of the Newton-Raphson algorithm. A less obvious disadvantage is that in our experiments, this algorithm shows worse numerical stability than the algorithms built on the constraint functions in situations when the features are very close to triple degeneracy.

A useful form of 3D tensor is the *deviator*. It is simply a 3D tensor whose trace is zero, which implies that the sum of the eigenvalues is also zero. We can obtain the deviator part of any 3D tensor T by subtracting one third of its trace from its three diagonal components. Since this is a linear operation, the zero-trace property is preserved on a discrete grid using tri-linear interpolation.

One variation of the basic geometric algorithm is to consider only the deviator field of the original tensors. For the case of extracting type P degenerate features, it is easy to get,

$$s = \frac{V_x^2 + V_y^2 + V_z^2}{3} \tag{14.14}$$

Substituting this term back into (14.11) and throwing away any redundant diagonal equation, we get a system with five equations and five unknowns.

In our experiments, we found that this variation is almost equivalent to the original algorithm in terms of numerical stability and convergence speed.

14.5 Topological Feature Lines

Now that we have obtained the degenerate points using one of the methods described in the two previous sections, the next step is to form the topological feature lines. The general idea is to connect the degenerate points on cell faces with those at neighboring cell faces. However, as we can clearly see in Fig. 14.2, some cells may have more than one degenerate point, and hence more than one feature line going though them. We therefore use a multi-pass approach to connect these degenerate points. The procedure proceeds by examining only those candidate cells that contain degenerate points (i.e. intersection points of feature lines with the face) on at least one of their six faces. In the first pass, all candidate cells containing exactly two intersection points are processed by: (a) simply connecting those two points, (b) recording the orientation of the line segment as tangents at the end points, and (c) marking the cell as processed. In each subsequent pass, the number of candidate cells is further reduced by connecting the remaining intersection point(s) to points in neighboring cells that have been processed earlier, and therefore have tangent information. If a face has multiple degenerate points, we select the point that minimizes the angle between the resulting feature line and the previously computed tangent. Each candidate cell is marked as processed, and the procedure continues until there are no more candidate cells.

In our current implementation, we use this iterative method to generate the tangent lines on topological feature points and ultimately resolve the line connections between multiple points. In the future, we plan to calculate the tangent of the degenerate tensor line at a specific feature point analytically instead of this post-processing method.

14.6 Results

We experimented with four data sets to test out our degenerate tensor extraction algorithm using the geometric approach. In the experiments, we use a pre-filtering algorithm that is similar to the one used in [8]. The first is a 2D rectangular patch with randomly set symmetric 3D tensor values at the four corners (see Fig. 14.2). The tensor values within the patch are obtained through linear interpolation. This synthetic data corresponds to tensors on a face of a 3D cell. The second is a 3D hexahedral cell also with randomly set symmetric 3D tensors values at its eight corners (see Fig. 14.4). It is resampled into a finer resolution for smoother features lines. The third is the stress tensor data in a semi-infinite volume with two point loads (see Fig. 14.5). The fourth is the deformation tensors in the computed flow past a cylinder with hemispherical cap

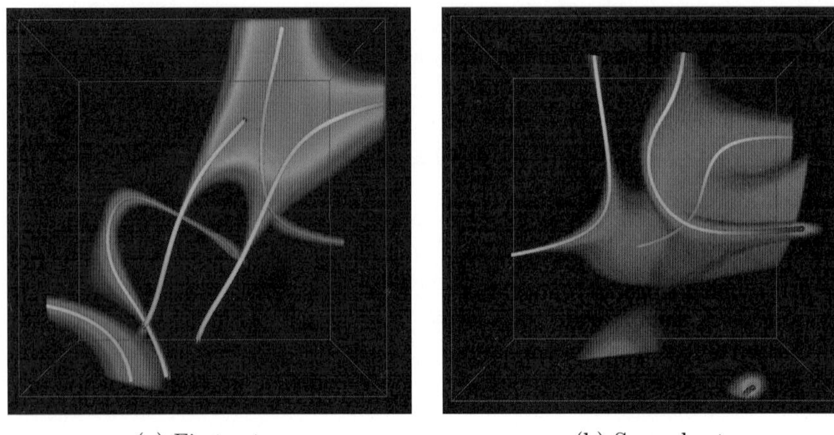

(a) First set   (b) Second set

Fig. 14.4. Randomly generated 3D tensors. Warmer line colors are closer to type P degenerate points where major and medium hyperstreamlines intersect, while cooler line colors are closer to type L degenerate points where medium and minor hyperstreamlines intersect. The rest of the volume is pseudo-colored by the discriminant using cool colors for low discriminant values (closer to feature lines) and warm transparent colors for distant values. See color plates

(see Fig. 14.6). From Figs. 14.4 to 14.5, the colors of the volumes are mapped to the tensor discriminant (14.6) with blue mapped with lower transparency to zero and warmer colors with higher transparency mapped to higher values. Degenerate tensors can be found in the blue regions. Additional digital images can be accessed online at: www.cse.ucsc.edu/research/avis/tensortopo.html.

Figure 14.4 shows degenerate tensors in a 3D cell form feature lines (rendered as tubes). Note that the feature lines are *not* hyperstreamlines, rather

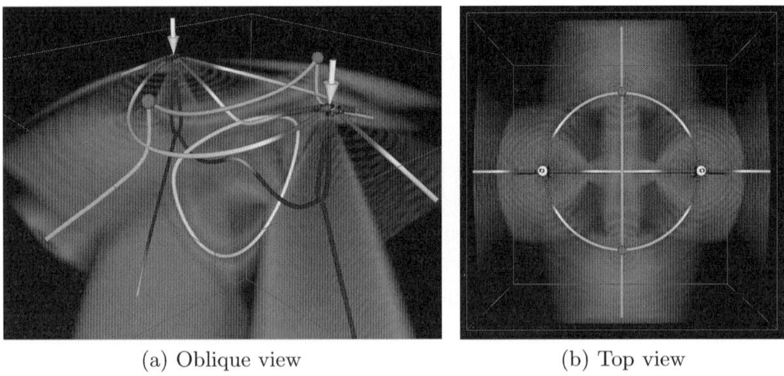

(a) Oblique view   (b) Top view

Fig. 14.5. Double point load data. Arrows indicate point load, while the 2 magenta spheres show the location of the triple degenerate points. Color scheme is the same as Fig. 14.4. See color plates they are where the major and medium, or the medium and minor, or all three hyperstreamlines intersect each other. Only the faint green is visible in the vicinity of the tubes because the tubes are in the blue regions. The color of the tubes are such that type P points with very different minor value are mapped to warmer colors, and type L points with very different major value are mapped to cooler colors. The milder colors are where the other eigenvalue is not as different as the degenerate pair. We see that complex feature lines can form even from a simple linearly interpolated random tensor field.

Figure 14.5 shows the double point load stress tensors. The yellow arrows indicate the two point loads, and the two magenta spheres are the triple degenerate points. We can see the line of double degeneracy connecting these two stress-free points as alluded to in [2]. Other very interesting feature lines are also extracted: (1) a vertical loop that lies directly under the double degenerate feature line connecting the two triple degenerate points. This feature is not present in the single point load data. This loop feature is also stable in the sense that it persists even as the relative magnitudes of the two point loads are varied. (2) how the blue feature line below each of the point load bifurcate and then reconnect. These two structures and the vertical loop are connected together by a type P feature line running between the two point loads. Looking from the top view in (b), we see another interesting feature which is the circular feature line that connects the two point loads and the two triple degenerate points. It is worth noting that in the vicinity below each load point, the stress tensors are similar to those found in single point load data sets where we have observed the degenerate tensors to form a conical *surface*. One can also make out these degenerate conical surfaces, particularly the one under the more distant point load in (a). Since our algorithm is designed for extracting features lines, it produces artifacts when the features form a surface or subvolume.

Figure 14.6 shows degenerate lines in the deformation tensors of the computed flow at an angle past a cylinder with a hemispherical cap. Only a portion of the data close to the cap is shown because most of the interesting features are found there. A little bit of asymmetry is apparent on the left side of Fig. 14.6(b) where the seam of the curvilinear grid wraps around. We see a curved line on the cap shown by the black arrow. It matches some of the patterns of the velocity topology from the same data set. There are more features at the upper half of the data because the flow there is more turbulent. Figure 14.6(a) is from an oblique view. Most of the features are close to the geometry of the object except a complicated branch structure which extends away from the geometry. It contains a small cyan horn shape pointed by the pink arrow, two green ring shapes, and a bifurcating structure. Figure 14.6(b) is from a top view. Recall that lines with cool colors have type L degeneracies while lines with cool colors have type P degeneracies. While we can see some lines that are greenish in color, we did not find any triple degeneracies. Also, while we can see very interesting complicated line structures, we have

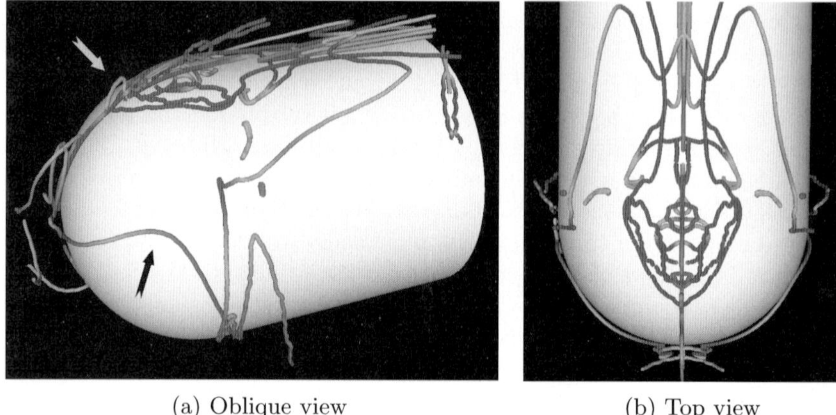

(a) Oblique view   (b) Top view

Fig. 14.6. Degenerate lines in deformation tensors of flow past a cylinder with a hemispherical cap. Feature lines are colored as in Fig. 14.4. See color plates

yet to explore their full significance as we still need to develop methods for extracting the separating surfaces in order to describe the full topology.

The time statistics for the different data sets are summarized in Table 14.1. All the results are generated on a Dell Dimension 8100 with a single 1.5 GHz Pentium 4, 1Gb of memory, and an nVidia GeForce2 Ultra.

14.7 Open Problems

There are many open problems that need to be investigated. We highlight a few of them here.

First, since all the algorithms are built on extracting lines, they have problems dealing with features that form surfaces and volumes. Finding the separatrices of these features would also need to be addressed.

Second, in our numerical algorithms, we define the degenerate tensors as points with two equal eigenvalues without considering the eigenvectors. But we are originally interested in these points because they are where hyperstreamlines can cross each other, and hyperstreamlines are defined on eigenvectors.

Table 14.1. Time to extract degenerate tensors in different datasets

Data Set	Time
2D Random Patch (1×1)	0.05 (millisec)
3D Random Cell ($32 \times 32 \times 32$)	0.9 (sec)
Double Point Load ($64 \times 64 \times 64$)	4.2 (sec)
Hemisphere ($72 \times 110 \times 84$)	23 (sec)

Therefore, a proper definition or an extraction algorithm based on both eigenvalues and eigenvectors could provide more insight into this problem. This is possible through a quantity solely defined on eigenvectors and is similar to the index of 2D critical points.

At each point along the degenerate lines, we can project the 3D tensors onto a 2D plane perpendicular to the eigenvector with distinct eigenvalue [7]. The projected 2D tensors also show a degenerate pattern. One can extract the separatrix of the 3D tensor field by calculating the separatrices of the projected 2D tensors at each point and connecting them together. With the 3D degenerate tensors and their separatrix surfaces, we will have a complete topological structure of 3D tensor fields.

Simplification and tracking of the topological structure proved to be useful for 2D tensor fields (see Chap. 13). In 3D, they are more difficult since the degenerate features become lines instead of points.

Finally these techniques should be extended to other application domains such as diffusion tensor (DT) MRI data described in other chapters of this book. While the main attribute of interest is usually the path of the fibers, highly linear fibers are where we would likely find feature lines. Hence, it is possible that topological visualization of DT-MRI data would also be beneficial. For this approach to be of real practical interest, the issue of topological artifacts induced by noisy data must be addressed as well. DT-MRI data are considered as typical tensor fields since there is no inherent constraint on the eigenvalues that may result in different codimensions. Although it could have large regions where the tensors are close to degeneracy, if one examines those points with very high precision and checks their persistence against noise, the results still form lines. That is, the topological features in such tensor fields form feature lines that are stable even in the presence of noise [8]. In practice, if an algorithm detects these nearly degenerate regions, such as in isotropic regions, it can mark off that region and skip the subsequent topological analysis because these regions contain very little topological information. Alternatively, those regions can be removed by post-processing or simplification. While we have found that feature lines are stable even in noisy environment, the topological structure (both for vectors and tensors) is quite sensitive. This can be used to our advantage, for example, when comparing topological structures from two tensor fields.

14.8 Conclusion

Double degenerate points in 3D real symmetric tensor fields form lines. These are the stable features. In this chapter, we presented an intuitive geometric approach used in extracting these feature lines. It provides an alternative to the constraint functions and the discriminant function formulations. In all these three approaches, degenerate points are first extracted on each face of a candidate hexahedral cell. These points are then connected in an iterative fashion to generate feature lines. We applied this algorithm on several data sets including randomly generated tensor fields, the analytic double point load data set, and the computational data set on a flow past a cylinder with a hemispherical cap. The results from the double point load stress tensor field reveals new insight on a thoroughly studied data set by Hesselink et al. At the same time, the results also point to several areas that require further investigation such as studying the correlation between the interesting patterns we saw in the real data sets and the underlying physics. These new insights will be useful in designing strategies for seeding hyperstreamlines, topology simplification, and tracing topology in time-varying data.

Acknowledgment

This work is supported by NSF ACI-9908881. The flow data is courtesy of NASA. We would also like to thank Peter Lax and Beresford Parlett for their correspondence.

References

1. T. Delmarcelle and L. Hesselink. The topology of second-order tensor fields. In R.D. Bergeron and A.E. Kaufman, editors, *Proceedings IEEE Visualization '94*, pp. 140–148. IEEE Computer Society Press, 1994.
2. L. Hesselink, Y. Levy, and Y. Lavin. The topology of symmetric, second-order 3D tensor fields. *IEEE Transactions on Visualization and Computer Graphics*, 3(1):1–11, Jan-Mar 1997.
3. D. Hilbert. Über die Darstellung definiter Formen als Summen von Formenquadraten. *Math. Annalen*, 32:342–350, 1888.
4. P. D. Lax. On the discriminant of real symmetric matrices. *Communications on Pure and Applied Mathematics*, 51(11-12):1387–1396, 1998.
5. Peter Lax. *Linear Algebra*. Wiley, 1996.
6. B. N. Parlett. The (matrix) discriminant as a determinant. *Linear Algebra and its Applications*, 355:85–101, 2002.
7. Wei Shen. Seeding strategries for hyperstreamlines. Master's thesis, University of California, Santa Cruz, 2004.
8. Xiaoqiang Zheng and Alex Pang. Topological lines in 3D tensor fields. In *Proceedings of Visualization 04*, pp. 313–320, Austin, 2004.
9. Xiaoqiang Zheng and Alex Pang. Topological lines in 3D tensor fields and discriminant hessian factorization. *IEEE Transactions on Visualization and Computer Graphics*, 2005. to appear.

15

Locating Closed Hyperstreamlines in Second Order Tensor Fields

Thomas Wischgoll and Joerg Meyer

University of California at Irvine, Irvine, CA 92697-2625, USA
{twischgo,jmeyer}@uci.edu

Summary. The analysis and visualization of tensor fields is an advancing area in scientific visualization. Topology-based methods that investigate the eigenvector fields of second order tensor fields have gained increasing interest in recent years. Most algorithms focus on features known from vector fields, such as saddle points and attracting or repelling nodes. However, more complex features, such as closed hyperstreamlines are usually neglected. In this chapter, a method for detecting closed hyperstreamlines in tensor fields as a topological feature is presented. The method is based on a special treatment of cases where a hyperstreamline reenters a cell and prevents infinite cycling during hyperstreamline calculation. The algorithm checks for possible exits of a loop of crossed edges and detects structurally stable closed hyperstreamlines. These global features cannot be detected by conventional topology and feature detection algorithms used for the visualization of second order tensor fields.

15.1 Introduction

Many problems in natural science and engineering involve tensor fields. For example, stresses, viscous stresses, rate-of-strain, and momentum flux density are described as symmetric tensor fields. Due to the multivariate nature of tensor fields, appropriate methods for visualization are required in order to investigate the data. This, of course, includes the detection of special properties of a tensor field, for instance topological features, that can be emphasized on in the visualization to reduce visual clutter.

The topological analysis of tensor fields as described by Hesselink et al. [DH94] focuses on degenerate points and their topological meaning. A special type of degenerate point, the trisector point, corresponds to saddle points in vector fields from a topological point of view. Hyperstreamlines, that follow the vectors in a particular, previously chosen eigenvector field, lead to separatrices inside a 2-D tensor field. Similarly, a detailed analysis of the degenerate points [HLL97] in a symmetric, second order 3-D tensor field leads to hyperstreamlines [HD93] depicting parts of the topology of the tensor field. To incorporate the two remaining eigenvector fields that are not used for integrating the hyperstreamline, an ellipse spanned by those two eigenvectors is used, resulting in a tube-shaped representation that follows the main eigenvector field.

Obviously, integrating curves inside an eigenvector field plays an important role in such a visualization. The qualitative nature of these curves can be studied with topological methods developed originally for dynamical systems. Especially in the area of fluid mechanics, topological analysis and visualization have been used with success [GLL91, HH91, Ken98, SHJK00].

Besides point-shaped singularities, other topological features exist in tensor fields. Similar to closed streamlines in vector fields [WS01, WS02], closed hyperstreamlines can be found in tensor fields. These integral curves within an eigenvector field are closed, therefore forming a loop. Their importance stems from the fact that quite often neighboring integral curves either tend to bend toward the loop or originate from the loop (i.e. tend to move toward the loop after reversing the direction of time). This is a well established result from dynamical systems theory [GH83, HS74]. Consequently, being able to determine closed hyperstreamlines in tensor fields is an important addition to tensor field topology.

Several publications have dealt with related topics in vector fields. Hepting et al. [HDER95] study invariant tori in four-dimensional dynamical systems by using suitable projections into three dimensions to enable detailed visual analysis of the tori. Wegenkittel et al. [WLG97] present visualization techniques for known features of dynamical systems. Bürkle et al. [BDJ$^+$99] use a numerical algorithm developed by some of the coauthors [DJ99] to visualize the behavior of more complicated dynamical systems. In the literature on numerical methods, one can find several algorithms for the calculation of closed curves in dynamical systems [Jea80, vV87], but these algorithms are tailored to dealing with smooth dynamical systems where a closed form solution is given.

In most cases, visualization deals with piecewise linear, bilinear or tri-linear data. In this chapter, a suitable algorithm for this situation is presented which can be integrated into a computational algorithm for standard hyperstreamlines. While computing a hyperstreamline, the algorithm tracks the visited cells and checks for repetition. Upon revisiting a cell, the algorithm tests if the hyperstreamline stays in the same cell cycle indefinitely. For this purpose, the boundary of the current cell cycle is investigated to determine if the integral curve can cross this boundary.

The structure of the remainder of this chapter is as follows. First, a short description of the mathematical background is given. Subsequently, the algorithm for detecting closed hyperstreamlines is discussed. Finally, results of the algorithm are presented and concluding remarks are given.

15.2 Mathematical Background

This section provides the necessary theoretical background and the mathematical terms used in the algorithm. The scope of this chapter is restricted to steady, linearly interpolated three-dimensional second order tensor fields defined on a tetrahedral grid:

$$t : \mathbb{R}^3 \supset D \to Mat(3 \times 3, \mathbb{R}), \quad (x, y, z) \mapsto \begin{pmatrix} t_{11} & t_{12} & t_{13} \\ t_{21} & t_{22} & t_{23} \\ t_{31} & t_{32} & t_{33} \end{pmatrix} =: (t_{ij}) \ .$$

D is assumed to be bounded. This is the case for almost every experimental or simulated tensor field that has to be visualized. A tensor described as a three-by-three matrix can be decomposed into two matrices $S = (s_{ij})$ and $A = (a_{ij})$ such that the equation $T = A + S$ holds where $s_{ij} = \frac{1}{2}(t_{ij} + t_{ji})$ and $a_{ij} = \frac{1}{2}(t_{ij} - t_{ji})$. Then S is called the symmetric part of the tensor T since the equation $s_{ij} = s_{ji}$ holds for every i and j, while A is the antisymmetric part of the tensor T with $a_{ij} = -a_{ji}$. Since the antisymmetric part of a tensor basically describes a rotation only, this chapter focuses on symmetric, second order tensors. For these, the eigenvalues exist and are real. The corresponding eigenvectors form an orthogonal basis of $\mathbb{R}^3$. This allows the computation of hyperstreamlines by using one eigenvector field for calculating integral curves, while the remaining two eigenvalues can be used to span an ellipse resulting in a tube that follows the direction of the followed eigenvector field [HD93]. In addition, the ellipse can be scaled using the remaining eigenvalues.

According to the definition by Hesselink et al. [DH94], the topology of a tensor field is the topology of its eigenvector fields. Consequently, critical points known from vector fields, such as saddles, nodes, and foci, occur as singularities in tensor fields as well. Due to the way hyperstreamlines are defined, an additional kind of topological feature results from that definition. In the case of two or more eigenvalues being identical, only two or one eigenvector(s) can be determined. As a consequence, hyperstreamlines end at such a point, since there is no unique way to continue. Therefore, these locations are usually referred to as degenerate points. Recent studies as described in Chap. 14 by Zheng et al. show that these points form lines instead of individual points. Consequently, this type of singularity occurs more often compared to vector field singularities. However, with respect to hyperstreamlines, degenerate points play only a minor role since a hyperstreamline that is terminated by a degenerate point can no longer be a closed hyperstreamline.

Since hyperstreamlines follow one of the eigenvector fields, the behavior of integral curves $h_a : \mathbb{R} \to Mat(3 \times 3, \mathbb{R}), \tau \mapsto h_a(\tau)$ can be described by their properties $h_a(0) = a$ and $\frac{\partial h_a}{\partial \tau}(\tau) = t(h_a(\tau))$. For a Lipschitz continuous eigenvector field, one can prove the existence and uniqueness of integral curves h_a through any point $a \in D$, see [HS74, Lan95]. The actual computation of integral curves is usually done by numerical algorithms, such as Euler methods, Runge-Kutta-Fehlberg methods or Predictor/Corrector methods [SB90].

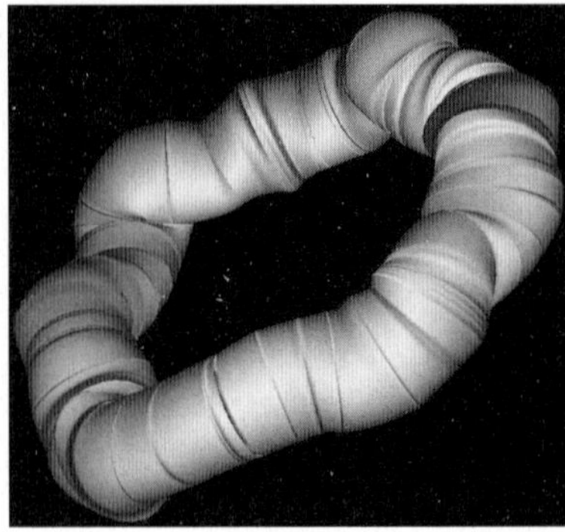

Fig. 15.1. Example of a closed hyperstreamline in a 3D tensor field. See color plates

The topology of a tensor field is defined as the topology of its eigenvector fields. Thus, the topological analysis considers asymptotic behavior of integral curves in these different eigenvector fields. In order to be able to clearly identify where integral curves are coming from and where they are going, one can define two different sets describing the area covered by the integral curve for approaching a positive or a negative infinite parameter value resulting in the α- and ω-limit set, respectively. The α-limit set of an integral curve h is defined by $\{p \in \mathbb{R}^3 | \exists (\tau_n)_{n=0}^{\infty} \subset \mathbb{R}, \tau_n \to -\infty, \lim_{n \to \infty} h(\tau_n) \to p\}$. The ω-limit set of an integral curve h is defined by $\{p \in \mathbb{R}^3 | \exists (\tau_n)_{n=0}^{\infty} \subset \mathbb{R}, \tau_n \to \infty, \lim_{n \to \infty} h(\tau_n) \to p\}$. If the α- or ω-limit set of an integral curve consists of only one point, this point is a critical point or a point on the boundary ∂D. (It is usually assumed that the integral curve stays at the boundary point indefinitely.)

The most common case of an α- or ω-limit set in an eigenvector field containing more than one inner point of the domain is a closed hyperstreamline [HS74]. This is an integral curve h_a with the property that there is a $\tau_0 \in \mathbb{R}$ with $h_a(\tau + n\tau_0) = h_a(\tau) \quad \forall n \in \mathbb{N}$. Consequently, for every closed hyperstreamline there exists a hyperstreamline that converges to this closed hyperstreamline when integrating in positive or in negative direction. This fact will be exploited later in the algorithm for detecting this topological feature.

Figure 15.1 shows a typical example of a closed hyperstreamline in a three-dimensional tensor field. Such a closed hyperstreamline is called *structurally stable* if, after small changes in the tensor field, the closed hyperstreamline remains.

15.3 Detection of Closed Hyperstreamlines

The concept of detecting closed hyperstreamlines in a three-dimensional second order tensor field is similar to the three-dimensional vector case [WS02], because a hyperstreamline follows one of the eigenvector fields. Once such a closed hyperstreamline is detected in one of the eigenvector fields a tubular structure can be built around the closed curve in a fashion similar to regular hyperstreamlines.

Since the algorithm for detecting closed hyperstreamlines in symmetric, second order 3-D tensor fields is very similar to the 3-D vector case it will be repeated here only briefly. Details can be found in [WS02]. Before the algorithm itself is explained, a few notations need to be defined. We use the term *current hyperstreamline* to describe the hyperstreamline currently under testing for the loop condition.

To reduce computational cost, the hyperstreamline is first integrated using a Runge-Kutta method of fourth order with an adaptive step size control. In order to determine eigenvectors required for this step, the tensors are interpolated tri-linearly inside the cells. Using the interpolated tensors, eigenvalues and eigenvectors can then be calculated. This is known to be numerically more stable. Otherwise, large numerical errors have the potential to modify the topology of the tensor field in such a way that singularities do not form lines any more. Further information about tensor interpolation is described by Kindlmann et al. [KWH00].

During this integration step, every cell that is crossed by the current hyperstreamline is stored in a list. If a hyperstreamline approaches a loop it reenters the same cell. This results in a *cell cycle* consisting of a finite sequence of neighboring cells $c_0, \ldots, c_n$ with $c_0 = c_n$ crossed by the current hyperstreamline.

This cell cycle identifies a region where it needs to be determined if the current hyperstreamline can escape that cycle. To check this, every backward integrated hyperstreamline starting at an arbitrary point on a face of the boundary of the cell cycle has to be considered. Looking at the edges of a face it can be seen directly that it is not sufficient to just integrate hyperstreamlines backward which originate at the vertices of that edge. This is due to the fact that individually started hyperstreamlines only cover a discrete portion of the edge. Instead, a hyperstreamsurface has to be computed with the edge in question as initial condition. Figure 15.2 shows an example where a single cell and a backward integration is depicted. A hyperstreamsurface is started at the rear left vertical edge and turns inside the cell towards the rear lower right corner of the cell. The parts of the hyperstreamsurface that are outside the cell are drawn as dashed lines. The two edges of the hyperstreamsurface which are identical with a backward integrated hyperstreamline started at the vertices of the rear left edge of the cell leave the cell at the lower and rear face, respectively. However, a hyperstreamline started at the center of the rear left edge of the cell (drawn in red) leaves the cell at the right face. If the cell cycle continuous at the right face the backward integration would be considered as leaving the cell if only the backward integrated hyperstreamlines starting at the vertices of an edge would have been considered. As a consequence, we have to find another definition for exits as in the two-dimensional vector case [WS01]. Thus, *potential exit edges*, which are the starting points of the

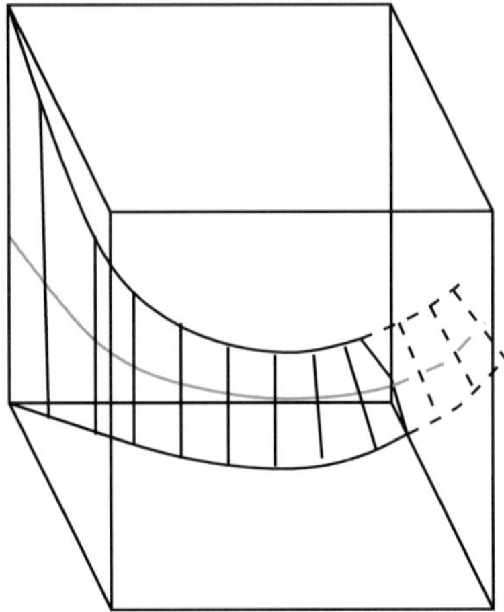

Fig. 15.2. Backward integrated hyperstreamsurface. See color plates

backward integration step, are defined as the edges on the boundary of the cell cycle. In analogy to the two-dimensional case, curves on a boundary face of a cell contained in the cell cycle where the eigenvector field is tangential to the face is identified as a *potential exit edge* as well.

Due to the nature of the interpolation inside the tetrahedral grid, it can be shown that there will be at most a two-dimensional curve on the face of a tetrahedron of that grid where the eigenvector field is tangential to the face, the whole face is tangential to the eigenvector field, or there is no tangential area at all. An isolated point on the face where the eigenvector field is tangential to the face cannot occur and do not need to be considered as a potential exit.

The potential exit edges as previously defined then serve as initial conditions for the backward integration step. Hyperstreamlines are computed originating at the potential exit edges. These hyperstreamsurfaces are then called *backward integrated hyperstreamsurface*. In case part of the hyperstreamline leaves the cell cycle the current hyperstreamline can leave at the cell cycle at that location and there is no closed hyperstreamline present in the current cell cycle. Hence, this exit edge is referred to as a *real exit edge*. It is worthwhile noting that the backward integrating step is insensitive to degenerate points. On encounter of a degenerate point, a hyperstreamsurface may separate into two parts, but can still be computed. For the backward integrated hyperstreamsurface the streamsurface algorithm introduced by Hultquist [Hul92] is used. Further details about the described methodology can be found in [WS02] due to its similarity to the vector case.

Applying this motivation to symmetric, second order 3-D tensor fields, an algorithm for detecting closed hyperstreamlines can be described. First, a hyperstreamline is integrated using a standard integration method. During that process the cells covered by the current hyperstreamline are traced to check if a cell cycle is reached. Then, all potential exit edges are identified by going backward through the crossed cells. As a final step, all exit edges are validated by integrating a hyperstreamsurface backward from every potential exit edge through the whole cell cycle. If there is no real exit edge, meaning that no backward integrated hyperstreamline left the cell cycle, the current hyperstreamline cannot leave the cell cycle. Consequently, there exists a closed hyperstreamline within the cell cycle on condition that there is no singularity contained in the cell cycle. On the other hand, if a real exit edge exists, then there is no closed hyperstreamline present in the current cell cycle. Consequently, the criterion serves as both a necessary as well as a sufficient condition. The proof for this algorithm is similar to the vector case and can be found in [WS02].

15.4 Results

To test the implementation, a synthetic data set was created which includes one closed hyperstreamline in the minor eigenvector field. To compute this data set, a two-dimensional vector field which contains two sinks and is symmetrical with respect to the y-axis is used as a starting point. In addition, all vectors residing at the y-axis are zero in this vector field. By rotating this two-dimensional vector field about the y-axis, a three-dimensional flow is created. To convert each vector v in this vector field into a tensor, basic linear algebra methods are used. First, two vectors v_1 and v_2 are determined in such a way that these two vectors in combination with the one from the vector field form an orthonormal basis of $\mathbb{R}^3$. Defining a matrix $T = (v, v_1, v_2)$ yields to a tensor $t = T \cdot E \cdot T^{-1}$, where E is a matrix defined as

$$E = \begin{pmatrix} 1 & 0 & 0 \\ 0 & 2 & 0 \\ 0 & 0 & 3 \end{pmatrix} .$$

Determining the minor eigenvector in a tensor field that was created in such a way, results in exactly the same vector that was plugged in initially. Consequently, the tensor field contains a single closed minor hyperstreamline. Figure 15.3 shows the hyperstreamline that was detected by the algorithm. The wavy appearance of the closed hyperstreamline is due to the way this data set was generated; the location of the closed hyperstreamline is determined very accurately by the algorithm. The hyperstreamline is drawn only as the center line without considering the medium and major eigenvectors. In addition, a hyperstreamline which was computed by a regular hyperstreamline algorithm was started in the vicinity of the closed hyperstreamline. The segments of this hyperstreamline are colored according to the minor eigenvalue. Due to the attracting nature of this closed hyperstreamline, the regularly

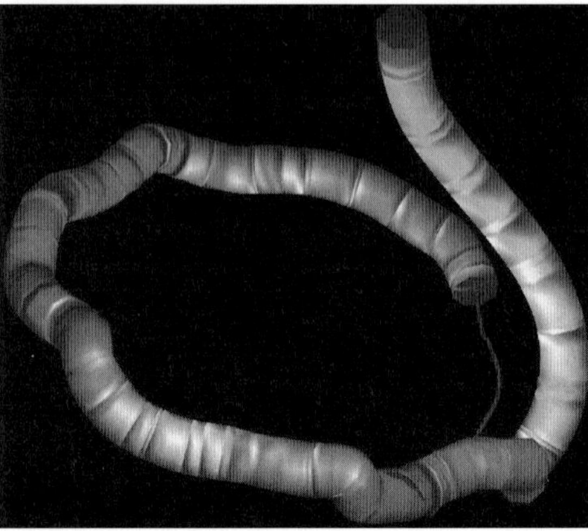

Fig. 15.3. Closed hyperstreamline (minor eigenvector field) in combination with a regular hyperstreamline. See color plates

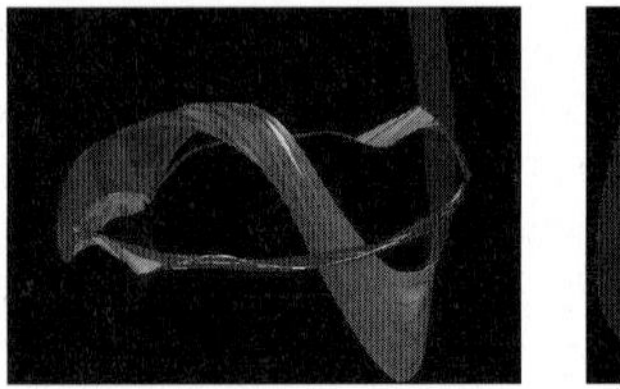 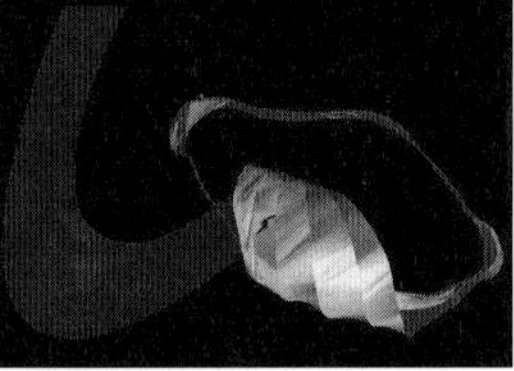 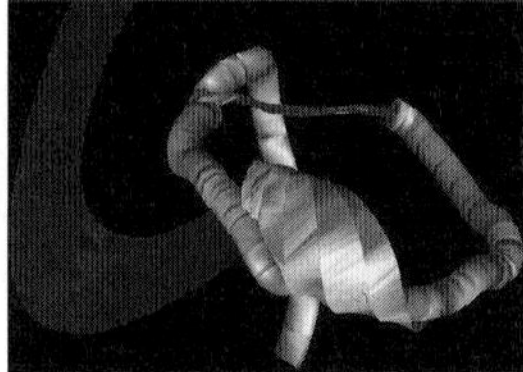

Fig. 15.4. Closed hyperstreamline including hyperstreamsurfaces exposing the surrounding tensor field (minor eigenvector field). See color plates

computed hyperstreamline approaches it and eventually merges with the first as can be seen in the figure.

Figure 15.4 shows the same closed hyperstreamline with two hyperstreamsurfaces. The hyperstreamsurfaces – just like the hyperstreamline – are attracted by this closed hyperstreamline. The hyperstreamsurface becomes smaller and smaller while it spirals around the closed hyperstreamline. After a few turns around the closed hyperstreamline, the ellipses are only slightly wider than the closed hyperstreamline itself, finally causing the hyperstreamsurface to completely merge with the hyperstreamline. A rather arbitrary color scheme is used for the hyperstreamsurfaces to enhance the three-dimensional impression.

To apply the algorithm to a more common data set, a single point load data set was used. Here, a force is applied to an infinite half space. The stress-strain tensor field is determined to describe the pressure inside that infinite half space. Figure 15.5 shows the result of the algorithm. Two major hyperstreamlines were computed, starting at the top of the figure and ending at the lower left corner. The force acting on the infinite half space is attached to the center of the funnel-shaped end of the larger hyperstreamline in the

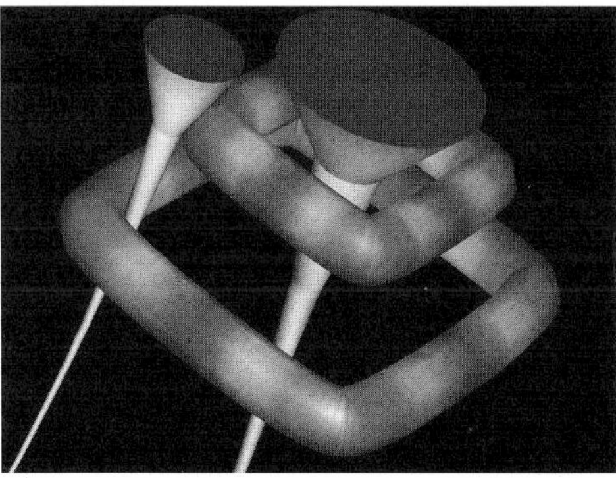

Fig. 15.5. Closed hyperstreamlines in single point load data set. See color plates

figure. Several closed hyperstreamlines can be found in the minor eigenvector field of this data set. In fact, there is a complete surface totally covered by closed hyperstreamlines. Figure 15.5 shows just two of these hyperstreamlines to avoid visual clutter. Due to the interpolation used for computing the tensors in the data set, the closed hyperstreamlines do not appear as perfect circles as would be expected from the simulation. Similar to the previous example, the segments of all hyperstreamlines are colored according to the eigenvalue whose eigenvector is used to follow the hyperstreamline.

15.5 Conclusion

A method for detecting closed hyperstreamlines in symmetric, second order tensor fields was presented. It was found that most methods that have been established for vector fields can be applied to tensor fields as well. As can be seen in the first example of Sect. 15.4, closed hyperstreamlines can have an attracting property and therefore form a topological feature. Consequently, this feature, which is missing in topological analysis algorithms, was added.

Acknowledgments

This research was supported by the National Institute of Mental Health (NIMH), the National Partnership for Advanced Computational Infrastructure (NPACI), and the Electrical Engineering and Computer Science Department of the University of California, Irvine. Further, the authors like to thank Gerik Scheuermann at the University of Leipzig, Germany, and the visualization team in Kaiserslautern, Germany for providing the single point load data set.

References

[BDJ$^+$99]   D. Bürkle, M. Dellnitz, O. Junge, M. Rumpf, and M. Spielberg. Visualizing complicated dynamics. In A. Varshney, C. M. Wittenbrink, and H. Hagen, editors, *IEEE Visualization '99 Late Breaking Hot Topics*, pp. 33–36, San Francisco, 1999.

[DH94]   T. Delmarcelle and L. Hesselink. The topology of symmetric, second-order tensor fields. In *IEEE Visualization '94 Proceedings*, pp. 140–147, Los Alamitos, 1994. IEEE Computer Society.

[DJ99]   M. Dellnitz and O. Junge. On the Approximation of Complicated Dynamical Behavior. *SIAM Journal on Numerical Analysis*, 36(2):491–515, 1999.

[GH83]   J. Guckenheimer and P. Holmes. *Dynamical Systems and Bifurcation of Vector Fields*. Springer, New York, 1983.

[GLL91]   A. Globus, C. Levit, and T. Lasinski. A Tool for Visualizing the Topology of Three-Dimensional Vector Fields. In G. M. Nielson and L. Rosenblum, editors, *IEEE Visualization '91*, pp. 33–40, San Diego, 1991.

[HD93]   L. Hesselink and T. Delmarcelle. Visualizing second order tensor fields with hyperstreamlines. *IEEE Computer Graphics and Applications*, 13(4):25–33, 1993.

[HDER95]   D. H. Hepting, G. Derks, D. Edoh, and R. D. Russel. Qualitative analysis of invariant tori in a dynamical system. In G. M. Nielson and D. Silver, editors, *IEEE Visualization '95*, pp. 342–345, Atlanta, GA, 1995.

[HH91]   J. L. Helman and L. Hesselink. Visualizing Vector Field Topology in Fluid Flows. *IEEE Computer Graphics and Applications*, 11(3):36–46, May 1991.

[HLL97]   L. Hesselink, Y Lavin, and Y. Levy. Singularities in nonuniform tensor fields. In *IEEE Visualization '97*, pp. 59–66. IEEE Computer Society, July 10 1997.

[HS74]   M. W. Hirsch and S. Smale. *Differential Equations, Dynamical Systems and Linear Algebra*. Academic Press, New York, 1974.

[Hul92]   J. P. M. Hultquist. Constructing Stream Surface in Steady 3D Vector Fields. In *Proceedings IEEE Visualization '92*, pp. 171–177. IEEE Computer Society Press, Los Alamitos CA, 1992.

[Jea80]   M. Jean. Sur la méthode des sections pour la recherche de certaines solutions presque périodiques de systèmes forces periodiquement. *International Journal on Non-Linear Mechanics*, 15:367–376, 1980.

[Ken98]   D. N. Kenwright. Automatic Detection of Open and Closed Separation and Attachment Lines. In D. Ebert, H. Rushmeier, and H. Hagen, editors, *IEEE Visualization '98*, pp. 151–158, Research Triangle Park, NC, 1998.

[KWH00]   G. Kindlmann, D. Weinstein, and D. Hart. Strategies for direct volume rendering of diffusion tensor fields. *IEEE Transactions on Visualization and Computer Graphics*, 6(2):124–138, 2000.

[Lan95]   S. Lang. *Differential and Riemannian Manifolds*. Springer, New York, third edition, 1995.

[SB90]   J. Stoer and R. Bulirsch. *Numerische Mathematik 2*. Springer, Berlin, 3 edition, 1990.

[SHJK00]   G. Scheuermann, B. Hamann, K. I. Joy, and W. Kollmann. Visualizing local Vector Field Topology. *Journal of Electronic Imaging*, 9(4):356–367, 2000.

[vV87]   M. van Veldhuizen. A New Algorithm for the Numerical Approximation of an Invariant Curve. *SIAM Journal on Scientific and Statistical Computing*, 8(6):951–962, 1987.

[WLG97]   R. Wegenkittl, H. Löffelmann, and E. Gröller. Visualizing the Behavior of Higher Dimensional Dynamical Systems. In R. Yagel and H. Hagen, editors, *IEEE Visualization '97 Proceedings*, pp. 119–125, Phoenix, AZ, 1997.

[WS01]   T. Wischgoll and G. Scheuermann. Detection and Visualization of Closed Streamlines in Planar Flows. *IEEE Transactions on Visualization and Computer Graphics*, 7(2):165–172, 2001.

[WS02]   T. Wischgoll and G. Scheuermann. 3D Loop Detection and Visualization in Vector Fields. In *Visualization and Mathematics 2002*, pp. 151–160, Berlin, Germany, 2002.

Tensor Field Visualization
Using a Metric Interpretation

Ingrid Hotz[1], Louis Feng[1], Hans Hagen[2], Bernd Hamann[1], and Kenneth Joy[1]

[1] Institute for Data Analysis and Visualization, (IDAV), Department of Computer
Science, University of California, Davis CA 95616, USA
{ihotz,zfeng}@ucdavis.edu, {hamann,joy}@cs.ucdavis.edu
[2] Computer Graphics and Visualization Group, Technical University of
Kaiserslautern, PO Box 3049, 67653 Kaiserslautern, Germany
hagen@informatik.uni-kl.de

Summary. This chapter introduces a visualization method specifically tailored to
the class of tensor fields with properties similar to stress and strain tensors. Such
tensor fields play an important role in many application areas such as structure
mechanics or solid state physics. The presented technique is a global method that
represents the physical meaning of these tensor fields with their central features: regions of compression or expansion. The method consists of two steps: first, the tensor
field is interpreted as a distortion of a flat metric with the same topological structure; second, the resulting metric is visualized using a texture-based approach. The
method supports an intuitive distinction between positive and negative eigenvalues.

16.1 Introduction

Since the physical interpretation of mathematical features of tensor fields is
highly application-specific it is important that visualization techniques are
closely driven by the special application. In this chapter, we focus on symmetric tensor fields of second order that are similar to stress strain tensor fields,
or the symmetrical part of the gradient tensor. These tensor fields are characterized by the property that they have positive and negative eigenvalues.
The sign of the eigenvalues indicates regions of expansion and compression,
and it is therefore of special interest. To understand the field behavior, it is
important to express these features in an intuitive way. The underlying idea
of our visualization method is to transform the tensor field into a metric. This
metric is represented using a texture that is aligned to the eigenvector fields,
similarly to line integral convolution (LIC) [CL93, SH95]. The eigenvalues are
included using the free parameters in the texture generation: the convolution
filter length, and parameters of an input noise texture. This approach leads
to a fabric-like texture that is dense in regions of compression and sparse in
regions of expansion.

16.2 Related Work

Even though several good visualization techniques exist for tensor fields, they only cover a few specific applications. Many of these methods are extensions of vector field visualization methods, which focus on a technical generalization without providing an intuitive physical interpretation of the resulting images. They often concentrate on the representation of eigendirections and neglect the importance of the eigenvalues. Therefore, in many application areas traditional two-dimensional plots are still used, which represent the interaction of two scalar variables.

One way to represent a tensor field is based on using icons. They illustrate the characteristics of a field at some selected points (see, for example, [Hab90, KGM95, LW93]). Even though these icons represent the tensor value at one point well they fail to provide a global view of the tensor field. A more advanced but still discrete approach uses hyperstreamlines. This approach is strongly related to streamline methods used for vector fields. They were introduced by Delmarcelle and Hesselink [DH92] and have been utilized in a geomechanical context by Jeremic et al. [JSchF02]. Given a point in the field, one eigenvector field is used to generate a vector field streamline. The other two eigendirections and eigenvalues are represented by the cross section along the streamline. This method extracts more information than icons, but it still leaves the problem of choosing appropriate seed points to the user. Thus, both methods have limited usage in exploring complete data sets and are limited to low-resolution due to cluttering.

To generate a more global view, a widely accepted solution for vector fields is the reduction of the field to its topological structure. These methods generate topologically similar regions that lead to a natural separation of a field domain. The concept of topological segmentation was also applied to two-dimensional tensor fields [HD95]. The topological skeleton consists of degenerated points and connecting separatrices. Degenerated points are where the tensor has multiple eigenvalues and the eigenvectors are not uniquely defined. Although the tensor field can be reconstructed on the basis of its topological structure, physical interpretation is difficult.

Following an approach of Pang et al. [BP98, ZP02] a tensor field is considered as a force field that deforms an object placed inside it. The local deformation of probes, such as planes and spheres, illustrate the tensor field. This method only displays a part of the information because it reduces the tensor field to a vector field. To avoid visual clutter only a small number of probes can be included in one picture. Zheng et al. [ZPa03] extended this method by applying it to light rays that are bended by the local tensor value.

Another class of visualization methods provides a continuous representation, based on textures. The first ones to use a texture to visualize a tensor field in a medical context were Ou and Hsu [OH01]. An approach based on the adaptation of LIC to tensor fields by Zheng et al. [ZP03]. Here, a white-noise texture is blurred according to the tensor field. In contrast to LIC images, the convolution filter is a two-dimensional or three-dimensional volume determined by the local 2D or 3D tensor field respectively. This visualization is especially good for showing the anisotropy of a tensor field. However, one problem of this method is the integration of the sign of the eigenvalues. Points with the same eigenvalues but with opposite sign are illustrated as isotropic.

There exist some other techniques designed especially for the visualization of diffusion tensors that only have positive eigenvalues. But they are not appropriate for stress, strain or gradient tensor fields.

16.3 Metric Definition

To motivate our approach we discuss an example for the kind of tensor fields we are interested in. These are stress tensor fields and gradient tensor fields whose behavior is very similar, as a stress tensor is often computed as gradient of a virtual displacement field. It can be observed that for gradient fields or stress and strain tensors, positive eigenvalues lead to a separation of particles or expansion of a probe. Eigenvalues equal to zero imply no change in distances, and negative eigenvalues indicate a convergence of the particles or compression of the probe.

For the symmetric part of a gradient tensor $\mathbf{S}$ of a vector field $\mathbf{v} = (v_1, v_2, v_3)$ with $s_{ij} = \frac{1}{2}\left(v_{i,j} + v_{j,i}\right)$ this behavior is expressed by (16.1). Here, $v_{i,j}$ denotes the partial derivative of the ith component of $\mathbf{v}$ with respect to coordinate x_j.

$$\frac{\mathrm{d}}{\mathrm{d}t}(\mathrm{d}s^2) = \sum_{i,k=1}^{3} s_{ik}\,\mathrm{d}x_i\,\mathrm{d}x_k = \sum_{j=1}^{3} \lambda_j\,\mathrm{d}u_j^2 \ . \tag{16.1}$$

Here, $\mathrm{d}s = (\mathrm{d}x_1,\mathrm{d}x_2,\mathrm{d}x_3)$ and $\mathrm{d}s^2$ is the quadratic distance of two neighboring points, $\lambda_j, j = 1, 2, 3$ are the eigenvalues of $\mathbf{S}$, and $\mathrm{d}u_j$ are the components of $\mathrm{d}x$ corresponding to the eigenvector basis $\{\mathbf{w}_j, j = 1, 2, 3\}$. If we focus on just one eigendirection $\mathbf{w}_i$, the change of $\mathrm{d}s^2$ is defined by the corresponding eigenvalue λ_i:

$$\lambda_i > 0 \rightarrow \frac{\mathrm{d}}{\mathrm{d}t}\,\mathrm{d}s^2 > 0 \ , \quad \lambda_i = 0 \rightarrow \frac{\mathrm{d}}{\mathrm{d}t}\,\mathrm{d}s^2 = 0 \ , \quad \lambda_i < 0 \rightarrow \frac{\mathrm{d}}{\mathrm{d}t}\,\mathrm{d}s^2 < 0 \ . \tag{16.2}$$

A similar behavior can be observed for the deformation of a probe in a stress field (see Fig. 16.1).

Considering a time-independent vector field, a formal integration of (16.1) results in the following expression for $\mathrm{d}s^2$:

$$\mathrm{d}s^2(t) = \mathrm{d}s^2(0) + \sum_{ik}(s_{ik} \cdot t)\,\mathrm{d}x_i\,\mathrm{d}x_k \ . \tag{16.3}$$

Using $\quad \mathrm{d}s^2(0) = a \cdot \sum_i \mathrm{d}x_i\,\mathrm{d}x_i \quad$ we obtain:

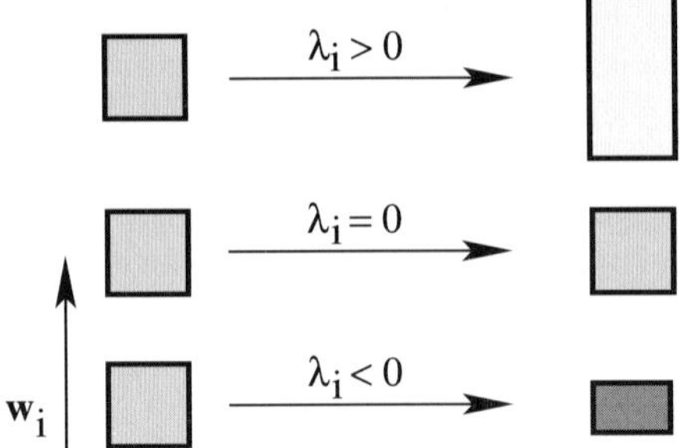

Fig. 16.1. Deformation of a unit probe under influence of a stress tensor in direction of eigenvector $\mathbf{w}_i$. Eigenvalues larger than zero correspond to a tensile, and eigenvalues smaller than zero to a compressive force in the direction of the eigenvector

$$\mathrm{d}s^2(t) = \sum_{ik} \underbrace{\left(a\delta_{ik} + s_{ik} \cdot t\right)}_{=: \, g_{ik}} \mathrm{d}x_i \, \mathrm{d}x_k, \qquad (16.4)$$

where δ_{ik} is the Kronecker-delta. The tensor $\mathbf{g}$ with components $g_{ik} = a\delta_{ik} + s_{ik} \cdot t$ can be interpreted as a time-dependent metric of the underlying parameter space D. The constant a plays the role of a unit length, and t is a time variable that can be used as a scaling factor. This metric definition is the basis of our tensor field visualization method.

16.3.1 The Transformation

Based on the observations made in Sect. (16.3), we define a transformation of the tensor field into a metric. We do not exactly follow the motivating (16.4) but use a more flexible approach.

Let $\mathbf{T}$ be a tensor field defined on a domain D. The tensor at a point $P \in D$ is given by $\mathbf{T}(P)$. For each point P, the tensor $\mathbf{T}(P)$ is mapped to a metric tensor $\mathbf{g}(P)$ describing the metric in P. In the most general form, the assignment is achieved by the following three steps:

1. Diagonalization of the tensor field:
   Switching from the original coordinate basis to the eigenvector basis $\{\mathbf{w}_1, \mathbf{w}_2, \mathbf{w}_3\}$, we obtain a diagonal tensor $\mathbf{T}'$ having the eigenvalues of $\mathbf{T}$ on its diagonal:
   $$\mathbf{T} \mapsto \mathbf{T}' = U \cdot \mathbf{T} \cdot U^T = \mathrm{diag}\left(\lambda_1, \lambda_2, \lambda_3\right) , \qquad (16.5)$$

   where U is the diagonalization matrix.

2. Transformation and scaling of the eigenvalue, to define the metric $\mathbf{g}'$ according to the eigenvector basis:

   $$\mathbf{T}' \mapsto \mathbf{g}' = \mathrm{diag}\left(F(\lambda_1), F(\lambda_2), F(\lambda_3)\right) , \qquad (16.6)$$

where $F : [-\lambda_{max}, \lambda_{max}] \rightarrow I\!\!R^+$ is a positive monotone function, with $\lambda_{max} = max\{|\lambda_i(P)|; P \in D, i = 1, 2, 3\}$.

3. Definition of the metric g in the original coordinate system by inverting the diagonalization defined in (16.5):

$$\mathbf{g} = U^T \cdot \mathbf{g}' \cdot U. \tag{16.7}$$

If the mapping F is linear, the three steps can be combined into one step, and F can be applied to the tensor components, independently of the chosen basis. The resulting metric $\mathbf{g}$ has the following properties:

- It is positive definite and symmetric.
- Its eigenvector field corresponds to the original eigenvector field of $\mathbf{T}$. Thus, the tensor field topology in the sense of Delmarcelle et al. [HD95] is preserved.
- Its eigenvalues are given by $F(\lambda_j)$. Positive eigenvalues are mapped to values greater than a, negative eigenvalues to values smaller than a but larger then zero. The zero tensor is mapped to a multiple of the unit matrix.
- Since the transformation is invertible, we get a one-to-one correspondence of the metric and the tensor field.

16.3.2 Examples for Transformation Functions F

In this paragraph we suggest some explicit definitions for the function F. Except from the first example all these functions are nonlinear and therefore cannot be directly applied to the tensor components. The functions we discuss can be classified in two groups:

1. Anti-symmetric Treatment of the Eigenvalues
To underline the motivation defined by (16.4), we can define the transformation function as:

$$F(\lambda) = a + \sigma f(\lambda) . \tag{16.8}$$

Here, $a = F(0)$ defines the unit length, and $\sigma \neq 0$ is an appropriate scaling factor that guarantees that the resulting metric is positive definite. The function $f : I\!\!R \rightarrow I\!\!R$ is a monotone function with $f(0) = 0$. If we want to treat positive and negative eigenvalues symmetrically it is $f(-\lambda) = -f(\lambda)$. From the large class of functions satisfying this condition we have considered three examples:

a. Identity: $f = id$, $f(\lambda) = \lambda$.
Since f is linear, the metric g is defined by $g_{ij} = F(t_{ij}) = a + \sigma \cdot t_{ij}$. This equation corresponds exactly to our motivating (16.4), where σ plays the role

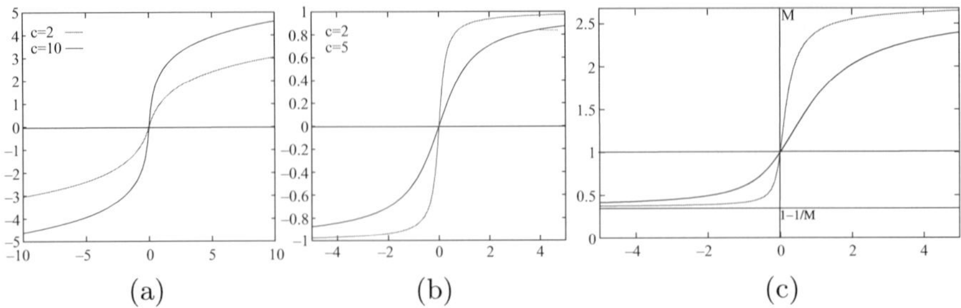

(a)   (b)   (c)

Fig. 16.2. Figures (a) and (b) are examples for an anti-symmetric transformation function f. **(a)** Logarithmic function; **(b)** arc-tangent for two different slopes for $\lambda = 0$. **(c)** is an example of a non-symmetric transformation function F for two different slopes at the origin

of the time variable t. With $\sigma < a/\lambda_{max}$ we can guarantee that the metric is positive definite.

b. Anti-symmetric logarithmic function.

To emphasize regions where the eigenvalues change sign one can choose a function f with a larger slope in the neighborhood of zero.

$$f(\lambda; c) = \begin{cases} \log(c \cdot \lambda + 1) \text{ for } \lambda \geq 0 \\ -\log(1 - c \cdot \lambda) \text{ for } \lambda < 0 \end{cases} . \tag{16.9}$$

If we require $\sigma < a/\log(c \cdot \lambda_{max} + 1)$ the resulting metric is positive definite.

c. Asymptotic function.

A function where the limitation of the scaling factor σ is independent of λ_{max} is

$$f(\lambda; c) = \arctan(c \cdot \lambda), \tag{16.10}$$

with $\sigma < 2a/\pi$. For both functions, the constant c controls the 'sharpness' at the zero crossing. For higher values of c the function becomes steeper, see Fig. 16.2.

2. Non-symmetric Function

As the visual perception of texture attributes is nonlinear, an anti-symmetric approach is not always the best choice. An alternative that takes care of this aspect is defined by the class of functions $F[-\lambda_{max}, \lambda_{max}] \rightarrow [\frac{a}{M}, a \cdot M]$, where

$$F(-\lambda) = \frac{a^2}{F(\lambda)} . \tag{16.11}$$

The constant a defines again the unit, aM the maximum, and $\frac{a}{M}$ the minimum value for F satisfying $M > 1$. Functions with this property can be obtained by using anti-symmetric functions f as exponent:

$$F(\lambda) = a \cdot \exp(\sigma \cdot f(\lambda)) \text{ where } f(-\lambda) = -f(\lambda) \ . \qquad (16.12)$$

An example for such a function with $a = 1$ is $F(\lambda; c, \sigma) = \exp(\sigma \arctan(c \cdot \lambda))$. The constant c determines the slope of the function in the origin, see Fig. 16.2. The second class of functions produces much better results because the differences in the density of the resulting structure is more obvious. The special choice of the function f does not have a significant influence on the result. Another advantage of this class of functions F is that the resulting metric is always positive definite and therefore, the scaling factor σ is not limited. By an animation of this parameter we can enhance the impression of stretching and compression.

16.3.3 Visualization

We now have transformed the problem of visualizing a tensor field to the problem of visualizing an abstract metric. One way to solve this problem is an isometric embedding of the metric [Hot02]. The disadvantage of this approach is that it is restricted to two dimensions, and its existence is only guaranteed locally. In general, several patches are needed to cover a field's entire domain. Since we want to produce a global representation of a field we decided to follow a different approach: Our basic idea is to use a texture that resembles a piece of fabric to express the characteristic properties of the metric. The texture is stretched or compressed and bended according to the metric. Large values of the metric, which indicate large distances, are illustrated by a texture with low density or a stretched piece of fabric. We use a dense texture for small values of the metric. One can also think of a texture as probe inserted into the tensor field.

We generate the texture using LIC, a very popular method for vector field visualization. LIC blurs a noise image along the vector field or integral curves. Blurring results in a high correlation of the pixel along field lines, whereas almost no correlation appears in direction perpendicular to the field lines. The resulting image leads to a very effective depiction of flow direction everywhere, even in a dense vector field. LIC was introduced in 1993 by Cabral and Leedom [CL93]. Since the method was introduced, several extensions and improvements were made to make it faster [SH95] and more flexible.

We compute one LIC image for every eigenvector field to illustrate the eigendirections of the tensor field. For the integration of the integral curves we use a Runge-Kutta method of fourth order, the LIC image is computed using Fast-LIC as proposed in [SH95]. In each LIC image the eigenvalues of every eigenvector field are used to define the free parameters of the underlaying noise image and the convolution. Finally, we overlay all resulting LIC images to obtain the fabric-like texture.

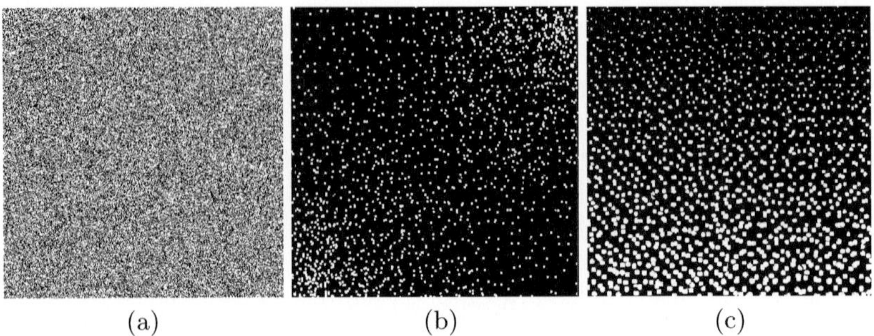

Fig. 16.3. Example for different input images. (**a**) White noise image with maximum resolution; (**b**) spot noise image with changing density; (**c**) spot noise image with changing spot size

Input Noise Image

We use the free parameters of this input image to encode properties of the metric. Three basic parameters are changed according to the eigenvalues. They are: density, spot size, and color intensity of the spots. Considering these parameters, the standard white-noise image is the noise image with maximum density, minimal spot size, and constant color intensity. It allows one to obtain a very good overall impression of the field; its resolution is only limited by pixel size. Unfortunately, it is not flexible enough to integrate the eigenvalues which represent fundamental field properties besides the directions. For this reason, we use sparse noise input images, with lower density and larger spot size even if we obtain a lower resolution. Some examples for different input images with changing density and spot size are shown in Fig. 16.3. The connection of these parameters to the eigenvalues is explained in the following paragraphs:

Density. For each direction field $\mathbf{w}_i$, we define a specific density d_i depending on the orthogonal eigenvalues. A compression orthogonal to fibers leads to increasing density, and an expansion to decreasing density. For two-dimensional textures this approach leads to the following definition of a one-dimensional density d_i [spots/cm]:

$$d_i(\lambda) = d_0 \cdot \frac{1}{F(\lambda_j)}, \ \text{with } j = \begin{cases} 2 & \text{if} \quad i = 1 \\ 1 & \text{if} \quad i = 2 , \end{cases} \qquad (16.13)$$

where F is defined by (16.6), and d_0 defines the 'unit-density,' $d(0) = d_0/F(0)$. In three dimensions, we have two orthogonal eigenvalues and thus obtain a direction-dependent density $d_{i,j}$ for each direction $\mathbf{w}_j$:

$$d_{i,j}(\lambda) = d_0 \cdot \frac{1}{F(\lambda_j)} \ . \qquad (16.14)$$

Table 16.1. Assignment of eigenvalues to free parameters for a three-dimensional texture.

Free Parameters		Eigenvector Field		
		$i = 1$	$i = 2$	$i = 3$
density value	$d_{i,j}$	$\frac{1}{\lambda_2}$	$\frac{1}{\lambda_1}$	$\frac{1}{\lambda_1}$
	$d_{i,k}$	$\frac{1}{\lambda_2}$	$\frac{1}{\lambda_1}$	$\frac{1}{\lambda_1}$
color intensity	I_i	$\frac{1}{\lambda_1}$	$\frac{1}{\lambda_2}$	$\frac{1}{\lambda_3}$
convolution length	l_i	λ_1	λ_2	λ_3
spot diameter	$r_{i,j}$	λ_2	λ_3	λ_1
	$r_{i,k}$	λ_3	λ_1	λ_2

Spot Size. Increasing the radius of the underlying noise image leads to thicker, decreasing the radius leads to thinner fibers. This value is controlled by the orthogonal eigenvalues. In three dimensions, we define ellipsoids with three different diameters according to the three eigenvalues:

$$r_{i,j} = \frac{r_0}{d_{i,j}} \ .$$

(16.15)

Convolution Length. The defined noise image only uses the eigenvalues orthogonal to the actual eigendirection field. A stretching or compressing in the direction of the integral lines changes the length of the fibers. Fiber length is directly correlated to the length of the convolution filter l_i, i.e.,

$$l_i = l_0 \cdot F(\lambda_i) \ .$$

(16.16)

Color and Color Intensity. In addition to these three 'structure' parameters, color intensity can be used to enhance the impression of compression and stretching. We use red for compression and green for tension. We apply a continuous color mapping from red for the smallest negative eigenvalues, white for zero eigenvalues, and green for positive eigenvalues. The definition of the different parameters for three dimensions is summarized in Table 16.1.

16.4 Results and Conclusions

We have evaluated our method using synthetic and real data sets. Simple tensor fields, where the eigenvector fields are aligned to the coordinate axes, have allowed us to validate the effect of changing texture parameters. We have obtained similar results for datasets where the eigenvector fields are rotated by 90 degrees. Results where only one eigenvector field is used are shown in Fig. 16.4. Images for the same datasets showing both eigendirections are shown in Fig. 16.5. We have used different input textures and parameter mappings.

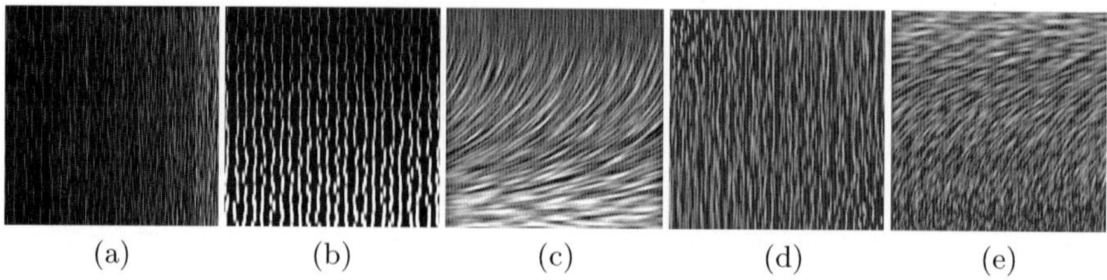

(a)   (b)   (c)   (d)   (e)

Fig. 16.4. Effect of changing image parameters for one eigenvector field of different simple synthetic tensor fields. In (a)–(c), only the input image is changed corresponding to the eigenvalues of the orthogonal eigenvector field; (**a**) change of density; (**b**) change of spot size; (**c**) change of density and spot size. Images (**d**) illustrates the effect of changing the convolution length, where the parameters of the input noise image are constant. Image (**e**) shows a combination of the three parameters (density, spot size, and convolution length)

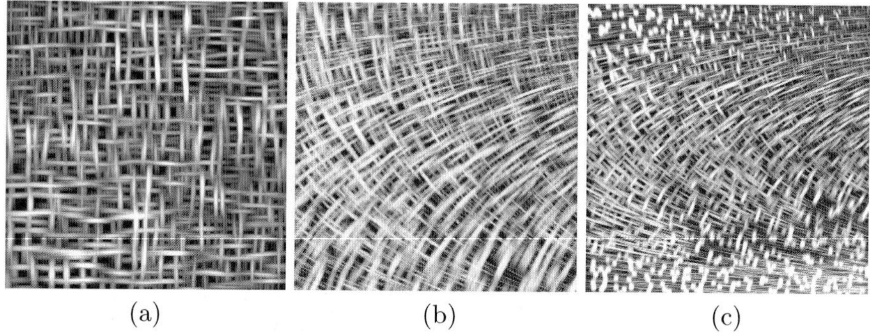

(a)   (b)   (c)

Fig. 16.5. Combination of two eigenvector fields, each representing both eigenvalues. In (**a**) and (**b**), only density and spot size are changed; (**c**) shows a combination of the three parameters

The next examples are results for simulated finite element data sets of the stress field resulting from applying different load combinations to a solid block. These datasets are well-studied and therefore appropriate to evaluate our method. For the simulation, a ten-by-ten-by-ten grid had been used. The tensor field resulting from the simulation is continuous inside each cell, but not on cell boundaries. This fact can be observed in our images. Figure 16.6 and Fig. 16.7 (see color plates) show different slices of the three-dimensional dataset from a single point load. Figure 16.8 (see color plates) represents a block where two forces with opposite sign were applied. These images provide a good visual segmentation of regions of compression and expansion.

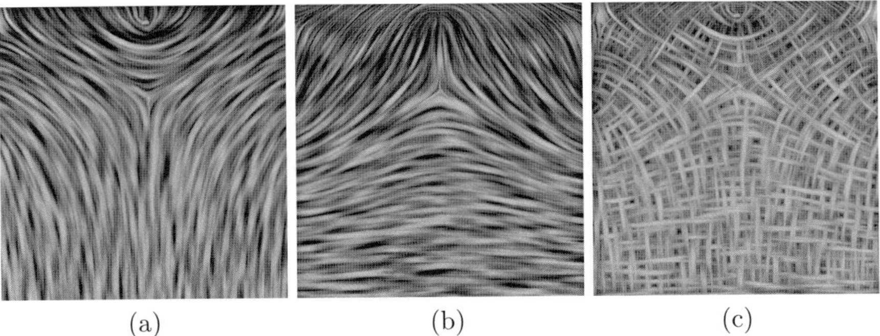

Fig. 16.6. Images showing a yz-plane slice of single top-load data set, where a force is applied in z-direction. (a) and (b) illustrate the two eigenvector fields separately; in (c) they are overlaid. In all images, spot size and density are changed according to eigenvalues

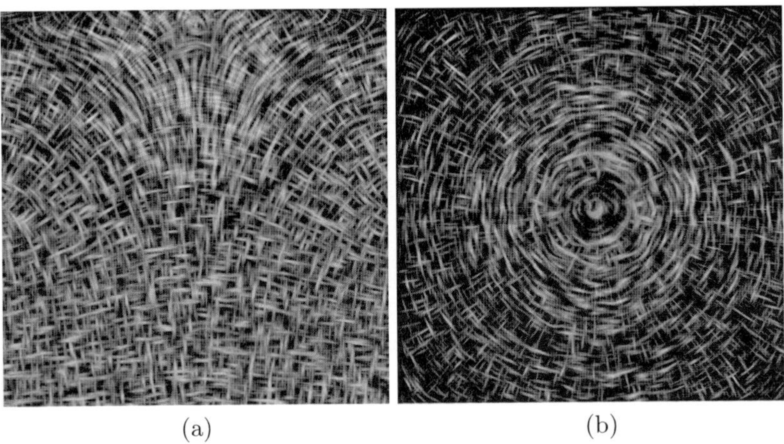

Fig. 16.7. See color plates. This figure shows a single-top-load. Spot size and density of the input images are adapted to the corresponding eigenvectors. Red shows regions of compression, green expansion according the respective eigenvector field: the images are planar slices along the (a) yz-plane and (b) xy-plane slice orthogonal to the force

The interpretation of a tensor field as a distortion of a flat metric can be used to produce a visualization based on the real physical effect of the tensor field. The distortion of the texture according to the metric supports a flexible representation of two-dimensional slices of a tensor field, which is easy to understand. An extension to three dimensions is possible but there is still the problem of cluttering which must be solved.

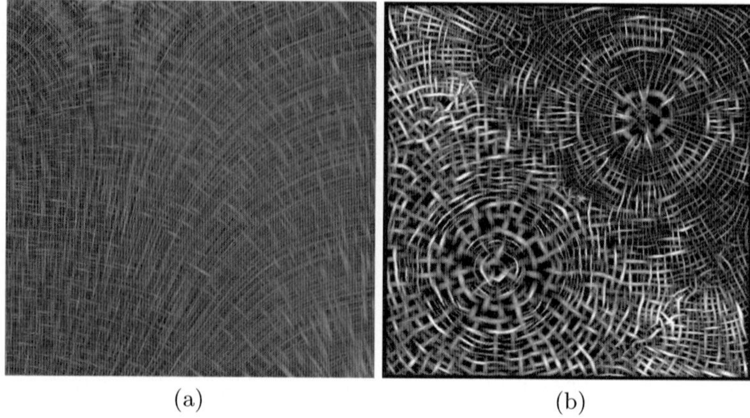

(a)   (b)

Fig. 16.8. See color plates. The images represents a yz-plane (a) and xz-plane (b) slice of a two-force dataset. (**a**): In the lower-left corner we see a region of compression, a result mainly due to the pushing force on the left; in the upper-right corner expansion dominates as a result of the right pulling force. (**b**): The *left circle* corresponds to the pushing and the right to the pulling force. The fluctuation of the color is a result of the low resolution of the simulation

References

[BP98]   Ed Boring and Alex Pang. Interactive Deformations from Tensor Fields. Proceedings of the Visualization '98 Conference, 1998, pp. 297–304.

[CL93]   Brian Cabral and Leith Leedom. Imaging Vector Fields Using Line Integral Convolution. In SIGGRAPH '93 Conference Proceedings, 1993, pp. 263–272.

[DH92]   Thierry Delmarcelle and Lambertus Hesselink. Visualization of second order tensor fields and matrix data. Proceedings of the Visualization '92 Conference, 1992, pp. 316–323.

[Hab90]   Robert B. Haber. Visualization Techniques for Engineering Mechanics. In Computing Systems in Engineering, 1990, pp. 37–50.

[HD95]   Lambertus Hesselink, Thierry Delmarcelle and James L. Helman. Topology of Second-Order Tensor Fields. In Computers in Physics, 1995, pp. 304–311.

[Hot02]   Ingrid Hotz. Isometric Embedding by Surface Reconstruction from Distances. Proceedings of the IEEE Visualization '02 Conference, 2002, pp. 251–258.

[HFHHJ04]   Ingrid Hotz, Louis Feng, Hans Hagen, Bernd Hamann, Boris Jeremic, and Kenneth Joy. Physically Based Methods for Tensor Field Visualization. Proceedings of the IEEE Visualization '04 Conference, 2004, pp. 123–130.

[JSchF02]   Boris Jeremic, Gerik Scheuermann and Jan Frey et al. Tensor Visualization in Computational Geomechanics. In International Journal for Numerical and Analytical Methods in Geomechanics, 2002, pp. 925–944.

[KGM95]   Ron D. Kriz, Edward H. Glaessgen and J.D. MacRae. Visualization Blackboard: Visualizing gradients in composite design and fabrication. IEEE Computer Graphics and Applications, vol 15, 1995, pp. 10–13

[LW93]   W. C. de Leeuw and J. J. van Wijk. A Probe for Local Flow Field Visualization. Proceedings of the Visualization '93 Conference, 1993, pp. 39–45.

[OH01]   J. Ou and E. Hsu. Generalized Line Integral Convolution Rendering of Diffusion Tensor Fields. Proceedings of the 9th Scientific Meeting and Exhibition of the International Society for Magnetic Resonance in Medicine (ISMRM), p. 790, 2001.

[SH95]   Detlev Stalling and Hans-Christian Hege. Fast and Resolution Independent Line Integral Convolution. In SIGGRAPH '95 Conference Proceedings, 1995, pp. 149–256.

[ZP02]   Xiaoqiang Zheng and Alex Pang. Volume Deformation For Tensor Visualization. Proceedings of the Visualization '02 Conference, 2002, pp. 379–386.

[ZPa03]   Xiaoqiang Zheng and Alex Pang. Interaction of Light and Tensor Field. Proceedings of VISSYM '03, 2003, pp. 157–166.

[ZP03]   Xiaoqiang Zheng and Alex Pang. HyperLIC, Proceedings of the IEEE Visualization '03 Conference, 2003, pp. 249–256.

Part IV

Tensor Field Transformations

Symmetric Positive-Definite Matrices: From Geometry to Applications and Visualization

Maher Moakher[1] and Philipp G. Batchelor[2]

[1] Laboratory for Mathematical and Numerical Modeling in Engineering Science, National Engineering School at Tunis, ENIT-LAMSIN, B.P. 37, 1002 Tunis Belvédère, Tunisia
`maher.moakher@enit.rnu.tn`
[2] Imaging Sciences Division, 5th floor Thomas Guy House, Guy's Hospital, King's College London, London SE1 9RT, UK
`philipp.batchelor@kcl.ac.uk`

Summary. In many engineering applications that use tensor analysis, such as tensor imaging, the underlying tensors have the characteristic of being positive definite. It might therefore be more appropriate to use techniques specially adapted to such tensors. We will describe the geometry and calculus on the Riemannian symmetric space of positive-definite tensors. First, we will explain why the geometry, constructed by Emile Cartan, is a natural geometry on that space. Then, we will use this framework to present formulas for means and interpolations specific to positive-definite tensors.

17.1 Introduction

Symmetric positive-definite (SPD) matrices arise in many physical and mathematical contexts. This is not surprising as the set of SPD matrices has a very rich structure and possesses many interesting features. Recent years have seen an increasing demand for a rigorous framework for dealing with different operations on the set of SPD matrices such as regularization, interpolation, and averaging of SPD matrices data sets.

In this work we exploit the differential geometric structure of the set of SPD matrices and use analogy with Euclidean space to give precise definitions for means of SPD matrices. We also discuss various anisotropy measures as well as methods for constructing multivariate interpolations of SPD matrices.

17.2 Geometry of the Space of SPD Matrices

In this section we fix notations and briefly recall some differential-geometric properties of the space of symmetric positive-definite matrices. Further details can be found in standard texts such as [4, 6, 13].

Let $\mathcal{M}(n)$ denote the space of $n \times n$ real matrices. On $\mathcal{M}(n)$ we have the Frobenius inner product $\langle \mathbf{A}, \mathbf{B} \rangle_F = \mathrm{tr}(\mathbf{A}^T \mathbf{B})$ and the associated norm $\|\mathbf{A}\|_F = [\mathrm{tr}(\mathbf{A}^T \mathbf{A})]^{1/2}$. On $\mathcal{M}(n)$ we define the Euclidean metric by

$$d_F(\mathbf{A}, \mathbf{B}) = \|\mathbf{A} - \mathbf{B}\| . \tag{17.1}$$

Let $GL(n)$ be the general linear group of all nonsingular matrices in $\mathcal{M}(n)$. The exponential of a matrix $\mathbf{A} \in \mathcal{M}(n)$ is given as usual by the power series $\exp \mathbf{A} = \sum_{k=0}^{\infty} \mathbf{A}^k / k!$, which converges for all $\mathbf{A} \in \mathcal{M}(n)$. The exponential is a differentiable map from $\mathcal{M}(n)$ onto $GL(n)$.

The vector space of symmetric matrices in $\mathcal{M}(n)$ is denoted by $\mathcal{S}(n)$. For $\mathbf{P} \in \mathcal{S}(n)$ we say that $\mathbf{P}$ is positive semidefinite if $\mathbf{x}^T \mathbf{P} \mathbf{x} \geq 0$ for all $\mathbf{x} \in \mathbb{R}^n$. If $\mathbf{P}$ is positive semidefinite and invertible we say that $\mathbf{P}$ is symmetric positive definite. The subset of $\mathcal{S}(n)$ consisting of all positive-definite matrices is a convex cone whose interior consists of all positive-definite matrices and is denoted by $\mathcal{P}(n)$. While in most applications $n = 3$ (or $n = 2$), the different notions dealt with in this work are introduced for arbitrary $n > 0$. The graphical illustrations presented here are for the interesting case $n = 3$.

17.2.1 Riemannian Structure of $\mathcal{P}(n)$

The set $\mathcal{P}(n)$ is a manifold whose tangent space at any of its points $\mathbf{P}$ is the space $T_{\mathbf{P}}\mathcal{P}(n) = \{\mathbf{P}\} \times \mathcal{S}(n)$. The infinitesimal arclength

$$ds := (\mathrm{tr}(\mathbf{P}^{-1}d\mathbf{P})^2)^{1/2} = \|\mathbf{P}^{-1/2}d\mathbf{P}\mathbf{P}^{-1/2}\|_F \tag{17.2}$$

defines a Riemannian metric on $\mathcal{P}(n)$. The general linear group $GL(n)$ acts transitively on the manifold $\mathcal{P}(n)$ by congruent transformations defined for $\mathbf{S} \in GL(n)$ by $[\mathbf{S}]\mathbf{P} = \mathbf{S}^T\mathbf{P}\mathbf{S}$. Using properties of the trace one can easily verify that for any curve $\mathbf{P}(t)$ in $\mathcal{P}(n)$ we have

$$\|([\mathbf{S}]\mathbf{P}(t))^{-1/2}[\mathbf{S}]d\mathbf{P}(t)([\mathbf{S}]\mathbf{P}(t))^{-1/2}\|_F = \|(\mathbf{P}(t))^{-1/2}d\mathbf{P}(t)(\mathbf{P}(t))^{-1/2}\|_F,$$

and hence, $[\mathbf{S}]$ is an isometry for the Riemannian metric.

The exponential of a symmetric matrix is a symmetric positive-definite matrix. The inverse map, i.e., the principal logarithm, which we denote by Log, of a symmetric positive-definite matrix is a symmetric matrix. The geodesic distance between $\mathbf{P}$ and $\mathbf{Q}$ in $\mathcal{P}(n)$ is given by [6, p. 326]

$$d_R(\mathbf{P}, \mathbf{Q}) = \|\mathrm{Log}(\mathbf{P}^{-1}\mathbf{Q})\|_F = \left[\sum_{i=1}^{n} \log^2 \lambda_i(\mathbf{P}^{-1}\mathbf{Q})\right]^{1/2}, \tag{17.3}$$

where $\lambda_i(\mathbf{P}^{-1}\mathbf{Q})$, $1 \le i \le n$ are the eigenvalues of the matrix $\mathbf{P}^{-1}\mathbf{Q}$. Because $\mathbf{P}^{-1}\mathbf{Q}$ is similar to $\mathbf{P}^{-1/2}\mathbf{Q}\mathbf{P}^{-1/2}$, the eigenvalues $\lambda_i(\mathbf{P}^{-1}\mathbf{Q})$ are all positive and hence (17.3) is well defined for all $\mathbf{P}$ and $\mathbf{Q}$ of $\mathcal{P}(n)$. The unique geodesic joining $\mathbf{P}$ and $\mathbf{Q}$ is the curve

$$[0,1] \ni t \mapsto \mathbf{P}^{1/2}(\mathbf{P}^{-1/2}\mathbf{Q}\mathbf{P}^{-1/2})^t\mathbf{P}^{1/2} \ . \tag{17.4}$$

It follows from (17.3) that $\mathrm{d}_R(\mathbf{P}^{-1}, \mathbf{Q}^{-1}) = \mathrm{d}_R(\mathbf{P}, \mathbf{Q})$. Hence, the inversion $\mathbf{P} \mapsto \mathbf{P}^{-1}$ is an involutive isometry on $\mathcal{P}(n)$ for this metric, and therefore, $\mathcal{P}(n)$ becomes a Riemannian symmetric space. It is in fact a typical example of a symmetric space of non-compact type as classified by E. Cartan [13]. It is also an example of a Riemannian manifold of nonpositive curvature [6].

17.2.2 The Kullback-Leibler Divergence

In information geometry, closeness between two probability distributions p and q on an event space Ω is usually measured by the Kullback-Leibler divergence or 'relative entropy' [1],

$$KL(p, q) = \int_\Omega p(\mathbf{x}) \log \frac{p(\mathbf{x})}{q(\mathbf{x})} \, d\mathbf{x} \ . \tag{17.5}$$

Recall that a divergence on a space X is a non-negative function $J(\cdot, \cdot)$ on the Cartesian product space $X \times X$ which is zero only on the diagonal, i.e., $J(x, y) \ge 0$ for all x and y in X and that $J(x, y) = 0$ if and only if $x = y$. We mention here that a symmetrized form of this divergence has been recently used by Lenglet et al. [7] for the segmentation of probability density fields in the context of diffusion MRI.

The Kullback-Leibler divergence between the two zero-mean Gaussian distributions

$$p(\mathbf{x}|\mathbf{P}) = \frac{1}{\sqrt{(2\pi)^n \det \mathbf{P}}} \exp\left(-\frac{1}{2}\mathbf{x}^T\mathbf{P}^{-1}\mathbf{x}\right) \ ,$$

$$q(\mathbf{x}|\mathbf{Q}) = \frac{1}{\sqrt{(2\pi)^n \det \mathbf{Q}}} \exp\left(-\frac{1}{2}\mathbf{x}^T\mathbf{Q}^{-1}\mathbf{x}\right) \ ,$$

whose covariant matrices are $\mathbf{P}$ and $\mathbf{Q}$ gives rise to the Kullback-Leibler divergence for the two SPD matrices $\mathbf{P}$ and $\mathbf{Q}$

$$KL(\mathbf{P}, \mathbf{Q}) = \mathrm{tr}(\mathbf{Q}^{-1}\mathbf{P} - \mathbf{I}) - \log \det(\mathbf{Q}^{-1}\mathbf{P}) \ . \tag{17.6}$$

If λ_i, $i = 1, \ldots, n$ denote the (positive) eigenvalues of $\mathbf{Q}^{-1}\mathbf{P}$ then

$$KL(\mathbf{P}, \mathbf{Q}) = \sum_{i=1}^{n}(\lambda_i - \log \lambda_i - 1) \ . \tag{17.7}$$

From this expression, as $x - \log x - 1 \geq 0$ for all $x > 0$ with equality holding only when $x = 1$, it becomes clear that $KL(\cdot, \cdot)$ defines a divergence on the space of SPD matrices.

We emphasize here the fact that the Kullback-Leibler divergence (17.6) does not define a distance on the space of positive-definite matrices as it is neither symmetric with respect to its two arguments nor does it satisfy the triangle inequality. Its symmetrized form $KL_s(\mathbf{P}, \mathbf{Q}) = \frac{1}{2}(KL(\mathbf{P}, \mathbf{Q}) + KL(\mathbf{Q}, \mathbf{P}))$ can be expressed as

$$KL_s(\mathbf{P}, \mathbf{Q}) = \tfrac{1}{2}\operatorname{tr}(\mathbf{Q}^{-1}\mathbf{P} + \mathbf{P}^{-1}\mathbf{Q} - 2\mathbf{I}), \qquad (17.8)$$

or, in terms of the λ_i's, as

$$KL_s(\mathbf{P}, \mathbf{Q}) = \frac{1}{2}\sum_{i=1}^{n}\left(\sqrt{\lambda_i} - \frac{1}{\sqrt{\lambda_i}}\right)^2. \qquad (17.9)$$

By construction, the symmetrized Kullback-Leibler divergence (17.8) is invariant under inversion, i.e., $KL_s(\mathbf{P}^{-1}, \mathbf{Q}^{-1}) = KL_s(\mathbf{P}, \mathbf{Q})$. It is easy to see that it is also invariant under congruent transformations, i.e.,

$$KL_s(\mathbf{P}, \mathbf{Q}) = KL_s(\mathbf{S}^T\mathbf{P}\mathbf{S}, \mathbf{S}^T\mathbf{Q}\mathbf{S}), \qquad \text{for all } \mathbf{S} \in GL(n).$$

From (17.9) it becomes clear that the symmetrized Kullback-Leibler divergence (17.8) behaves as the square of a distance. For comparison of the distance measures $d_F(\cdot, \cdot)$, $d_R(\cdot, \cdot)$ and $KL_s(\cdot, \cdot)$ in Fig. 17.1 we show 'spheres' centered at the identity tensor and with radii $r = 0.1$, 0.5 and 1: (a) $d_F(\mathbf{I}, \mathbf{P}) = \|\mathbf{I} - \mathbf{P}\|_F = r$, (b) $d_R(\mathbf{I}, \mathbf{P}) = \|\operatorname{Log}\mathbf{P}\|_F = r$, and (c) $\sqrt{KL_s(\mathbf{I}, \mathbf{P})} = \frac{1}{\sqrt{2}}\|\mathbf{P}^{1/2} - \mathbf{P}^{-1/2}\|_F = r$, where $\mathbf{P} \in \mathcal{P}(3)$.

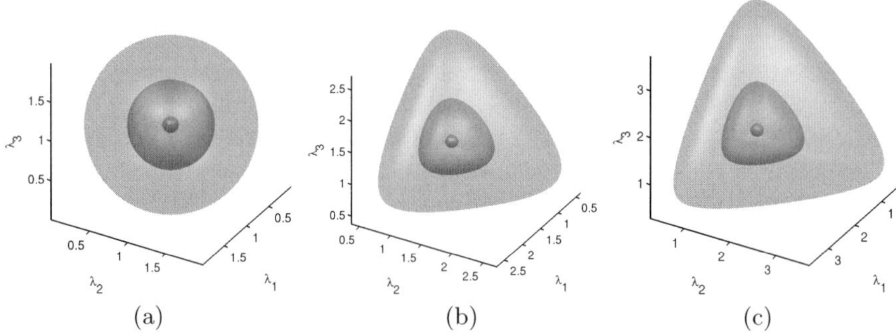

(a)   (b)   (c)

Fig. 17.1. *'Spheres':* Isosurfaces of the distance measure between a SPD tensor in $\mathcal{P}(3)$ with eigenvalues $(\lambda_1, \lambda_2, \lambda_3)$ and the identity tensor; (a) Euclidean distance, (b) geodesic distance, and (c) square root of the Kullback-Leibler symmetrized divergence

17.3 Anisotropy Indices

In this section we are going to use the distance and divergence functions discussed above to define properly invariant measures of anisotropy of SPD tensors. Such measures are a useful tool for the identification of changes in tissue structure from diffusion tensor magnetic resonance imaging (DT-MRI) data sets, see for example [2, 10, 11].

Definition 17.3.1 *We define the anisotropy index of a matrix relative to a distance (or a divergence) to be its distance (or square root of the divergence) to its closest isotropic matrix.*

This definition guarantees that the anisotropy index is a non-negative quantity that is zero only for isotropic matrices and that it inherits all the invariance properties of the distance (or divergence) it is induced from.

Proposition 17.3.2 *Let $\mathbf{P}$ be a SPD matrix with eigenvalues $\lambda_1, \ldots, \lambda_n$.*

- *The anisotropy index relative to the Euclidean distance is*

$$A_F(\mathbf{P}) = \mathrm{d}_F\left(\mathbf{P}, \frac{\mathrm{tr}\,\mathbf{P}}{n}\mathbf{I}\right) = \sqrt{\mathrm{tr}\,\mathbf{P}^2 - \frac{1}{n}\mathrm{tr}^2\,\mathbf{P}}$$

$$= \sqrt{\frac{n-1}{n}\sum_{i=1}^{n}\lambda_i^2 - \frac{2}{n}\sum_{1\leq i<j\leq n}\lambda_i\lambda_j}\;.$$

- *The anisotropy index relative to the Riemannian distance is*

$$A_R(\mathbf{P}) = \mathrm{d}_R\left(\mathbf{P}, \sqrt[n]{\det\mathbf{P}}\,\mathbf{I}\right) = \sqrt{\mathrm{tr}\,\mathrm{Log}^2\,\mathbf{P} - \frac{1}{n}\mathrm{tr}^2\,\mathrm{Log}\,\mathbf{P}}$$

$$= \sqrt{\frac{n-1}{n}\sum_{i=1}^{n}\ln^2\lambda_i - \frac{2}{n}\sum_{1\leq i<j\leq n}\ln\lambda_i\ln\lambda_j}\;.$$

- *The anisotropy index relative to the symmetrized Kullback-Leibler divergence is*

$$A_{KL}(\mathbf{P}) = \sqrt{\mathrm{d}_{KL}\left(\mathbf{P}, \sqrt{\mathrm{tr}\,\mathbf{P}/\mathrm{tr}\,\mathbf{P}^{-1}}\,\mathbf{I}\right)} = \sqrt{2(\sqrt{\mathrm{tr}\,\mathbf{P}\,\mathrm{tr}\,\mathbf{P}^{-1}} - n)}$$

$$= \sqrt{2\sqrt{\sum_{i=1}^{n}\lambda_i\sum_{i=1}^{n}1/\lambda_i} - 2n}\;.$$

Proof. By straightforward computations we first determine the positive number α such that the isotropic matrix $\alpha\mathbf{I}$ is closest (relative to the distance or divergence in question) to $\mathbf{P}$, then we compute the corresponding distance or divergence.

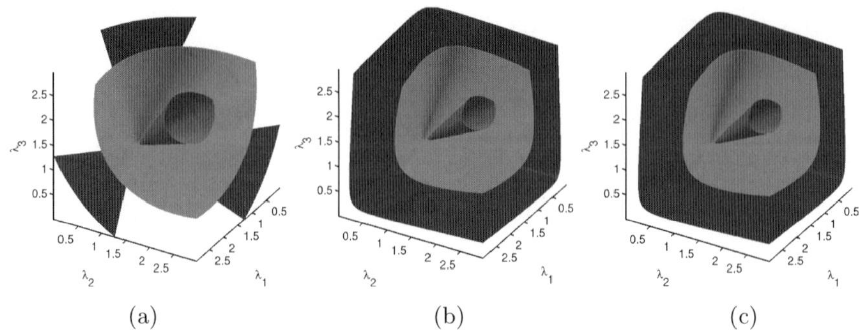

Fig. 17.2. *Anisotropy indices:* Isosurfaces of the anisotropy index of SPD tensors in $\mathcal{P}(3)$ represented in the space $(\lambda_1, \lambda_2, \lambda_3)$ of eigenvalues; (**a**) Fractional anisotropy, (**b**) geodesic anisotropy, and (**c**) Kullback-Leibler anisotropy

Note that $A_R(\cdot)$ has the same functional form in terms of the eigenvalues as $A_F(\cdot)$ but on a logarithmic scale. We remark that $A_R(\cdot)$ and $A_{KL}(\cdot)$ are invariant under matrix inversion while $A_F(\cdot)$ is not.

The range of all of the above anisotropy indices is $[0, \infty)$. In order to compare these indices with other anisotropy indices with range $[0, 1)$ used in the literature, we normalize these indices in the following way

$$FA(\mathbf{P}) = A_F(\mathbf{P})/\|\mathbf{P}\|_F \ ,$$
$$GA(\mathbf{P}) = A_R(\mathbf{P})/(1 + A_R(\mathbf{P})) \ ,$$
$$KLA(\mathbf{P}) = A_{KL}(\mathbf{P})/(1 + A_{KL}(\mathbf{P})) \ .$$

The normalized anisotropy index relative to the Euclidean distance coincides with the fractional anisotropy index (FA) commonly used in the DT-MRI community [2, 10, 11]. The geodesic anisotropy (GA) was recently introduced in [3] and applied to a DT-MRI data set.

Figure 17.2 gives isosurfaces for the (normalized) anisotropy index[1] with respect to the Euclidean distance, Riemannian distance, and the Kullback-Leibler divergence for SPD matrices in $\mathcal{P}(3)$. The fractional anisotropy is defined for all symmetric tensors but only the parts of the isosurfaces that are inside the positive orthant of the $(\lambda_1, \lambda_2, \lambda_3)$-space are shown. Both the geodesic and the Kullback-Leibler anisotropies are defined only for SPD tensors. Their isosurfaces always stay inside the positive orthant. For the geodesic and the Kullback-Leibler anisotropies, the limiting value 1 corresponds to singular matrices (i.e., the boundary of the positive orthant), whereas for the fractional anisotropy this value is attained when at least one eigenvalue is infinite. For nearly isotropic tensors, the geodesic and the Kullback-Leibler anisotropies are similar to the fractional anisotropy. However, for tensors relatively far form being isotropic the behavior of the geodesic anisotroppy is similar to that of

---

[1] From now on we will consider only the normalized anisotropy indices.

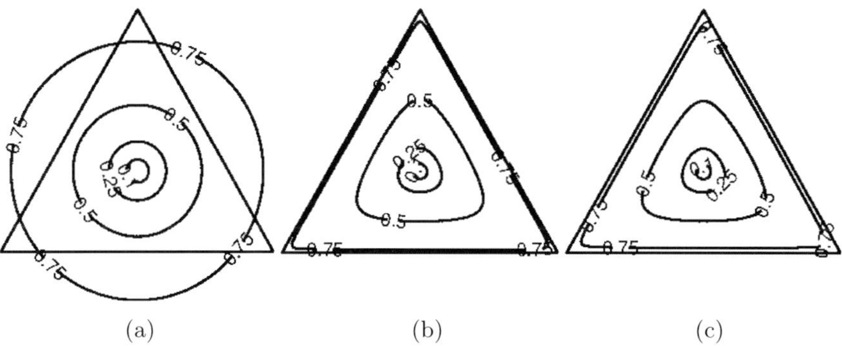

Fig. 17.3. *Anisotropy indices:* Contours of the anisotropy index of SPD tensors in $\mathcal{P}(3)$ with eigenvalues $(\lambda_1, \lambda_2, \lambda_3)$ on an octahedral plane; (**a**) Fractional anisotropy, (**b**) geodesic anisotropy, and (**c**) Kullback-Leibler anisotropy.

the Kullback-Leibler anisotropy, and both behave quite differently than the fractional anisotropy.

The set of all symmetric tensors in $\mathcal{S}(3)$ with a given trace is a plane in the $(\lambda_1, \lambda_2, \lambda_3)$-space, called an octahedral plane, which is perpendicular to the line of isotropic tensors (or in the language of plasticity theory, the line of hydrostatic pressure). The intersection of this plane with the positive orthant of SPD tensors is an equilateral triangle. In Fig. 17.3, contours of the anisotropies on the octahedral plane that passes through the identity tensor, i.e., plane of tensors with trace equal 3, are presented. Once again, the fractional anisotropy does not see the boundary of the set of SPD tensors: for relatively large values of the anisotropy the contour lines go over the limiting equilateral triangle. The contour lines for the geodesic and Kullback-Leibler anisotropies, on the other hand, stay inside this triangle and follow it closely for large values of the anisotropy index.

We recall that the spectral decomposition of a SPD matrix $\mathbf{P}$ in $\mathcal{P}(3)$ is $\mathbf{P} = \mathbf{R}\mathbf{D}\mathbf{R}^T$, where $\mathbf{D} = \mathrm{diag}(\lambda_1, \lambda_2, \lambda_3)$ are the eigenvalues of $\mathbf{P}$ and $\mathbf{R}$ is an orthogonal matrix whose columns are the eigenvectors of $\mathbf{P}$. The set of (positive) eigenvalues $\lambda_1, \lambda_2, \lambda_3$ and the orthogonal matrix $\mathbf{R}$ provide a parametrization for the elements of $\mathcal{P}(3)$. It has been customary to use this parametrization to visualize a SPD matrix $\mathbf{P}$ as an ellipsoid whose principal directions are parallel to the eigenvectors of $\mathbf{P}$ and axes proportional to the eigenvalues of $\mathbf{P}$. Thus the methods discussed in this chapter such as averaging, interpolation can also be used to perform these operations for ellipsoids. In Fig. 17.4 we use this representation to visualize the diffusion tensors of a brain region and we use color for representing the indicated anisotropy index.

17.4 Means

The arithmetic and geometric means, usually used to average a finite set of positive numbers, generalize naturally to a finite set of SPD matrices. This

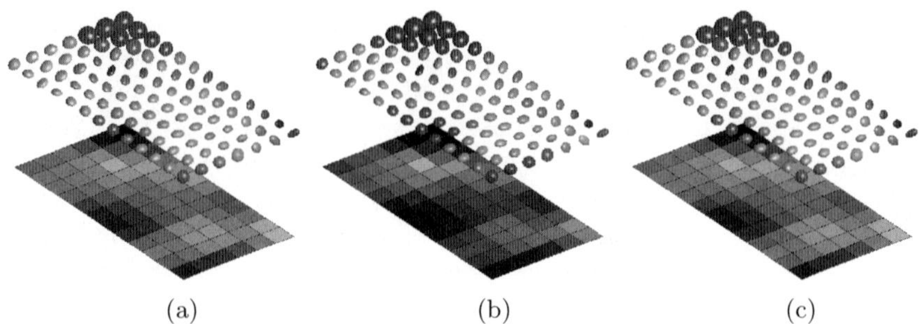

Fig. 17.4. *Anisotropies:* Diffusion ellipsoids of a brain region colored by the FA (**a**), the GA (**b**) and the KLA (**c**). (See color plates)

generalization is based on the key observation that a mean has a variational characterization [8]. The arithmetic mean minimizes the sum of the squared Euclidean distances to given positive numbers x_k, $k = 1, \ldots, m$

$$\bar{x} = \arg\min_{x>0} \sum_{k=1}^{m} |x - x_k|^2.$$

Likewise, the geometric mean, $\tilde{x} = \sqrt[m]{x_1 x_2 \cdots x_m}$, minimizes the sum of the squared hyperbolic distances to the given positive numbers x_k

$$\tilde{x} = \arg\min_{x>0} \sum_{k=1}^{m} |\log x - \log x_k|^2.$$

By analogy with the set of positive numbers we define means of symmetric positive-definite matrices as follows:

Definition 17.4.1 *We define a mean relative to a distance (or a divergence) of a finite set of SPD matrices* $\mathbf{P}_1, \ldots, \mathbf{P}_m$ *to be the SPD matrix* $\mathbf{P}$ *that minimizes*

$$\sum_{i=1}^{m} \mathrm{d}(\mathbf{P}_i, \mathbf{P})^2 \,,$$

where $\mathrm{d}(\cdot, \cdot)$ *designates the distance (or the square root of the divergence).*

17.4.1 Metric-Based Means

Using the Euclidean distance (17.1) and the Riemannian distance (17.3) on $\mathcal{P}(n)$ in Definition 17.4.1 we obtain the arithmetic and geometric means.

Proposition 17.4.2 *Given a set of SPD matrices* $\mathbf{P}_1, \ldots, \mathbf{P}_m$.

- *Their mean relative to the Euclidean distance (17.1) is the arithmetic mean given by*

$$\mathcal{A}(\mathbf{P}_1,\ldots,\mathbf{P}_m) = \frac{1}{m}\sum_{i=1}^{m}\mathbf{P}_i\,. \qquad (17.10)$$

- *Their mean relative to the Riemannian distance (17.3) is the geometric mean $\mathcal{G}(\mathbf{P}_1,\ldots,\mathbf{P}_m)$ which is the unique solution of the nonlinear matrix equation*

$$\sum_{i=1}^{m}\mathrm{Log}(\mathbf{P}_i^{-1}\mathbf{P}) = \mathbf{0}\,. \qquad (17.11)$$

We note that, in general, equation (17.11) can not be solved in closed forms. This is basically due to the non-commutative nature of matrix multiplication. However, the geometric mean of two matrices $\mathbf{P}_1$ and $\mathbf{P}_2$ is given explicitly by

$$\mathcal{G}(\mathbf{P}_1,\mathbf{P}_2) = \mathbf{P}_1(\mathbf{P}_1^{-1}\mathbf{P}_2)^{1/2} = \mathbf{P}_2(\mathbf{P}_2^{-1}\mathbf{P}_1)^{1/2}. \qquad (17.12)$$

We remark that the arithmetic and geometric means are invariant under congruent transformations, and that the geometric mean is invariant under inversion. We refer the reader to [8] for further details on the geometric mean and a proof of its characterization (17.11). Solution of the nonlinear matrix equation (17.11) can be obtained numerically by different methods. For instance, one can use Newton's method on general Riemannian manifolds which is similar to the classical Newton's method on a Euclidean space but with the substitution of straight lines by geodesics and vector addition by the exponential map, see e.g., [12]. We also point out the fixed point algorithm proposed in [9] specifically to solve (17.11).

17.4.2 Kullback-Leibler Divergence-Based Means

In the previous section we showed that arithmetic and geometric means are defined, and arise naturally, as the unique minimizers of the sum of squared distances from a given set of SPD matrices. The following Lemma shows that the arithmetic and harmonic means arise as minimizers of functions defined by the Kullback-Leibler divergence and that the geometric mean of those two means arise as the unique minimizer of a function defined by the symmetrized Kullback-Leibler divergence.

Lemma 17.4.3 *Let $\mathbf{Q}_i$, $i = 1,\ldots,m$ be m given SPD matrices.*

1. The function

$$A(\mathbf{P}) := \sum_{k=1}^{m} KL(\mathbf{Q}_i,\mathbf{P})$$

is minimized by $\mathcal{A}(\mathbf{Q}_1,\ldots,\mathbf{Q}_m)$, i.e., the arithmetic mean of $\mathbf{Q}_1,\ldots,\mathbf{Q}_m$.

2. *The function*

$$B(\mathbf{P}) := \sum_{k=1}^{m} KL(\mathbf{P}, \mathbf{Q}_i)$$

is minimized by $\mathcal{H}(\mathbf{Q}_1, \ldots, \mathbf{Q}_m) := m \left(\sum_{i=1}^{m} \mathbf{Q}_i^{-1} \right)^{-1}$, *i.e., the harmonic mean of* $\mathbf{Q}_1, \ldots, \mathbf{Q}_m$.

3. *The function*

$$C(\mathbf{P}) := \sum_{k=1}^{m} KL_s(\mathbf{P}, \mathbf{Q}_i)$$

is minimized by $\mathcal{G}(\mathcal{A}(\mathbf{Q}_1, \ldots, \mathbf{Q}_m), \mathcal{H}(\mathbf{Q}_1, \ldots, \mathbf{Q}_m))$, *i.e., the geometric mean of the arithmetic mean of* $\mathbf{Q}_1, \ldots, \mathbf{Q}_m$ *and the harmonic mean of* $\mathbf{Q}_1, \ldots, \mathbf{Q}_m$.

Proof. With the help of the formula $\dfrac{\partial \det \mathbf{X}}{\partial \mathbf{X}} = (\det \mathbf{X})(\mathbf{X}^{-1})^T$, we have

$$\nabla A(\mathbf{P}) = m\mathbf{P}^{-1} - \mathbf{P}^{-1} \sum_{i=1}^{m} \mathbf{Q}_i \mathbf{P}^{-1},$$

$$\nabla B(\mathbf{P}) = -m\mathbf{P}^{-1} + \sum_{i=1}^{m} \mathbf{Q}_i^{-1},$$

$$\nabla C(\mathbf{P}) = \tfrac{1}{2} \left(\sum_{i=1}^{m} \mathbf{Q}_i^{-1} - \mathbf{P}^{-1} \sum_{i=1}^{m} \mathbf{Q}_i \mathbf{P}^{-1} \right).$$

Equating these gradients to zero and solving for $\mathbf{P}$ yield the results.

The following Lemma shows that the mean based on the symmetrized Kullback-Leibler divergence of two matrices coincides with their geometric mean.

Lemma 17.4.4 *The geometric mean satisfies the identity*

$$\mathcal{G}(\mathbf{P}, \mathbf{Q}) = \mathcal{G}(\mathcal{A}(\mathbf{P}, \mathbf{Q}), \mathcal{H}(\mathbf{P}, \mathbf{Q}))$$

for any two matrices $\mathbf{P}$, $\mathbf{Q}$ *in* $\mathcal{P}(n)$.

Proof. By invariance of the arithmetic, geometric and harmonic means under congruent transformations it suffices to prove this Lemma for the case $\mathbf{P} = \mathbf{I}$. In fact, we have

$$\begin{aligned}
\mathcal{G}(\mathcal{A}(\mathbf{I}, \mathbf{Q}), \mathcal{H}(\mathbf{I}, \mathbf{Q})) &= \mathcal{G}(\tfrac{1}{2}(\mathbf{I} + \mathbf{Q}), 2(\mathbf{I} + \mathbf{Q}^{-1})^{-1}) \\
&= (\mathbf{I} + \mathbf{Q}^{-1})^{-1}((\mathbf{I} + \mathbf{Q}^{-1})(\mathbf{I} + \mathbf{Q}))^{1/2} \\
&= (\mathbf{I} + \mathbf{Q}^{-1})^{-1}(\mathbf{Q} + 2\mathbf{I} + \mathbf{Q}^{-1})^{1/2} \\
&= (\mathbf{I} + \mathbf{Q}^{-1})^{-1}(\mathbf{Q}^{1/2} + \mathbf{Q}^{-1/2}) \\
&= (\mathbf{I} + \mathbf{Q}^{-1})^{-1}(\mathbf{I} + \mathbf{Q}^{-1})\mathbf{Q}^{1/2} = \mathbf{Q}^{1/2} = \mathcal{G}(\mathbf{I}, \mathbf{Q}) .
\end{aligned}$$

Before we close this section we note that weighted means can also be defined by analogy with means of positive numbers.

Definition 17.4.5 *We define a weighted mean relative to a distance (or a divergence) of a finite set of SPD matrices* $\mathbf{P}_1,\ldots,\mathbf{P}_m$ *with (non-negative) weights* $w_1,\ldots,w_m$ *to be the SPD matrix* $\mathbf{P}$ *that minimizes*

$$\sum_{i=1}^{m} w_i \, \mathrm{d}(\mathbf{P}_i,\mathbf{P})^2 \,,$$

where $\mathrm{d}(\cdot,\cdot)$ *designates the distance (or the square root of the divergence).*

Among the applications of weighted means we can cite their use as a smoothing filter for denoising measured SPD data, see e.g., Chap. 21 by Welk et al. In the next section we are going to use weighted means to define interpolation of scattered SPD data.

17.5 Interpolation

One of the emerging problems from the DT-MRI community is the interpolation of scattered diffusion tensor data, see for example Chap. 18 by Pajevic et al. and Chap. 19 by Weickert and Welk. Given the values of a symmetric positive-definite matrix field at some points of space what is the natural way to evaluate the tensor field at some other points? We present here several methods of multivariate interpolation of SPD tensor data over simplicial domains. These interpolation methods are analogous to multivariate Lagrange interpolation of scalar or vector data. The main ingredients are the use of weighted means and barycentric coordinates.

17.5.1 Univariate Interpolation

We start by discussing the univariate interpolation. Given two symmetric positive-definite matrices $\mathbf{P}_1$ and $\mathbf{P}_2$, as the set of SPD matrices $\mathcal{P}(n)$ is subset of the Euclidean space of real matrices $\mathcal{M}(n)$, one can define the function

$$\lambda \mapsto \mathbf{P}(\lambda) = \lambda\mathbf{P}_1 + (1-\lambda)\mathbf{P}_2, \quad 0 \le \lambda \le 1 \,, \tag{17.13}$$

as the linear interpolation of the two tensors $\mathbf{P}_1$ and $\mathbf{P}_2$. Indeed, as $\mathcal{P}(n)$ is an open convex cone, the tensor $\mathbf{P}(\lambda)$ is SPD for all $\lambda \in [0,1]$. We remark in passing that if λ is outside of the interval $[0,1]$, the matrix $\mathbf{P}(\lambda)$ can leave the set $\mathcal{P}(n)$, which means that linear extrapolation of SPD matrices might not be possible.

Another way to look at $\mathbf{P}(\lambda)$ is that it is the weighted arithmetic mean of $\mathbf{P}_1$ and $\mathbf{P}_2$ with weights λ and $1-\lambda$. Note that the weights are exactly the barycentric coordinates on the line segment (simplex of dimension one) $[0,1]$.

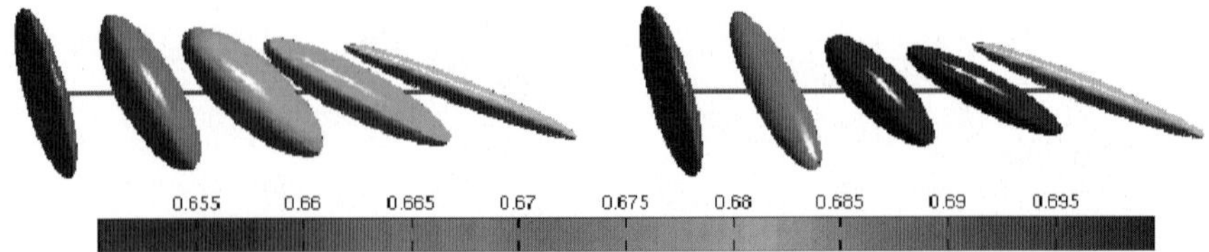

Fig. 17.5. *Univariate interpolation:* Ellipsoidal representation of linear interpolation (*left*) and geodesic interpolation (*right*) between two SPD tensors. In both cases, the colors are based on the values of the geodesic anisotropy index. (See color plates)

This property of the linear interpolation on the line segment $[0, 1]$, which also holds true for simplices of higher dimension, can be generalized by replacing the weighted arithmetic mean by other weighted means. For example, if we use the weighted geometric mean we obtain the geodesic interpolation given explicitly by

$$\lambda \mapsto \mathbf{G}(\lambda) = \mathbf{P}_1(\mathbf{P}_1^{-1}\mathbf{P}_2)^{\lambda} = \mathbf{P}_2(\mathbf{P}_2^{-1}\mathbf{P}_1)^{1-\lambda}, \quad 0 \leq \lambda \leq 1 . \tag{17.14}$$

The geodesic interpolation naturally takes into account the positive-definite character of the involved matrices. Furthermore, the matrix $\mathbf{G}(\lambda)$ is always in $\mathcal{P}(n)$ even if λ falls outside the interval $[0, 1]$ (extrapolation). If the matrices $\mathbf{P}_1$ and $\mathbf{P}_2$ commute then $\mathbf{G}(\lambda) = \mathbf{P}_1^{\lambda}\mathbf{P}_2^{1-\lambda}$. Figure 17.5 shows diffusion ellipsoids for linear interpolation based on (17.13) and geodesic interpolation based on (17.14) between two SPD tensors.

17.5.2 Multivariate Interpolation

Given $d + 1$ SPD matrices $\mathbf{P}_1, \ldots, \mathbf{P}_{d+1}$ that are the values of a SPD matrix field at the $d + 1$ vertices of a d-dimensional simplex, the linear Lagrange interpolation at a point with barycentric coordinates $(\lambda_1, \ldots, \lambda_{d+1})$ is given by

$$(\lambda_1, \ldots, \lambda_{d+1}) \mapsto \mathbf{P}(\lambda_1, \ldots, \lambda_{d+1}) = \sum_{i=1}^{d+1} \lambda_i \mathbf{P}_i , \tag{17.15}$$

where the λ_i's satisfy $0 \leq \lambda_i \leq 1$, for $1 \leq i \leq d + 1$ and $\lambda_1 + \cdots + \lambda_{d+1} = 1$.

Once again, $\mathbf{P}(\lambda_1, \ldots, \lambda_{d+1})$ can be seen as the weighted arithmetic mean of the SPD matrices $\mathbf{P}_1, \ldots, \mathbf{P}_{d+1}$. Similar to the univariate case, we can also define the geodesic interpolation of $\mathbf{P}_1, \ldots, \mathbf{P}_{d+1}$ at a point with barycentric coordinates $(\lambda_1, \ldots, \lambda_{d+1})$ as the weighted geometric mean of $\mathbf{P}_1, \ldots, \mathbf{P}_{d+1}$ with weights $\lambda_1, \ldots, \lambda_{d+1}$. However, unlike the univariate case, for $d > 1$ this weighted geometric mean cannot be given explicitly and one has to numerically solve the nonlinear matrix equation

$$\sum_{i=1}^{d+1} \lambda_i \, \mathrm{Log}(\mathbf{P}_i^{-1}\mathbf{X}) = \mathbf{0} . \tag{17.16}$$

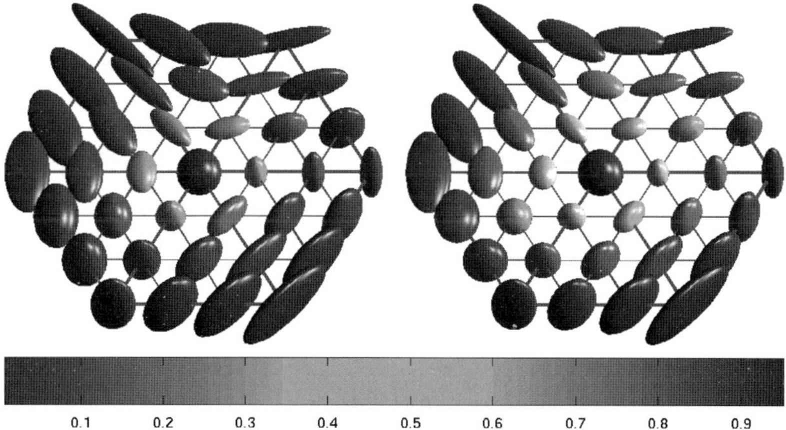

Fig. 17.6. *Bivariate interpolation:* Ellipsoidal representation of the interpolation of a 3D tensor field over a 2-dimensional hexagonal region: Euclidean interpolation (*left*) and geodesic interpolation (*right*). In both cases, the colors correspond to the values of the geodesic anisotropy index. (See color plates)

In the case where all $\mathbf{P}_i$'s commute this equation yields the solution

$$\mathbf{P}_1^{\lambda_1} \cdots \mathbf{P}_{d+1}^{\lambda_{d+1}} \ .$$

Otherwise, (17.16) is solved numerically, e.g., by the fixed point algorithm described in [9].

As an illustration of multivariate interpolation we visualize in Fig. 17.6 the result of a bivariate interpolation of SPD tensors on a hexagonal region. A tensor field given by its values at the vertices of the blue triangles is interpolated based on both the Euclidean and geodesic methods.

References

1. Amari, S. (1985) Differential-Geometrical Methods in Statistics. Springer-Verlag, Berlin Heidelberg.
2. Basser, P. and Pierpaoli, C. (1996) *Microstructural and physiological features of tissues elucidated by quantitative-diffusion-tensor MRI*, J. Magn. Reson. B **111**/3, pp. 209–219.
3. Batchelor, P. G., Moakher, M., Atkinson, D., Calamante, F., Connelly, A. (2004) A rigorous framework for diffusion tensor analysis using Riemannian geometry. Magn. Reson. Med., in press.
4. Helgason, S. (1978) Differential Geometry, Lie Groups, and Symmetric spaces. Academic Press, New York.
5. Kullback, S. L. (1959) Information Theory and Statistics. Wiley, New York.
6. Lang, S. (1999) Fundamentals of Differential Geometry. Springer-Verlag, New York.

7. Lenglet, C., Rousson, M., Deriche, R. (2004) *Segmentation of 3D Probability Density Fields by Surface Evolution: Application to Diffusion MRI*, in: MICCAI 2004, Part I, C. Barillot, D. R. Haynor, P. Hellier, eds. Lecture Notes in Computer Science, Vol. 3216, Springer-Verlag, Berlin, pp. 18–25.
8. Moakher, M. (2003) A differential geometric approach to the geometric mean of symmetric positive-definite matrices. SIAM J. Matrix Anal. Appl., in press.
9. Moakher, M. (2004) On the averaging of symmetric positive-definite tensors, submitted to: J. Elasticity.
10. Papadakis, N. G., Xing, D., Houston, G. C., Smith, J. M., Smith, M. I., James, M. F., Parsons, A. A., Huang, C. L.-H., Hall, L. D., Carpenter, T. A. (1999) *A study of rotationally invariant and symmetric indices of diffusion anisotropy*, Magn. Reson. Imag., **17**/6, pp. 881–892.
11. Pierpaoli, C. and Basser, P. J. (1996) *Toward a quantitative assessment of diffusion anisotropy*, Magn. Reson. Med., **36**/6, pp. 893–906.
12. Smith, S. T. (1993) *Geometric optimization methods for adaptive filtering*. Ph.D. thesis, Harvard University, Cambridge, Massachussetts.
13. Terras, A. (1988) Harmonic Analysis on Symmetric Spaces and Applications II. Springer-Verlag, New York.

Continuous Tensor Field Approximation of Diffusion Tensor MRI data

Sinisa Pajevic[1], Akram Aldroubi[2], and Peter J. Basser[3]

[1] National Institutes of Health, MSCL/CIT, Bethesda, MD 20892-5620, USA
`pajevic@nih.gov`
[2] Dept. of Mathematics, Vanderbilt University, Nashville, TN 37240-0001, USA
`aldroubi@math.vanderbilt.edu`
[3] National Institutes of Health, STBB/NICHD, Bethesda, MD 20892-5772, USA
`pjbasser@helix.nih.gov`

Summary. Diffusion Tensor MRI (DT-MRI) measurements are a discrete noisy sample of an underlying macroscopic effective diffusion tensor field, $\underline{D}(\mathbf{x})$, of water. This field is presumed to be piecewise continuous/smooth at a gross anatomical length scale. Here we describe a mathematical framework for obtaining an estimate of this tensor field from the measured DT-MRI data using a spline-based continuous approximation. This methodology facilitates calculation of new structural quantities and provides a framework for applying differential geometric methods to DT-MRI data. A B-spline approximation has already been used to improve robustness of DT-MRI fiber tractography. Here we propose a piecewise continuous approximation based on Non-Uniform Rational B-Splines (NURBS), which addresses some of the shortcomings of the previous implementation.

18.1 Introduction

Diffusion tensor MRI provides a measurement of an effective diffusion tensor of water, $\underline{D}^{\text{eff}}$, in each voxel within an imaging volume [1]. These diffusion measurements are inherently discrete, noisy and voxel-averaged. Here we treat DT-MRI data as discrete noisy samples of an underlying macroscopic piecewise continuous diffusion tensor field, $\underline{D}(\mathbf{x})$, where, $\mathbf{x} = (x, y, z)$ are the spatial coordinates in the laboratory frame of reference. This field is presumed to be piecewise continuous or smooth at a gross anatomical length scale, an assumption based on the known anatomy of many soft fibrous tissues, including white matter, muscles, ligaments, and tendons. One of our objectives is to develop a mathematical framework to estimate this piecewise continuous field, $\underline{D}(\mathbf{x})$, from discrete noisy DT-MRI measurements. A reliable estimate of this field enables us to use differential geometric methods directly. Additionally, it enables computation and display of intrinsic architectural or microstructural

MRI features based upon tissue fiber geometry [2, 2]. Some previously suggested characteristics are curvature and torsion of the individual fiber tracts, as well as the properties of the tangent field, e.g. twisting, bending, and diverging [4]. Here we focus on estimating curvature of the fiber tracts (tangent field) but also show the architectural features of the tensor field itself. Estimating such quantities accurately using measured diffusion tensor data and interpolation is difficult, since their evaluation requires spatial differentiation of noisy tensor quantities. Below we show that they can be calculated more reliably and robustly using continuous tensor field approximation.

Originally, estimating the tensor field from sample tensor data was performed using B-spline approximation [5]. It was used with DT-MRI data to elucidate fiber tract trajectories, which can be done by integrating the fiber direction (vector) field [9]. Other methods for fiber tracking at the time utilized interpolation or directly followed the local fiber orientation [6, 7, 8], with exception of Poupon et al. [11] who used a regularization method. Integrating a noisy direction vector field can result in fiber trajectories that wander off course. Using a smoothed representation of the direction field, obtained from the continuous representation of $\mathbf{D}(\mathbf{x})$, however, can improve the fidelity of tract following [9]. Establishing connectivity and continuity of neural pathways can also benefit from the development of this specialized tensor field processing methodology. These tasks require determining continuous links between different regions of the brain, or assessing disjunctions between them. Finally, there are a number of generic image processing tasks one would like to perform on high dimensional DT-MRI data, since no signal processing framework currently exists for these. These include: filtering noise, sharpening edges, detecting boundaries; compressing, storing and transmitting large image files; interpolating and extrapolating tensor data; resampling data at different resolutions (e.g., rebinning); extracting textural features, segmenting images, clustering data, and classifying tissues; and detecting statistical outliers. The B-spline approximation provides the mathematical underpinnings for performing these tasks both rapidly and efficiently [10]. However, the problem with it is that it introduces smoothing in the data uniformly and isotropically and is incapable of dealing with discontinuities. The smaller structures as well as sudden or rapid changes (edges, high curvatures, etc.) will be distorted at the levels of approximation/smoothing required to alleviate the noise effects. To achieve a more efficient approximation we use Non-Uniform Rational B-Splines (NURBS). They allow for discontinuities and can describe complex piecewise continuous geometrical shapes with many fewer parameters than the original B-spline approximation.

Although there are other approaches for finding an approximate tensor field, in this chapter we focus on a mathematical framework for continuous approximation based on splines. A number of other methods for tensor field approximation exist, for example see references [11, 12, 13, 14]. Also, Chap. 17 by Moakher and Batchelor and Chap. 19 by Weickert and Welk present novel and sophisticated ways of interpolating and regularizing tensor fields.

However, the goal of this chapter is not to review comprehensively the tensor field approximation methods, instead, we describe and compare two different spline methods for computing approximated tensor fields: (i) the previously proposed method using B-splines and (ii) a new method that uses NURBS.

18.2 Continuous Approximation and Representation of Discrete Tensor Data

The two approximation methods we focus on, (i) and (ii), have many common features which we generalize here. In both, to construct a continuous approximation to a diffusion tensor field, we start with a set of basis functions (approximants) whose linear combinations define an approximation space. In [5], to make the approximation scheme practicable, we required it possess the following properties: (P1) The set of basis functions must be sufficiently rich to represent the diffusion tensor field precisely and accurately; (P2) The mathematical description of the approximation space is computationally tractable; (P3) The approximation of the diffusion tensor field is implemented using algorithms that are fast, robust, and accurate. In this chapter we also require (P4) the approximation scheme must be able to produce a piecewise continuous representation. We will see later that this can be done using NURBS, which will provide even richer set of basis functions (strengthening P1), however, the requirement for speed in P3 will have to be relaxed.

To meet these requirements in general, we use atomic spaces [16], which are a generalization of shift invariant spaces. In particular, we choose an atomic space, $S_A(\mathbf{x}, \underline{B})$, such that any function in that space, $\underline{T}(\mathbf{x})$ is of the form

$$\underline{T}(\mathbf{x}) = \sum_{i=1}^{N_r} \sum_{i=1}^{N_x} \sum_{j=1}^{N_y} \sum_{k=1}^{N_z} P^m(i,j,k) \times \underline{B}^m(\mathbf{x}, \mathbf{Q}_{i,j,k}) \qquad (18.1)$$

In other words, each approximant in the approximation space, $\underline{T}(\mathbf{x})$, is a weighted sum of a finite number of tensor field generators , $\underline{B}^m(\mathbf{x}, \mathbf{Q}_{i,j,k})$, $m = 1, \ldots, N_r$. The $P^m(i,j,k)$ are the coefficients for the total of $N_r N_x N_y N_z$ basis functions and are the first set of parameters of the approximation model. The other parameters that describe the basis functions are lumped into $\mathbf{Q}_{i,j,k}$, and can be different for different basis functions as indicated.

We showed previously that finding the tensor field generator could be reduced to finding a continuous representation of each of its individual tensor components [10]. To represent the field of the symmetric diffusion tensor, we proposed the following six orthogonal tensor-field generators used in (18.1) to define the tensor approximation space:

$$\underline{B}^1(\mathbf{x}) = b^1(\mathbf{x})\begin{bmatrix} 1 & 0 & 0 \\ 0 & 0 & 0 \\ 0 & 0 & 0 \end{bmatrix}, \ \underline{B}^2(\mathbf{x}) = b^2(\mathbf{x})\begin{bmatrix} 0 & 0 & 0 \\ 0 & 1 & 0 \\ 0 & 0 & 0 \end{bmatrix}, \ \underline{B}^3(\mathbf{x}) = b^3(\mathbf{x})\begin{bmatrix} 0 & 0 & 0 \\ 0 & 0 & 0 \\ 0 & 0 & 1 \end{bmatrix}$$

$$\underline{B}^4(\mathbf{x}) = b^4(\mathbf{x})\begin{bmatrix} 0 & 1 & 0 \\ 1 & 0 & 0 \\ 0 & 0 & 0 \end{bmatrix}, \ \underline{B}^5(\mathbf{x}) = b^5(\mathbf{x})\begin{bmatrix} 0 & 0 & 1 \\ 0 & 0 & 0 \\ 1 & 0 & 0 \end{bmatrix}, \ \underline{B}^6(\mathbf{x}) = b^6(\mathbf{x})\begin{bmatrix} 0 & 0 & 0 \\ 0 & 0 & 1 \\ 0 & 1 & 0 \end{bmatrix}$$

$$(18.2)$$

Each tensor field generator $\underline{B}^m(x)$, can now be expressed in terms of a single function, $b^m(\mathbf{x})$, which now serves as a basis for the ith component of the tensor field. Based on the choice for this function we distinguish between two implementations for the field generators; the original one that used B-splines [5] and the new one that uses NURBS.

18.3 B-Spline Approximation

With the B-splines we choose $b^m(\mathbf{x})$ to be a product of one-dimensional functions, i.e., $b^m(\mathbf{x}) = f^m(x)g^m(y)h^m(z)$. The basis functions are now separable in two ways, first with respect to the components of the tensor, and second with respect to the coordinates. Finding the continuous field $\mathbf{D}(\mathbf{x})$ can be reduced to applying a one dimensional approximation algorithm along x, y and z coordinates sequentially within the imaging volume for each component [10].

The $f^m(x), g^m(y), h^m(z)$ are B-spline functions [17, 19] which are obtained by repeated convolutions of the simple box function (Fig. 18.1a) The number of convolutions determines the order of the B-spline, i.e., linear, quadratic, cubic, etc. The use of the separable basis function provides also an easy way to account for the nonuniform resolutions in x, y, and z directions in some DT-MRI acquisitions.

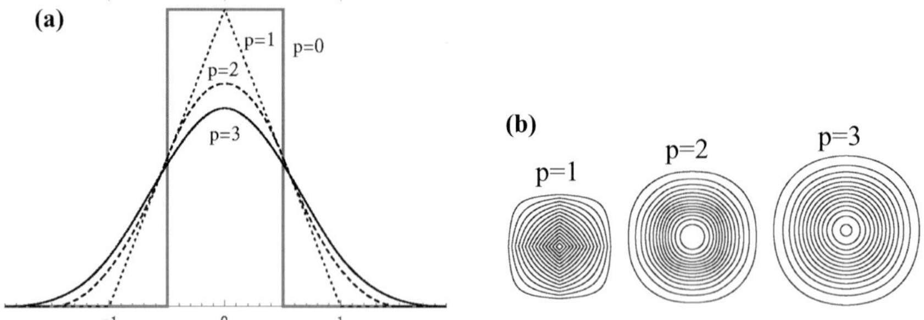

Fig. 18.1. (a) 1-D B-spline functions of degree $p = 0$ through 3. The B-spline of degree n is obtained by n-fold convolutions of the box function ($p = 0$) as indicated. (b) 2-D separable B-spline basis functions with degrees $p = 1$, 2, and 3

Using B-spline functions has several advantages: B1) the generators have finite spatial extent (i.e., finite support), which speeds up and simplifies digital processing algorithms; B2) they can be evaluated fast in a recursive fashion (as well as analytically, faster) in terms of splines of lower degree; B3) the derivatives of B-splines can be expressed recursively in terms of the original B-splines; B4) by changing the polynomial order or degree of the B-spline functions, we can control the degree of smoothness and differentiability of our continuous approximation; B5) by adjusting the (scale) parameters of the B-spline representation we can choose between interpolation (fitting data points exactly) and approximation (fitting data points approximately); B6) invariant representation under affine as well as perspective transformations; B7) possess the convex-hull property; and B8) B-spline functions naturally generate multi-resolution structures that are useful in analyzing signals and images at different length scales.

Additionally, the separable multi-dimensional spline functions behave well for the cubic and higher order splines as demonstrated in Fig. 18.1b. It shows that the two-dimensional spline function $b^m(\mathbf{x})$ constructed as a product of linear one-dimensional B-splines is anisotropic (i.e., shows preferential directions) and will produce artifacts when used for scaling (i.e., smoothing) a general tensor field. However, when the cubic B-splines are used these artifacts are negligibly small and the $b^m(\mathbf{x})$ constructed in this way perform nearly as well as the true two-dimensional isotropic basis functions, but are much more computationally efficient to implement. In our application we use mainly the cubic B-splines. If higher order derivatives are needed, it is advisable to use B-splines of higher polynomial order than three to preserve the isotropic properties of the multidimensional basis functions.

Another advantage of using B-splines is that they need very few additional parameters. In fact the simplest implementation can consist of only one parameter, the scale parameter, Δ, which controls the smoothness of the model, and indicates the degree of parameter reduction in the model. For example, when the scaling parameter Δ equals 0.25, the B-spline model is a projection of the original data to a 4-fold smoother space and in 1-D case requires 4 times less parameters. Typically, we use three scale parameters, Δ_x, Δ_y, and Δ_z, which control the degree of smoothness along each direction. The shifts on a uniform grid within the imaging volume, are indicated by k, l, and m. The generator for B-splines in this case is written as

$$\underline{B}^m(\mathbf{x}, \mathbf{Q}_{i,j,k}) = \underline{B}^m(\mathbf{x}, \mathbf{\Delta}) = \underline{B}^m(x\Delta_x - i, y\Delta_y - j, z\Delta_z - k) \tag{18.3}$$

The optimal choice of the coefficients, $P^m(i, j, k)$, for a given choice of the B-spline and scale parameters is the one that minimizes the least-squared difference between the original tensor data and the approximated diffusion tensor field [10].

18.3.1 Implementing B-Spline Approximation

Once the polynomial order of the B-spline is chosen (generally cubic), then for a given DT-MRI data set, we calculate B-spline coefficients in the x, y, and z-directions for each of the six independent diffusion tensor elements using the spatial separability property described above. Thus, we perform 18 1-D transforms on the tensor data set. The 1-D B-spline approximation we use is based on a scale conversion algorithm which finds the optimal approximation of the original signal at a given scale Δ [15, 17, 18, 19]. The only difference in our implementation is the exclusion of the post-filtering step, as described in the block diagram of the algorithm in [20]. The task of this algorithm is to find the minimal least square approximation of the original signal in the space scaled down by factor Δ. This algorithm efficiently obtains the B-spline coefficients by projecting the B-spline expansion of the original signal onto the scaled space basis. This algorithm is not exact, i.e., it does not provide a mathematically precise projection between the two spaces. However, the deviations from the exact solution are mostly formal in nature. In practice, the performance of this algorithm is nearly optimal, while gaining in speed and efficiency. This and other details of our implementation are described in the Appendix of [5].

An important step in the implementation is also to choose the appropriate scale parameters. If the scale parameters equal 1, the continuous representation becomes interpolation; if one or more of the Δ_i is less than 1, the continuous representation becomes a data reduction technique that approximates or fits the discrete tensor data. Since the Δ is the ratio of the number of unknown parameters to the number of measured data points for the 1-D approximation the scale parameters can only take on specific rational values, $\{\Delta\}_N$, which designates the rational number closest to Δ that contains N in the denominator. For DT-MR images N is usually large enough to allow sufficient precision in the range of the scale parameter values between 0 and 1. We reduce the number of scale parameters by choosing only one Δ and by assigning the three values of the model as $\{\Delta\}_{N_x}, \{\Delta\}_{N_y}, \{V_r\Delta\}_{N_z}$, where V_r is the voxel aspect ratio ($V_r \approx 2$) in our case), thus making the grid of B-spline coefficients more uniform. Ideally, the value of Δ should be twice the ratio of the maximal spatial frequency of the pure (noise-free) signal and the sampling frequency. Note, however, that our approximation method is not a simple low-pass filter and the projecting onto a smoother space is *not* the same as smoothing. The first one provides the least square fit while the latter does not, in general. In cases where structures within the image appear at all length scales, the choice of Δ is empirical as the structures on the small scales (single or a few voxels) must be blurred in order to improve estimates of large structures of the diffusion tensor field elsewhere.

The B-spline approximation, although successfully applied to the fiber tracking application [9] (see Fig. 18.2), does not provide a reliable framework for applying general methods of differential geometry to DT-MRI data.

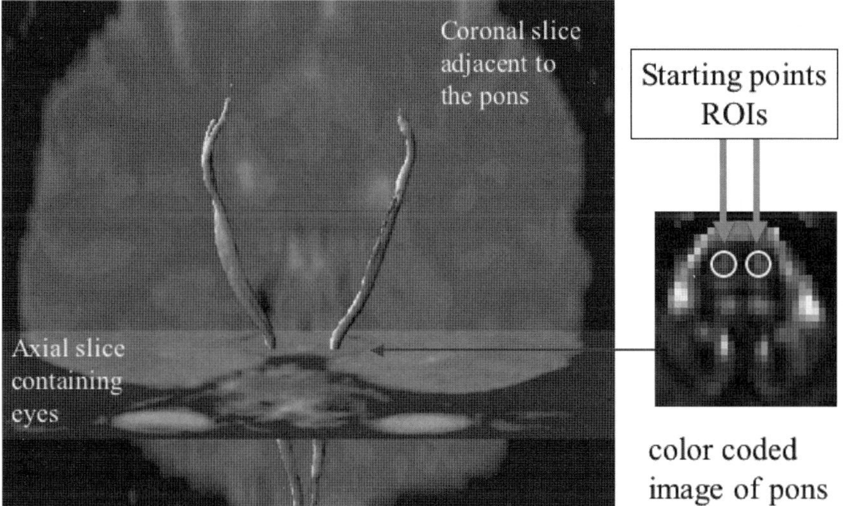

Fig. 18.2. Fiber tracts result from integrating along the tangent direction of the B-spline approximated tensor field, and with starting points chosen from the two circular regions in the area of pons. The obtained result agrees well with known anatomical data. (See colour plates.)

Calculations of curvature, torsion and other differential geometric quantities were highly unreliable [5].

18.4 Non-Uniform Rational B-Splines (NURBS)

Non-Uniform Rational B-Splines, or NURBS as they are widely known, are a powerful tool to describe and model complex curves and surfaces using a small number of parameters [21]. It is a much richer set of basis functions which generalize many concepts of ordinary B-splines. To introduce the NURBS model we focus on the 1-D model, since here too the multidimensional models are derived using products of basis functions.

There are three main groups of parameters that describe a NURBS model. The first is the knot vector, U, which controls the non-uniformity along a particular dimension, the second is a set of weights, $\mathbf{W}$, one for each basis functions, and the third are the 'control points', which correspond to the B-spline coefficients of our model, but we adopted this commonly used jargon.

The knot vector is a set of monotonically nondecreasing numbers in the real interval $[a, b]$ which parametrizes a given curve, i.e.,

$$U = \{\underbrace{a, \ldots, a}_{p+1}, u_{p+1}, \ldots, u_{i-1}, u_i, u_{i+1}, \ldots, u_{m-p-1}, \underbrace{b, \ldots, b}_{p+1}\} \qquad (18.4)$$

As can be seen some values can be repeated and an important quantity is the multiplicity of the knot, n_m, which is equal to the number of times a given value is repeated. In this way it is possible to control the continuity of the curve. Each basis function is C^k-continuous, $k = p - n_m$ at a knot with multiplicity n_m, and C^∞ continuous elsewhere. The $p + 1$ repetition of the end points of the interval is just a statement that at the edges the curve is discontinuous. Alternatively, one can lower the multiplicity at the end points by using boundary conditions.

The set of basis functions is obtained using the recursive structure of the B-splines except that now the factors in front of the interacting B-splines of lower order are not constant but are functions of the knot vector. They are called Non-Uniform B-Splines (NUBS). The NUBS basis functions are obtained using the following recursion:

$$B_{i,p}(u) = \left(\frac{u - u_i}{u_{i+p} - u_i} \right) B_{i,p-1}(u) - \left(\frac{u - u_{i+p+1}}{u_{i+p+1} - u_{i+1}} \right) B_{i+1,p-1}(u)$$

$$B_{i,0}(u) = \begin{cases} 1 & u \in [u_i, u_{i+1}) \\ 0 & \text{otherwise} \end{cases} \tag{18.5}$$

and the kth derivate at point u can be obtained using

$$B_{i,p}^{(k)}(u) = p \left(\frac{B_{i,p-1}^{(k-1)}(u)}{u_{i+p} - u_i} - \frac{B_{i+1,p-1}^{(k-1)}(u)}{u_{i+p+1} - u_{i+1}} \right) \tag{18.6}$$

Figure 18.3a shows a set of NUBS for the given values of spline degree and the knot vector. Once a set of NUBS is obtained we use the second set of parameters, $\mathbf{W}$, which are the weights associated with each of the NUB basis

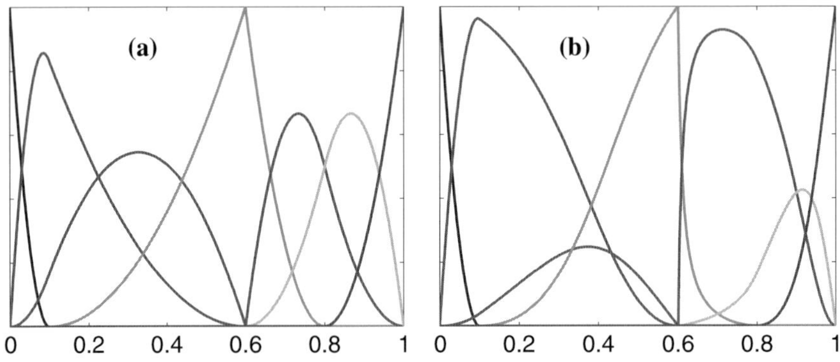

Fig. 18.3. (a) A set of 1-D NUB-basis functions with $p = 2$ and the knot vector $U = [0\ 0\ 0\ 0.1\ 0.6\ 0.6\ 0.8\ 1\ 1\ 1]$. (b) A set of rational basis functions (NURBS) obtained using the NUBs in (a) and by changing the weights for the 3rd, 4th and 5th basis function to 0.2, 0.5 and 5, respectively. The remaining NUBs had weights $w = 1$. (See colour plates)

functions, to obtain the *rational basis* functions (Fig. 18.3b). The rational basis function $R_{i,p}(u)$ corresponding to the ith NUB basis function, $B_{j,p}$, is obtained as

$$R_{i,p}(u) = \frac{B_{i,p}(u)w_i}{\sum\limits_{j=0}^{n} B_{j,p}(u)w_j} \tag{18.7}$$

The third set of parameters are the coefficients P^m of the spline model, or in NURBS parlance, *control points*. The control points are actually tuplets of B-spline coefficients grouped together to reflect the geometry of the model. For example, for a 3-D space curve the B-spline coefficients of the $x(u)$, $y(u)$ and $z(u)$ functions are grouped together to form a 3-D control point, $\mathbf{P}_i = (P^i_x, P^i_y, P^i_z)$. The NURBS curve model $\mathbf{C}(u)$ can now be written as

$$\mathbf{C}(u) = \sum_{i=0}^{n} R_{i,p}(u)\mathbf{P}_i \tag{18.8}$$

Once the weights and the knot vector are chosen, which we discuss below, the rational basis functions $R_{i,p}(u)$ are determined, and the model in (18.8) is linear. Thus, when solving this linear system for control points, here too we can choose between interpolation (number of control points is the same as the number of data points) or the least square fit (fewer control points). The NURBS curve model can be extended using the function products, as described in Sect. 18.2, to surfaces, volumes and ultimately to tensor fields. Here we finally write our NURBS tensor model in terms of *control tensors*, $\mathbf{D}^c_{i,j,k}$,

$$\mathbf{D}(x,y,z) = \sum_{i=0}^{n}\sum_{j=0}^{m}\sum_{k=0}^{l} R_{i,j,k}(x,y,z)\mathbf{D}^c_{i,j,k} \tag{18.9}$$

where $R_{i,j,k}(x,y,z)$ is a new 3-D rational function defined from NUBS, which now require three different knots vectors U, V, and S and can be of different degree in each dimension (p,q,r), i.e.,

$$R_{i,j,k}(x,y,z) = \frac{B_{i,p}(x)B_{j,q}(y)B_{k,r}(z)w_{i,j,k}}{\sum\limits_{i'=0}^{n}\sum\limits_{j'=0}^{m}\sum\limits_{k'=0}^{l} B_{i',p}(x)B_{j',q}(y)B_{k',r}(z)w_{i',j',k'}} \tag{18.10}$$

Equation (18.9) is equivalent to (18.1), except that here the N_r independent components of the tensor field are lumped together into a control tensor. This geometric interpretation can be very useful. For example, since the convex hull property has much tighter bounds in the case of the NURBS model we can use positive semidefiniteness of the control tensors to enforce the same property for the tensor field at any point in space.

The NURBS model shares all the good properties of the B-spline model (B1-B8) but has important additional advantages: (N1) precisely represents a large family of mathematical curves, piecewise polynomials, conic sections (circles, ellipses, hyperbolas, parabolas), Bezier curves, and very efficiently arbitrary shapes (N2) can control the degree of smoothness and continuity, including discontinuous functions, thus suitable for piecewise continuous representation.

However, although they enable fast evaluation in a recursive fashion at any point in the space (like B-spline), obtaining the appropriate parameters of the model is much harder now. We assume here that one wants to use the properties N1-N2, otherwise the NURBS model can be simplified. After all, the B-splines are a special case of NURBS with uniformly spaced knot vector and all weights equal. Here we mainly refer to NURBS as model that requires non-uniform knots and varying weights.

As mentioned above, we obtained the control points by solving the linear system in (18.8). The knot vector is initially chosen based on the spacing between the data (1-D case), but later knots are randomly added or removed. The most difficult part in fitting the NURBS model is to determine the optimal set of weights. Here, we initially set the weights to 1 and after obtaining the desired set of control points we use simulated annealing to obtain the new set of weights, keeping control points and the knot vector fixed. After randomly adding or removing a single knot we obtain a new knot vector and with the new weights calculate the new set of rational basis functions, $R_{i,p}(u)$. This procedure is repeated until satisfactory solution is obtained.

In the case of one dimensional data one can still obtain useful NURBS fits relatively quickly. Figure 18.4a shows a fit to synthetic 2-D data (noisy samples of two different 2-D curves were joined together to create an apparent discontinuity). The solid line indicates the fit to a NURBS model and one can see that even with a discontinuity, the NURBS describes the curve very well with only 14 control points. The B-spline model was incapable of describing such curve.

The image inset in Fig. 18.4b shows a 2D-projection of a tract (solid yellow line) onto a slice of DT-MRI volume with color coded orientations. The tract

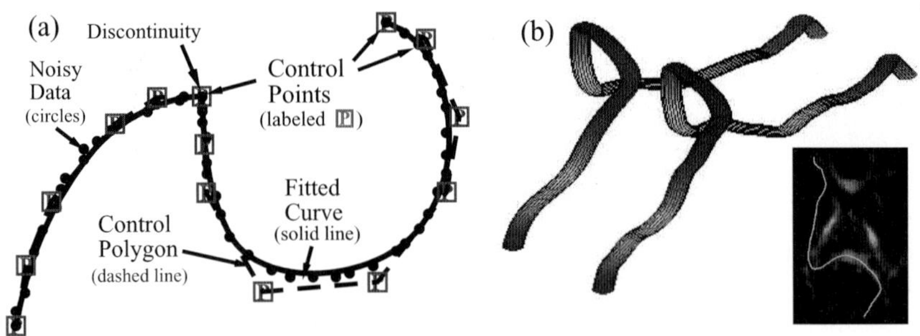

Fig. 18.4. (a) 2-D curve NURBS model fit to noisy data (b) 3-D curve NURBS model fit to fiber tracking data, indicated on the inset image. (See colour plates)

passes through the corpus callosum and spans from one end of the brain to the other. Figure 18.4b shows side by side the same tract in 3-D described with NURBS model (left) and B-spline model (right). The B-spline model, parameterized with B-spline coefficients needs a total of $3*130 = 390$ parameters to produce as faithful representation of the space curve as the NURBS model did with only 15 control points (total of 60 parameters). Such a sparser parameter space enables more efficient explorations of connectivity, and more importantly can significantly alleviate the noise effects. In the next section we compare B-spline and NURBS models on the important example of estimating local curvature of the fiber tract.

18.5 B-spline vs NURBS Comparison on Curvature Estimation

Estimating curvature is problematic for noisy data. The curvature of a fiber tract, or a space curve, is defined as

$$\kappa(u) = \left| \frac{d\mathbf{t}(u)}{du} \right| = \frac{|\dot{\mathbf{r}} \times \ddot{\mathbf{r}}|}{|\dot{\mathbf{r}}|^3} \qquad (18.11)$$

where $\mathbf{r} = \mathbf{r}(u)$ is the position vector parameterized by u, and $\mathbf{t}(u)$ is the tangent of the space curve at $\mathbf{r}(u)$. Since higher derivatives are involved, this estimate is very sensitive to noise (each derivation acts as a linear ramp high pass filter). Another look at the problem is that the fiber tracts are not polynomial and their estimates are noisy. Thus in order to faithfully depict a given curve one has to represent curves with a relatively high number of B-spline coefficients, thus sampling the noise often. The curvature of noise is infinite and thus the local estimates of the radius will be biased towards zero, besides being also very noisy. We reported previously that the B-spline approximation did not produce satisfactory results in this regard. Here we compare B-spline estimates with NURBS estimates.

We test curvature estimation on a simulated space curve consisting of four circular arcs with radii $R_c = 100,10,5,35$ in arbitrary units. We then sampled 50 points with sampling error of 1%, which are indicated as solid black circles on the inset in upper right corner of Fig. 18.5. The inset also shows the 15 control points of the fit, together with the 'ideal' control points (light blue circles) which could describe such curve exactly. There are total of 10 'ideal' points but not all are shown since in many cases they are very close to the control points obtained from the fit. We see that the NURBS fitting routine can be improved further, however, even this imperfect fit provides significant improvement over the B-spline approximation. The solid black line in Fig. 18.5a indicates the true radius, with the exception of the three inflection points where the curvature is infinite. The solid blue line indicates the NURBS estimates outperforms the B-spline approximation for any level of smoothness,

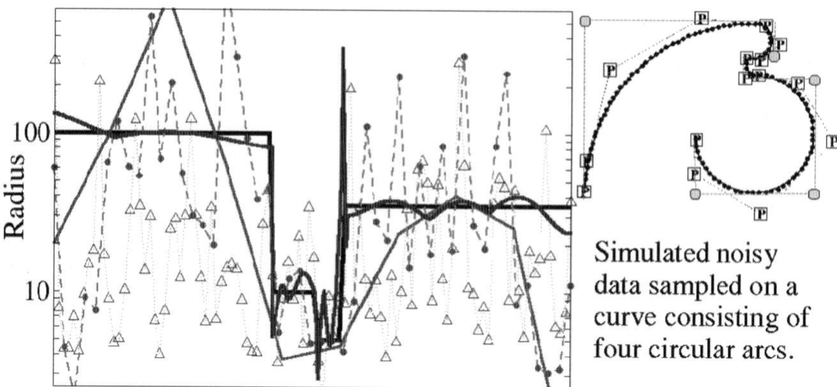

Fig. 18.5. Radii of curvature obtained from a noisy data set of points sampled from a curve consisting of four circular arcs (see the inset in upper right corner) with radii 100,10,5,35. The sampling error was 1%. The *solid black* line indicates the true radius (at inflection points the radius is infinite). The *solid blue* line indicates the NURBS fit, while B-spline approximation estimates are labeled as follows: $\Delta = 1$, i.e., interpolation (*green triangles*), $\Delta = 0.5$ (*purple dots*), or $\Delta = 0.2$ (*red solid line*). Note that the original curve could have been described with only 10 control points (the *light blue* circles, not all shown). (See colour plates)

as described in the caption. The spike in the NURBS estimate occurs at the inflection point where the radius of curvature is infinite.

In Fig. 18.6 we determined the radius of curvature for every voxel in one of the slices using both NURBS estimate and the B-spline approximation with $\Delta = 0.2$ (since such choice produced relatively stable estimates in Fig. 18.5, however with significant loss in resolution. This loss of resolution is evident in Fig. 18.6a, where it appears that very little variation of the radius of curvature is occurring, for example, in the splenium of the corpus callosum. The NURBS estimate in 18.6b does show significant variation. Even though the lower curvature structures appear 'spotty' in the NURBS estimate they indicate errors of only 20 % (a good precision for the curvature radius).

18.6 Discussion and Conclusion

The continuous approximation methodology takes noisy, voxel-averaged, and discrete statistical samples of an underlying macroscopic effective diffusion tensor field as its input, and produces a piecewise continuous, smooth tensor field approximation as its output. Besides being able to recover the original noiseless tensor field reliably, the approximation schemes substantially reduces bias of the mean and variance of various quantities derived from the tensor field, e.g., $\text{Trace}(\underline{\mathbf{D}}(\mathbf{x}))$. This new methodology also facilitates following nerve and other fiber tract trajectories in vivo. New MR features or parameters

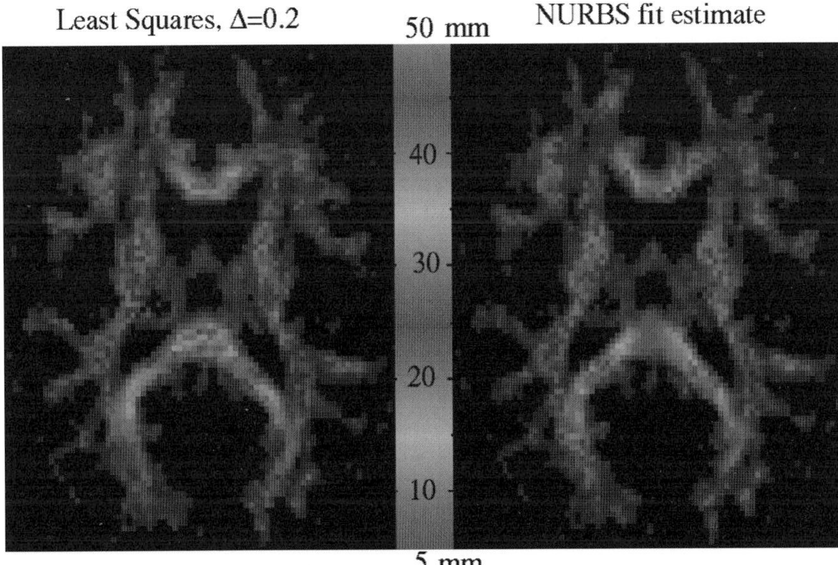

Fig. 18.6. Color coded images of the radius of curvature obtained at the center of each voxel for the given slice using B-spline approximation with $\Delta = 0.2$ (*left*) and NURBS (*right*), with colorbar indicating the scales. We see that the NURBS estimates are capable of showing the spatial variation of the fiber curvature. Note, that although the models are continuous, the estimates obtained from them are not necessarily smooth. The pixelization in the image, however, is arbitrary and we could have obtained the estimates at any point in space with the continuous models. (See colour plates)

that characterize structure, architecture, and functional assessment of tissues can be developed from this continuous representation of DT-MRI data. As analytical functions are used to approximate the diffusion tensor field, we can evaluate and display quantities such as the gradient tensors [5], which cannot be evaluated accurately from noisy DT-MRI data.

18.6.1 Microscopic Field (Underlying) vs Macroscopic Field (Voxel Averaged)

The microscopic tensor field is one that describes water diffusion on a microscopic scale, whereas the macroscopic effective tensor field describes the tensor field on a voxel scale. If we assume no intercompartmental mixing of spins, the measured macroscopic tensor field is just the voxel-average of this microscopic tensor field. While these macro and micro fields should be similar in regions containing tissue whose distribution of fiber direction is uniform within the voxel, in tissues whose distribution of fiber direction is non-uniform, such as regions where fibers diverge or converge (splay), bend or twist, branch or merge, a significant disparity may exist between these fields. Generally, in these regions, the macroscopic field will be a powder average of the heterogeneous microscopic tensor field within a voxel. An important long-term goal is to develop techniques to identify regions in which such powder averaging occurs, and then attempt to infer the microscopic tensor field from macroscopic voxel-scale measurements there using additional information from other sources [22] (see also Chap. 5 by Alexander).

18.6.2 NURBS vs B-Spline

The B-spline approximation is not nearly as efficient as the NURBS model. Its estimation of quantities involving higher derivatives is inaccurate and thus the model is not adequate for applying differential geometric methods. Another shortcoming of the B-spline approximation method is that it forces continuity of the tensor field at boundaries or interfaces, where there is no physical requirement to impose continuity. This results in high approximation errors at the edges of the structures.

NURBS can account for piecewise continuity by modifying knot vector. NURBS produce promising results for 1-D curves, and to some extent with surfaces. However, to date, we have been unable to obtain an efficient tensor model, mainly due to an extremely large parameter space and the very rich model, which is difficult to fit (many local minima). It appears that the NURBS methodology will have to be used differently than the B-spline approximation, and a long computation will be required to obtain the model, using various stochastic fitting methods (simulated annealing, genetic algorithms, etc.) Once the model is obtained it will be possible to explore its geometry, tract fibers, and run various differential geometric models with almost the same efficiency as with B-splines. Work is underway to improve NURBS fitting and at the same time to generalize this continuous tensor field approximation to treat internal boundaries and discontinuities in the tensor field more naturally and robustly by using control tensors that do not use the actual coordinates x, y, and z for parameterization. In other words the control tensor will contain information about its position in space. The tensor model is now written as

$$\mathbf{D}(u,v,s) = \sum_{i=0}^{n}\sum_{j=0}^{m}\sum_{k=0}^{l} R_{i,j,k}(u,v,s)\mathbf{D}_{i,j,k}^{c}(\mathbf{r}_{i,j,k}) \qquad (18.12)$$

Effectively, the control tensor is now a 9-dimensional quantity (6 independent tensor components plus 3 spatial dimensions).

References

1. P.J. Basser, J. Mattiello, and D. Le Bihan. MR diffusion tensor spectroscopy and imaging. Biophysical Journal 66(1), 259-67 (1994).

2. P.J. Basser. Inferring microstructural features and the physiological state of tissues from diffusion-weighted images. NMR in Biomedicine, 8(7-8), 333-44 (1995).
3. P.J. Basser, and C. Pierpaoli. Microstructural and physiological features of tissues elucidated by quantitative-diffusion-tensor MRI. Journal of Magnetic Resonance B 111(3), 209-19 (1996).
4. P.J. Basser. New histological and physiological stains derived from diffusion-tensor MR images. Annals New York Acad Sci 820, 123-38 (1997).
5. S. Pajevic, A. Aldroubi and P.J. Basser. A continuous tensor field approximation of discrete DT-MRI data for extracting microstructural and architectural features of tissue. Journal of Magnetic Resonance, 154, 85-100 (2002).
6. T. E. Conturo, N. F. Lori, T. S. Cull, E. Akbudak, A. Z. Snyder, J. S. Shimony, R. C. McKinstry, H. Burton, M. E. Raichle, Tracking neuronal fiber pathways in the living human brain, Proceedings National Acad Sci USA 96, 10422-7 (1999).
7. S. Mori, B. J. Crain, V. P. Chacko, P. C. M. van Zijl, Three-dimensional tracking of axonal projections in the brain by magnetic resonance imaging, Annals of Neurology, 45, 265-269 (1999).
8. S. Mori, W. E. Kaufmann, G. D. Pearlson, B. J. Crain, B. Stieltjes, M. Solaiyappan, P. C. van Zijl, In vivo visualization of human neural pathways by magnetic resonance imaging, Annals of Neurology 47, 412-4 (2000).
9. P.J. Basser, S. Pajevic, C. Pierpaoli, A. Aldroubi, and J. Duda. In Vivo Fiber-Tractography in Human Brain Using Diffusion Tensor MRI (DT-MRI) Data, Magnetic Resonance in Medicine, 44:625-632 (2000).
10. A. Aldroubi and P.J. Basser, Reconstruction of vector and tensor fields from sampled discrete data. in 'Contemporary Mathematics'. (L.W. Baggett, D.R. Larson, editors) pp. 1-15, American Math. Society, Providence, RI (1999).
11. C. Poupon, C. A. Clark, V. Frouin, J. Régis, I. Bloch, D. L. Bihan, J.-F. Mangin, Regularization of diffusion-based direction maps for the tracking of brain white matter fascicles, Neuroimage 12 (2), 184-195 (2000).
12. G. Parker, J. A. Schnabel, M. R. Symms, D. J. Werring, G. J. Barker, Nonlinear smoothing for reduction of systematic and random errors in diffusion tensor imaging, Journal of Magnetic Resonance Imaging, 11, 702–710 (2000).
13. J.-F. Mangin, C. Poupon, C. Clark, D. Le Bihan and I. Bloch, Eddy-Current Distortion Correction and Robust Tensor Estimation for MR-Diffusion Imaging, Lecture Notes in Computer Science, 2208, 186 (2001).
14. C.F. Westin, S.E. Maier, H. Mamata, A. Nabavi, F.A., Jolesz, R. Kikinis, Processing and visualization for diffusion tensor MRI. Medical Image Analysis, 6, 93-108 (2002).
15. A. Aldroubi, M. Eden, and M. Unser. Discrete spline filters for multiresolutions and wavelets of L2, SIAM Journal on Mathematical Analysis, 25, 1412-1432 (1994).
16. A. Aldroubi. Oblique projections in atomic spaces. Proceedings of the American Math. Society 124, 2051-2060 (1996).
17. M. Unser, A. Aldroubi, and M. Eden. B-Spline Signal Processing: Part II-Efficient Design and Implementation. IEEE Transactions on Signal Processing 41(2), 834-848 (1993).
18. C. DeBoor, A Practical Guide to Splines, Springer-Verlag Telos, 1994
19. M. Unser, A. Aldroubi, and M. Eden. B-Spline Signal Processing: Part I-Theory. IEEE Transactions on Signal Processing 41(2), 821-833 (1993).

20. M. Unser, A. Aldroubi, and M. Eden. Enlargment or reduction of digital images with minimum loss of information, IEEE Transactions on Image Processing 4, 247-258 (1995).
21. L. Piegl, W. Tiller, The NURBS Book, Springer-Verlag, 1997
22. D.S. Tuch and T.G. Reese and M.R. Wiegell and N.G. Makris and J.W. Belliveau and V.J. Wedeen. High angular resolution diffusion imaging reveals intravoxel white matter fiber heterogeneity, Magnetic Resonance in Medicine, 48, 577-582 (2002).

Tensor Field Interpolation with PDEs

Joachim Weickert and Martin Welk

Mathematical Image Analysis Group, Faculty of Mathematics and Computer Science, Saarland University, Building 27, 66041 Saarbrücken, Germany
{weickert,welk}@mia.uni-saarland.de

Summary. We present a unified framework for interpolation and regularisation of scalar- and tensor-valued images. This framework is based on elliptic partial differential equations (PDEs) and allows rotationally invariant models. Since it does not require a regular grid, it can also be used for tensor-valued scattered data interpolation and for tensor field inpainting. By choosing suitable differential operators, interpolation methods using radial basis functions are covered. Our experiments show that a novel interpolation technique based on anisotropic diffusion with a diffusion tensor should be favoured: It outperforms interpolants with radial basis functions, it allows discontinuity-preserving interpolation with no additional oscillations, and it respects positive semidefiniteness of the input tensor data.

19.1 Introduction

Many tasks in image processing, computer vision and computer graphics require to interpolate or resample images in order to obtain data at locations that do not coincide with the grid points where the digital image values are known. Classical methods to achieve this goal are linear interpolation, cubic or quintic splines, radial basis functions and sinc-based interpolation techniques; see e.g. [10, 13]. If the data are not available on a regular grid, scattered data interpolation techniques have been proposed [7, 14]. More recently, also interpolation methods based on variational formulations and nonlinear partial differential equations (PDEs) have been advocated [4, 11], in particular for so-called inpainting methods [5, 9, 12], where the image data are only corrupted in specific areas. Nonlinear PDEs allow to design discontinuity-preserving interpolants.

While image interpolation is fairly well-understood for scalar images, not much research has been done so far with respect to interpolation of matrix fields. Aldroubi and Basser [1] have proposed sampling in shift invariant amalgam spaces, while Pajevic et al. study in Chap. 18 of this volume B-splines and non-uniform rational B-splines for interpolating tensor fields. In Chap. 17,

Moakher and Batchelor investigate the Riemannian symmetric space of positive definite tensors and propose interpolation strategies that respect positive definiteness. In Chap. 23, Suarez-Santana et al. use a convolution-based interpolation with structure-adaptive weights. No attempts, however, have been made so far to study nonlinear PDE-based interpolation schemes for tensor fields. This is the goal of the present chapter.

The chapter is organised as follows. In Sect. 19.2 we first consider the scalar case. We review splines as minimisers of suitable energy functionals whose Euler–Lagrange equations lead to elliptic PDEs. By showing that variational image restoration methods lead to similar PDEs, we derive a novel unified model for image approximation and interpolation. This unified model is extended to the tensor framework in Sect. 19.3. It covers linear and nonlinear PDEs of arbitrary order. Experiments are presented with data sets from DT-MRI and computational fluid dynamics that demonstrate the properties of the different PDE interpolants. The chapter is concluded with a summary in Sect. 19.4.

19.2 Scalar Interpolation

19.2.1 Spline Interpolation

Let us start our considerations with one of the most important scalar interpolation methods: spline interpolation in 1-D. Assume we are given some interpolation points $0 = x_1 < x_2 < \cdots < x_n = 1$ with function values $f(x_1), \ldots, f(x_n)$. For performing spline interpolation we are seeking a smooth function $u(x) : [0, 1] \to \mathbb{R}$ that minimises

$$E(u) = \int_0^1 (\partial_x^m u)^2 \, dx \tag{19.1}$$

subject to

$$u(x_i) = f(x_i) \qquad (i = 1, \ldots, n). \tag{19.2}$$

It is well-known that this gives linear interpolation for $m = 1$. In this case we have continuity, i.e. C^0-smoothness at the interpolation points. For $m = 2$ we obtain cubic spline interpolation, with C^2-smoothness at the interpolation points, and $m = 3$ gives quintic spline interpolation with C^4-smoothness. In general, we get spline interpolation of degree $2m-1$ with C^{2m-2}-smoothness.

A necessary condition for minimising (19.1) is given by the Euler–Lagrange equation $(-1)^{m+1} \partial_{xx}^m u = 0$. Together with the interpolation constraints (19.2), we can cast both conditions in a single equation:

$$c(x) \cdot \underbrace{(u(x) - f(x))}_{\text{interpolation}} - (1 - c(x)) \cdot \underbrace{(-1)^{m+1} \partial_{xx}^m u}_{\text{smoothness}} = 0 \tag{19.3}$$

with

$$c(x) := \begin{cases} 1 & \text{if } x \in \{x_0, \ldots, x_n\} \\ 0 & \text{else}. \end{cases} \tag{19.4}$$

This is a linear PDE of order $2m$. For large m, we obtain a very smooth solution, but in general we can expect no maximum–minimum principle for $m > 1$. As a consequence, the interpolating spline may give over- and under-shoots, i.e. there is no guarantee that it remains within the convex hull of the data. This can be very undesirable in a number of applications. The case $m = 1$, on the other hand, is not very exciting since it leads to simple linear interpolations which are not sufficiently smooth for many purposes. However, later on we shall see that it can be attractive to stick to the case $m = 1$, if we permit *nonlinear anisotropic* PDEs instead of *linear* ones.

19.2.2 Regularisation

It is instructive to complement our considerations on *interpolation* by an important *approximation* paradigm, namely variational regularisation methods. In 1-D, they can be introduced as follows. Given some noisy signal $f : [0,1] \to \mathrm{I\!R}$, we want to find a signal u that minimises an energy functional that rewards similarity between $u(x)$ and $f(x)$, as well as smoothness of $u(x)$:

$$E(u) = \int_0^1 \left(c \cdot \underbrace{(u - f)^2}_{\text{similarity}} + (1 - c) \cdot \underbrace{\Psi(u_x^2)}_{\text{smoothness}} \right) dx \tag{19.5}$$

with some weight $0 < c < 1$ and an increasing penalising function $\Psi : [0, \infty) \to \mathrm{I\!R}$. This leads to the Euler–Lagrange equation

$$c \cdot (u - f) - (1 - c) \cdot \partial_x\left(\Psi'(u_x^2)\, u_x\right) = 0 \tag{19.6}$$

with homogeneous Neumann boundary conditions. In general, this is a non-linear PDE of order 2 that satisfies a maximum–minimum principle. The non-linear penaliser $\Psi(u_x^2)$ allows discontinuity-preserving smoothing. The total variation (TV) penaliser [15] e.g. is given by $\Psi(u_x^2) = 2|u_x|$. It leads to an Euler–Lagrange equation with the TV diffusivity $g(u_x^2) := \Psi'(u_x^2) = \frac{1}{|u_x|}$. It reduces smoothing at locations where the gradient magnitude is large.

19.2.3 A Unified Model

The PDE interpretation of spline interpolation and regularisation allows us now to study a unified model for image interpolation and approximation. Let $\Omega \subset \mathrm{I\!R}^n$ denote our n-dimensional image domain and assume we are given some incomplete or noisy scalar image data $f : \Omega \to \mathrm{I\!R}$. Then we propose to obtain an interpolated or processed image u that satisfies

$$c(x) \cdot (u - f) - (1 - c(x)) \cdot Lu = 0 \tag{19.7}$$

with a *confidence function* $c(x) : \Omega \to [0, 1]$, some elliptic differential operator L, and homogeneous Neumann boundary conditions.

Let us first analyse the confidence function $c(x)$. This function allows to fill in missing data at locations x where $c(x) = 0$, while $u(x)$ reproduces $f(x)$ at locations where $c(x) = 1$. Consequently, we can use this model for interpolation by simply setting c to 0 or 1. It should be noted that the locations x where $c(x) := 1$ do not necessarily have to be on a regular grid: The model is equally valid for scattered data interpolation and inpainting. At locations where we choose $0 < c(x) < 1$, we obtain an approximation by regularisation. For classical regularisation, c is fixed. However, $c(x)$ expresses the confidence in the data. It can be chosen e.g. such that it is inversely proportional to the local noise variance of f, if there are indications that the data are not equally reliable at different locations. Hence we have a very flexible method for denoising (approximation) with simultaneous filling-in of data (interpolation).

Regarding the elliptic differential operator L, many possibilities exist. Inspired from spline interpolation, a suitable n-dimensional generalisation of (19.3) would use the Laplacian operator (also called harmonic or linear diffusion operator) $Lu := \Delta u$ for $m = 1$, the biharmonic operator $Lu := -\Delta^2 u$ for $m = 2$, or the triharmonic operator $Lu := \Delta^3 u$ for $m = 3$. These linear operators correspond to interpolation with radial basis functions [3]. From the theory of nonlinear diffusion filtering, on the other side, it would be interesting to use the isotropic nonlinear operator $Lu := \mathrm{div}\,(g(|\nabla u|^2)\,\nabla u)$ or its anisotropic counterpart[1] $Lu := \mathrm{div}\,(g(\nabla u_\sigma \nabla u_\sigma^\top)\,\nabla u)$, where u_σ is a Gaussian-smoothed version of u, and g is a decreasing positive diffusivity function. The isotropic operator reduces diffusion at edges of u_σ, while the anisotropic one permits diffusion along edges of u_σ and reduces diffusion across edges of u_σ. For more details on nonlinear diffusion the reader is referred to [17]. Note that only the second-order differential operators allow a maximum–minimum principle, where the values of u stay within the range of the values that f takes at locations where $c(x) > 0$. One should also note that all these differential operators are rotationally invariant, unlike a number of popular interpolation techniques such as multivariate spline interpolation.

19.2.4 Experiments

Let us now evaluate the quality of our unified model (19.7) in the case of scalar image interpolation. To this end we extract the solutions of the elliptic PDEs as steady states of corresponding parabolic evolutions that are discretised by an explicit (Euler forward) finite difference scheme.

Figure 19.1 shows a test image and a sparsified version where only 1 out of 64 pixels is used. Based on this sparsified image, interpolation with various

---

[1] A scalar-valued function $g(x)$ is extended to a matrix-valued function $g(A)$ by applying g to the eigenvalues on A and leaving the eigenvectors unchanged.

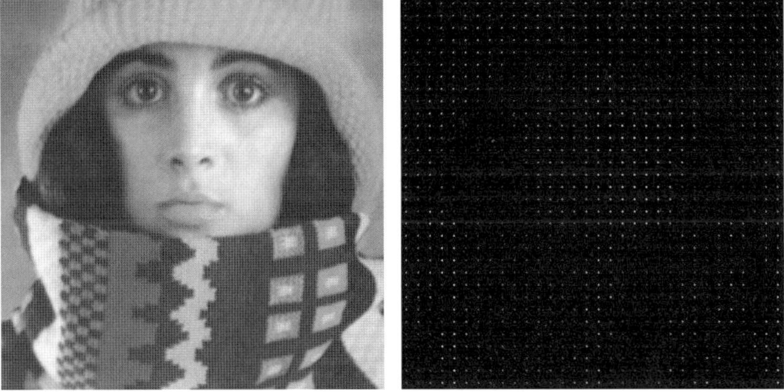

Fig. 19.1. (a) *Left*: Original image. (b) *Right*: Data points for interpolation. Only 1 out of 64 points is used

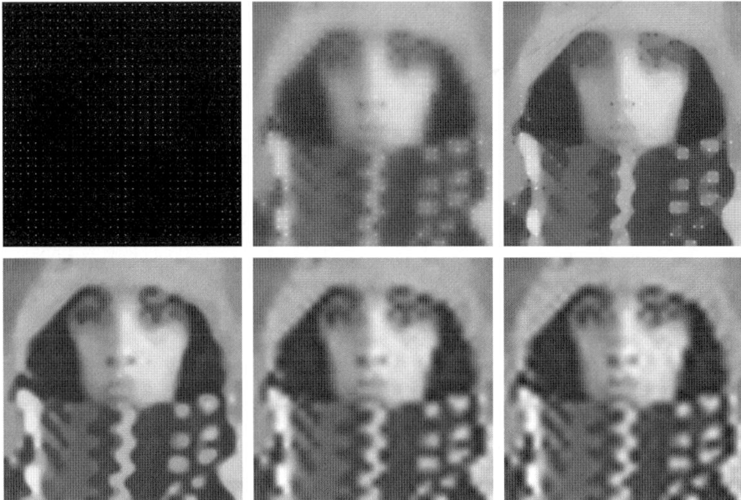

Fig. 19.2. Scalar-valued interpolation of Fig. 19.1(b). (a) *Top Left*: Interpolation data. (b) *Top Middle*: Interpolation with linear diffusion. (c) *Top Right*: Isotropic nonlinear diffusion. (d) *Bottom Left*: Anisotropic nonlinear diffusion. (e) *Bottom middle*: Biharmonic smoothing. (f) *Bottom right*: Triharmonic smoothing

differential operators and optimised parameters is shown in Fig. 19.2. In the nonlinear diffusion cases, a Charbonnier diffusivity [6] is used:

$$g(s^2) = \frac{1}{1 + s^2/\lambda^2} \tag{19.8}$$

with some contrast parameter $\lambda > 0$. Quantitative results in terms of the average Euclidean distance

Table 19.1. Interpolation quality of the scalar-valued methods from Fig. 19.2. AED = average Euclidean distance to the correct image

Smoothing Operator	AED	Max.–Min. Principle
linear diffusion	19.80	yes
isotropic nonlinear diffusion	18.42	yes
anisotropic nonlinear diffusion	15.16	yes
biharmonic smoothing	15.76	no
triharmonic smoothing	16.36	no

$$\text{AED}\,(u, v) \; := \; \left(\frac{1}{|\Omega|} \int_\Omega (u(x) - v(x))^2 \, dx \right)^{1/2} \tag{19.9}$$

between the interpolated image u and its ground truth v are given in Table 19.1. We observe that linear diffusion performs worst and is significantly worse than isotropic nonlinear diffusion. Biharmonic and triharmonic smoothing give fairly good results, but blur image edges and show oscillations near them. They also violate a maximum–minimum principle. Anisotropic diffusion performs best: It gives the highest SNR. It also obeys a maximum–minimum principle, respects discontinuities and does not suffer from visible oscillations.

19.3 Tensor Interpolation

19.3.1 PDE Formulations

Let us now investigate how the scalar PDE-based interpolation techniques from the previous section can be extended to the tensor case.

For the linear PDEs, extensions to the tensor framework are straightforward: Harmonic (linear diffusion), biharmonic and triharmonic smoothing can be applied componentwise leading to

$$c(x)(u_{ij} - f_{ij}) \; - \; (1 - c(x)) \, \Delta^1 u_{ij} = 0 \quad \text{(harmonic)} \tag{19.10}$$

$$c(x)(u_{ij} - f_{ij}) \; + \; (1 - c(x)) \, \Delta^2 u_{ij} = 0 \quad \text{(biharmonic)} \tag{19.11}$$

$$c(x)(u_{ij} - f_{ij}) \; - \; (1 - c(x)) \, \Delta^3 u_{ij} = 0 \quad \text{(triharmonic)} \tag{19.12}$$

for a tensor image $F = (f_{ij}) : \Omega \to \mathbb{R}^{n \times n}$ and its interpolant $U = (u_{ij})$. The fact that biharmonic and triharmonic smoothing violate a maximum–minimum principle in the scalar setting has an interesting consequence in the tensor framework: The interpolated tensor field may not be positive semidefinite (PSD), even if all tensors at locations x with $c(x) > 0$ are positive semidefinite. This may be a drawback for applications such as diffusion tensor MRI.

In the nonlinear diffusion setting where discontinuities are to be preserved, a suitable channel coupling is natural. We can design interpolation methods by applying recent tensor-valued extensions of nonlinear diffusion filtering in the isotropic [16] and anisotropic case [18]: In the isotropic case, channel coupling is achieved by a joint diffusivity leading to

$$c(x)\,(u_{ij}-f_{ij}) \;-\; (1-c(x))\,\mathrm{div}\left(g\left(\sum_{k,l} |\nabla u_{kl}|^2 \right) \nabla u_{ij} \right) \;=\; 0 \,. \qquad (19.13)$$

In the anisotropic case, a joint diffusion tensor is used:

$$c(x)\,(u_{ij}-f_{ij}) \;-\; (1-c(x))\,\mathrm{div}\left(g\left(\sum_{k,l} \nabla u_{kl,\sigma} \nabla u_{kl,\sigma}^\top \right) \nabla u_{ij} \right) \;=\; 0 \,. \qquad (19.14)$$

Interestingly, one can show that such a channel coupling allows PSD preservation for these second-order PDEs, both in the continuous [2] and the discrete setting [18]. An intuitive explanation for this fact is given by the observation that coupled nonlinear diffusion can be regarded as a weighted averaging of matrices where identical (but space-variant) weights are used for all channels. If the matrices are positive semidefinite, then their weighted average is also positive semidefinite.

19.3.2 Experiments

For our experiments on tensor field interpolation we have created a synthetic 2-D test image that is depicted in Fig. 19.3(a). The positive definite tensors are visualised by ellipses. Their colour is a function of the orientation of the ellipse and its anisotropy, such that an isotropic ellipse (a disk) appears white.

We perform two experiments where we evaluate the interpolation quality of the different tensor-valued PDEs: a zooming experiment where the interpolation points are equidistant, and a tensor-valued scattered data interpolation

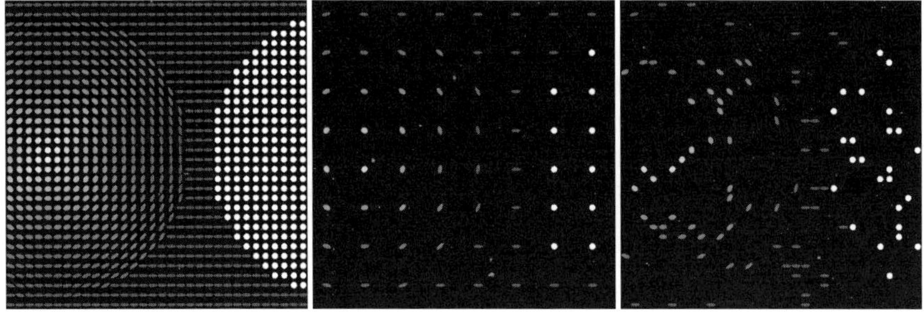

Fig. 19.3. (a) *Left*: Synthetic 2-D tensor test image, 32 × 32 pixels. (b) *Middle*: Regular interpolation data where every fourth pixel in each direction is given. (c) *Right*: Scattered interpolation data where 10 percent of all pixels have been selected randomly. See colour plates

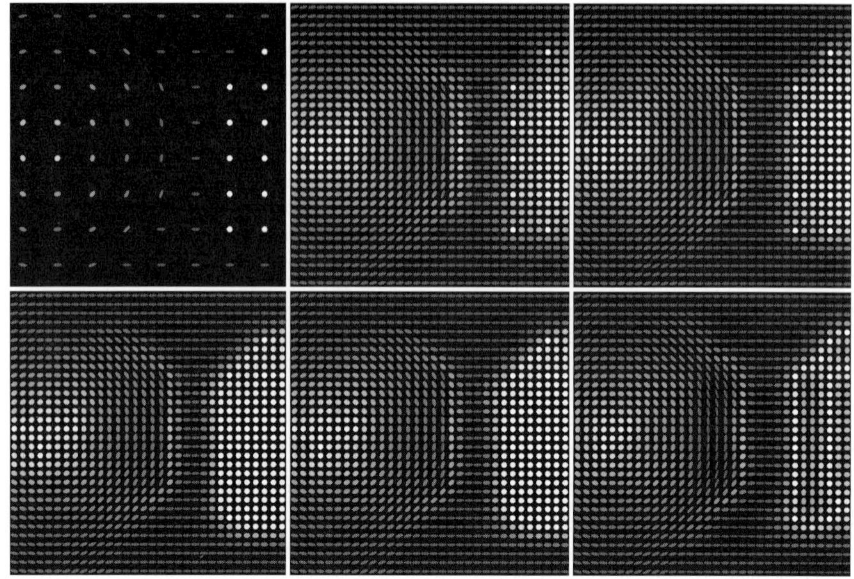

Fig. 19.4. Tensor-valued interpolation of Fig. 19.3(b). (**a**) *Top Left*: Interpolation data. (**b**) *Top Middle*: Interpolation with linear diffusion. (**c**) *Top Right*: Isotropic nonlinear diffusion. (**d**) *Bottom Left*: Anisotropic nonlinear diffusion. (**e**) *Bottom middle*: Biharmonic smoothing. (**f**) *Bottom right*: Triharmonic smoothing. See colour plates

experiment. The corresponding interpolation data are given in Figs. 19.3(b) and (c), respectively.

For the zooming experiment the results for the different PDE-based interpolation methods are depicted in Fig. 19.4. We observe that linear and isotropic nonlinear diffusion may create singularities at interpolation points near discontinuities. Biharmonic and in particular triharmonic interpolation, on the other hand, lead to visible oscillations. This is most evident in the white region where incorrect colours are created at the incorrect colours that are created in the white region. These artifacts reflect the fact that these equations are not PSD-preserving. Anisotropic nonlinear diffusion interpolation appears to be the best of both worlds: Since it is PSD-preserving, it does not introduce oscillatory artifacts. Moreover, it seems that is suffers less from singularities at interpolation points than linear and isotropic nonlinear diffusion interpolation.

The scattered data experiment in Fig. 19.5 allows qualitatively similar observations: Linear and isotropic nonlinear diffusion can exhibit singularities at interpolation points, while biharmonic and triharmonic interpolation create very disturbing oscillations. Once again, anisotropic nonlinear diffusion performs best.

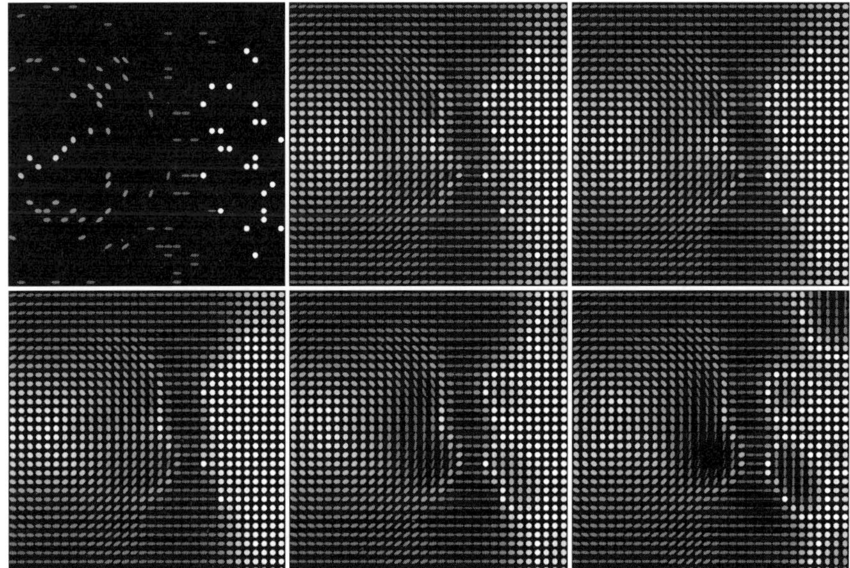

Fig. 19.5. Tensor-valued scattered data interpolation of Fig. 19.3(c). (**a**) *Top Left*: Interpolation data. (**b**) *Top Middle*: Interpolation with linear diffusion. (**c**) *Top Right*: Isotropic nonlinear diffusion. (**d**) *Bottom Left*: Anisotropic nonlinear diffusion. (**e**) *Bottom middle*: Biharmonic smoothing. (**f**) *Bottom right*: Triharmonic smoothing. See colour plates

In Table 19.2 we measure the difference between the interpolated tensor field $U = (u_{ij})$ and the ground truth $V = (v_{ij})$ for both experiments. This is done by computing the average Frobenius distance

$$\mathrm{AFD}\,(u,v) \; := \; \left(\frac{1}{4\,|\Omega|} \sum_{i,j=1}^{2} \int_{\Omega} (u_{ij}(x) - v_{ij}(x))^2 \, dx \right)^{1/2} , \qquad (19.15)$$

the tensorial analogue to the average Euclidean distance (19.9). The results confirm in both cases the visual impression that anisotropic nonlinear diffusion is the favourable interpolant for tensor fields.

19.4 Summary

We have presented a unified PDE model for regularisation and interpolation, both for scalar- and tensor-valued data. This framework allows rotationally invariant models and is not restricted to regular grids: It can also be used for scattered data interpolation and inpainting. Our experiments have shown that the use of a novel interpolation technique based on anisotropic nonlinear

Table 19.2. Interpolation quality of the tensor-valued interpolation experiments from Fig. 19.4 (zoom) and Fig. 19.5 (scattered data). Criteria are the average Frobenius difference (AFD) and preservation of positive semidefiniteness (PSD)

Smoothing Operator	AFD (Zoom)	AFD (Scattered)	PSD
linear diffusion	8.78	9.85	yes
isotropic nonlinear diffusion	8.03	9.59	yes
anisotropic nonlinear diffusion	7.25	9.19	yes
biharmonic smoothing	8.10	9.47	no
triharmonic smoothing	8.54	12.92	no

diffusion with a diffusion tensor gives the most favourable results: It outperforms interpolation techniques based on radial basis functions, linear diffusion and isotropic nonlinear diffusion, Moreover, it allows discontinuity-preserving interpolation without visible oscillations. Provided that the tensor input data are positive semidefinite, this property is naturally inherited to its diffusion interpolant. This renders anisotropic nonlinear diffusion interpolation a highly interesting tool for applications such as diffusion tensor MRI.

In our future work, we head for a detailed theoretical analysis of these methods. We also plan to implement numerical methods with high efficiency, and study possible extensions. We will also investigate the usefulness of anisotropic nonlinear diffusion interpolation for lossy image compression. First results are reported in [8].

Acknowledgements

We thank Mila Nikolova (ENS Cachan), Gabriele Steidl (University of Mannheim), and Vicent Caselles (University Pompeu Fabral, Barcelona) for fruitful discussions on PDE-based interpolation.

References

1. A. Aldroubi and P. Basser. Reconstruction of vector and tensor fields from sampled discrete data. In D. Larson and L. Baggett, editors, *The Functional and Harmonic Analysis of Wavelets*, volume 247 of *Contemporary Mathematics*, pp. 1–15. AMS, Providence, 1999.
2. T. Brox, J. Weickert, B. Burgeth, and P. Mrázek. Nonlinear structure tensors. Technical Report 113, Dept. of Mathematics, Saarland University, Saarbrücken, Germany, October 2004.
3. M. D. Buhmann. *Radial Basis Functions*. Cambridge University Press, Cambridge, UK, 2003.
4. V. Caselles, J.-M. Morel, and C. Sbert. An axiomatic approach to image interpolation. *IEEE Transactions on Image Processing*, 7(3):376–386, March 1998.

5. T. F. Chan and J. Shen. Non-texture inpainting by curvature-driven diffusions (CDD). *Journal of Visual Communication and Image Representation*, 12(4):436–449, 2001.

6. P. Charbonnier, L. Blanc-Féraud, G. Aubert, and M. Barlaud. Two deterministic half-quadratic regularization algorithms for computed imaging. In *Proc. 1994 IEEE International Conference on Image Processing*, volume 2, pp. 168–172, Austin, TX, November 1994. IEEE Computer Society Press.

7. R. Franke. Scattered data interpolation: Tests of some methods. *Mathematics of Computation*, 38:181–200, 1982.

8. I. Galić, J. Weickert, M. Welk, A. Bruhn, A. Belyaev, and H.-P. Seidel. Towards PDE-based image compression. Manuscript, June 2005. Submitted.

9. H. Grossauer and O. Scherzer. Using the complex Ginzburg–Landau equation for digital impainting in 2D and 3D. In L. D. Griffin and M. Lillholm, editors, *Scale-Space Methods in Computer Vision*, volume 2695 of *Lecture Notes in Computer Science*, pp. 225–236, Berlin, 2003. Springer.

10. T. Lehmann, C. Gönner, and K. Spitzer. Survey: Interpolation methods in medical image processing. *IEEE Transactions on Medical Imaging*, 18(11):1049–1075, November 1999.

11. F. Malgouyres and F. Guichard. Edge direction preserving image zooming: A mathematical and numerical analysis. *SIAM Journal on Numerical Analysis*, 39(1):1–37, 2001.

12. S. Masnou and J.-M. Morel. Level lines based disocclusion. In *Proc. 1998 IEEE International Conference on Image Processing*, volume 3, pp. 259–263, Chicago, IL, October 1998.

13. E. Meijering. A chronology of interpolation: From ancient astronomy to modern signal and image processing. *Proceedings of the IEEE*, 90(3):319–342, March 2002.

14. G. M. Nielson and J. Tvedt. Comparing methods of interpolation for scattered volumetric data. In D. F. Rogers and R. A. Earnshaw, editors, *State of the Art in Computer Graphics: Aspects of Visualization*, pp. 67–86. Springer, New York, 1994.

15. L. I. Rudin, S. Osher, and E. Fatemi. Nonlinear total variation based noise removal algorithms. *Physica D*, 60:259–268, 1992.

16. D. Tschumperlé and R. Deriche. Orthonormal vector sets regularization with PDE's and applications. *International Journal of Computer Vision*, 50(3):237–252, December 2002.

17. J. Weickert. *Anisotropic Diffusion in Image Processing*. Teubner, Stuttgart, 1998.

18. J. Weickert and T. Brox. Diffusion and regularization of vector- and matrix-valued images. In M. Z. Nashed and O. Scherzer, editors, *Inverse Problems, Image Analysis, and Medical Imaging*, volume 313 of *Contemporary Mathematics*, pp. 251–268. AMS, Providence, 2002.

20

Diffusion-Tensor Image Registration

James C. Gee[1] and Daniel C. Alexander[2]

[1] Department of Radiology, University of Pennsylvania, 3600 Market Street, Suite 370, Philadelphia, PA 19104, USA
`GeeJames@uphs.upenn.edu`
[2] Department of Computer Science, University College London, Gower Street, London, WC1E 6BT, UK
`D.Alexander@cs.ucl.ac.uk`

Summary. In this chapter, we introduce the problem of registering diffusion tensor magnetic resonance (DT-MR) images. The registration task for these images is made challenging by the orientational information they contain, which is affected by the registration transformation. This information about orientation and other aspects of the diffusion tensor are exploited in the development of similarity measures with which to guide DT-MR image registration, and the current state-of-the-art is reviewed. The chapter concludes with a discussion of some outstanding issues and future avenues for research in diffusion tensor registration.

20.1 Introduction

Image registration is a process by which a geometric (and possibly signal) transformation of an image is obtained that brings its features into alignment with those of a second image with similar content. Algorithms of this type have numerous applications [1]. Relevant to diffusion tensor magnetic resonance imaging (DT-MRI), registration can be used to spatially normalize ensembles of brain images acquired from different subjects, thus enabling accurate mapping of characteristics of the DT, such as diffusion anisotropy, within the brain in order to assist clinical studies into the variation of measurements derived from the DT over normal and patient population groups. Development of multi-modality atlases for surgical planning and teaching is another valuable application.

The next section introduces the special characteristics of DT-MRI data, the general problem of image registration and some particular challenges when specializing to diffusion tensor registration. The first of these challenges, warping of DT images, is discussed in Sect. 20.3. The second challenge, that of developing appropriate similarity measures with which to drive DT-MRI registration, is considered within the context of a brief literature review in

Sect. 20.4. We conclude in Sect. 20.5 with a summary of the state-of-the-art and some future avenues for research in diffusion tensor registration.

20.2 Background

20.2.1 Diffusion MRI

Diffusion-tensor MRI [2] determines the apparent diffusion tensor of water molecules in each voxel of an MRI volume. The method assumes that water molecules move according to a simple anisotropic diffusion process so that the distribution p of displacements $\mathbf{x}$ over a fixed time t is a zero-mean Gaussian with covariance $2t\mathsf{D}$, where D is the diffusion tensor. The apparent diffusion tensor is the best fit D to a set of diffusion-weighted MRI measurements; see Chap. 5 by Alexander.

The Gaussian function has ellipsoidal contours. The lengths of the major axes of the ellipsoidal contours are in the same proportions as the square roots of the eigenvalues $\lambda_1 \geq \lambda_2 \geq \lambda_3$ of D. The eigenvectors $\mathbf{e}_1$, $\mathbf{e}_2$ and $\mathbf{e}_3$, where $\mathbf{e}_i$ has eigenvalue λ_i, of D are the directions of the major axes of the ellipsoid. The eigenvalues provide simple scalar indices of the size and shape of p. The trace of the diffusion tensor $\mathrm{Tr}(\mathsf{D}) = \sum_{i=1}^{3} \lambda_i$ is proportional to the mean squared displacement of water molecules. The fractional anisotropy ν (see [3] and Chap. 5) is the normalized standard deviation of the λ_i and indicates the directional dependence of p.

Biological tissue contains microstructural barriers, such as cell walls and membranes, to the movement of water molecules. The barriers are sparser in fluid-filled regions, such as the ventricles in the brain, than in dense tissue, such as white matter and gray matter. Microstructural barriers reduce the average length of displacements. Thus $\mathrm{Tr}(\mathsf{D})$ is lower in white-matter and gray-matter regions than in fluid-filled regions. In gray matter, the microstructural barriers usually have no preferred orientation and hinder water movement equally in all directions. Thus p is isotropic in most gray-matter regions and $\lambda_1 \approx \lambda_2 \approx \lambda_3$. White matter consists of bundles of parallel axon fibers. The axon cell walls hinder water movement perpendicular to the fibers, but not along the fiber axis. Thus displacements are larger on average in the direction of the fibers and p is anisotropic with a ridge in the fiber direction so that $\lambda_1 \geq \lambda_2 \approx \lambda_3$ and $\mathbf{e}_1$ is the fiber direction.

A well documented drawback of DT-MRI is that it provides only a single fiber-orientation estimate in each voxel and fails at fiber crossings. At fiber crossings, tissue microstructure has multiple dominant fiber orientations and p has ridges in each. When the microstructure contains two orthogonal and equally weighted dominant fiber orientations, p has two orthogonal ridges with equal size. The best-fit Gaussian model then has disc-shaped contours and $\lambda_1 \approx \lambda_2 > \lambda_3$. With three orthogonal fibers, $\lambda_1 \approx \lambda_2 \approx \lambda_3$ and the apparent diffusion tensor is indistinguishable from that observed in isotropic tissue.

The literature now contains a variety of alternative reconstruction algorithms that can extract multiple fiber directions from diffusion MRI measurements. Chap. 10 by Ozarslan describes one such method and Chap. 5 reviews the others.

20.2.2 Image Registration

Underlying every registration task is an associated optimization problem, the solution of which optimizes a measure of similarity, $\phi(I(\mathbf{x}), J(\mathbf{v}(\mathbf{x})))$, of two images, I, J, within the constraints of an image transformation model $\mathbf{v}$. A numerical measure of similarity is obtained by comparing the data values at corresponding points in the two images. For single component intensity images, the simplest approach is to use the difference in scalar intensity at corresponding image locations. However, neighborhood measures such as the cross correlation provide more information and generally produce better results. Many other similarity measures have been proposed, relying on particular assumptions about the data appearance, statistical relationships between measurements or detailed anatomical information gained from medical expertise [4]. In the case of DT imagery, a comparative measure of similarity between diffusion tensors is required to drive the registration algorithm.

The registration problem requires a nonlinear optimization regardless of the similarity measure employed, and thus iterative methods are necessary to solve for $\mathbf{v}$. When the number of parameters that specify the unknown transformation is small, it is common to code the algorithm using optimization routines, such as conjugate gradients, from available numerical libraries [5]. Nonlinear optimization is generally more accurate when the objective function has analytic derivatives that we can implement explicitly to guide the optimization.

In contrast to the low-dimensional methods above, techniques for highly non-rigid or deformable registration typically involve transformation models with orders of magnitude more degrees of freedom [6]. These transformations allow modeling and quantification of image differences that arise from highly complex motion, development, or anatomical variability. They also entail different approaches to the optimization, since the similarity functional ϕ is fundamentally under-constrained and the solution space contains many indistinguishably good answers. The standard solution to ill-posedness is Tikhonov regularization. By constraining the energy of the solution's derivatives through the introduction of a stabilizing functional, $\psi(\mathbf{v})$, one is restricted to a computable subspace and provable uniqueness. This strategy is also useful in ensuring that solutions are physically meaningful, a motivation for using continuum mechanical models in some of the non-rigid algorithms. The resulting optimization problem may be formulated with classical variational (or control or Bayesian) theory [8]: $E(\mathbf{v}) = \int_{\Omega} \phi(\mathbf{v}) + \psi(\mathbf{v})d\Omega$, where E is the global variational energy to be optimized over image domain Ω.

The variational framework permits three equivalent views of the regularized optimization that constitutes the non-rigid registration problem [7]. The equation for E is the first, a global potential energy, from which the weak equation follows that in turn leads to the Euler-Lagrange (E-L) differential equations. The variational or weak form, as in classical elastic matching [8], may be used in the finite element method, while the E-L equations, including versions of optical flow [7], are associated with finite difference techniques.

A special issue that arises in the registration of diffusion tensors and detailed in the next section is the effect of image transformations on the voxel data in a DT image. Specifically, J warped into register with I becomes $R(\mathbf{v})(J(\mathbf{v}^{-1}))$, and ϕ must be adjusted accordingly. This transformation of the voxel's data as well as its location has significant implications for solution of the corresponding diffusion tensor registration problem.

20.2.3 DT-MRI Registration

Diffusion-tensor images contain orientational information not present in other structural images. The motivation for using diffusion-tensor data to drive the registration is that the orientational information potentially provides powerful new cues for matching. Matching orientations can clamp otherwise poorly defined transformations in homogeneous regions. To see this, we shall first consider two new challenges that are particular to registration of diffusion-tensor images.

The first challenge of diffusion-tensor-image registration lies in warping a diffusion tensor image. Image transformations change the orientation of diffusion tensors as well as their location. We must ensure that the DT orientations remain consistent with the anatomy after an image transformation. Figure 20.1(a) shows $\mathbf{e}_1$ in anisotropic voxels of an axial slice of a DT-MR image of a healthy human brain. Figures 20.1(b) and (c) show the same slice after a 45° rotation. To generate Fig. 20.1(b), we transform the image in the standard way. The rotation of the image is R and we copy the value in voxel $\mathbf{x}$ of the transformed image directly from $R^{-1}(\mathbf{x})$ in the untransformed image. However, because of the image rotation, $\mathbf{e}_1$ no longer points along the white-matter fibers. To maintain consistency between the diffusion-tensor orientations and the fibers in the image, the diffusion tensors must undergo the same rotation as the image, as in Fig. 20.1(c). In Fig. 20.1(c), the value in voxel $\mathbf{x}$ is $R^T D R$, where D is the value at $R^{-1}(\mathbf{x})$ in the untransformed image. More complex image transformations affect the image orientation differently at different points. The reorientation of the diffusion tensors must depend on the local reorientation of the image. Note that an additional challenge in warping diffusion-tensor images lies in interpolation strategies for this data. Here, we use linear interpolation of the tensor elements, but Chap. 17 by Moakher and Batchelor discusses a more principled approach.

The second challenge lies in finding similarity measures to drive the registration process. We need similarity measures for diffusion-tensor data. The

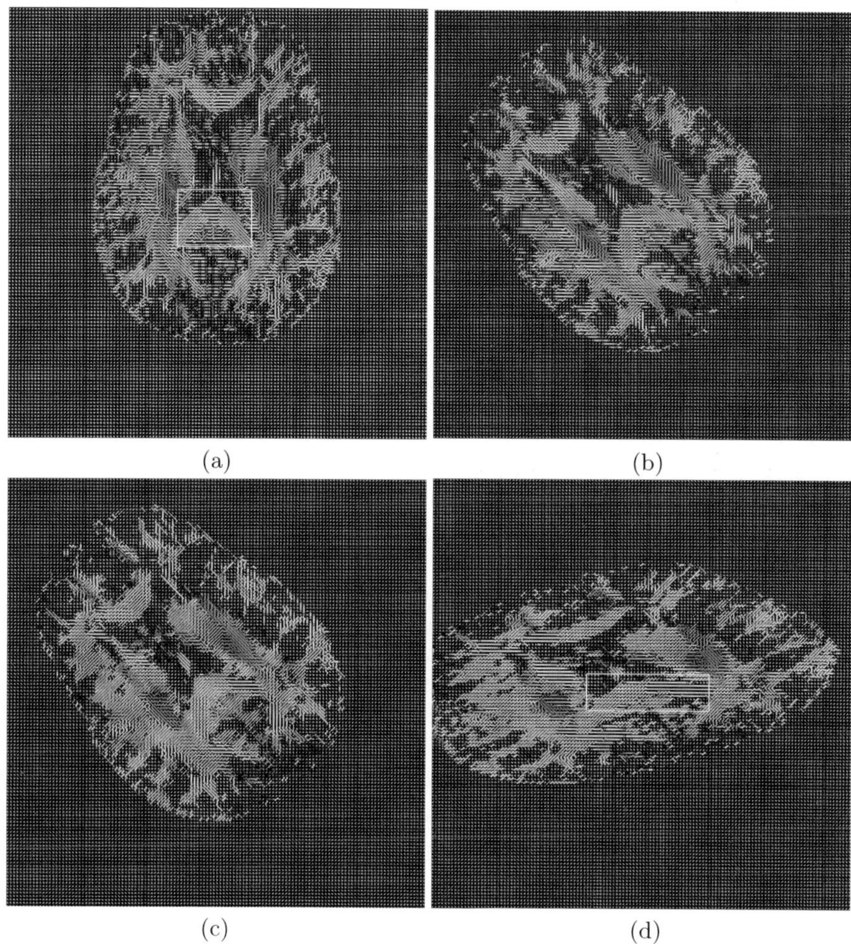

Fig. 20.1. Diffusion tensor reorientation. Panel (**a**) shows $\mathbf{e}_1$ in anisotropic regions of an axial slice of a DT-MR image of a healthy human brain. Panel (**b**) shows the same slice after a $45°$ rotation about the z-axis with no reorientation of the apparent diffusion tensors. Panel (**c**) shows the slice after the same rotation, but with each tensor transformed by the same rotation. Panel (**d**) shows the slice after an affine transformation with PPD reorientation (see Sect. 20.3). The regions of interest in panels (a) and (d) show part of the corpus callosum

diffusion tensor within a tissue is independent of the measurement process. Errors in the apparent diffusion tensor measured using DT-MRI may depend to some extent on the scanner and the parameters of the imaging sequence. However, these differences should be minor compared to differences in the apparent diffusion tensor in different kinds of brain tissue. Furthermore, most often we register images acquired from the same scanner using the same imaging sequence. Thus, direct comparisons, such as the least-squares difference,

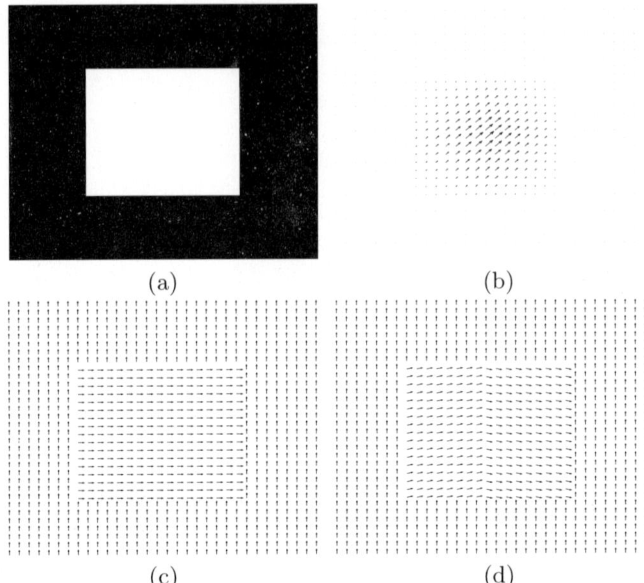

Fig. 20.2. Illustrates the need for orientation matching on two example images, one scalar image, panel (a), and one vector image, panel (c). The scalar image in panel (a) does not change under the transformation in panel (b). The vector image in panel (c) is homogeneous in the same regions as the scalar image in (a). Panel (d) shows the image in (c) after the transformation in (b). The transformation changes the vector image, but not the scalar image

should produce better results than information-theoretic statistics, such as the mutual information [4], which are designed to match images with significantly different values in corresponding regions. To exploit the information in DT-MRI fully, we need similarity measures that are sensitive to all aspects of the diffusion tensor including the size, shape and orientation.

Matching orientations, instead of or as well as intensity values, reduces the number of plausible transformations between two images. Consider the image in Fig. 20.2(a). Clearly the identity transformation transforms Fig. 20.2(a) to itself. However, since the foreground and background regions of Fig. 20.2(a) are homogeneous, many other transformations also transform Fig. 20.2(a) to itself, such as the transformation in Fig. 20.2(b). Now consider a similar image with homogeneous regions of directions (or tensors) as in Fig. 20.2(c). The identity transformation retains the homogeneity of the foreground and background regions of Fig. 20.2(c). However, the transformation in Fig. 20.2(b) causes local changes in the image orientation. With a warping algorithm that updates the orientation of the diffusion tensors to reflect changes in image orientation, we obtain the result in Fig. 20.2(d). A major motivation for using diffusion-tensor data to drive registration algorithms is that we can avoid spurious kinks and whorls in homogeneous regions by searching for transformations that match orientations in these regions.

20.3 Warping DT-MRIs

Alexander et al. [9] outline simple 'reorientation strategies' to determine the effect of an image transformation on the diffusion tensor in each voxel. They show how to reorient diffusion tensors under an affine transformation of the image. The reorientation strategies extend easily to more flexible transformation groups by using the Jacobian of the transformation at each voxel as a local affine model. With the local affine model, the same reorientation strategies derived for global affine transformations provide the diffusion tensor transformation to accompany any image transformation.

Alexander et al. make the fundamental assumption that image transformations affect only the orientation (eigenvectors) of the diffusion tensor. The shape (eigenvalues) of the diffusion tensor remains unchanged. They argue that the apparent diffusion tensor is a property of the tissue microstructure and independent of the shape or extent of the tissue region within the image. For example, tissue in the corpus callosum has a particular density of axon fibers. We expect that the density of fibers in two different sized and different shaped corpus callosa is approximately equal and, thus, the apparent diffusion tensors within the two corpus callosa have approximately the same shape. If we double the size of the corpus callosum region in an image, we do not double the size of the average particle displacement, but rather double the number of barriers to water mobility so that p, and hence D, remains unchanged.

From an affine or local affine transformation, consisting of a linear transformation F and a translation, reorientation strategies determine a rotation R to update the orientation of the diffusion tensor. The first reorientation strategy in [9], the 'finite strain' reorientation strategy, uses the polar decomposition of F. The polar decomposition separates F into a pure rotation R and a pure deformation U, where $F = UR$. In finite-strain reorientation, the pure rotation component, $R = (FF^T)^{-1/2}F$, reorients the diffusion tensor.

For a global affine transformation, the finite-strain reorientation strategy uses the same rotation for every tensor in the image. However, the required rotation depends on the original orientation of the tensor. Consider the schematic fibers and apparent diffusion tensors in Fig. 20.3. A horizontal shear transforms Fig. 20.3(a) to Fig. 20.3(b). The horizontal shear does not affect the orientation of the horizontal fiber, but does change the orientation of the vertical and diagonal fibers. The reorientation of the apparent diffusion tensors in those fibers must reflect the reorientation of the fibers themselves, which finite-strain reorientation fails to do. The second reorientation strategy in [9], the 'preservation of principal directions' (PPD) algorithm, uses the original orientation of the apparent diffusion tensor to select the rotation in each voxel.

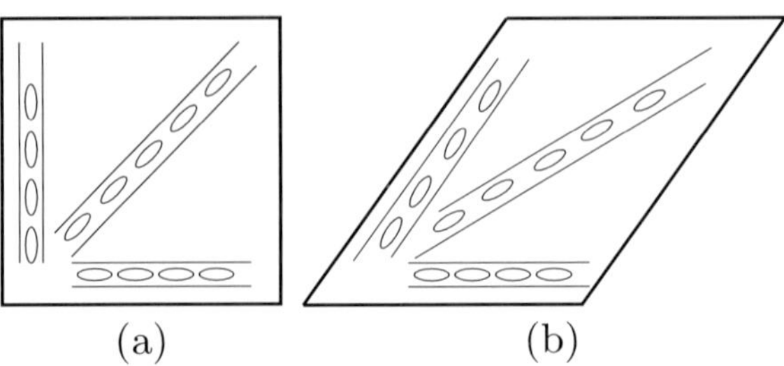

(a)   (b)

Fig. 20.3. Schematic diagrams of white-matter fibers and the diffusion tensors in each before (**a**) and after (**b**) a horizontal shear of the region

The PPD algorithm determines a rotation to match the eigenvectors of D with their image under F. Suppose that $\mathbf{n}_i = F\mathbf{e}_i/|F\mathbf{e}_i|$ is the normalized image of $\mathbf{e}_i$ under F. First, the algorithm finds a rotation R_1 for which $R_1\mathbf{e}_1 = \mathbf{n}_1$. Then the algorithm finds the rotation R_2 about $\mathbf{n}_1$ that maximizes $\mathbf{n}_2 \cdot (R_2R_1\mathbf{e}_2)$. The rotation $R = R_2R_1$ reorients the diffusion tensor. The PPD algorithm thus maps $\mathbf{e}_1$, which is the local fiber-orientation estimate, directly to $F\mathbf{e}_1$, the transformed fiber-orientation estimate, and $\mathbf{e}_2$ as close as possible to $F\mathbf{e}_2$ in the plane perpendicular to $\mathbf{e}_1$.

Figure 20.4 compares the outputs of the reorientation strategies in [9] on a region of a human brain image. Figure 20.1(a) highlights a region of the corpus callosum containing an inverted-V-shaped fiber in the plane of the image slice. Figure 20.1(d) shows the same slice after a shear along one arm of the highlighted fiber chosen to make the other arm approximately horizontal in the image. Figure 20.4(a) shows the apparent diffusion tensors in the region highlighted in Fig. 20.1(a). Figures 20.4(b), (c) and (d) show the apparent diffusion tensors in the same region after the shearing transformation, as highlighted in Fig. 20.1(d), using no reorientation, finite-strain reorientation and PPD, respectively. With no reorientation, the apparent diffusion tensors no longer point along the fiber after the shear. The differences in the results from finite-strain reorientation and PPD are minor, but the tensors in the PPD result point more consistently along the horizontal arm of the fiber. The most noticeable difference is at the right-hand end of the fiber, where finite-strain rotates the tensors too much, but with PPD the tensors show the correct horizontal fiber direction.

When the deformation component of the image transformation is small, finite-strain reorientation is a good approximation to PPD. The finite-strain method is computationally simpler than PPD, particularly for global affine transformations where it only requires one rotation for the whole image rather than a separate rotation in each voxel. Furthermore, the finite-strain expression for R is analytic and differentiable unlike PPD, which is algorithmic. For these reasons, the finite-strain reorientation strategy is sometimes preferred to the more accurate PPD method.

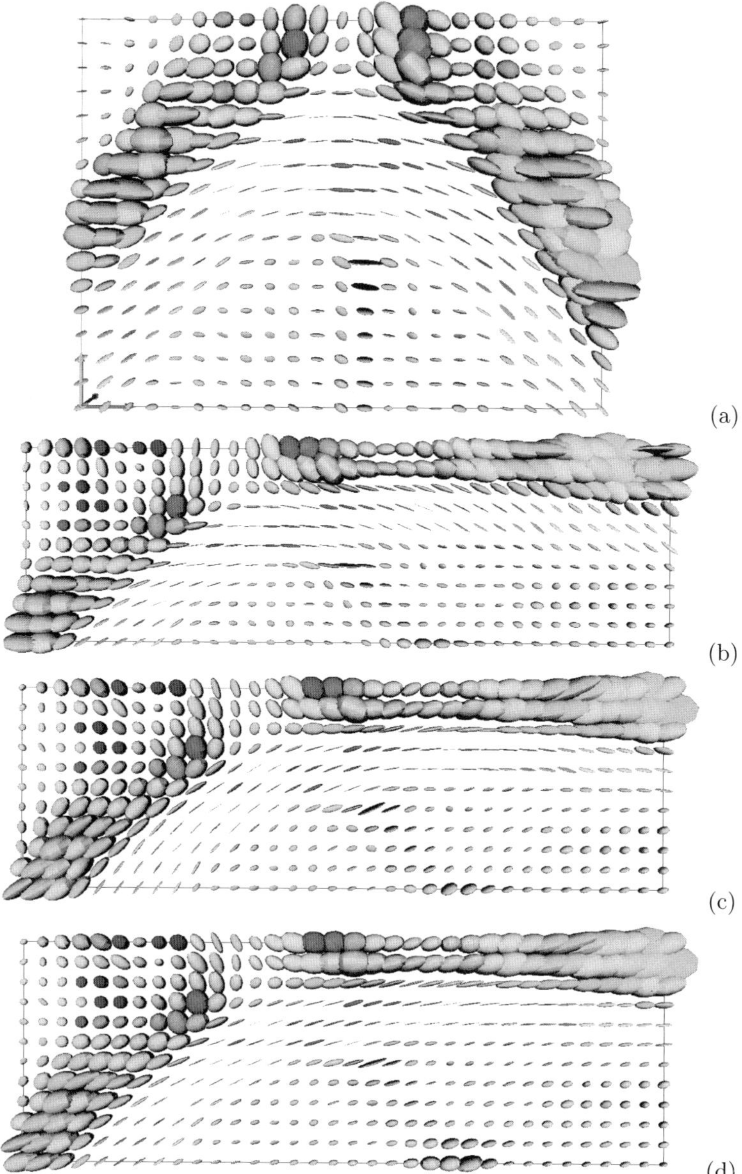

Fig. 20.4. Compares the results of Alexander's reorientation strategies. (See color plates.) Panel (**a**) shows the apparent diffusion tensors in the region of interest in Fig. 20.1(a). Panels (**b**), (**c**) and (**d**) show the apparent diffusion tensors in the same region after a shear along the left-hand arm of the corpus callosum fiber in the region, as highlighted in Fig. 20.1(d), using no reorientation, finite-strain reorientation and PPD, respectively

Xu et al. [10] note that PPD assumes $\mathbf{e}_1$ is the fiber orientation. Since $\mathbf{e}_1$ is only an estimate subject to measurement noise, they suggest a variation that uses a statistical estimate of the fiber orientation from the voxel neighborhood.

Other variations on the PPD method are simple to imagine. For example, we might compute the rotation of D that matches its eigenvectors to those of the transformed tensor $F^T D F$. The problem of associating the eigenvectors of D and $F^T D F$ can become significant for large deformations, but solutions are simple to devise. It is not clear whether this approach, or Xu et al.'s algorithm, is better or worse than PPD and the literature contains no conclusive comparisons.

The assumption that the diffusion-tensor shape is fixed is only an approximation. The assumption breaks down in, for example, tissues containing crossing or diverging fibers. Consider a fiber-crossing region containing equal densities of axons in two orthogonal orientations. The apparent diffusion tensor in the region is oblate with $\lambda_1 \approx \lambda_2$. A shear along the direction of one of the fiber orientations leaves the orientation of one fiber fixed, but changes the orientation of the other. This reduces the angle between the two fibers so that the apparent diffusion tensor is no longer oblate but elongated in the direction between the two fiber orientations. In brain imaging, these effects are usually minor so that the fixed shape assumption is reasonable.

20.4 Review of Current DT-MRI Registration Literature

Alexander and Gee [11, 12] use the elastic matching algorithm of Gee et al. [8, 13] for matching DT-MR images. They propose a variety of comparative statistics for diffusion tensor data. They compare the statistics as similarity measures for driving the registration. The statistics they propose include correlation of $\mathrm{Tr}(D)$ or ν over small image neighborhoods, direct tensor comparisons such as the tensor difference, $\Delta(D_1, D_2) = \mathrm{Tr}\left[(D_1 - D_2)^2\right]$, and the tensor scalar product, $D_1 : D_2 = \mathrm{Tr}(D_1 D_2)$, and principal direction comparisons, such as $(\nu_1 \nu_2)^{1/2}(\mathbf{e}_{11} \cdot \mathbf{e}_{21})$, where ν_i is the fractional anisotropy of D_i and $\mathbf{e}_{i1}$ is the principal eigenvector of D_i. They also suggest using the tensor difference and tensor scalar product with the deviatoric tensors $\tilde{D} = D - 1/3 I$, where I is the identity tensor, and normalizing both $\Delta(D_1, D_2)$ and $D_1 : D_2$ by $\mathrm{Tr}(D_1)\mathrm{Tr}(D_2)$. Alexander and Gee do not include tensor reorientation in the optimization of their elastic transformation and thus do not match orientations.

Curran and Alexander [14] optimize an affine transform to match DT-MR images with no reorientation, finite-strain reorientation and PPD. On a single example run, they recover synthetic transformations more accurately using PPD and finite-strain reorientation than using no reorientation. In later work [15], they highlight added difficulties in orientation matching over scalar image matching caused by more severe local minima in the objective function optimized to compute the registration.

Ruiz-Alzola et al. [16] formally generalize the standard scalar measures of similarity, such as sum of squared differences and correlation, for application to tensor data, and develop a novel tensor measure of 'cornerness' [17, 18] to identify candidates with highly distinguishing features for robust template matching – registration performance is further improved by implementing a multi-resolution optimization strategy. The resultant sparse correspondences are interpolated over the entire image domain using a newly introduced Kriging estimator, and finite-strain reorientation is performed subsequent to matching. The method should run faster than those that implement global optimization, its speed gained from the uncoupling of the correspondence calculation and displacement interpolation procedures, each of which can then be optimized separately for efficient implementation.

Guimond et al. [19] take note of the computational complexity introduced by tensor reorientation and adapt their multi-channel version of the demons deformable registration algorithm to use the set of rigid-invariant tensor eigenvalues along with the T2-weighted intensity as the features with which image similarity is determined. They show that this orientation independent approach qualitatively compares in performance with an implementation of full-tensor (plus T2-weighted intensity) registration with finite-strain reorientation and outperforms scalar registration using only the T2-weighted information. In preliminary studies, an order of magnitude speedup is obtained by matching rigid-invariant tensor features over that using the full tensor, with both operating in multi-resolution fashion.

In one of the most comprehensive studies in the field to date, Park et al. [20] further examined Guimond's multi-channel method and find instead that the use of all tensor components together with PPD reorientation yields the most reliable registration results, particularly, for atlas construction. Their study introduces task-specific evaluation measures based on alignment of extracted fiber bundles from the registered data. The comparison included registration of real and synthetic DT imagery based on: T2-weighted intensity alone; fractional anisotropy alone; difference of the first and second tensor eigenvalues; fractional anisotropy together with trace of the tensor; all three tensor eigenvalues; and the 6 independent tensor components. The newly proposed performance indices characterize the alignment along the length of corresponding fiber bundles in the registered data as well as the disparity between their endpoints. By examining the correspondence of reconstructed fiber bundles, errors in both gross anatomic and voxelwise tensor alignment can be effectively detected. These task-specific measures were complemented with additional voxel-based indices of tensor overlap and alignment.

Rohde et al. [21] similarly construct vectors of DT-derived indices or features, $\mathbf{I} = \{I_i(\mathbf{x})\}$, at each image voxel $\mathbf{x}$, whose similarity is evaluated with the multivariate version of mutual information for normally distributed data. This multi-channel measure is shown to approximate the linear correlation coefficient between the same features of two images, I, J, and additionally takes into account the correlation between the images' non-corresponding features $\{I_i, J_j\}$, where $i \neq j$. Rohde et al. incorporate the measure into an existing non-rigid registration algorithm that iteratively refines an adaptive radial-basis representation of the transformation solution. Finite-strain reorientation of the warped diffusion tensors is applied, but only after the initial affine alignment and as a postprocessing step of the non-rigid method. The simultaneous use of multiple indices, particularly those encoding directional information, is shown to be advantageous in experiments over real and simulated data [22].

Verma and Davatzikos [23] in preliminary work also propose a multi-channel characterization of the DT-MRI data at a voxel to facilitate correspondence detection, where the features are obtained by applying a novel Gabor filter bank with different scales and frequencies that are all oriented along the dominant direction of the tensors in a neighborhood about the voxel.

Duda et al. [24] propose a similarity measure ϕ for non-rigid registration with two terms, the first comparing tensor eigenvalues to quantify shape differences between diffusion ellipsoids and the second, a novel region-based measure for orientation matching. Specifically, the relative pattern of pairwise orientation differences between the voxel of interest located at $\mathbf{x}$ and every voxel within a neighborhood centered at $\mathbf{x}$ is proposed as a more robust and accurate replacement of the usual voxelwise comparison of orientation information, either at a voxel or over a region (see Fig. 20.5). The similarity optimization is regularized, and its solution obtained by iteratively linearizing via first order Taylor series expansion of E. Preliminary results indicate the new orientation measure may reduce the number of local minima typically observed in tensor registration.

Zhang et al. [25] match general apparent diffusion coefficient (ADC) profiles rather than diffusion tensors. The ADC profile, defined in [26] and Chap. 5, is the value of the ADC in each direction and is thus a function of the sphere. When p is Gaussian, the ADC in direction $\hat{\mathbf{x}}$ is proportional to $\hat{\mathbf{x}}^T D \hat{\mathbf{x}}$. At fiber crossings, the ADC profile can depart significantly from this model [26]. The naturally induced L^2 distance between positive-valued spherical functions is specialized to the case of diffusion tensors, which differs from Δ by an additional term that effectively accounts for differences in mean diffusivity and in practice appears to afford more robust registration performance over small regions. Zhang et al. couple this statistic with a non-standard affine parameterization that allows an analytic formulation of the finite strain-based reorientation of tensors adopted in their work. Preliminary results are shown demonstrating the piecewise affine extension to high dimensional non-rigid registration of DT-MRI data.

20.5 Discussion

The development of DT-MRI registration is at a relatively early stage, as evidenced by the small number of available methods and the paucity of

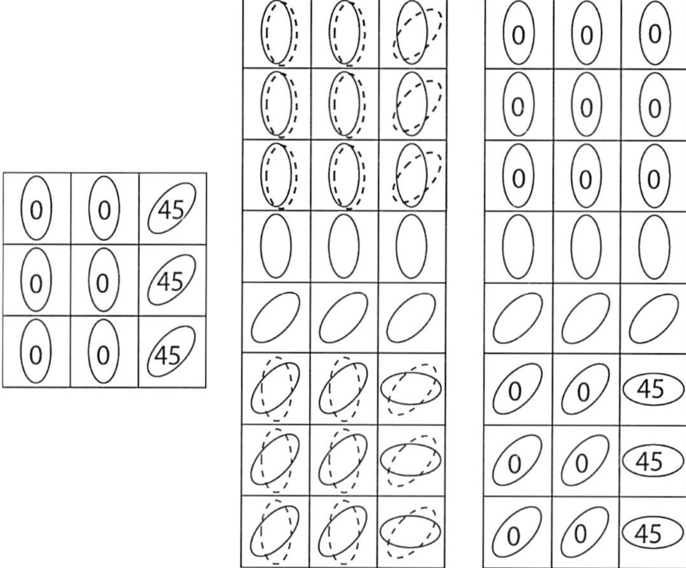

Fig. 20.5. Matching diffusion orientation patterns in Duda et al. (*Left*) A neighborhood of interest. The number shown in each square/voxel is the angle difference between the principal eigenvector of the tensor located at the voxel and that of the tensor at the center voxel. (*Middle*) The neighborhood of interest (in dashed outline) is overlain onto two different regions of a larger neighborhood (image strip). The voxelwise orientation difference is much larger for the lower region. (*Right*) The orientation patterns are shown for the same two regions. Note that the orientation pattern in the lower region is the same as in the original neighborhood of interest, while the pattern in the upper region is different. The orientation pattern measure would match the original neighborhood with the lower region, whereas a voxelwise measure of orientation would match to the upper region

comprehensive performance evaluation studies. Intense interest in clinical and research application of DT-MRI, however, is sure to dramatically accelerate further innovation in the field. Current approaches have mostly examined general or diffusion-tensor-specific features and their optimal combination in multi-valued measures of similarity. Awareness of the unique requirement for tensor reorientation during DTI warping has not, however, translated to routine integration within algorithms because of the computational challenges presented by existing reorientation strategies.

Furthermore, although the idea is seductive, the registration and diffusion MRI communities are yet to demonstrate improvements to registration from orientation matching. Park et al. show only that the information in the off-diagonal tensor components improves matching over using just the tensor eigenvalues, but do not show explicitly that the improvement comes from orientation matching. Curran and Alexander and Zhang et al. show improvements from orientation matching only in simulation or on very limited sets of examples. It seems likely that we can expect only minor improvements from orientation matching with low dimensional transformations. Reports of authors in the field support this supposition. The true power of orientation matching will come from harnessing the flexibility of high dimensional transformations. These are also the most difficult to validate, but progress in performance evaluation is required before results can be transferred to the clinical workplace.

There are various other avenues for research. In Chap. 17, Moakher and Batchelor present a framework for diffusion tensor analysis using Riemannian geometry that takes into account the positive definiteness of true diffusion tensors [27]. They use the framework to define a distance between diffusion tensors, which could be used as a similarity measure for registration. Related work can be found in [28].

If Curran's initial findings about the increased local minima in tensor registration objective functions over scalar registration prove to be a general feature of the problem, we may require more sophisticated optimization algorithms to get the best out of DT-MRI data for registration.

An obvious extension of current work on DT-MRI registration is to use the extra information in the output of the multiple-fiber reconstructions, such as those described in Chaps. 5 and 10. However, we still require considerable research to optimize registration methods for DT-MRI and confine, for now, registration of multiple-fiber reconstructions to future work.

References

1. Hajnal, J., Hill, D.L.G., Hawkes, D.J.: Medical Image Registration. CRC Press, London (2001)
2. Basser, P.J., Matiello, J., Le Bihan, D.: MR diffusion tensor spectroscopy and imaging. Biophysical Journal, **66**, 259–267 (1994)
3. Basser, P.J., Pierpaoli, C.: Microstructural and physiological features of tissues elucidated by quantitative diffusion tensor MRI. Journal of Magnetic Resonance Series B, **111**, 209–219 (1996)
4. Maintz, J.B.A., Viergever, M.A.: A survey of medical image registration. Medical Image Analysis, **2**, 1–36 (1998)
5. Ibanez, L., Ng, L.: Basic registration. In: Yoo, T.S. (ed) Insight into Images: Principles and Practice for Segmentation, Registration, and Image Analysis. A.K. Peters, Wellesey (2004)
6. Lester, H., Arridge, S.R.: A survey of hierarchical non-linear medical image registration. Pattern Recognition, **32**, 129–149 (1999)
7. Avants, B., Sundaram, T., Duda, J., Ng, L., Gee, J.: Non-rigid image registration. In: Yoo, T.S. (ed) Insight into Images: Principles and Practice for Segmentation, Registration, and Image Analysis. A.K. Peters, Wellesey (2004)
8. Gee, J.C., Bajcsy, R.K.: Elastic matching: Continuum mechanical and probabilistic analysis. In: Toga, A.W. (ed) Brain Warping. Academic Press, San Diego (1998)

9. Alexander, D.C., Pierpaoli, C., Basser, P.J., Gee, J.C.: Spatial transformation of diffusion tensor magnetic resonance images. IEEE Transactions on Medical Imaging, **20**, 1131–1139 (2001)

10. Xu, D., Mori, S., Shen, D., van Zijl, P.C.M., Davatzikos, C.: Spatial normalization of diffusion tensor fields. Magnetic Resonance in Medicine, **50**, 175–182 (2003)

11. Alexander, D.C., Gee, J.C.: Elastic matching of diffusion tensor MRIs. Computer Vision and Image Understanding, **77**, 233–250 (2000)

12. Alexander, D.C., Gee, J.C., Bajcsy, R.K.: Similarity measures for matching diffusion tensor images. In: Proc. British Machine Vision Conference. BMVA, Worcs (1999)

13. Gee, J.C., Haynor, D.R.: Numerical methods for high dimensional warps. In: Toga, A.W. (ed) Brain Warping. Academic Press, San Diego (1998)

14. Curran, K.M., Alexander, D.C.: Orientation matching for registration of diffusion tensor images. In: Sonka, M., Fitzpatrick, J.M. (ed) Proc. SPIE Medical Imaging: Image Processing. SPIE, Bellingham (2003)

15. Curran, K.M., Alexander, D.C.: Orientation coherence optimization in tensor image registration. In: Proc. Medical Imaging Understanding and Analysis. BMVA, Worcs (2004)

16. Ruiz-Alzola, J., Westin, C.F., Warfield, S.K., Alberola, C., Maier, S., Kikinis, R.: Nonrigid registration of 3D tensor medical data. Medical Image Analysis, **6**, 143–161 (2002)

17. Ruiz-Alzola, J., Westin, C.F., Warfield, S.K., Nabavi, A., Kikinis, R.: Nonrigid registration of 3D scalar, vector and tensor medical data. In: Delp, S.L., DiGioia, A.M., Jaramaz, B. (ed) Medical Image Computing and Computer-Assisted Intervention. Springer-Verlag, Berlin (2000)

18. Ruiz-Alzola, J., Kikinis, R., Westin, C.F.: Detection of point landmarks in multidimensional tensor data. Signal Processing, **81**, 2243–2247 (2001)

19. Guimond, A., Guttmann, C.R.G., Warfield, S.K., Westin, C.F.: Deformable registration of DT-MRI data based on transformation invariant tensor characteristics. In: Proc. IEEE International Symposium on Biomedical Imaging. IEEE Press, Piscataway (2002)

20. Park, H.J., Kubicki, M., Shenton, M.E., Guimond, A., McCarley, R.W., Maier, S.E., Kikinis, R., Jolesz, F.A., Westin, C.F.: Spatial normalization of diffusion tensor MRI using multiple channels. NeuroImage, **20**, 1995–2009 (2003)

21. Rohde, G.K., Pajevic, S., Pierpaoli, C., Basser, P.J.: A comprehensive approach for multi-channel image registration. In: Gee, J.C., Maintz, J.B.A., Vannier, M.W. (ed) Proc. 2nd International Workshop on Biomedical Image Registration. Springer-Verlag, Berlin (2003)

22. Rohde, G.K., Pajevic, S., Pierpaoli, C.: Multi-channel registration of diffusion tensor images using directional information. In: Proc. IEEE International Symposium on Biomedical Imaging. IEEE Press, Piscataway (2004)

23. Verma, R., Davatzikos, C.: Matching of diffusion tensor images using Gabor features. In: Proc. IEEE International Symposium on Biomedical Imaging. IEEE Press, Piscataway (2004)

24. Duda, J.T., Rivera, M., Alexander, D.C., Gee J.C.: A method for nonrigid registration of diffusion tensor magnetic resonance images. In: Sonka, M., Fitzpatrick, J.M. (ed) Proc. SPIE Medical Imaging: Image Processing. SPIE, Bellingham (2003)

25. Zhang, H., Yushkevich, P.A., Gee, J.C.: Registration of diffusion tensor images. In: Proc. Computer Vision and Pattern Recognition. IEEE Press, Piscataway (2004)
26. Alexander, D.C., Barker, G.J., Arridge, S.R.: Detection and modeling of non-Gaussian apparent diffusion coefficient profiles in human brain data. Magnetic Resonance in Medicine, **48**, 331–340 (2002)
27. Batchelor, P.G., Calamante, F., Moaker, M., Atkinson, D., Connelly, A., Hill, D.: A rigorous method for calculus on diffusion tensors: Taking into account positivity of eigenvalues. In: Proc. 12th Scientific Meeting ISMRM. ISMRM, Berkeley (2004)
28. Fletcher, P.T., Joshi, S.: Principal geodesic analysis on symmetric spaces: Statistics of diffusion tensors. In: Sonka, M., Kakadiaris, I.A., Kybic, J. (ed) Proc. Workshop on Computer Vision Approaches to Medical Image Analysis. Springer-Verlag, Berlin (2004)

Part V

Image Processing Methods for Tensor Fields

21

Tensor Median Filtering and M-Smoothing

Martin Welk, Christian Feddern, Bernhard Burgeth, and Joachim Weickert

Mathematical Image Analysis Group, Faculty of Mathematics and Computer
Science, Saarland University, Building 27, 66041 Saarbrücken, Germany
{welk,feddern,burgeth,weickert}@mia.uni-saarland.de

Summary. Median filters for scalar-valued data are well-known tools for image
denoising and analysis. They preserve discontinuities and are robust under noise.
We generalise median filtering to matrix-valued data using a minimisation approach.
Experiments on DT-MRI and fluid dynamics tensor data demonstrate that tensor-
valued median filtering shares important properties of its scalar-valued counterpart,
including the robustness as well as the existence of non-trivial steady states (root
signals).

A straightforward extension of the definition allows the introduction of matrix-
valued mid-range filters and, more general, M-smoothers. Mid-range filters can also
serve as a building block in constructing further (e.g. supremum-based) tensor image
filters.

21.1 Introduction

Matrix-valued data generated from measurements are often polluted by noise.
It is therefore a necessity to design filters which allow to denoise matrix data
without eliminating valuable information. Particularly in the context of DT-
MRI data processing intensive research has attacked this problem recently.
One class of approaches is based on manipulating the matrix components directly. Sometimes the components are treated independently, thereby reducing
matrix-valued image processing directly to the scalar-valued case, cf. [20] for
linear or [9] for nonlinear techniques. Particularly for nonlinear filters, channel coupling as e.g. in [15] and [17] respects better the inherent relations of
matrix-valued data. In [17], a nonlinear structure tensor has been introduced
which has also been applied successfully in the context of optic flow estimation [5]. Other proposed smoothing techniques work on derived quantities like
eigendecompositions of diffusion tensors [6, 13, 15] or the fractional anisotropy
[12].

Median filtering has been introduced first in signal processing by Tukey
[16]. In the meantime, it has become an established technique in image
processing [7, 10] which is attractive especially for its ability to cope with

extreme noise such as uniform or salt-and-pepper noise, and its discontinuity-preserving properties. A remarkable relation between median filtering and PDE-based techniques has been brought up by Guichard and Morel [8].

Medians have early been noted to be part of a more general class of averaging operators [4] which are now known as M-estimators and which also comprise the arithmetic mean, mid-range and mode; in image processing, they underly the M-smoother techniques.

In this contribution, we present a generalisation of median filtering along with mid-range filtering and general M-smoothers to tensor-valued data. The key to this generalisation is the transfer of the minimisation property from scalar to matrix data. Matrix-valued medians using the Frobenius norm have first been introduced in [19]. They stand in a close relation to the vector-valued median notion that goes back to Austin [2]. Other attempts to design multivariate median filters for vector-valued data are described in [3, 11].

21.2 Scalar-Valued Median Filters

The median of a finite set of real numbers is the middle element in the sequence that contains the given numbers ordered by size. This type of average displays a high robustness against outliers in the data set. Besides that, taking the median commutes with monotonic transformations of the data.

An interesting characterisation of the median of a set X is that it is a minimiser of the convex function

$$E_X(y) := \sum_{x \in X} |y - x| \tag{21.1}$$

where $|y - x|$ is the Euclidean distance on real numbers.

Median filtering for greyscale images is done by assigning each pixel the median of all grey values within a certain neighbourhood of the pixel as its new grey value. The neighbourhood is commonly taken to be either a square-shaped $((2k + 1) \times (2k + 1))$ or disk-shaped stencil centered at the pixel. Iterations of the median filter often lead to a non-trivial steady state, a so-called root signal. Although for discrete median filtering not each initial image converges to a root signal – a counter-example is given by an image made up of alternating black and white rows of pixels – the ability of iterated median filtering to preserve discontinuities is one of its most interesting properties. Moreover, the robustness of the median causes the pronounced denoising capability of median filters for extreme noise.

Guichard and Morel [8] have established an interesting link to PDE-based image filters by proving that in a continuous setting iterated median filtering approximates mean curvature flow.

21.3 Tensor-Valued Median Filters

The excellent properties of median filters make it highly desirable to provide a similar tool for the processing of matrix-valued images. The filtering process is the same as in the scalar-valued case once a suitable median definition for matrix data is found. We therefore aim at establishing such a notion.

21.3.1 Requirements for Tensor-Valued Medians

In the absence of a linear ordering for matrices, the original order-based definition does not support a generalisation to matrices. Instead, we start by listing properties that a matrix-valued median should possess to enable a similar range of applications as in the scalar-valued case.

First, the median of a given set of symmetric matrices must itself be a symmetric matrix. Moreover, in application contexts like DT-MRI positive semidefiniteness is a natural property of the tensor data; in these cases, the median of positive semidefinite matrices should be positive semidefinite, too.

While general monotonic transformations don't make sense in the matrix-valued setting, it is still natural to demand invariance of the median w.r.t. scaling, i.e. for a real number λ

$$\operatorname{med}(\lambda A_1, \dots, \lambda A_n) = \lambda \operatorname{med}(A_1, \dots, A_n) \ . \tag{21.2}$$

Crucial in image processing applications is the requirement of rotational invariance. Applying the same rotation R to all input matrices should imply the same rotation of the median:

$$\operatorname{med}(R^{\mathrm{T}} A_1 R, \dots, R^{\mathrm{T}} A_n R) = R^{\mathrm{T}} \operatorname{med}(A_1, \dots, A_n)\, R \ . \tag{21.3}$$

The constraints of positive semidefiniteness preservation and rotational invariance narrow considerably the range of possible definitions[1].

Finally, a matrix-valued generalisation of medians should reproduce the scalar median if all input values are multiples of one and the same matrix A:

$$\operatorname{med}(\lambda_1 A, \dots, \lambda_n A) = \operatorname{med}(\lambda_1, \dots, \lambda_n)\, A \ . \tag{21.4}$$

21.3.2 Definition of Matrix-Valued Medians

Adapting (21.1) to the matrix-valued setting, we define the median of a matrix set $X = \{A_1, \dots, A_n\}$ as the minimiser of

$$E_X(Y) = \sum_{i=1}^{n} \|Y - A_i\| \tag{21.5}$$

---

[1] In particular, taking the scalar median in each matrix component violates both conditions. For $\left(\begin{smallmatrix} 5 & 2 \\ 2 & 1 \end{smallmatrix}\right)$, $\left(\begin{smallmatrix} 1 & 2 \\ 2 & 5 \end{smallmatrix}\right)$, and $\left(\begin{smallmatrix} 1 & 0 \\ 0 & 1 \end{smallmatrix}\right)$ one obtains $\left(\begin{smallmatrix} 1 & 2 \\ 2 & 1 \end{smallmatrix}\right)$, which is indefinite. A rotation gives $\left(\begin{smallmatrix} 5 & -2 \\ -2 & 1 \end{smallmatrix}\right)$, $\left(\begin{smallmatrix} 5 & 2 \\ 2 & 1 \end{smallmatrix}\right)$, and $\left(\begin{smallmatrix} 1 & 0 \\ 0 & 1 \end{smallmatrix}\right)$ with componentwise median $\left(\begin{smallmatrix} 5 & 0 \\ 0 & 1 \end{smallmatrix}\right)$.

where $\|\cdot\|$ is a matrix norm which needs to be specified; its choice is confined by rotational invariance and semidefiniteness preservation where required. We discuss two possibilities: the Frobenius norm and the spectral norm[2].

First, the Frobenius norm of a matrix $A \in \mathbb{R}^{m \times m}$ is defined by

$$\|A\| = \|A\|_{\mathrm{F}} := \left(\sum_{j,k=1}^{m} a_{jk}^2 \right)^{1/2} .$$

Note that this is also the Euclidean norm of A considered as a vector in m^2-dimensional vector space. The resulting median definition is therefore quite general – it carries over verbatim to non-square matrices, including vectors as special case. For the latter, the multivariate median introduced by Austin [2] is recovered. At last, the Frobenius norm is easy to compute from the matrix components and differentiable except at 0.

Second, the spectral norm $\|A\|_{\mathrm{S}}$ of a symmetric square matrix $A \in \mathbb{R}^{m \times m}$ is the largest absolute value of an eigenvalue of A. Its computation is more costly than that of the Frobenius norm. The spectral norm is non-differentiable at all matrices having eigenvalues of multiplicity greater than one; in 2D these are exactly the multiples of the unit matrix.

The rotational invariance of both the Frobenius and spectral norm guarantee the rotational invariance property (21.3) for the median. The scaling property (21.2) and the embedding of the scalar median (21.4) follow directly from the scaling property $\|\lambda A\| = |\lambda| \, \|A\|$ holding for every norm $\|\cdot\|$.

To prove that the median defined via the Frobenius norm preserves positive semidefiniteness, we prove that it is always a convex combination of the given matrices $A_1, \ldots, A_n$. Assume X is a matrix outside the convex hull of $A_1, \ldots, A_n$. Then there exists a hyperplane h separating X from $A_1, \ldots, A_n$. Let Y be the point of h closest to X; then $X - Y$ is perpendicular to h. Moreover, $\langle X - Y, Y - A_i \rangle$ is positive for all $i = 1, \ldots, n$ which implies

$$\begin{aligned}
\langle X - A_i, X - A_i \rangle &- \langle Y - A_i, Y - A_i \rangle \\
&= \langle X, X \rangle - 2\langle X, A_i \rangle - \langle Y, Y \rangle + 2\langle Y, A_i \rangle \\
&= 2\langle X - Y, Y - A_i \rangle + \langle X - Y, X - Y \rangle > 0
\end{aligned}$$

i.e. X can't be a minimiser of (21.5). Preservation of positive semidefiniteness follows since convex combinations of positive semidefinite matrices are also positive semidefinite.

With the spectral norm, positive semidefiniteness is also preserved in most cases. There exist, however, cases in which this is not true.

We point out that the matrix median is not bound by its definition to select values among the given data. However, it still does so in many cases – new values are generated only if none of the given matrices is located well enough amidst the entire set.

---

[2] The L^1 norm which sums up the absolute values of all matrix entries cannot be used since it would lead to component-wise median, compare footnote 1.

21.4 Mid-Range Filters and M-Smoothers

The use of the minimiser property of the median as the base of its generalisation encourages an extension of this principle to further image filters which can be described in terms of similar minimisations.

21.4.1 Mid-Range Values and Mid-Range Filtering

The mid-range value of a set X of real numbers is usually defined as the arithmetic mean of their maximum and minimum. Like the median, it is turned into a local image filter simply by application to the grey-values within a suitable neighbourhood of a pixel.

To define a matrix-valued mid-range value, we note that the scalar mid-range value is the minimiser of the convex function

$$E_X(y) := \max_{x \in X} |y - x| \ \ .$$

Replacing again $|y - x|$ with a matrix norm, we introduce the mid-range value for a set $X = \{A_1, \ldots, A_n\}$ of matrices as the minimiser of the convex function

$$E_X(Y) := \max_{i=1,\ldots,n} \|Y - A_i\| \ \ .$$

The minimiser definition of scalar mid-range values does not rely on the extrema of X themselves; instead, these are recovered by adding or subtracting from the midrange $\mathrm{mid}\,(X)$ the corresponding value of the objective function,

$$\max(X) = \mathrm{mid}\,(X) + \max_{x \in X} |\mathrm{mid}\,(X) - x| \ , \tag{21.6}$$

for the minimum, $+$ has to be replaced by $-$ on the right-hand side.

Using these identities to *define* extrema of X would be circular in the scalar setting; yet rewriting (21.6) for matrices reveals an interesting relation. Namely, when $\mathrm{mid}\,(X)$ is defined via the spectral norm, a supremum of the matrix set X can be introduced by

$$\sup(X) := \mathrm{mid}\,(X) + \max_{i=1,\ldots,n} \|\mathrm{mid}\,(X) - A_i\|_{\mathrm{S}} \, I$$

where the scalar-valued maximum on the right-hand side is converted into a matrix simply by multiplication with the unit matrix I. It can be proven that this supremum definition is equivalent to that introduced in Chap. 22 by Burgeth et al. via the so-called Loewner ordering of matrices.

21.4.2 M-Estimators and M-Smoothers

A more general class of nonlinear averages for real numbers is established by replacing the distances $|y - x|$ by their p-th powers, $p > 0$. Minimisers of

$$E_X(y) := \sum_{x \in X} |y - x|^p \tag{21.7}$$

belong to the class of *M-estimators* [4]; the corresponding local image filters are *M-smoothers* [14, 21]. Besides the median ($p = 1$), the family of M-estimators also contains the arithmetic mean ($p = 2$) and as limit case for $p \to \infty$, the mid-range value. The analog of this concept for continuous distributions of data values incorporates another remarkable limit case: By sending p to zero, the mode of the distribution is obtained, i.e. the maximum of its density. Generally, M-smoothers for $p < 1$ are attractive for applications because of their higher robustness and ability to *enhance* edges.

For $p \geq 1$ the objective function E_X is convex. For $p < 1$ it has local minima at all $x \in X$ and is strictly concave in the remaining intervals.

Adapting (21.7), we define matrix-valued M-estimators as minimisers of

$$E_X(Y) := \sum_{i=1}^{n} \|Y - A_i\|^p \,, \quad p > 0 \,,$$

where $\|\cdot\|$ again denotes Frobenius or spectral norm. For $p = 1$, we obtain the median; for $p > 1$, the strict convexity of E_X guarantees uniqueness of the minimiser. In the non-convex case $p < 1$, the situation becomes tremendously more complex. We restrict our discussion to the Frobenius norm. Analog to the scalar case, all matrices from X are local minima but unlike there, additional minima can exist in regions where E_X is smooth. These minima cannot come arbitrarily close to the input values: Since the gradient magnitude $|\nabla(\|Y - A_j\|^p)|$ grows over all limits when Y approaches the singularity at A_j, there exists for each $p < 1$ and given data set X a radius $\varrho = \varrho(p, X)$ such that within a ϱ-neighbourhood of A_j, the gradient $\nabla(\|Y - A_j\|^p)$ dominates $\sum_{i \neq j} \nabla(\|Y - A_i\|^p)$ guaranteeing A_j to be the only local minimum of E_X within that neighbourhood.

In the design of an M-smoother with $p < 1$, the crucial question therefore arises which minimum of E_X should be chosen as the value of the M-estimator. We present two alternatives. The global minimum with its advantage of avoiding any artificial assumptions has the drawback of being highly sensitive to changes in the input data. An alternative is a focussing strategy that starts with the unique minimum at $p = 1$ and tracks its drifting while p decreases. Although this method reduces the set of minima to be considered, instabilities of two kinds are still introduced into it by the way how minima evolve with decreasing p. First, minima can split by bifurcations where no obvious criterion tells which branch to follow. Second, minima can vanish; then the focussing must jump into another minimum, chosen e.g. by gradient descent. Besides that, the focussing method applied in the scalar setting would just trivially lock in at the median.

21.5 Algorithmic Aspects

In computing medians defined via the Frobenius norm, the convexity of $E_X(Y)$ and its differentiability except at $Y = A_i$ legitimate the use of gradient descent techniques[3]. One difficulty is encountered: the gradient vector $\nabla\|A_i - Y\|$ has equal length for all $Y \neq A_i$ and thus contains no information on the distance to A_i. Consequentially, the gradient of E_X, too, though indicating a descent direction, is of no use in determining an appropriate step size. This problem is solved by an adaptive step-size control based on the over- and undershoots encountered in the subsequent iteration steps.

The algorithm starts by identifying the $A_j \in X$ for which $E(A_j)$ is smallest. If $\left\|\nabla\sum_{i\neq j}\|A_i - A_j\|\right\| \leq 1$, we have found the minimiser of $E_X(Y)$ and stop. Otherwise we proceed by gradient descent in the direction of $-\nabla E_X(Y)$ with some arbitrary initial step size $s_0 > 0$. If in step k the matrix Y_{k-1} was replaced by $Y_k = Y_{k-1} - s_k\nabla E(Y_{k-1})$, the projection of $\nabla E(Y_k)$ onto $\nabla E(Y_{k-1})$ is compared with $\nabla E(Y_{k-1})$ to estimate over- and undershoots. To this end, we compute $r = \frac{\langle\nabla E(Y_{k-1}),\nabla E(Y_k)\rangle}{\langle\nabla E(Y_k),\nabla E(Y_k)\rangle}$. A ratio $r < 0$ indicates an overshoot while $r \gg 0$ signals an undershoot. According to this ratio, s_{k+1} is adapted. The simplest way to do so is to set $s_{k+1} = s_k/(1 - r)$. In practice we limit the adaptation factor per iteration step, e.g. to $[1/2, 2]$. In case of extreme overshoots, i.e. $r < r_{\mathrm{o}}$ with a constant $r_{\mathrm{o}} \in (-1, 0)$, the last step is rolled back and repeated with smaller step size.

M-smoothers with $1 < p < \infty$ for the Frobenius norm are computed analogously. In the mid-range computation however, singularities show up along the bisector hyperplanes between certain data points. All filters based on the spectral norm inherit also its singularities which appear along the hypersurfaces of matrices Y for which the differences $Y - A_i$ have multiple eigenvalues. Both types of hypersurface-singularities arise from maximum operations between differentiable functions $f_1(Y)$ and $f_2(Y)$ of Y. In the mid-range computation these are $f_1(Y) = \|Y - A_i\|$ and $f_2(Y) = \|Y - A_j\|$ for two data matrices A_i, A_j while in computing the spectral norm $\|Y - A_i\|_S$ the maximum of two eigenvalues $f_1(Y) = \lambda_1(Y - A_i)$ and $f_2(Y) = \lambda_2(Y - A_i)$ is to be determined. These singularities are therefore regularised by replacing $\max(f_1(Y), f_2(Y))$ with $wf_1(Y) + (1 - w)f_2(Y)$ where the weight function $w = w(f_1(Y) - f_2(Y))$ is a smoothed Heaviside function.

For $p < 1$ the missing convexity is the dominating problem. Improving the numerics in the nonconvex case is a topic of our ongoing research. In our experiments, we use two approaches: a grid search within the convex hull of the input data for the global minimum and the focussing strategy.

---

[3] An alternative approach to the computation of matrix-valued median and mid-range filters via convex optimisation is described in [18]

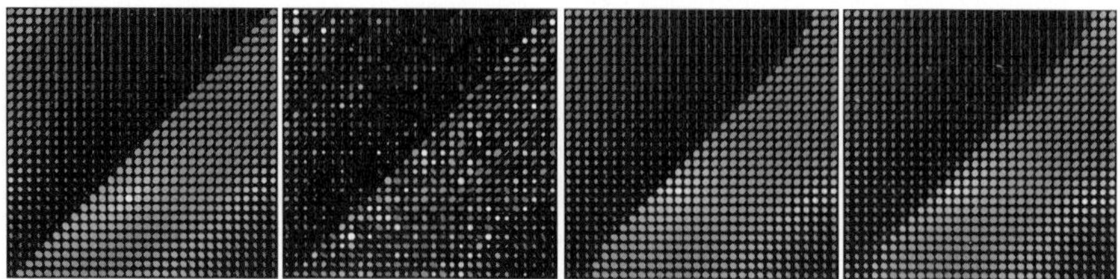

Fig. 21.1. Edge preserving tensor denoising. See colour plates. *Left* to *right*: (**a**) Positive semidefinite matrix field, 29×30. (**b**) Eigenvalues perturbed by Gaussian noise. (**c**) Median filtering of (**a**), 5×5 stencil, Frobenius norm, 5 iterations. (**d**) Same for (**b**). Adapted from [19]

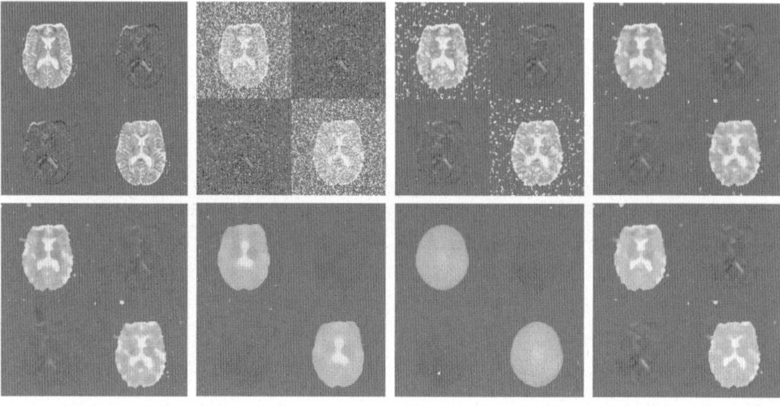

Fig. 21.2. Median filtering of 2D DT-MRI data. *Top, left* to *right*: (**a**) 2D DT-MRI data set (128×128). (**b**) 30% of all pixels replaced by uniform noise. (**c**) The noisy image after one iteration of median filtering, 3×3 stencil, Frobenius norm. (**d**) 5 iterations. *Bottom, left* to *right*: (**e**) Median filtering, 25 iterations, 3×3 stencil, Frobenius norm. (**f**) 5×5 stencil, 25 iterations. (**g**) 9×9 stencil, 25 iterations. (**h**) 25 iterations of median filtering with 3×3 stencil using spectral norm

21.6 Experiments

In the figures, we use two visualisations of symmetric 2×2 matrices. In Figs. 21.2, 21.3 and 21.5, matrix components are depicted by separate grey-value images where middle grey corresponds to zero; the colour Figs. 21.1, 21.4 and 21.6 show matrices represented by ellipses. In the positive semidefinite data sets (Figs. 21.1 and 21.4), each matrix A is first transformed into the ellipse $x^{\mathrm{T}} A^{-2} x = 1$ which has principal axes in the directions of the eigenvectors of A with lengths equal to the eigenvalues of A; in Fig. 21.4 the size variation among the ellipses is then reduced by rescaling each matrix with $(\det A)^{-1/3}$. For the fluid dynamics data which contain indefinite matrices (Fig. 21.6), the lengths of principal axes are set to the eigenvalues of $I + \varepsilon A$ instead, $\varepsilon \approx 0.22$, such that a zero matrix is represented by a unit circle. Again, rescaling is used

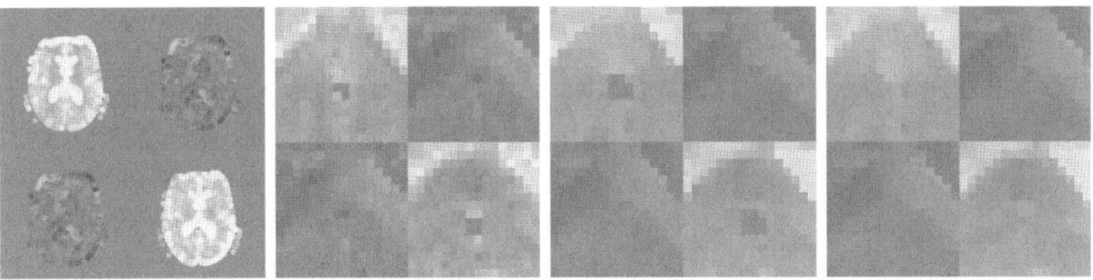

Fig. 21.3. Filtering of 2D DT-MRI data. *Left* to *right*: (**a**) Mid-range filtering of Fig. 21.2(a), 5×5 stencil, Frobenius norm. (**b**) Detail (16×16 pixels) from Fig. 21.2(a), corpus callosum region below ventricle. (**c**) Same detail M-smoothed with $p = 0.1$, 3×3 stencil, Frobenius norm, using grid search. (**d**) M-smoothed with same parameters as in (c) but using focussing strategy

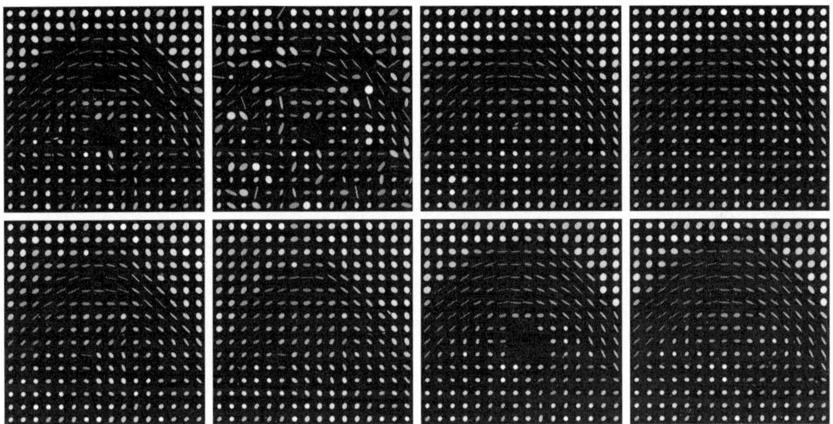

Fig. 21.4. Filtering of 2D DT-MRI data. See colour plates. *Top, left* to *right*: (**a**) Corpus callosum detail, cf. Fig. 21.3(b), represented by ellipses. Missing ellipses result from outliers with negative eigenvalues. (**b**) Same with noise, cf. Fig. 21.2(b). (**c**) Median filtering of noisy image, 3×3 stencil, Frobenius norm, 1 iteration. (**d**) Same as (c) but 5 iterations. *Bottom, left* to *right*: (**e**) Mid-range filtering of the original image, 3×3 stencil, Frobenius norm. (**f**) Same but with 5×5 stencil. (**g**) M-smoothed ($p = 0.1$, 3×3 stencil, Frobenius norm) using grid search. (**h**) Same with focussing strategy

to reduce the size variations. The colouring of the ellipses is determined by the principal axes directions.

Figure 21.1 demonstrates particularly the discontinuity preservation and robustness of median filtering. To this end, we use a synthetic set of positive semidefinite 2×2 matrices containing a straight line discontinuity (a). After five iterations of median filtering, the straight edge is very well preserved, with a notable distortion only near the image boundaries. The latter results from the reflecting boundary conditions that treat the edge–boundary junction like a corner which is consequentially rounded. At the same time, the noise from

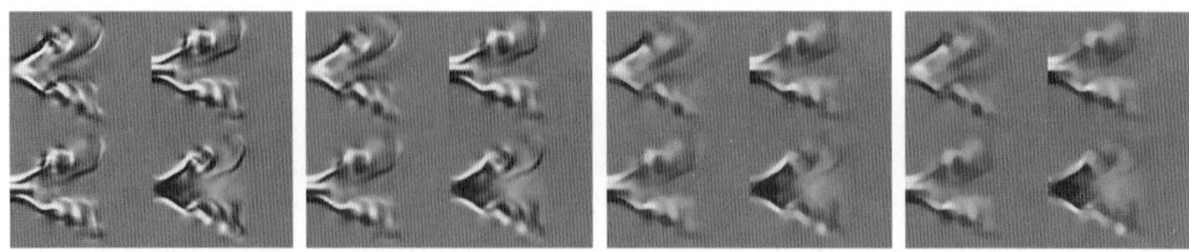

Fig. 21.5. Median filtering of a tensor field containing indefinite matrices. The data are deformation tensors originating from a fluid dynamics simulation. *Left* to *right*: (**a**) Initial data, 124×101 pixels. (**b**) 10 iterations, 3×3 stencil, Frobenius norm. (**c**) 100 iterations. (**d**) 1000 iterations

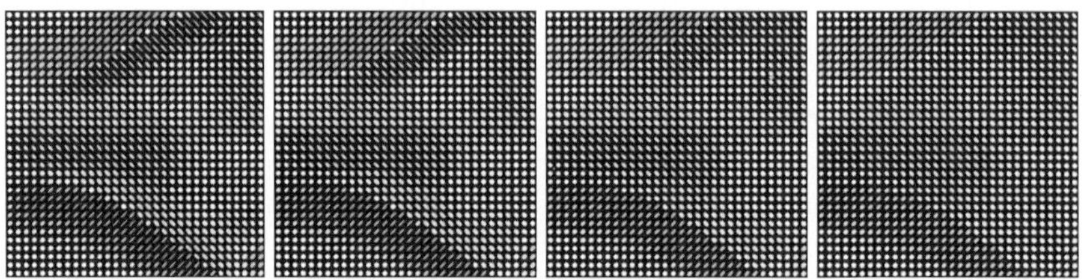

Fig. 21.6. Median filtering of fluid dynamics data. See colour plates. *Left* to *right*: (**a**) Detail (32×32) from Fig. 21.5(a). (**b**) Median filtering, 3×3 stencil, Frobenius norm, 10 iterations. (**c**) 100 iterations. (**d**) 1000 iterations

image (b) has almost completely been removed in image (d) which is hardly to distinguish from (c), the filtered version of the original image (a).

In Figs. 21.2–21.4 we demonstrate our filtering methods on a set of positive semidefinite 2×2 matrices. The original image, Fig. 21.2(a) has been extracted from a human brain DT-MRI scan. The iterated median filtering experiments (Fig. 21.2) have been performed on a noisy version (b) where 30% of all matrices were replaced by uniform noise (uniform in orientation and uniform in the eigenvalues). Images (c–e) show the effect of increased iterations of a 3×3 stencil; the filtering result for higher numbers of iterations does hardly change any more – evidence that root signals exist even in the matrix-valued case. The effect of stencil size is illustrated in (e–g). The shape of objects as it develops under median filtering with spectral norm (h) hardly differs from that obtained with the Frobenius norm (e). Figure 3 shows mid-range filtering (a) and M-smoothing with $p = 0.1$ (c, d). Both are not iterated and applied to the original image, Fig. 21.2(a). To contrast better the grid search (c) and focussing strategy (d) for the M-smoothers, an enlarged detail (b) is used for their demonstration. Selected detail views from Fig. 21.2 and 21.3 are visualised by ellipses in Fig. 21.4.

Median filtering of indefinite matrix data is illustrated in Figs. 21.5 and 21.6 using a set of data set from fluid dynamics simulations.

21.7 Conclusion

Median filtering, mid-range filtering and M-smoothers have been extended to matrix data. To achieve this, a minimisation property was transferred from the scalar- to the matrix-valued setting. In the definitions, a degree of freedom remains in the choice of the matrix norm to be used; Frobenius and spectral norm were discussed as possibilities. Numerics for medians, mid-range filters and M-smoothers with $p > 1$ have been sketched. For $p < 1$ the non-uniqueness of minimisers constitutes a serious problem. Improving the numerics in this case is a subject of ongoing research.

Acknowledgements

We thank Anna Vilanova i Bartrolí (Biomedical Imaging Group, TU Eindhoven) and Carola van Pul (Maxima Medical Center, Eindhoven) for providing us with the DT-MRI data set and for discussing questions involving data conversion. The fluid dynamics data set is owed to Wolfgang Kollmann (MAE Department, UC Davis) and Gerik Scheuermann (Department of Computer Science, Leipzig University). Susanne Biehl and Stephan Zimmer helped us by writing conversion tools.

References

1. Astola, J., Haavisto, P., Neuvo, Y. (1990) Vector median filters. Proceedings of the IEEE **78(4)**, 678–689
2. Austin, T. L., Jr. (1959) An approximation to the point of minimum aggregate distance. Metron **19**, 10–21
3. Barnett, V. (1976) The ordering of multivariate data. Journal of the Royal Statistical Society A, **139 (3)**, 318–355
4. Barral Souto, J. (1938) El modo y otras medias, casos particulares de una misma expresión matemática. Cuadernos de Trabajo No. 3, Instituto de Biometria, Universidad Nacional de Buenos Aires, Argentina
5. Brox, T., Weickert, J. (2002) Nonlinear matrix diffusion for optic flow estimation. In: Van Gool, L. (Ed.) Pattern Recognition. Lecture Notes in Computer Science, Vol. 2449, Springer, Berlin, 446–453
6. Coulon, O., Alexander, D. C., Arridge, S. A. (2001) A regularization scheme for diffusion tensor magnetic resonance images. In: Insana, M. F., Leahy, R. M. (Eds.) Information Processing in Medical Imaging – IPMI 2001. Lecture Notes in Computer Science, Vol. 2082, Springer, Berlin, 92–105
7. Dougherty, E. R., Astola, J. (Eds.) (1999) Nonlinear Filters for Image Processing. SPIE Press, Bellingham
8. Guichard, F., Morel, J.-M. (1997) Partial differential equations and image iterative filtering. In: Duff, I. S., Watson, G. A. (Eds.) The State of the Art in Numerical Analysis, no. 63 IMA Conference Series (New Series), Clarendon Press, Oxford, 525–562

9. Hahn, K., Pigarin, S., Pütz, B. (2001) Edge preserving regularization and tracking for diffusion tensor imaging. In: Niessen, W. J., Viergever, M. A. (Eds.) Medical Image Computing and Computer-Assisted Intervention – MICCAI 2001. Lecture Notes in Computer Science, Vol. 2208, Springer, Berlin, 195–203

10. Klette, R., Zamperoni, R. (1996) Handbook of Image Processing Operators. Wiley, New York

11. Koschan, A., Abidi, M. (2001) A comparison of median filter techniques for noise removal in color images. In: Proc. Seventh German Workshop on Color Image Processing, Erlangen, Germany, 69–79

12. Parker, G. J. M., Schnabel, J. A., Symms, M. R., Werring, D. J., Barker, G. J. (2000) Nonlinear smoothing for reduction of systematic and random errors in diffusion tensor imaging. Journal of Magnetic Resonance Imaging 11, 702–710

13. Poupon, C., Mangin, J., Frouin, V., Régis, J., Poupon, F., Pachot-Clouard, M., Le Bihan, D., Bloch, I. (1998) Regularization of MR diffusion tensor maps for tracking brain white matter bundles. In: Wells, W. M., Colchester, A., Delp, S. (Eds.) Medical Image Computing and Computer-Assisted Intervention – MICCAI 1998. Lecture Notes in Computer Science, Vol. 1496, Springer, Berlin, 489–498

14. Torroba, P. L., Cap, N. L., Rabal, H. J., Furlan, W. D. (1994) Fractional order mean in image processing. Optical Engineering 33 (2), 528–534

15. Tschumperlé, D., Deriche, R. (2001) Diffusion tensor regularization with constraints preservation. In: Proc. 2001 IEEE Computer Society Conference on Computer Vision and Pattern Recognition, Vol. 1, Kauai, HI, Dec. 2001. IEEE Computer Society Press, 948–953

16. Tukey, J. W. (1971) Exploratory Data Analysis. Addison-Wesley, Menlo Park

17. Weickert, J., Brox, T. (2002) Diffusion and regularization of vector- and matrix-valued images. In: Nashed, M. Z., Scherzer, O. (Eds.) Inverse Problems, Image Analysis, and Medical Imaging. Contemporary Mathematics, Vol. 313, AMS, Providence, 251–268

18. Welk, M., Becker, F., Schnörr, C., Weickert, J. (2005) Matrix-valued filters as convex programs. In Kimmel, R., Sochen, N., Weickert, J. (Eds.) Scale-Space and PDE Methods in Computer Vision. Lecture Notes in Computer Science, Springer, Berlin, to appear.

19. Welk, M., Feddern, C., Burgeth, B., Weickert, J. (2003) Median filtering of tensor-valued images. In: Michaelis, B., Krell, G. (Eds.) Pattern Recognition. Lecture Notes in Computer Science, Vol. 2781, Springer, Berlin, 17–24

20. Westin, C., Maier, S. E., Khidhir, B., Everett, P., Jolesz, F. A., Kikinis, R. (1999) Image processing for diffusion tensor magnetic resonance imaging. In: Taylor, C., Colchester, A. (Eds.) Medical Image Computing and Computer-Assisted Intervention – MICCAI 1999. Lecture Notes in Computer Science, Vol. 1679, Springer, Berlin, 441–452

21. Winkler, G., Aurich, V., Hahn, K., Martin, A. (1999) Noise reduction in images: some recent edge-preserving methods. Pattern Recognition and Image Analysis 9 (4), 749–766

Mathematical Morphology on Tensor Data Using the Loewner Ordering

Bernhard Burgeth, Martin Welk, Christian Feddern, and Joachim Weickert

Mathematical Image Analysis Group, Faculty of Mathematics and Computer Science, Saarland University, Building 27, 66041 Saarbrücken, Germany
{burgeth,welk,feddern,weickert}@mia.uni-saarland.de

Summary. The notions of maximum and minimum are the key to the powerful tools of greyscale morphology. Unfortunately these notions do not carry over directly to tensor-valued data. Based upon the Loewner ordering for symmetric matrices this chapter extends the maximum and minimum operation to the tensor-valued setting. This provides the ground to establish matrix-valued analogues of the basic morphological operations ranging from erosion/dilation to top hats. In contrast to former attempts to develop a morphological machinery for matrices, the novel definitions of maximal/minimal matrices depend continuously on the input data, a property crucial for the construction of morphological derivatives such as the Beucher gradient or a morphological Laplacian. These definitions are rotationally invariant and preserve positive semidefiniteness of matrix fields as they are encountered in DT-MRI data. The morphological operations resulting from a component-wise maximum/minimum of the matrix channels disregarding their strong correlation fail to be rotational invariant. Experiments on DT-MRI images as well as on indefinite matrix data illustrate the properties and performance of our morphological operators.

Key words: mathematical morphology, dilation, erosion, matrix-valued images, positive definite matrix, indefinite matrix, diffusion tensor MRI

22.1 Introduction

Since the late sixties mathematical morphology has proven itself a very valuable source of techniques and methods to process images: The path-breaking work of Matheron and Serra [12, 13] started a fruitful and extensive development of morphological operators and filters. Morphological tools have been established to perform noise suppression, edge detection, shape analysis, and skeletonisation for applications ranging from medical imaging to geological sciences, as it is documented in monographs [8, 14, 15, 16] and conference proceedings [6, 17]. It would be desireable to have the tools of morphology at our disposal to process tensor-valued images since nowadays the notion of image encompasses this data type as well. The variety of appearances of tensor fields clearly calls for the development of appropriate tools for the analysis of such data structures because, just as in the scalar case, one has to remove noise and to detect edges and shapes by appropriate filters.

Median filtering [21], Chap. 21 by Welk et al., active contour models and mean curvature motion [4], Chap. 25 by Weickert et al., nonlinear regularisation methods and related diffusion filters [2, 18, 20], Chap. 22 by Suarez-Santana et al., Chap. 23 by Westin et al., Chap. 25 by Weickert et al., also Chap. 19 by Weickert and Welk, exist for matrix-valued data that genuinely exploit the interaction of the different matrix-channels.

First successful steps to extend morphological operations to matrix-valued data sets have been made in [3] where the basic operations dilation and erosion as well as opening and closing are transfered to the matrix-valued setting. However, the proposed approaches lack the continuous dependence on the input matrices. This makes the meaningful construction of morphological derivatives impossible.

The goal of this chapter is to present an alternative approach to morphological operators for tensor-valued images based on the Loewner ordering. This offers a greater potential for extensions and brings expedient notions of morphological derivatives within our reach. The morphological operations to be defined should work on the set $\mathrm{Sym}(n)$ of real symmetric $n \times n$ matrices and have to satisfy conditions such as:

i)   Continuous dependence of the basic morphological operations on the matrices used as input for the aforementioned reasons.
ii) Rotational invariance.
iii) Preservation of the positive semidefiniteness of the matrix field since DT-MRI data sets, for instance, posses this property, see e.g. Chap. 5 by Alexander, Chap. 7 by Vilanova et al., Chap. 17 by Moakher and Batchelor.

Remarkably, the requirement of rotational invariance rules out the straightforward component-wise approach, as is shown in [3]. In this chapter we will introduce a novel notion of the minimum/maximum of a finite set of symmetric, not necessarily positive definite matrices. These notions will exhibit the above mentioned properties.

The chapter is structured as follows: The next section is devoted to a brief review of the greyscale morphological operations we aim to extend to the matrix-valued setting, starting from the basic erosion/dilation and reaching to the morphological equivalents of gradient and Laplacian. In Sect. 3 we present the crucial maximum and minimum operations for matrix-valued data and investigate some of their relevant properties. We report the results of our experiments with various morphological operators applied to real DT-MRI images as well as indefinite tensor fields from fluid mechanics in Sect. 4. Section 5 offers concluding remarks.

22.2 Brief Review of Scalar Morphology

In grey scale morphology an image is represented by a scalar function $f(x,y)$ with $(x,y) \in \mathbb{R}^2$. The so-called *structuring element* is a set B in $\mathbb{R}^2$ determining the neighbourhood relation of pixels. In this chapter we restrict ourselves to flat greyscale morphology where this binary type of structuring element is used. Then greyscale *dilation* $\oplus$, resp., *erosion* $\ominus$ replaces the greyvalue of the image $f(x,y)$ by its supremum, resp., infimum within the mask B:

$$(f \oplus B)(x,y) := \sup \{ f(x-x', y-y') \mid (x',y') \in B \} ,$$
$$(f \ominus B)(x,y) := \inf \{ f(x+x', y+y') \mid (x',y') \in B \} .$$

By concatenation other operators are constructed such as *opening* and *closing*,

$$f \circ B := (f \ominus B) \oplus B , \qquad f \bullet B := (f \oplus B) \ominus B ,$$

the *white top-hat* and its dual, the *black top-hat*

$$\mathrm{WTH}(f) := f - (f \circ B) , \qquad \mathrm{BTH}(f) := (f \bullet B) - f ,$$

finally, the *self-dual top-hat,*

$$\mathrm{SDTH}(f) := (f \bullet B) - (f \circ B) .$$

In an image the boundaries or edges of objects are the loci of high grey-value variations and those can be detected by gradient operators. Erosion and dilation are also the elementary building blocks of the basic morphological gradients. The so-called *Beucher gradient*

$$\varrho_B(f) := (f \oplus B) - (f \ominus B)$$

is an analog to the norm of the gradient $\|\nabla f\|$ if an image is considered as a differentiable function. Other useful approximations to $\|\nabla f\|$ are the *internal* and *external gradient,*

$$\varrho_B^-(f) := f - (f \ominus B) , \qquad \varrho_B^+(f) := (f \oplus B) - f .$$

We also present a morphological equivalent for the Laplace operator $\Delta f = \partial_{xx} f + \partial_{yy} f$ suitable for matrix-valued data. The *morphological Laplacian* has been introduced in [19]. We consider a variant given by the difference between external and internal gradient:

$$\Delta_m f := \varrho_B^+(f) - \varrho_B^-(f) = (f \oplus B) - 2 \cdot f + (f \ominus B) .$$

This form of a Laplacian represents the second derivative $\partial_{\eta\eta} f$ where η denotes the direction of the steepest slope. $\Delta_m f$ is matrix-valued, but $\mathrm{trace}(\Delta_m f)$ provides us with useful information: Regions where $\mathrm{trace}(\Delta_m f) \leq 0$ can be viewed as the influence zones of maxima while those areas with trace$(\Delta_m f) \geq 0$ are influence zones of minima. It therefore allows us to distinguish between influence zones of minima and maxima in the image f. This is crucial for the design of so-called *shock filters*.

The basic idea underlying shock filtering is applying either a dilation or an erosion to an image, depending on whether the pixel is located within the influence zone of a minimum or a maximum [10]:

$$\delta_B(f) := \begin{cases} f \oplus B & \text{if} \quad \text{trace}(\Delta_m f) \leq 0 \,, \\ f \ominus B & \text{else} \,. \end{cases} \tag{22.1}$$

The shock filter expands local minima and maxima at the cost of regions with intermediate greyvalues. When iterated experimental results in greyscale morphology suggest that a non-trivial steady state exists characterised by a piecewise constant segmentation of the image.

In the scalar case the zero-crossings $\Delta f = 0$ can be interpreted as edge locations [7, 9, 11]. We will also use the trace of the morphological Laplacian in this manner to derive an edge map.

22.3 Extremal Matrices in the Loewner Ordering

There is a natural partial ordering on $\mathrm{Sym}(n)$, the so-called *Loewner ordering* defined via the cone of positive semidefinite matrices $\mathrm{Sym}^+(n)$ by

$$A, B \in \mathrm{Sym}(n) : \quad A \geq B :\Leftrightarrow A - B \in \mathrm{Sym}^+(n) \,,$$

i.e. if and only if $A - B$ is positive semidefinite.

This partial ordering is *not* a lattice ordering, that is, the notion of a unique supremum and infimum with respect to this ordering does not exist [1]. Nevertheless, given any finite set of symmetric matrices $\mathcal{A} = \{A_1, \dots, A_n\}$, we will be able to identify suitable maximal, resp., minimal matrices

$$\overline{A} := \max \mathcal{A} \quad \text{resp.,} \quad \underline{A} := \min \mathcal{A} \,.$$

For presentational reasons we restrict ourselves from now on to the case of 2×2-matrices in $\mathrm{Sym}(2)$. The 3×3-case is treated similarly but is technically more involved.

To find these extremal matrices for a set $\mathcal{A}$ we proceed as follows: The cone $\mathrm{Sym}^+(2)$ can be visualized in 3D using the bijection

$$\begin{pmatrix} \alpha & \beta \\ \beta & \gamma \end{pmatrix} \longleftrightarrow \frac{1}{\sqrt{2}} \begin{pmatrix} 2\beta \\ \gamma - \alpha \\ \gamma + \alpha \end{pmatrix} , \quad \text{resp.,} \quad \frac{1}{\sqrt{2}} \begin{pmatrix} z - y & x \\ x & z + y \end{pmatrix} \longleftrightarrow \begin{pmatrix} x \\ y \\ z \end{pmatrix} .$$

This mapping creates an isometrically isomorphic image of the cone $\mathrm{Sym}^+(2)$ in the Euclidean space $\mathrm{I\!R}^3$ given by $\{(x, y, z)^\top \in \mathrm{I\!R}^3 | \sqrt{x^2 + y^2} \leq z\}$ and

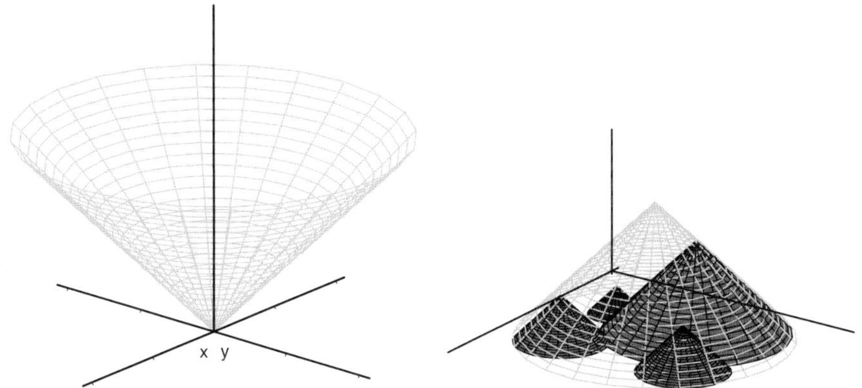

Fig. 22.1. (a) *Left*: Image of the Loewner cone $\mathrm{Sym}^{+}(2)$. (b) *Right*: Cone covering four penumbras of other matrices. The tip of each cone represents a symmetric 2×2 matrix in $\mathbb{R}^{3}$. For each cone the radius and the height are equal

depicted in Fig. 22.1(a). For $A \in \mathrm{Sym}(2)$ the set $P(A) = \{Z \in \mathrm{Sym}(2) | A \geq Z\}$ denotes the penumbra of the matrix A. It corresponds to a cone with vertex in A and a circular base in the x-y-plane:

$$P(A) \cap \{z = 0\} = \text{ circle with centre } \left(\sqrt{2}\beta, \frac{\gamma - \alpha}{\sqrt{2}} \right) \text{ and radius } \frac{\mathrm{trace}(A)}{\sqrt{2}} \; .$$

Considering the associated penumbras of the matrices in $\mathcal{A}$ the search for the *maximal matrix* $\overline{A}$ amounts to determine the smallest cone covering all the penumbras of $\mathcal{A}$; see Fig. 22.1(b). Note that the height of a penumbra in the x-y-plane is equal to the radius of its base, namely $\frac{\mathrm{trace}(A)}{\sqrt{2}}$. Hence a penumbra is already uniquely determined by the circle constituting its base. This implies that the search for a maximal matrix comes down to find the smallest circle enclosing the base-circles of the matrices in $\mathcal{A}$. This is a non-trivial problem in computer graphics. An efficient numerical solution for finding the smallest ball enclosing a given number of points has been implemented in C++ only recently by Gärtner [5].

By sampling the basis circles we use this implementation for the calculation of the smallest circle enclosing them. This gives us the smallest covering cone and hence the maximal matrix $\overline{A}$. A suitable *minimal matrix* $\underline{A}$ is obtained via the formula

$$\underline{A} = \left(\mathrm{max}(A_1^{-1}, \ldots, A_n^{-1}) \right)^{-1}$$

inspired by the well-known relation $\mathrm{min}(a_1, \ldots, a_n) = \left(\mathrm{max}(a_1^{-1}, \ldots, a_n^{-1}) \right)^{-1}$ valid for real numbers $a_1, \ldots, a_n$. Furthermore, inversion preserves positive definiteness as well as rotational invariance. For $i = 1, \ldots, n$ we have $\underline{A} \leq A_i \leq \overline{A}$ with respect to the Loewner ordering. We emphasise that $\overline{A}$ and $\underline{A}$ depend continuously on $A_1, \ldots, A_n$ by their construction. Also the rotational invariance is preserved, since the Loewner ordering is already rotational invariant: $A \geq B \iff UAU^\top \geq UBU^\top$ holds for any orthogonal matrix U. Finally it is important to note that if all the A_i are positive definite then so is $\overline{A}$ as well as $\underline{A}$.

Nevertheless, the definitions of the matrices $\overline{A}$ and $\underline{A}$ are still meaningful for matrices that are not positive definite as long as they have a nonnegative trace (since it corresponds to a radius in the construction above). It also becomes evident from their construction that in general neither $\overline{A}$ nor $\underline{A}$ coincide with any of the A_i: $\overline{A}, \underline{A} \notin \mathcal{A}$.

With these essential notions of suitable maximal and minimal matrices $\overline{A}$ and $\underline{A}$ at our disposal the definitions of the higher morphological operators carry over essentially verbatim, with one exception:

The morphological Laplacian Δ_m as defined in Sect. 2 is a matrix. In equation (22.1) we used the *trace* of the morphological Laplacian to steer the interwoven dilation-erosion process, and to create an edge map.

A word of care has to be stated: unlike in the scalar-valued setting the minimum/maximum are not associative, e.g. $\max(A_1, A_2, A_3)$ generally can not be obtained by evaluating $\max(\max(A_1, A_2), A_3)$. This entails a loss of the semi-group property of the derived dilation and erosion. Clearly this has no effects as long as these morphological operations are not iterated.

In the next section we will apply various morphological operators to positive definite DT-MRI images as well as to indefinite matrix fields representing a flow field.

22.4 Experimental Results

In our numerical experiments we use two data sets:

1) Positive definite data. A 128×128 field of 2-D tensors which has been extracted from a 3-D DT-MRI data set of a human head. Those data are represented as ellipses via the level sets of the quadratic form $\{x^\top A^{-2} x \,|\, x \in \mathbb{R}^2\}$ associated with a matrix $A \in \mathrm{Sym}(n)$. The exponent -2 takes care of the fact that the small, resp., big eigenvalue corresponds to the semi-minor, resp., semi-major axis of the ellipse. The color coding of the ellipses reflects the direction of their principle axes. Another technical issue is that our DT-MRI data set of a human head contains not only positive definite matrices. Because of the quantisation there are singular matrices (particularly, a lot of zero matrices outside the head segment) and even matrices with negative eigenvalues. The negative values are of very small absolute value, and they result from measurement imprecision and quantisation errors. While such values do not constitute a problem in the dilation process, the erosion, relying on inverses of positive definite matrices, has to be regularised. Instead of the exact inverse A^{-1} of a given matrix A we use therefore $(A + \varepsilon I)^{-1}$ with a small positive ε.

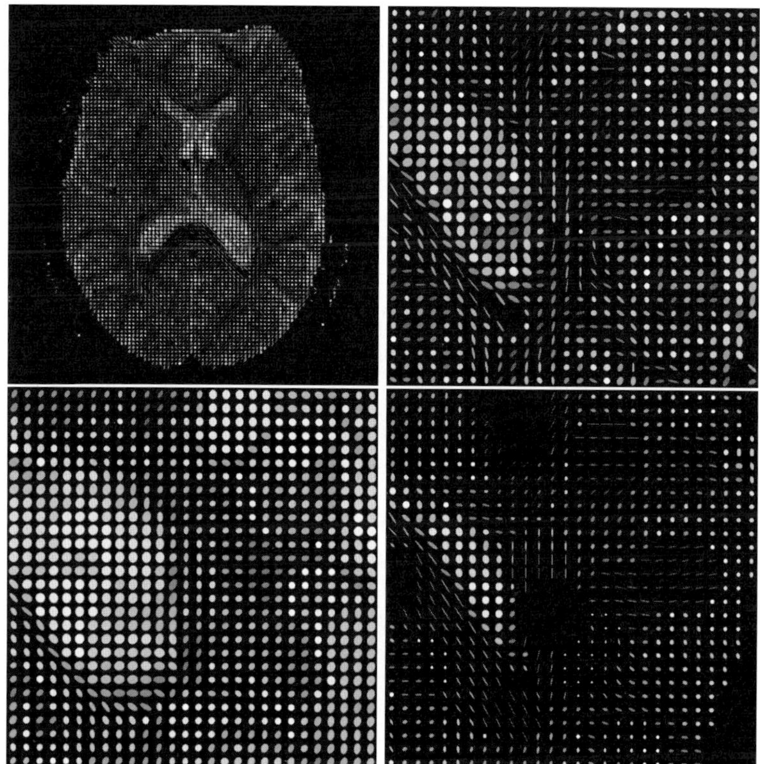

Fig. 22.2. (a) *Top left*: 2-D tensor field extracted from a DT-MRI data set of a human head. (b) *Top right*: enlarged section of left image. (c) *Bottom left*: dilation with DSE($\sqrt{5}$). (d) *Bottom right*: erosion with DSE($\sqrt{5}$)

2) Indefinite data. An image of size 248×202 containing indefinite matrices and depicting a rate-of-deformation tensor field from a experiment in fluid dynamics. Here tensor-valued data are represented in the figures by greyvalue images which are subdivided in four tiles. Each tile corresponds to one matrix entry. A middle grey value represents the zero value; *Magnitude* information of the matrix-valued signals is essentially encoded in the trace of the matrix and thus in the main diagonal. Instead, the off-diagonal of a symmetric matrix encode anisotropy.

Figure 22.2 displays the original head image and an enlarged section of it as well as the effect of dilation and erosion with a disk-shaped structuring element of radius $\sqrt{5}$. For the sake of brevity we denote in the sequel this element by DSE($\sqrt{5}$). We encounter the expected enhancement or suppression of features in the image. As known from scalar-valued morphology, the shape of details in the dilated and eroded images mirrors the shape of the structuring element.

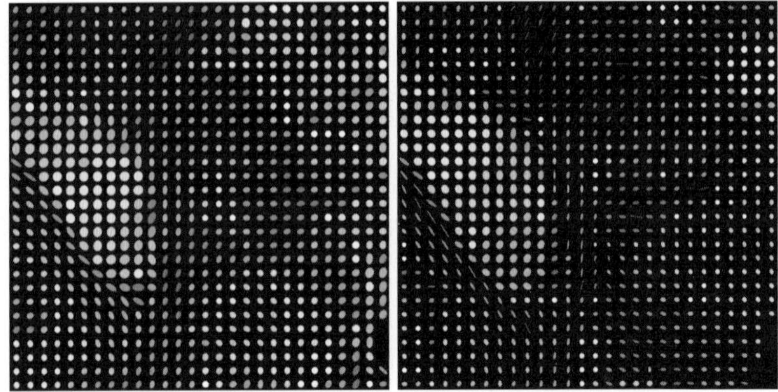

Fig. 22.3. (a) *Left*: closing with DSE($\sqrt{5}$). (b) *Right*: opening with DSE($\sqrt{5}$)

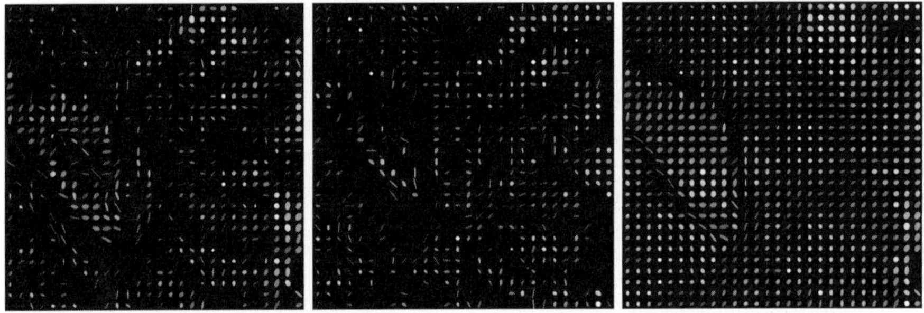

Fig. 22.4. (a) *Left*: white top hat with DSE($\sqrt{5}$). (b) *Middle*: black top hat with DSE($\sqrt{5}$). (c) *Right*: self-dual top hat with DSE($\sqrt{5}$)

In Figs. 22.3 and 22.7, the results of opening and closing operations are shown. In good analogy to their scalar-valued counterparts, both operations restitute the coarse shape and size of structures. Smaller details are eliminated by the opening operation, while the closing operation magnifies them. It also seems that the isotropy of the matrices is increased under both operations.

The top hat filters can be seen in Fig. 22.4. As in the scalar-valued case, the white top hat is sensitive for small-scale details formed by matrices with large eigenvalues, while the black top hat responds with high values to small-scale details stemming from matrices with small eigenvalues. The self-dual top hat as the sum of white and black top hat results in homogeneously high matrices rather evenly distributed in the image.

Figures 22.5 and 22.8 depict the internal and external morphological gradients and their sum, the Beucher gradient for positive and negative definite matrix-fields. It is no surprise that these operators respond to the presence of edges, the one-sided gradients more so than the Beucher gradient whose inertance is known. The images depicting the flow field show clearly that changes in the values of the matrices are well detected.

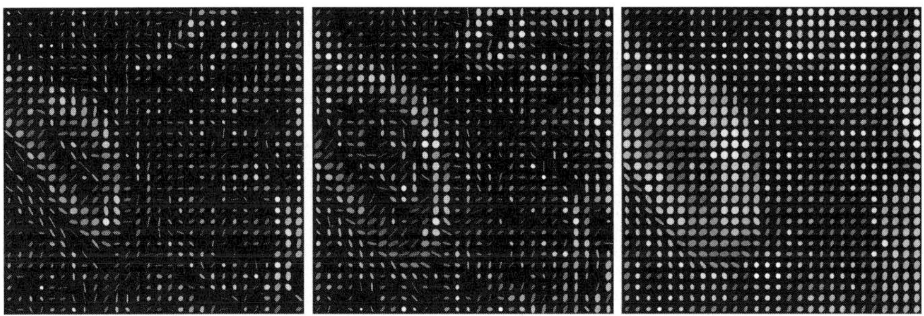

Fig. 22.5. (a) *Left*: external gradient with DSE($\sqrt{5}$). (b) *Middle*: internal gradient with DSE($\sqrt{5}$). (c) *Right*: Beucher gradient with DSE($\sqrt{5}$)

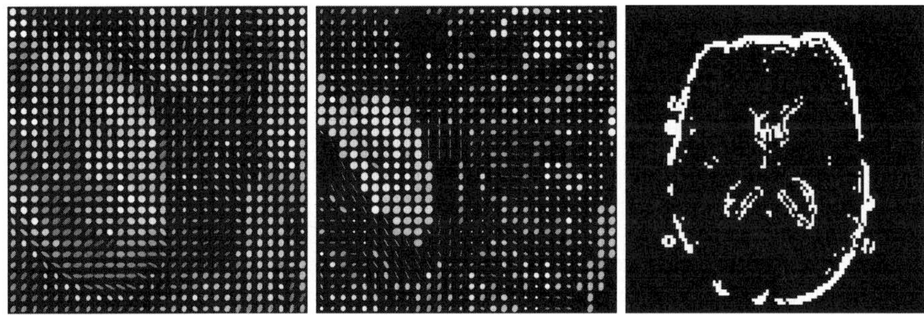

Fig. 22.6. (a) *Left*: morphological Laplacian with DSE($\sqrt{5}$). (b) *Middle*: result of shock filtering with DSE($\sqrt{5}$). (c) *Right*: edge map derived from zero crossings of the morphological Laplacian with DSE($\sqrt{5}$)

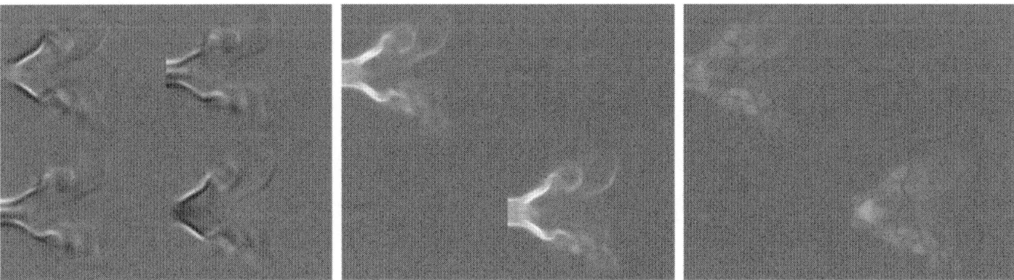

Fig. 22.7. (a) *Left*: original image of a flow field. (b) *Middle*: closing with DSE($\sqrt{5}$). (c) *Right*: opening with DSE($\sqrt{5}$)

The effect of the Laplacian Δ_m and its use for controlling a shock filter can be seen in Fig. 22.6: while applying dilation in pixels where the trace of the Laplacian is negative, it uses erosion wherever the trace of the Laplacian is positive. The result is an image in which regions with larger and smaller eigenvalues are sharper separated than in the original image. We also may concede some edge detection capabilities to the morphological Laplacian for tensor data. Image (c) in Fig. 22.6 displays an edge map derived by setting

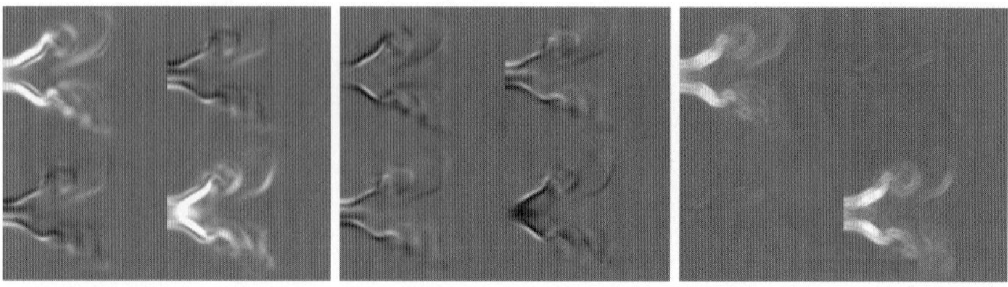

Fig. 22.8. (a) *Left*: external gradient with DSE($\sqrt{5}$). **(b)** *Middle*: internal gradient with DSE($\sqrt{5}$). **(c)** *Right*: Beucher gradient with DSE($\sqrt{5}$)

the pixel value to 255 if in that pixel the condition $-100 \leq \text{trace}(\Delta_m f) \leq 100$ is satisfied, and 0 if the absolute value of $\text{trace}(\Delta_m f)$ exceeds 100.

22.5 Conclusions

In this chapter we have extended fundamental concepts of mathematical morphology to the case of matrix-valued data. This has been achieved by determining maximal and minimal elements $\overline{A}$, $\underline{A}$ in the space of symmetric matrices $\text{Sym}(n)$ with respect to the Loewner ordering. These extremal elements serve as an suitable analogue for the continuous notion of maximum and minimum, which lie at the heart of mathematical morphology. As a consequence we were able not only to design the matrix-valued equivalents of basic morphological operations like dilation or erosion but also morphological derivatives and shock filters for tensor fields. In the experimental section the performance of the various morphological operations on positive definite as well as indefinite matrix-fields is documented.

Future work comprises the extension of the methodology to the demanding case of 3×3-matrix-fields as well a the development of more sophisticated morphological operators for matrix-valued data.

Acknowledgments

We are grateful to Anna Vilanova i Bartrolí (Eindhoven Institute of Technology) and Carola van Pul (Maxima Medical Center, Eindhoven) for providing us with the DT-MRI data set and for discussing questions concerning data conversion.

The fluid dynamics data set goes back to Wolfgang Kollmann (MAE Department, UC Davis) and has been kindly provided by Gerik Scheuermann (Institute for Computer Science, University of Leipzig). We would also like to thank Andrés Bruhn (Mathematical Image Analysis Group, Saarland University) for his valuable support in implementational issues.

References

1. J. M. Borwein and A. S. Lewis. *Convex Analysis and Nonlinear Optimization.* Springer, New York, 1999.
2. T. Brox, J. Weickert, B. Burgeth, and P. Mrázek. Nonlinear structure tensors. Technical report, Dept. of Mathematics, Saarland University, Saarbrücken, Germany, July 2004.
3. B. Burgeth, M. Welk, C. Feddern, and J. Weickert. Morphological operations on matrix-valued images. In T. Pajdla and J. Matas, editors, *Computer Vision – ECCV 2004, Part IV*, volume 3024 of *Lecture Notes in Computer Science*, pp. 155–167. Springer, Berlin, 2004.
4. C. Feddern, J. Weickert, B. Burgeth, and M. Welk. Curvature-driven PDE methods for matrix-valued images. *International Journal of Computer Vision*, 2005. In press.
5. B. Gärtner. http://www2.inf.ethz.ch/personal/gaertner/. WebPage last visited: July 2nd, 2004.
6. J. Goutsias, L. Vincent, and D. S. Bloomberg, editors. *Mathematical Morphology and its Applications to Image and Signal Processing*, volume 18 of *Computational Imaging and Vision*. Kluwer, Dordrecht, 2000.
7. R. M. Haralick. Digital step edges from zero crossing of second directional derivatives. *IEEE Transactions on Pattern Analysis and Machine Intelligence*, 6(1):58–68, 1984.
8. H. J. A. M. Heijmans. *Morphological Image Operators.* Academic Press, Boston, 1994.
9. R. Kimmel and A. M. Bruckstein. Regularized Laplacian zero crossings as optimal edge integrators. *International Journal of Computer Vision*, 53(3):225–243, 2003.
10. H. P. Kramer and J. B. Bruckner. Iterations of a non-linear transformation for enhancement of digital images. *Pattern Recognition*, 7:53–58, 1975.
11. D. Marr and E. Hildreth. Theory of edge detection. *Proceedings of the Royal Society of London, Series B*, 207:187–217, 1980.
12. G. Matheron. *Eléments pour une théorie des milieux poreux.* Masson, Paris, 1967.
13. J. Serra. *Echantillonnage et estimation des phénomènes de transition minier.* PhD thesis, University of Nancy, France, 1967.
14. J. Serra. *Image Analysis and Mathematical Morphology*, volume 1. Academic Press, London, 1982.
15. J. Serra. *Image Analysis and Mathematical Morphology*, volume 2. Academic Press, London, 1988.
16. P. Soille. *Morphological Image Analysis.* Springer, Berlin, 1999.
17. H. Talbot and R. Beare, editors. *Proc. Sixth International Symposium on Mathematical Morphology and its Applications.* Sydney, Australia, April 2002. http://www.cmis.csiro.au/ismm2002/proceedings/.
18. D. Tschumperlé and R. Deriche. Diffusion tensor regularization with constraints preservation. In *Proc. 2001 IEEE Computer Society Conference on Computer Vision and Pattern Recognition*, volume 1, pp. 948–953, Kauai, HI, December 2001. IEEE Computer Society Press.
19. L. J. van Vliet, I. T. Young, and A. L. D. Beckers. A nonlinear Laplace operator as edge detector in noisy images. *Computer Vision, Graphics and Image Processing*, 45(2):167–195, 1989.

20. J. Weickert and T. Brox. Diffusion and regularization of vector- and matrix-valued images. In M. Z. Nashed and O. Scherzer, editors, *Inverse Problems, Image Analysis, and Medical Imaging*, volume 313 of *Contemporary Mathematics*, pp. 251–268. AMS, Providence, 2002.
21. M. Welk, C. Feddern, B. Burgeth, and J. Weickert. Median filtering of tensor-valued images. In B. Michaelis and G. Krell, editors, *Pattern Recognition*, volume 2781 of *Lecture Notes in Computer Science*, pp. 17–24, Berlin, 2003. Springer.

A Local Structure Measure for Anisotropic Regularization of Tensor Fields

Suárez-Santana E.[1], Rodriguez-Florido M.A.[1], Castaño-Moraga C.[1], Westin C.-F.[1,2], and Ruiz-Alzola J.[1,2]

[1] Center for Technology in Medicine, University of Las Palmas de Gran Canaria, Campus de Tafira. Las Palmas de Gran Canaria. 35017, Spain
`{eduardo,marf,ccasmor,jruiz}@ctm.ulpgc.es`
[2] Laboratory of Mathematics in Imaging, Brigham & Women's Hospital and Harvard Medical School, Boston, MA 02115, USA
`westin@bwh.harvard.edu`

Summary. Acquisition systems are not fully reliable since any real sensor will provide noisy and possibly incomplete and degraded data. Therefore, in tensor measurements, all problems dealt with in conventional multidimensional statistical signal processing are present with tensor signals. In this chapter we describe some non-iterative approaches to tensor signal processing. Our schemes are achieved by the estimation of a local structure tensor, which is used as a key element in regularization. A stochastic point of view as well as a phase-invariant implementation are presented. This work also covers tensor extensions for common scalar operations such as anisotropic interpolation and filtering. An application of the structure tensor for regularization of deformation fields in tensor image registration is also shown. The techniques presented in this chapter suppose an alternative to variational and PDEs schemes, and another point of view of the tensor signal processing.

23.1 Introduction

The properties of uniqueness and stability of the solution are crucial in the formulation of problems in computer science. This is not always the case, so in these situations it becomes necessary the injection of ad-hoc constraints or a priori knowledge into the model. The modification of the computational theoretic model to enforce these properties is called regularization. It is important to realize that regularization applies to the model, not to the solution. So that, we may find on it dependence with respect to initial data. A singular example in signal processing is interpolation. In interpolation, values of a signal are known in several points of the space, and values in the rest of the points must be estimated. In this case it's common to step over the model directly to the algorithm. Nevertheless, implicit information is supplied as limited bandwidth requirement (sinc interpolation) or minimum squares derivatives (linear interpolation). Interpolation may be understood as regularization in this sense.

The way regularization is injected depends on the original formulation. For example, variational formulations are usually modified by the addition of a functional term. Under this framework, tasks in image processing such as interpolation, filtering or even registration may be regularized in very similar ways.

In this chapter, the structure tensor is presented as a valid key element in such tasks. Expressions to estimate the structure tensor are given not only for scalar fields, but also for general tensor valued images. Perhaps its most powerful application is in filtering, where it appears as an anisotropic weighting of the strength of the smoothing. A simpler approach is shown in interpolation, as an anisotropic weighting as well. Finally, extracting a scalar structure measure, it can steer the regularization of a deformation field in registration. In all cases, and as an alternative to variational, PDEs or other methods presented in different chapters of this book (see Chaps. 21, 22 and 25), our techniques follow non-iteratives and strictly anisotropic methods. The text is organized as follows. First, we present a stochastic interpretation of the local structure tensor as a generalized correlation matrix for general multidimensional tensor fields. An initial simple estimate is introduced, followed by a more advanced approach that guarantees phase invariance. In Sect. 23.3, this tensor is used to drive an anisotropic filtering technique based on a steerable filters decomposition. The application of the structure tensor for interpolation and for regularization of displacement fields in registration is shown in Sect. 23.4.

23.2 The Structure Tensor

23.2.1 A Stochastic Point of View

Consider a scalar random field $s(\mathbf{x})$ and the gradient vector random field $\nabla s(\mathbf{x})$, which can be represented *wrt* a basis by the component form[1] $s_{,k}$, where $k = 1 \ldots n$ and n is the dimension of the field. The correlation matrix of $\nabla s(x)$ is defined at each point by

$$\mathsf{T}(\mathbf{x}) = \mathbf{R}_\nabla(\mathbf{x}) = \mathrm{E}[\nabla s(\mathbf{x})\,\nabla s(\mathbf{x})^t] = \mathrm{E}[s_{,k}(\mathbf{x})\,s_{,l}(\mathbf{x})] \qquad (23.1)$$

and an initial estimate for it is given by

$$\hat{\mathsf{T}}(\mathbf{x}) = \hat{\mathbf{R}}_\nabla(\mathbf{x}) = \frac{1}{V(\mathcal{N}(\mathbf{x}))} \sum_{\mathbf{x}_i \in \mathcal{N}(\mathbf{x})} s_{,k}(\mathbf{x}_i)\,s_{,l}(\mathbf{x}_i) \;, \qquad (23.2)$$

where $\mathcal{N}(\mathbf{x})$ stands for the neighborhood of $\mathbf{x}$ and V for its number of samples.

---

[1] The *comma* convention has been used: $,k$ is an indexing of the partial derivatives, that is, $s_{,k} = \frac{\partial s(\mathbf{x})}{\partial x^k}$. Strictly, it corresponds to a covariant derivative.

The interpretation presented here (23.1) has been reported by [12]. Furthermore, it provides a theoretical background for the extension of the approach to the tensor case.

A tensor field is a function that assigns a tensor to each point of a domain, a surface, of more concrete, of a differential manifold. As shown in Chap. 1, tensor spaces are a generalization of vector spaces. Once a basis is set, tensors are expressed by means of their components that can be stored in multidimensional arrays $s_{i_1\ldots i_n}$. Therefore, a tensor field can be interpreted as a multichannel signal, where each channel corresponds to a different component of the tensor field. Analogous to scalar fields, gradient of a tensor field $s(\mathbf{x})$ can be defined as

$$\nabla \otimes s(\mathbf{x}) = s_{i_1\ldots i_n,k}(\mathbf{x}) \;, \tag{23.3}$$

again a tensor field, but of order $n+1$.

By means of tensor operations, it is possible to define the *correlation tensor* of the gradient of a tensor random field as

$$\mathbf{RT}_\nabla(\mathbf{x}) = \mathrm{E}\left[\nabla \otimes s(\mathbf{x}) \otimes \nabla \otimes s(\mathbf{x})\right] = \mathrm{E}\left[s_{i_1\ldots i_n,k}(\mathbf{x})\, s_{j_1\ldots j_n,l}(\mathbf{x})\right] \;. \tag{23.4}$$

We also define the *generalized correlation matrix* of the gradient of a tensor random field as the contraction (see Chap. 1 for details) of all indices in its correlation tensor (23.4) but those corresponding to the partial derivatives (comma indices):

$$\mathsf{T}(\mathbf{x}) = \mathbf{R}_\nabla(\mathbf{x}) = \mathrm{E}\left[\sum_{i_1\ldots i_n} s_{i_1\ldots i_n,k}(\mathbf{x})\, s_{i_1\ldots i_n,l}(\mathbf{x})\right] = \sum_{i_1\ldots i_n} \mathbf{R}_\nabla(\mathbf{x}; i_1\ldots i_n) \;,$$

$$\tag{23.5}$$

where $\mathbf{R}_\nabla(\mathbf{x}; i_1\ldots i_n) = \mathrm{E}\left[s_{i_1\ldots i_n,k}(\mathbf{x}) s_{i_1\ldots i_n,l}(\mathbf{x})\right]$ is the correlation matrix of the gradient field of the channel $i_1\ldots i_n$ of $s(\mathbf{x})$. Consequently, the generalized correlation matrix of the gradient of a tensor field is the sum of the correlation matrices of the gradient of each component of the tensor field. The properties of the correlation matrix (23.1) apply to the generalized correlation matrix (23.5).

Notice that its principal directions are obtained from contributions from each tensor component. The addition makes the ellipsoids associated with the generalized correlation matrices rounder than the ones associated with the correlation matrices of each component, which will tend to be more elongated, unless the correlation matrices of all tensor components have the same eigendecomposition.

23.2.2 A Phase-Invariant Estimate

Estimation of differential operators (e.g. gradient) has well-known practical implementations. However, they are highly sensitive to noise or they can produce double border detection. This is due to they are not independent to variations of phase in the signal (they provide different detections for lines and edges) [5], and are not idempotent operators [11].

In the scalar case, Knutsson et al. [4] proposed to obtain a phase-independent estimation of the local structure tensor $\hat{\mathsf{T}}$, by representing it with respect to a tensor basis $\{\mathsf{M}^k\}$ and selecting the coordinates as the magnitudes of the outputs of the original scalar field to a bank of multidimensional spherically separable quadrature filters, $||q_k||$: $\hat{\mathsf{T}} = \sum_k ||q_k|| \mathsf{M}^k$. The bank of quadrature filters have as transfer function:

$$Q(\omega)_k = \begin{cases} e^{(\frac{-4}{B^2 ln2})(ln^2(\frac{||\omega||}{||\omega_o||}))} \cdot (\hat{\omega}^t \hat{\mathbf{n}}_k)^2 & \text{if } \hat{\omega}^t \hat{\mathbf{n}}_k > 0 \\ 0 & \text{otherwise}, \end{cases} \qquad (23.6)$$

where $\hat{\mathbf{n}}_k$ is the unitary vector associated to the orientation of every quadrature filter in the bank. This kind of filters can be seen as an oriented Gaussian function in logarithmic scale, centered at $||\omega_o||$ and with bandwidth B. The tensor basis elements M^k represent the tensors associated to the quadrature filters orientations $\hat{\mathbf{n}}_k$, and they are obtained from the tensors resulted of the outer products of orientation vectors, $\{\mathsf{N}_k = \hat{\mathbf{n}}_k \hat{\mathbf{n}}_k^t\}$. The basis M^k is the dual basis of N_k, and can be obtained as: $\mathsf{M}^k = \langle \mathsf{N}_k, \mathsf{N}_l \rangle^{-1} \mathsf{N}_l$.

In order to cover all the local spectrum of the dataset, Knutsson proposed to use the directions pointing to the vertices of a regular polytope (an hexagon in 2-D, an icosahedron in 3-D, etc). For an n-dimensional dataset, by symmetry, the minimum number of elements in the tensor basis, and consequently the minimum number of orientations associated to the quadrature filters is $\frac{n(n+1)}{2}$. Hence, the local structure tensor can be written as

$$\hat{\mathsf{T}} = \sum_{k=1}^{n(n+1)/2} ||q_k|| \mathsf{M}^k \ . \qquad (23.7)$$

where the dual basis is given by a simple expression: $\mathsf{M}^k = C_1 \mathsf{N}_k + C_2 \mathsf{I}$, with C_1, C_2 scalars constants and I the identity tensor.

The extension of the previous approach to tensor fields is presented at [9]. This scheme uses the same representation (i.e., the same tensor basis and number of directions) of the local structure tensor, though a new method to compute the coordinates is needed. To this extent each quadrature filter is applied to every tensor component, and the magnitude of the outputs are used to compute a 2-norm. In a first order vector field, the Euclidean norm,

$$\hat{\mathsf{T}} = \sum_{k=1}^{n(n+1)/2} \underbrace{\sqrt{(||q_{[k]1}||^2 + ||q_{[k]2}||^2)}}_{\text{norm of } \left(\begin{array}{c} ||q_{[k]1}|| \\ ||q_{[k]2}|| \end{array}\right)} \mathsf{M}^k \ , \qquad (23.8)$$

while in the case of a 2D second order tensor field, resorting to the Frobenius norm,

$$\hat{\mathsf{T}} = \sum_{k=1}^{n(n+1)/2} \underbrace{(\|q_{[k]11}\|^2 + \|q_{[k]12}\|^2 + \|q_{[k]21}\|^2 + \|q_{[k]22}\|^2)^{\frac{1}{2}}}_{\text{Frob. norm of } \begin{pmatrix} \|q_{[k]11}\| & \|q_{[k]12}\| \\ \|q_{[k]21}\| & \|q_{[k]22}\| \end{pmatrix}} \mathsf{M}^k \, . \qquad (23.9)$$

For a tensor field of an arbitrary order:

$$\hat{\mathsf{T}} = \sum_{k=1}^{n(n+1)/2} \left(\sum_{i_1 \ldots i_n} \|q_{[k]i_1 \ldots i_n}\|^2 \right)^{\frac{1}{2}} \mathsf{M}^k \, , \qquad (23.10)$$

where subscripts $i_1 \ldots i_n$ are associated to the components of the tensor field.

This generalization is consistent with the fact that each component adds its own local structure (edges, lines, etc), and the sum of the filter responses only adds isotropic information unless they provide additional high structure.

23.3 Anisotropic Tensor Field Filtering

The Wiener filter is the optimal linear estimator that balances the trade-off between smoothing the signal discontinuities and removal of the noise. However, real signals are not Gaussian distributed and this technique produces an excessive blurring of high structure regions.

In this section, we present a general filtering technique that adapts spatially, following the local complexity coded by the structure tensor of the data field, a Wiener filter. This scheme enables filtering scalar, vector and higher order tensor fields [9]. The method is based on an extension of the classical unsharp masking [14], using the Wiener filter as the low-pass component, intended to get the coarse information, and the remaining as a set of high-pass filters oriented in different directions, that give the level of detail at each direction. The high-pass filters are obtained from the subtraction of the low pass filter to all-pass ones oriented in the corresponding directions. These components, the low-pass and high-pass ones, are balanced by a general local structure tensor for the tensor field that weights their importance (coarse and detail information). A previous version of this method, intended to be used on scalar data, along with a comparison with a state-of-the-art anisotropic diffusion technique was presented in [8]. Our method showed a better behavior enhancing closed structures like joints, while flux-diffusion worked better for thin structures as vessels. This result is due to the eigenvectors of the structure tensor respond better in regions of closed structures, where estimating the gradient and principal curvatures is more difficult.

The filtering scheme for tensor fields is based on the independent application of the same anisotropic scalar filter to every component, though the local structure measure is obtained from the whole input tensor field.

The scalar filter consists of a bank of steerable filters forming a basis:

$$s_r(\mathbf{x}) = s_{lp}(\mathbf{x}) + \sum_{k=1}^{n(n+1)/2} a_k(\mathbf{x})\, s_{hp_k}(\mathbf{x}) \ , \qquad (23.11)$$

where s_r denotes the global filter output of a n-dimensional dataset, s_{lp} and s_{hp_k}, the outputs to the low-pass and high-pass filters, respectively, and a_k the coefficients that weight the contribution of detail of every high-pass component. Obviously, these coefficients are related to the local complexity given by $\hat{\mathsf{T}}$ (23.7) and, hence, they can be obtained from the projection of $\hat{\mathsf{T}}$ onto every high-pass filter orientation $\hat{\mathbf{n}}_k$. Since we associate a basis tensor M^k to each orientation, the *dual tensors* associated to the outer products of the filter directions, $\{\hat{\mathbf{n}}_k \hat{\mathbf{n}}_k^t\}$, the coefficients a_k are obtained from the inner product of $\hat{\mathsf{T}}$ (normalized) and the basis tensors: $\langle \hat{\mathsf{T}}, \mathsf{M}^k \rangle$. This operation will yield a measure of the importance of the detail in each direction.

In the case of a tensor field of an arbitrary order, applying (23.11) to each tensor component $i_1 \ldots i_n$, and using the generalized local structure tensor $\hat{\mathsf{T}}$ (23.10), we obtain:

$$s_r(\mathbf{x})_{i_1 \ldots i_n} = s_{lp}(\mathbf{x})_{i_1 \ldots i_n} + \sum_{k=1}^{\frac{n\,(n+1)}{2}} < \hat{\mathsf{T}}, \mathsf{M}^k > s_{hp_k}(\mathbf{x})_{i_1 \ldots i_n} \ , \qquad (23.12)$$

where $s_{r\ i_1 \ldots i_n}$, $s_{lp_{i_1 \ldots i_n}}$ and $s_{hp_k\ i_1 \ldots i_n}$ follow the same interpretation than in the scalar case (23.11) for every tensor field component $i_1 \ldots i_n$. Note that this scheme is different of a multichannel filtering technique, because the high structure information of the tensor field is included in the general local structure tensor, and it affects to each tensor component taking in account the correlation between components.

In Fig. 23.1, some results applying this scheme to 2-D synthetic tensor data are presented.

One of the applications of this technique is regularizing the 3-D diffusion tensor field associated to the *diffusion tensor magnetic resonance imaging* (DT-MRI) modality. Our results with this type of data can be seen in Fig. 23.2. Although the estimated diffusion tensor should be positive semidefinite, our scheme doesn't guarantee this constraint, and to avoid small negatives eigenvalues, we set the negative eigenvalues to zero. It can be shown that this is optimal in a *least squares* sense, and equivalent to a projection onto the subspace of positive semidefinite tensors.

If we compare qualitatively our scheme with other approaches presented in Chaps. 21, 24 and 25, we can conclude that:

- Our scheme is non-iterative, and propose an alternative to PDEs techniques.
- Although the normalized convolution is non-iterative, it is not strictly anisotropic. Our technique uses the local structure tensor to drive the process.

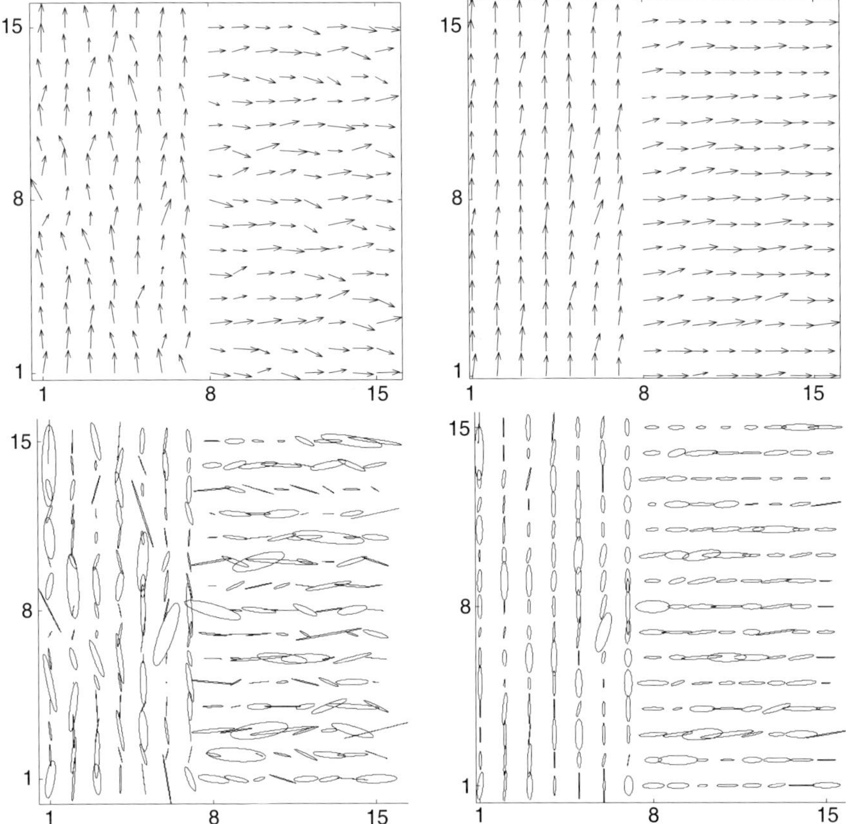

Fig. 23.1. (**a**) Synthetic random noisy 2-D vector field; (**b**) regularized vector field; (**c**) synthetic random noisy 2-D second-order tensor field represented as ellipses; (**d**) regularized tensor field. The noise is white, additive, and Gaussian with zero mean and 0.2 standard deviation. Notice how vectors and tensors are more aligned, while preserving the edge

- The design of our filtering scheme allows easier parallelization of the regularization process, compared to other techniques.

23.4 Applications

23.4.1 Structure Weighted Interpolation

Similarly to the scalar case, interpolating tensor data requires to estimate tensors at unsampled points in order to obtain an upsampled tensor field [7]. In this section a recently anisotropic interpolation technique for tensor data [2]

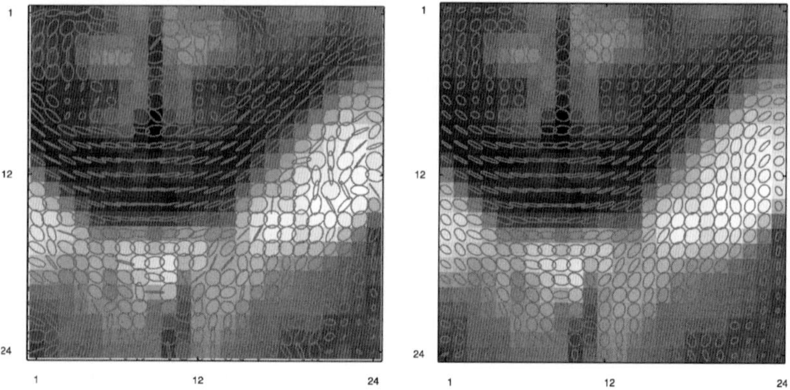

Fig. 23.2. *Left*: A 25×25 zoomed corpus callosum region of a slice in a DT-MRI dataset, overlapped by the 2D projections of the diffusion tensor (*ellipses*) in every point; *right*: the result after our filtering approach (see colour plates)

is presented, using the local structure tensor as a *metric tensor* to adaptively weight the samples.

This approach to interpolate assumes that the unknown tensor $\hat{D}$ in an upsampled point $\mathbf{x}$ can be estimated as a linear combination of tensor data sampled in a neighborhood $\mathcal{N}(\mathbf{x})$, as

$$\hat{D}(\mathbf{x}) = \frac{\sum_{i \in \mathcal{N}(\mathbf{x})} \omega_i \, D(\mathbf{x}_i)}{\sum_{i \in \mathcal{N}(\mathbf{x})} \omega_i} \; , \tag{23.13}$$

where ω_i denote the weights of each sample at $\mathbf{x}_i$.

Different interpolators and estimators assign different weights to samples. In some cases it is possible to obtain very efficient separable kernels. Nevertheless, in order to preserve edges, the local structure should be accounted for, and the estimator must be spatially adaptive.

Suppose, for example, that the weights are obtained as inversely proportional to the squared distance to the samples, $\omega_i = ||\mathbf{x} - \mathbf{x}_i||^{-2}$. This inverse squared distance interpolator is usual in many applications with conventional scalar images, but it smooths boundaries and other highly structured regions. Then, if only the distance between samples and the point to be estimated is considered, the estimator mixes high structure regions, i.e. edges, even though they are spatially close. Therefore an analysis of the local complexity of the signal is necessary prior to assigning weights to samples in order to avoid this behavior.

In order to simplify, and to keep the computational complexity as low as possible, the interpolation is based on the 4 nearest samples in 2-D and on the 8 nearest samples in 3-D; this could obviously be extended easily to larger neighborhoods. For regular discrete arrays, the interpolated point is located

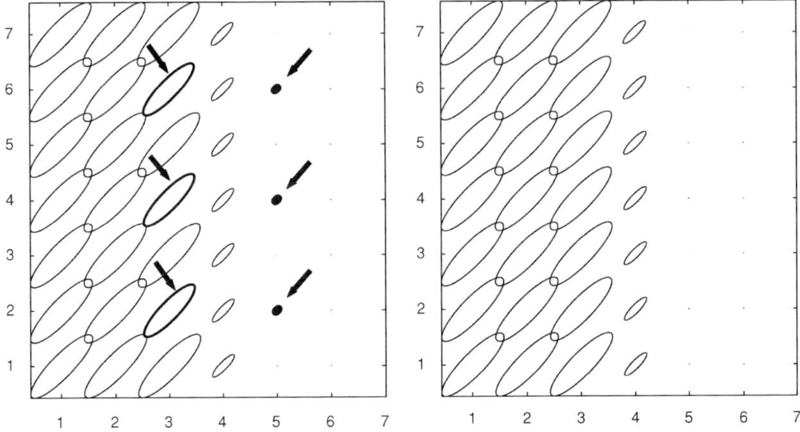

Fig. 23.3. Results from interpolation of tensor valued data. A constant tensor edge has been upsampled by a factor of two. *Left*: linear interpolation; *right*: anisotropic interpolation

in the center of the pixel/voxel, on an edge/side. The process is carried out in successive sweeps to interpolate in the centers, edges or sides.

The local structure tensor can be used to control how samples are weighted when building signal estimators. For instance, samples from two different sides of a strong edge should not be combined. Samples should be weighted along the direction of maximum signal variation less than those in the orthogonal one. Although the Euclidean distance between the interpolated point and data samples is the same, their contributions will be different. Hence, the weights for the linear combination in (23.13) are computed as

$$\omega_i = \frac{1}{(\mathbf{x} - \mathbf{x}_i)^t \, \hat{\mathsf{T}} \, (\mathbf{x} - \mathbf{x}_i)} \, , \tag{23.14}$$

with $\hat{\mathsf{T}}$ the local structure tensor of the tensor field. Since the weights are positive (the metric tensors are positive semidefinite), the interpolated tensors, if input tensors are PSDs (e.g. DT-MRI volume) will satisfy the PSD constraint.

In Fig. 23.3, we present a simple synthetic example that compares our approach with an isotropic one. Notice that the edge is smeared out further using linear interpolation compared to the method using the structure tensor as a local metric. Again, the main application to this scheme is the interpolation in DT-MRI modality. In Fig. 23.4 we present an interpolation test on the image presented before.

23.4.2 Structure Weighted Registration

Image registration consists of finding the coordinate transformation (also referred to as deformation or displacement field) that relates two different images: source and target. Hence when the transformation is applied to the

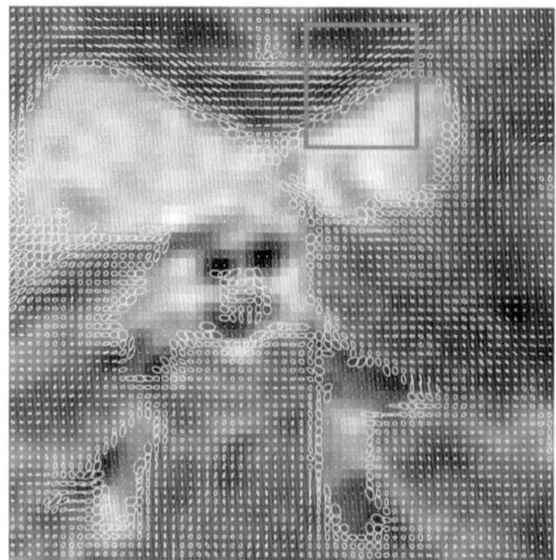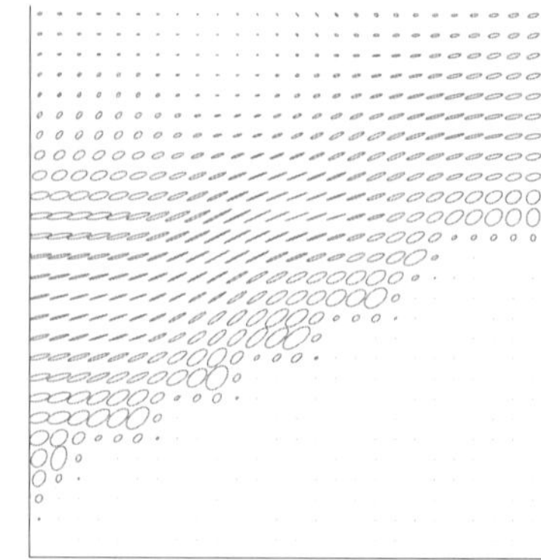

Fig. 23.4. *Left*: DT-MRI section of the *corpus callosum*; *right*: upsampling of the framed region (see colour plates)

source image, an image with the same geometry than the target one is obtained. In this case, regularization enforces the estimated field to fulfill the constraints of spatial coherence, smoothness and eventually invertibility of the estimated field.

Intensity based registration methods, usually correspond to one of two important families: template matching and variational. Template matching finds the displacement for every voxel in a source image by minimizing a local cost measure, obtained from a small neighborhood of the source image and a set of potential correspondent neighborhoods in a target image. In the case of template matching, regularization may be achieved by means of the *Normalized Convolution* [16], a refinement of weighted-least squares that explicitly deals with the so-called signal/certainty philosophy. Essentially, a scalar measure of local structure (the certainty), obtained from our structure tensor as [3, 10, 12, 13]

$$structure\,(\mathbf{x}) = \frac{\det \hat{\mathsf{T}}(\mathbf{x})}{\operatorname{trace}\,\hat{\mathsf{T}}(\mathbf{x})} \tag{23.15}$$

is incorporated as a weighting function in a least squares fashion. The field (the signal) obtained from template matching is then projected onto a vector space described by a non-orthogonal basis, i.e., the dot products between the field and every element of the basis provide covariant components that must be converted into contravariant by an appropriate metric tensor. Normalized convolution, explained in detail in Chap. 24 of this book, provides a simple and efficient implementation of this operation. Besides, an applicability function is enforced on the basis elements in order to guarantee a proper localization and avoid high frequency artifacts. This way the simplicity of template matching is kept while its drawbacks are addressed. Figure 23.5 shows a 2-D discrete deformation field that has been regularized using the certainty on the left side and a 2-D Gaussian applicability function with $\sigma = 0.8$.

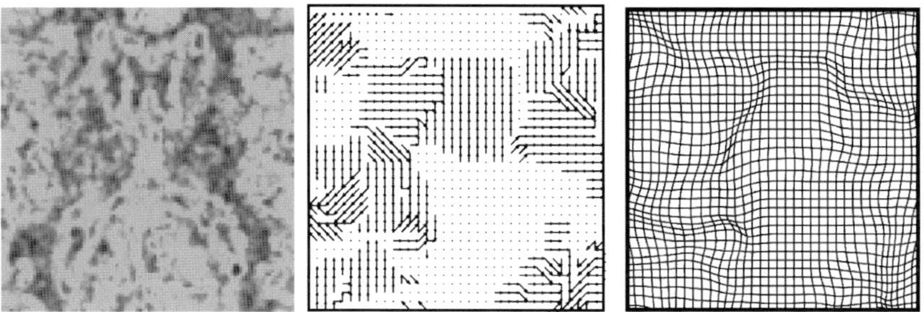

Fig. 23.5. *Left*: local structure from an axial section of the ventricles (certainty); *center*: discrete matching displacement (*signal*); *right*: weighted filtered deformation

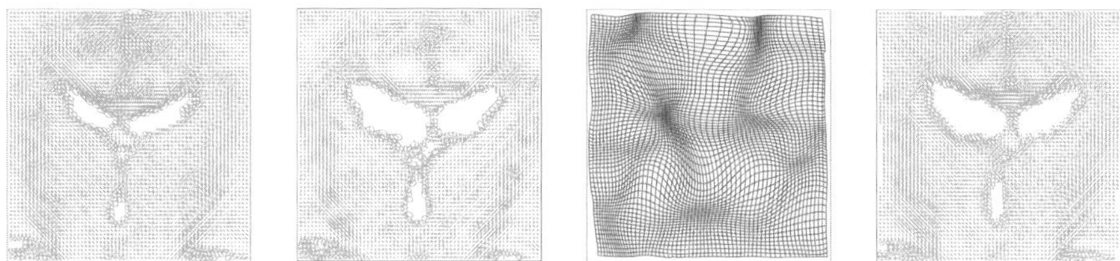

Fig. 23.6. Registration of two DT-MR images. (**a**) source tensor image; (**b**) target tensor image; (**c**) estimated deformation field, shown as a warping, from target to source; (**d**) source deformed (see colour plates)

This regularization technique has been implemented in a Gaussian pyramidal block-matching scheme [15], which works similarly to Kovačič and Bajcsy's [6]. In the highest level, the deformation field is estimated by template matching and regularized. In the next level, the source dataset is deformed with a displacement field obtained by spatial upsampling and interpolation of the one obtained in the previous level. The target and deformed source datasets are then registered to obtain the displacement field corresponding to the current level of resolution. This process is propagated to every level in the pyramid. Improvements may be found in literature.

Figure 23.6 shows the registration of two axial sections of DT-MR images of two different patients. Images have been registered using the norm of the difference [1] as the similarity measure, a Gaussian applicability of $\sigma = 1, 5$ and seven pyramidal levels.

Acknowledgment

The authors acknowledge the Spanish Comisión Interministerial de Ciencia y Tecnología for the project TIC2001-3808-C02-01.

References

1. D. C. Alexander, J.C. Gee, and R. K. Bajcsy. Similarity measures for matching diffusion tensor images. In *Proc. British Machine Vision Conference*, 1999.
2. Castaño-Moraga C.A., Rodriguez-Florido M.A., Alvarez L., Westin C.-F., Ruiz-Alzola J. Anisotropic interpolation of DT-MRI. In LNCS 3216, MICCAI. pp. 343–350, 2004.
3. C. Harris and M. Stephens. A combined corner and edge detector. In *Proceedings of the Fourth Alvey Vision Conference*, pp. 147–151, 1988.
4. Knutsson, H. Representing local structure using tensors. In *6th Scandinavian Conference on Image Analysis. Oulu, Finland*, pp. 244–251, 1989.
5. Knutsson H., and Andersson M. What's so good about quadrature filters? In *2003 IEEE International Conference on Image Processing*, 2003.
6. Stanislav Kovacic and R.K. Bajcsy. *Brain Warping*, chapter Multi-scale/Multiresolution Representations, pp. 45–65. Academic Press, 1999.
7. Pajevic S., Aldroubi A., and Basser P.J. A continuous tensor field approximation of discrete DT-MRI data for extracting microstructural and architectural features of tissue. *Journal of Magnetic Resonance*, 154:85–100, 2002.
8. Rodriguez-Florido M.A., Krissian K., Ruiz-Alzola J., Westin C.-F. Comparison between two restoration techniques in the context of 3d medical imaging. *LNCS – Springer-Verlag*, 2208:1031–1039, 2001.
9. Rodriguez-Florido M.A., Westin C.-F., and Ruiz-Alzola J. DT-MRI regularization using anisotropic tensor field filtering. In *2004 IEEE International Symposium on Biomedical Imaging*, pp. 336–339, 2004.
10. K. Rohr. On 3D differential operators for detecting point landmarks. *Image and Vision Computing*, 15:219–233, 1997.
11. Christian Ronse. On idempotence and related requirements in edge detection. *IEEE Transactions on Pattern Analysis and Machine Intelligence*, 15(5):484–490, 1993.
12. J. Ruiz-Alzola, R. Kikinis, and C.-F. Westin. Detection of point landmarks in multidimensional tensor data. *Signal Processing*, 81:2243–2247, 2001.
13. J. Ruiz-Alzola, C.F. Westin, S.K. Warfield, A. Nabavi, and R. Kikinis. Nonrigid registration of 3D scalar, vector and tensor medical data. In *MICCAI*, pp. 541–550, 2000.
14. Schriber,W.F. Wirephoto quality improvement by unsharp masking. *J.Pattern Recognition*, 2:117–121, 1970.
15. Eduardo Suárez, Carl-Fredrik Westin, Eduardo Rovaris, and Juan Ruiz-Alzola. Nonrigid registration using regularized matching weighted by local structure. In *MICCAI*, number 2 in LNCS, pp. 581–589, Tokyo, Japan, September 2002.
16. C-F. Westin. *A Tensor Framework for Multidimensional Signal Processing*. PhD thesis, Linköping University, Sweden, SE-581 83 Linköping, Sweden, 1994. Dissertation No 348, ISBN 91-7871-421-4.

Tensor Field Regularization using Normalized Convolution and Markov Random Fields in a Bayesian Framework

Carl-Fredrik Westin, Marcos Martin-Fernandez, Carlos Alberola-Lopez, Juan Ruiz-Alzola, and Hans Knutsson

Laboratory of Mathematics in Imaging, Brigham and Women's Hospital, Harvard Medical School, Boston, MA 02115, USA
{westin,marcma}@bwh.harvard.edu

Summary. This chapter presents two techniques for regularization of tensor fields. We first present a nonlinear filtering technique based on normalized convolution, a general method for filtering missing and uncertain data. We describe how the signal certainty function can be constructed to depend on locally derived certainty information and further combined with a spatially dependent certainty field. This results in reduced mixing between regions of different signal characteristics, and increased robustness to outliers, compared to the standard approach of normalized convolution using only a spatial certainty field. We contrast this deterministic approach with a stochastic technique based on a multivariate Gaussian signal model in a Bayesian framework. This method uses a Markov random field approach with a 3D neighborhood system for modeling spatial interactions between the tensors locally. Experiments both on synthetic and real data are presented. The driving tensor application for this work throughout the chapter is the filtering of diffusion tensor MRI data.

24.1 Introduction

Using conventional MRI, we can easily identify the functional centers of the brain (cortex and nuclei). However, with conventional anatomical MRI techniques, the white matter of the brain appears to be homogeneous without any suggestion of the complex arrangement of fiber tracts. Diffusion Tensor MRI (DT-MRI) is a relatively recent imaging modality that measures the diffusion of water in biological tissue. A common first order model of anisotropic diffusion is the Gaussian model that gives ellipsoidal isoprobability surfaces describing the diffusion. This then naturally leads to the tensor representation through the analogy between symmetric 3×3 tensors to the ellipsoidal representation. Within white matter, the mobility of the water is restricted by the axons that are oriented along the fiber tracts. Hence, the demonstration of anisotropic diffusion in the brain by MRI has paved the way for non-invasive exploration of the structural anatomy of the white matter in vivo [1, 12]. Alexander presents a good introduction to DT-MRI and the diffusion process in Chap. 5.

The diffusion weighted MRI images are corrupted by noise. There are many factors that contribute to the noise. One source is associated with the receiving coil resistance, others come from inductive losses. The major source of noise will depend on the strength of the static magnetic field and the volume sample size. In addition, the final image noise can also depend on other factors like the voxel size, the receiver bandwidth and the number of time averages in the acquisition process [4]. Hahn et al. discuss the origin of the noise and its impact in Chap. 6. By imposing smoothness or regularization constraints on the tensor field the amount of noise can be reduced. In this chapter we will present two different types of regularization approaches: one deterministic and one stochastic. An overview of other recent regularization methods can be found in [15].

24.2 Normalized Convolution

In this section we outline how normalized convolution (NC) can be used for regularizing scalar, vector, and higher order tensor fields. The method presented here closely follows the description in [17].

NC was introduced as a general method for filtering missing and uncertain data [7, 16]. This method can be viewed as locally solving a weighted least squares (WLS) problem. A local description of a signal, $\mathbf{f}$, can be defined using a weighted sum of basis functions stored as columns, $\mathbf{B}$. Minimizing[1]

$$||\mathbf{W}(\mathbf{B}\boldsymbol{\theta} - \mathbf{f})|| \tag{24.1}$$

with respect to the weights $\boldsymbol{\theta}$, which are the coordinates of the signal in the basis $\mathbf{B}$, results in the WLS solution [5]

$$\mathbf{f}_0 = \mathbf{B}\boldsymbol{\theta} = \mathbf{B}(\mathbf{B}^*\mathbf{W}^T\mathbf{W}\mathbf{B})^{-1}\mathbf{B}^*\mathbf{W}^T\mathbf{W}\mathbf{f} , \tag{24.2}$$

where $\mathbf{B}^*$ is the conjugate transpose of $\mathbf{B}$.

In NC the weights $\mathbf{W}$ are split into two parts. One that belongs to the basis functions and usually referred to as the applicability function a, a scalar windowing function that deals with spatial localization of the operators in $\mathbf{B}$. This provides an alternative to traditional windowing with the advantage of not changing the function values.

The second part belongs to the signal and is referred to as the signal certainty function c describing the credence of the signal samples. Missing

---

[1] The norm of a matrix $\mathbf{A}$ is the Frobenius norm given by $||\mathbf{A}|| = \sqrt{tr(\mathbf{A}^T\mathbf{A})}$, where $tr(\mathbf{A})$ is the trace and $\mathbf{A}^T$ the transpose of $\mathbf{A}$.

samples are handled by setting this function to zero. Note that handling missing data in a more traditional way by for example setting the signal values to zero would introduce artificial structures in the image. Further, the certainty function is usually set to zero outside the signal border reducing the impact of traditional edge effects.

The weight matrix $\mathbf{W}$ can be constructed by multiplying two diagonal matrices containing the applicability and the certainties in the diagonal respectively, $\mathbf{W}_a$ and $\mathbf{W}_c$. To keep in line with established notation [16] we define $\mathbf{W}^T\mathbf{W} = \mathbf{W}_a\mathbf{W}_c$ which will avoid squaring the weights in the calculations. Inserting this into equation (24.2) gives

$$\mathbf{f}_0 = \mathbf{B}\boldsymbol{\theta} = \mathbf{B}(\mathbf{B}^*\mathbf{W}_a\mathbf{W}_c\mathbf{B})^{-1}\mathbf{B}^*\mathbf{W}_a\mathbf{W}_c\mathbf{f} \ . \tag{24.3}$$

24.2.1 Certainty Measures

There are several ways to define signal certainty function c. For simplicity we here will use

$$c = c_v c_s \tag{24.4}$$

where c_v is the voxel certainty and c_s is the similarity certainty. The spatial voxel certainty measure c_v is defined by the input data. Further, the similarity certainty measure c_s has been constructed as:

$$c_s = c_m c_a \ , \tag{24.5}$$

where c_m and c_a are the magnitude and angular similarity measures, respectively. For the magnitude certainty c_m the following Gaussian magnitude function has been used

$$c_m = \exp\left[-\left(\frac{||\mathbf{T}_0|| - ||\mathbf{T}||}{\sigma}\right)^2\right], \tag{24.6}$$

where the norm of a tensor is given by $||\mathbf{T}|| = \sqrt{tr(\mathbf{T}^T\mathbf{T})}$, and $\mathbf{T}_0$ is a tensor calculated from a local neighborhood as explained in Sect. 24.2.3. The angular similarity measure, c_a, is based on the inner product between the normalized tensors and is given by

$$c_a = \langle\hat{\mathbf{T}}_0, \hat{\mathbf{T}}\rangle^\alpha = tr(\hat{\mathbf{T}}_0^T\hat{\mathbf{T}})^\alpha \tag{24.7}$$

where $\hat{\mathbf{T}} = \mathbf{T}/||\mathbf{T}||$. In general the spatial voxel certainty function, c_v, will be based on prior information about the data. The voxel certainty is set to zero outside the signal extent to reduce unwanted border effects. If no specific local information is available the voxel certainty is set to one. As described above, the second certainty component, c_s, is defined locally based on neighboring information. The idea here is to reduce the impact of outliers, where an outlier is defined in terms of the local signal neighborhood, and to reduce the blurring across interfaces between regions having very different signal characteristics.

24.2.2 Applicability Functions

The applicability function define the localization of the operator. The family of applicability functions used in the examples in this chapter is given by

$$a = \begin{cases} r^{-\alpha} \cos^{\beta}\left(\frac{\pi\ r}{2r_{\max}}\right) & r < r_{\max} \\ 0 & \text{otherwise} \end{cases} \tag{24.8}$$

where r denotes the distance from the neighborhood center and α, β and $r_{\max}$ are positive constants.

24.2.3 Simple Local Neighborhood Model

The simplest possible model in the NC framework is when using only one constant basis function, simplifying the expression for the NC (24.3) to a ratio of convolutions[2] [7]:

$$\mathbf{T}_0(m,n,p) = \frac{\sum\limits_{i,j,k} a(m+i, j+n, k+p)c_v(i, j, k)\mathbf{T}(i, j, k)}{\sum\limits_{i,j,k} a(m+i, j+n, k+p)c_v(i, j, k)} \tag{24.9}$$

where (m, n, p) are the indexes that correspond to each voxel. To focus on the power of introducing the signal/model similarity certainty measure, this simple local neighborhood model is used in our examples below.

24.2.4 Scalar Field Regularization

Before describing the tensor case (Sect. 24.2.5), we will first present a scalar example to show the effect of the the voxel and magnitude certainty functions. This concept can be seen as generalization of bilateral filtering [14] into the signal-certainty framework of normalized convolution.

Figure 24.1 shows the result of filtering a scalar signal using the proposed technique. Figure 24.1(a) shows the original scalar signal: a noisy step function. Figure 24.1(b) shows the result using standard NC demonstrating that reduction of noise is achieved at the expense of unwanted mixing of features from adjacent regions. The amount of border blurring can be controlled effectively by including the new magnitude certainty measure, c_m, given by equation (24.6). The smaller the σ value, the smaller the inter region averaging. The result for $\sigma = 2$ is shown in Fig. 24.1(c).

---

[2] Using correlation or convolution is a matter of preference since the applicability function is in general symmetric.

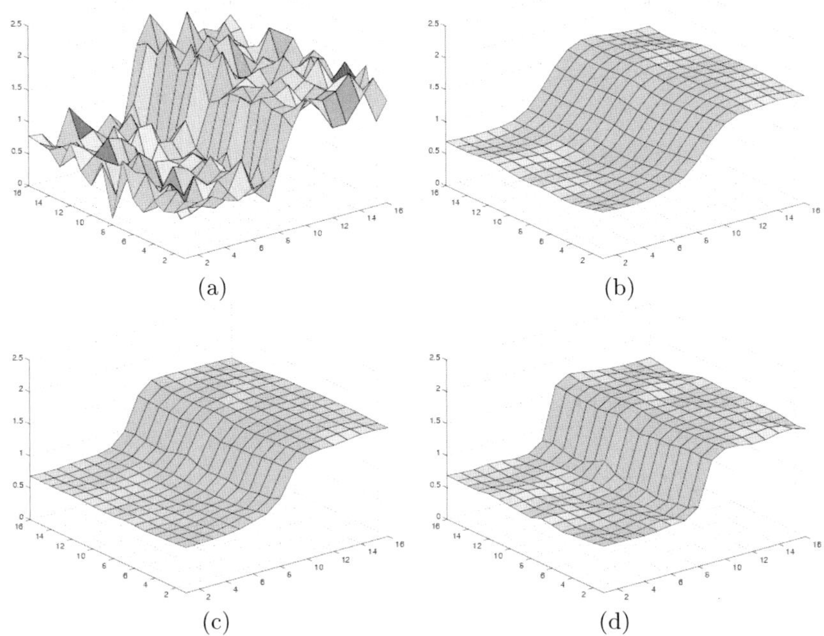

Fig. 24.1. Original scalar field (*step edge*) with added noise (**a**), the result without using the magnitude certainty measurement c_m (**b**), results using c_m with $\sigma = 1$ (**c**) and with $\sigma = 0.5$ (**d**). See appendix for color plates

24.2.5 Tensor Field Regularization

Figure 24.2 shows the result of filtering a synthetic 2D tensor field visualized using ellipses. The original tensor field with added noise is shown in Fig. 24.2(a) and the result in Fig. 24.2(b). In this example, the voxel certainty measure, c_v, was set to one except outside the signal extent where it was set to zero. When filtering tensor data, the angular measure c_a is important since it can be used to reduce mixing of information from regions having different orientations. This is demonstrated in Fig. 24.2(c) using $\alpha = 0$ and in Fig. 24.2(d) with $\alpha = 2$. Notice how the degree of mixing depends on the angular similarity measure.

Figure 24.3 shows a region of interest (ROI) for tensor field generated from DT-MRI data. Figure 24.3(b) shows the result of filtering the DT-MRI tensor field using the proposed method. In this example, the voxel certainty measure, c_v, was set to one except outside the signal extent where it was set to zero. An alternative to this is to use for example Proton Density MRI data defining where the MR signal is reliable. For the angular certainty function, c_a, $\alpha = 4$ was used.

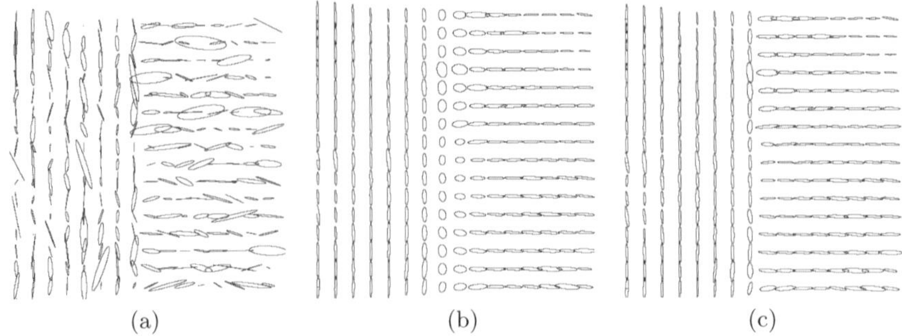

(a)   (b)   (c)

Fig. 24.2. Original synthetic tensor field with added noise (**a**) and the result using the proposed method using $\alpha = 0$ (**b**) and $\alpha = 2$ (**c**)

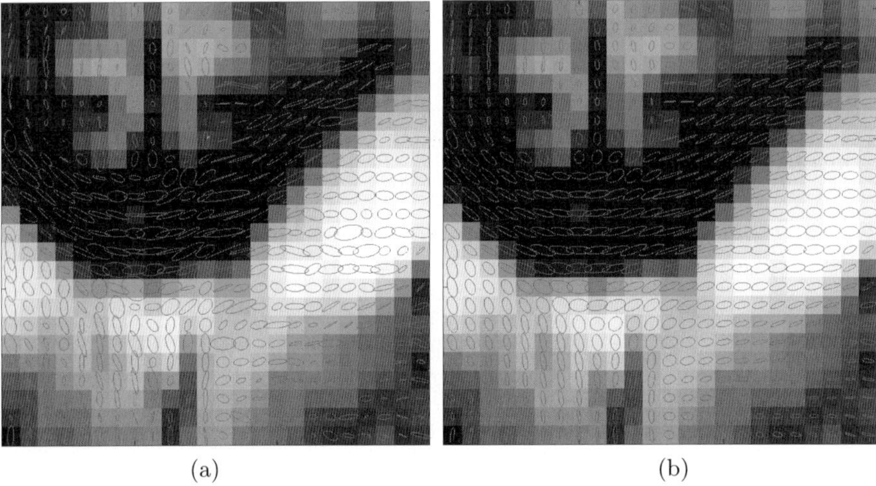

(a)   (b)

Fig. 24.3. Tensor field generated from noisy DT-MRI data (**a**) and result of filtering the tensor field using the NC method (**b**). The ROI is the corpus callosum, the dark bow-shaped region. See appendix for color plates

24.3 Bayesian Regularization using Multivariate Gaussian Markov Random Fields

The use of MRFs for regularization of tensor fields has gained interest in the last few years [13]. We will discuss a new approach for regularization of DT-MRI data using Markov Random Fields (MRFs) in a Bayesian framework [8, 9, 10]. The MRFs that are going to be described have Gaussian distribution [11]. A description of multivariate Gaussian distributed noise for tensors is presented in [2]. The concept of 'isotropic' noise is defined resulting in a distribution whose covariance has two parameters. Our noise model is not constrained to be isotropic so a non-constrained model for the covariance will be used. In this chapter we define a Bayesian model where MRFs are used for

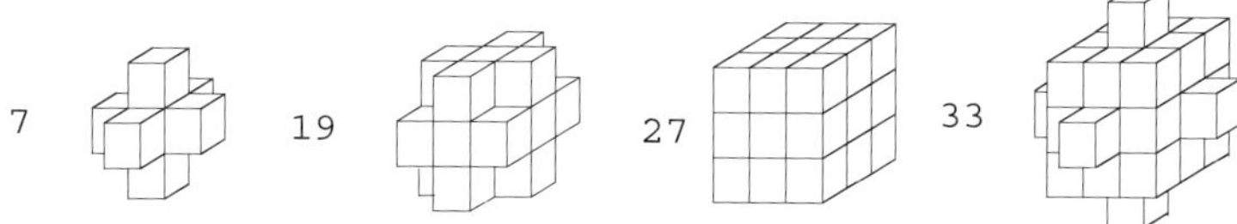

Fig. 24.4. Examples of 3D neighborhood systems $\delta(m, n, p)$ with different spatial extent. The numbers indicate the number of voxels L belonging to each system

achieving a global result from local interactions described by a simple neighborhood model [19]. We will first present a scalar version of the model and later extend this to the tensor case.

24.3.1 Prior Probability Model

Let the (non-observable) scalar volume that we want estimate be described by a random vector $\mathbf{X}$ with K elements. This vector is formed by rearranging the original data with dimensions $M \times N \times P$, and thus giving $K = MNP$ elements.

We assume that the prior probability density function (PDF) of the non-observable scalar field $\mathbf{X}$ is a K-dimensional multivariate Gauss-MRF [11] defined by a $K \times 1$ mean vector $\boldsymbol{\mu}$, and a $K \times K$ covariance matrix $\mathbf{C}$.

As the 3D spatial dependencies are assumed to be strictly local, the covariance matrix $\mathbf{C}$ will be sparse, and thus it will be more practical to work directly with the local characteristics of the field. This is achieved by defining a 3D neighborhood system $\delta(m, n, p)$ for each voxel. Each $\delta(m, n, p)$ is a set of L triplet indices. In Fig. 24.4, four different neighborhoods are shown. Using each index set (one for each voxel site) we can define the sets of neighboring random vectors $\delta X(m, n, p)$ with L elements as

$$\delta X(m, n, p) = \left\{ X(m', n', p'), (m', n', p') \in \delta(m, n, p) \right\} \tag{24.10}$$

and the same for the squared image values $\delta X^2(m, n, p)$,

$$\delta X^2(m, n, p) = \left\{ X^2(m', n', p'), (m', n', p') \in \delta(m, n, p) \right\} . \tag{24.11}$$

Under these assumptions the local characteristic of the field is given by the following conditional Gauss-MRF[3] [11]

$$p(X|\delta X) = \frac{1}{\sqrt{2\pi}\,\sigma_X} \exp\left\{ -\frac{(X - \mu_X)^2}{2\sigma_X^2} \right\} \tag{24.12}$$

---

[3] For simplicity we are omitting describing the dependence of the voxel indices (m, n, p), unless explicitly specified.

with

$$\mu_X = \frac{1}{L}\sum \delta X \qquad\qquad \sigma_X^2 = \frac{1}{L}\sum \delta X^2 - \mu_X^2 \qquad (24.13)$$

the prior local mean and variance, respectively, both estimated with the maximum likelihood (ML) method [5]. The summations in (24.13) is over the L elements of the sets $\boldsymbol{\delta}X$ and $\boldsymbol{\delta}X^2$ as defined in (24.10) and (24.11), respectively.

24.3.2 Likelihood Model

In this section we will define a likelihood model for the observed (noisy) signal. Let the observed scalar signal be defined by

$$\mathbf{Y} = \mathbf{X} + \mathbf{N} \qquad (24.14)$$

where $\mathbf{X}$ is the wanted (non-observable) signal, and where $\mathbf{N}$ denotes the noise. For simplicity we assume that the noise is independent of the signal $\mathbf{X}$ to be estimated. The likelihood model (also called transition model) is given by the conditional PDF of the observed signal $\mathbf{Y}$ given $\mathbf{X}$, which is assumed to be a K-dimensional multivariate Gauss-MRF with given $K \times 1$ mean vector $\mathbf{X}$ and $K \times K$ covariance matrix $\mathbf{C}_N$.

In the likelihood model we will exploit the spatial dependencies of the MRF to determine the local likelihood characteristic of the scalar data. This is achieved by assuming the following local conditional independence property for the PDF

$$p(Y|X, \boldsymbol{\delta}X) = p(Y|X) \qquad (24.15)$$

which is here described by a conditional Gauss-MRF

$$p(Y|X) = \frac{1}{\sqrt{2\pi}\sigma_N} \exp\left\{ -\frac{(Y-X)^2}{2\sigma_N^2} \right\}, \qquad (24.16)$$

where the local noise variance $\sigma_N^2 = \sigma_{Y|X}^2$ is assumed to be homogeneous, that is, independent of the spatial indices (m, n, p). This variance has to be estimated from the observed scalar volume $\mathbf{Y}$. The estimator for the noise variance used in the examples below is

$$\sigma_N^2 = \lambda \sigma_{N_{\text{ave}}}^2 + (1 - \lambda)\sigma_{N_{\text{min}}}^2 , \qquad (24.17)$$

where $0 \leq \lambda \leq 1$ is a free parameter defining the degree of regularization (low λ gives low regularization). The average local variance $\sigma_{N_{\text{mean}}}^2$ is given by

$$\sigma_{N_{\text{ave}}}^2 = \frac{1}{K} \sum_{m=1}^{M} \sum_{n=1}^{N} \sum_{p=1}^{P} \sigma_Y^2(m, n, p) , \qquad (24.18)$$

and where $\sigma_Y^2(m, n, p)$ is given by the ML method following the (24.13) replacing all the X variables with Y. The minimum local variance $\sigma_{N_{\text{min}}}^2$ is given by

$$\sigma^2_{N_{\min}} = \min_{m,n,p} \sigma^2_Y(m,n,p) \tag{24.19}$$

The reasoning for (24.17) is that as the signal and the noise are independent, and the total variance is given by adding the noise and the signal variance. A possible estimator for the noise variance would then be given by a total variance estimator in a region for which the signal is zero. If we consider the local variance as a realization for the total variance, then the minimum among this local variances will be a possible estimator for the noise variance (24.19). However, due to the presence of outliers and that the local variance has significant variability, this minimum will have a bias towards zero. An alternative estimator for the noise variance is given by the average of the local variances (24.18). In this case, due to the presence of signal components in the local variances, this estimator will have a bias towards infinity. A trade-off between these two estimators can be defined by introducing a regularization parameter λ ranging in the interval $(0,1)$ reducing the effect of these biases (24.17). The two estimators in (24.18) and (24.19) naturally define two bounds that can be used to define the maximum and minimum meaningful amount of regularization, and the parameter λ between 0 and 1 can be used as a regularization parameter to tune the desired amount of regularization.

24.3.3 Posterior Probability Modeling

This section describes how to combine the prior probability model for the estimated signal with the likelihood model for the observed signal. Bayes' theorem lets us write the posterior probability density function as

$$p(\mathbf{X}|\mathbf{Y}) = \frac{p(\mathbf{Y}|\mathbf{X})p(\mathbf{X})}{p(\mathbf{Y})}, \tag{24.20}$$

where $p(\mathbf{Y})$ depends only on the known signal $\mathbf{Y}$.

In the Gaussian case the maximum a posteriori (MAP) estimation is equal to the minimum mean square error (MMSE) estimation [5] given both by

$$\mathbf{X}_{\mathrm{MAP}} = \arg\max_{\mathbf{X}} p(\mathbf{X}|\mathbf{Y}) = \mathbf{X}_{\mathrm{MMSE}} = E[\mathbf{X}|\mathbf{Y}] = \boldsymbol{\mu}_{\mathbf{X}|\mathbf{Y}} \tag{24.21}$$

with $\boldsymbol{\mu}_{\mathbf{X}|\mathbf{Y}}$ defined by

$$\boldsymbol{\mu}_{\mathbf{X}|\mathbf{Y}} = \mathbf{C}_{\mathbf{N}}\left(\mathbf{C}_{\mathbf{X}} + \mathbf{C}_{\mathbf{N}}\right)^{-1}\boldsymbol{\mu}_{\mathbf{X}} + \mathbf{C}_{\mathbf{X}}\left(\mathbf{C}_{\mathbf{X}} + \mathbf{C}_{\mathbf{N}}\right)^{-1}\mathbf{Y}. \tag{24.22}$$

In general, it is not feasible to explicitly determine $\mathbf{C}_{\mathbf{X}}$, $\mathbf{C}_{\mathbf{N}}$ and $\boldsymbol{\mu}_{\mathbf{X}}$, and we will resort to either the Gibbs sampler (GS) algorithm to iteratively find a solution for the MMSE estimation or the simulated annealing (SA) algorithm for the MAP estimation [3, 19]. Those algorithms are based on iteratively visiting all the sites (voxels) by sampling the posterior local characteristic of the field directly (temperature parameter $T = 1$) for the GS algorithm and using a logarithmic cooling schedule defined by a temperature parameter T for the SA algorithm. The MMSE solution is given by the average of the solutions achieved after each iteration of the GS algorithm and the MAP solution is given by the last iteration of the SA algorithm (low temperature) [19]. In practice, 20 to 50 iterations are enough to get reasonable MMSE solutions and 10 to 20 for MAP solutions.

For determining the posterior local characteristic we will again resort to the Bayes' theorem:

$$p(X|Y,\delta X) = \frac{p(Y|X)p(X|\delta X)}{p(Y|\delta X)} \qquad (24.23)$$

where $p(Y|\delta X)$ depends only on the known signal Y. This posterior local characteristic is a Gauss-MRF given by [11]

$$p(X|Y,\delta X) = \frac{1}{\sqrt{2\pi T}\,\sigma_{X|Y}} \exp\left\{ -\frac{(X-\mu_{X|Y})^2}{2T\sigma_{X|Y}^2} \right\} \qquad (24.24)$$

with the following posterior local mean and variance

$$\mu_{X|Y} = \frac{\sigma_N^2\,\mu_X + \sigma_X^2 Y}{\sigma_X^2 + \sigma_N^2} \qquad\qquad \sigma_{X|Y}^2 = \frac{\sigma_N^2\,\sigma_X^2}{\sigma_X^2 + \sigma_N^2}. \qquad (24.25)$$

These expressions show that in the Gaussian case both the posterior local mean $\mu_{X|Y}$ and the posterior local variance $\sigma_{X|Y}^2$ can be obtained by closed form expressions, which greatly simplifies the implementation of the method, as well as reduces the computational burden. The proof for (24.25) is rather involved. Some hints on how to prove it can be found in [5], the core of the proof is that one quadratic form is to be constructed from a *summation* of two quadratic forms coming from the prior and likelihood PDFs.

To determine the performance of the described method a synthetic data volume was constructed. The volume is defined as a sphere with a one period sawtooth radial profile. Figure 24.5(a) shows the middle slice for this data, Fig. 24.5(b) the same volume with added noise, Fig. 24.5(c) the estimated MAP solution and Fig. 24.5(d) the MMSE solution. The regularization parameter λ was set to 0.5. Notice that as the method is designed for continuous signals, it cannot deal well with discontinuities. This is noticeable in Fig. 24.5(c) and 24.5(d) where the voxels close to the boundary have not been filtered. The use of an edge model as proposed in [19] may be helpful. Such models has the potential to filter the boundary voxels along the boundaries without inter region blurring. Comparing Fig. 24.5(c) to Fig. 24.5(d), we can see that the variability of the MAP solution is lower than the variability of the MMSE. However the bias of the MAP solution is greater than the bias for the MMSE. In general, the MAP method converges faster than the MMSE. To quantitatively compare these results, we have computed the signal to noise ratio (SNR). For the noisy data shown in Fig. 24.5(b) the SNR is 4.1, for the

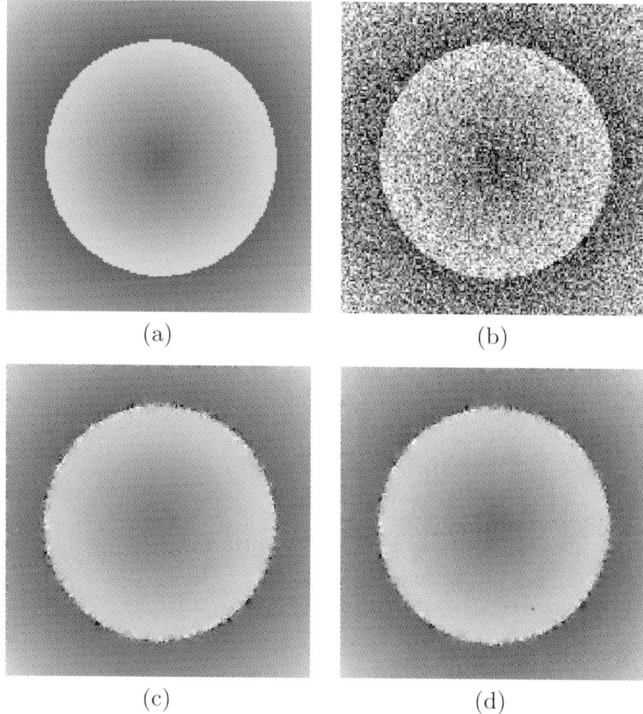

Fig. 24.5. Synthetic data volume (**a**), with added noise (**b**), the result using the MAP estimator (**c**) and the MMSE estimator (**d**)

MAP solution shown in Fig. 24.5(c) the SNR is 150.1 and for the MMSE solution shown in Fig. 24.5(d) the SNR is 184.6. Measuring the SNR only close to the discontinuity gives for the noisy data 4.8, for the MAP 18.6, and for the MMSE 21.7. The SNR values in the continuous areas are as follows: for the noisy 4.0, for the MAP 674.0 and for the MMSE 949.1. The SNR is better for the MMSE than for the MAP estimator due to the bias of the latter. As expected, the model performs better in the homogeneous areas.

Figure 24.6(a) shows a coronal view for MRI data set of a human brain and in Fig. 24.6(b) the result after applying the proposed regularization scheme. The regularization parameter λ was set to 0.2. The noise is reduced in the homogeneous regions without smoothing the boundaries.

24.3.4 Multi-Component Model Extension

In this section we extend the scalar case to multi-component case. For DT-MRI we have a second-rank tensor at each voxel position which is being represented by a symmetric 3×3 tensor matrix.

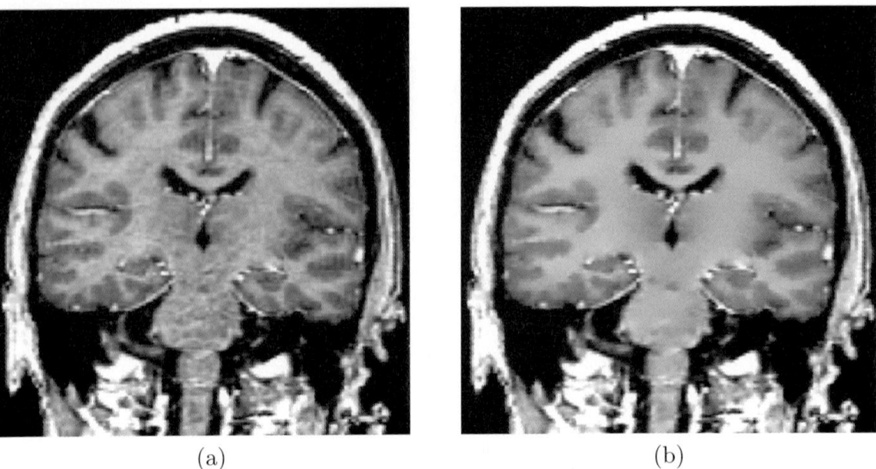

(a)   (b)

Fig. 24.6. A coronal slice of a MRI volume (**a**) and the result after applying the 3D Gaussian MRF scheme (**b**)

Let the non-observable tensor field be represented by a random matrix $\mathbf{X}$ with dimensions $3 \times 3 \times M \times N \times P$ of a volume of dimensions $M \times N \times P$, where each voxel is represented by a random tensor given by the 3×3 matrix

$$\mathbf{X}(m,n,p) = \begin{pmatrix} X_{11} & X_{12} & X_{13} \\ X_{21} & X_{22} & X_{23} \\ X_{31} & X_{32} & X_{33} \end{pmatrix} . \tag{24.26}$$

Each tensor matrix $\mathbf{X}(m,n,p)$ is symmetric so that $X_{ij} = X_{ji}$, and has 6 different random variables. The total number of different random variables is thus $K = 6MNP$. We further define a rearrangement matrix operator $\mathbf{LT}$ (lower triangular part) in order to extract the 6 different elements at each voxel position and to regroup them as a 6×1 column vector, $\mathbf{X}_{LT}(m,n,p)$ as

$$\mathbf{X}_{LT}(m,n,p) = \mathbf{LT}\big[\mathbf{X}(m,n,p)\big] = (X_{11} \ X_{21} \ X_{31} \ X_{22} \ X_{32} \ X_{33})^T . \tag{24.27}$$

By applying the rearrangement operator to each tensor, a 4D random matrix $\mathbf{X}_{LT}$ with dimensions $6 \times M \times N \times P$ is obtained without repeated elements. In order to formulate the probability density function of the tensor field we need to rearrange the tensor field $\mathbf{X}_{LT}$ as a column vector, we define a second rearrangement operator $\mathbf{CV}$ (column vector) as

$$\mathbf{X}_{CV} = \mathbf{CV}\big[\mathbf{X}_{LT}\big] \tag{24.28}$$

making $\mathbf{X}_{CV}$ a $K \times 1$ random vector which represents the whole tensor field.

In order to calculate the MAP or the MMSE estimator for the tensor field $\mathbf{X}_{CV}$ we need to extend the prior model presented in Sect. 24.3.1, the likelihood model in Sect. 24.3.2 and the posterior model in Sect. 24.3.3 by using

6-dimensional multivariate Gaussian distribution instead of the 1-dimensional Gaussian distribution explained for the scalar case. This should be done using the local characteristics of the field defined for each 6-component vector variable $\mathbf{X}_{LT}(m, n, p)$. A short list of what is needed to be estimated in the method follows:

– For the prior PDF we need to estimate the vector means $\boldsymbol{\mu}_{\mathbf{X}_{LT}}(m, n, p)$ and the covariance matrices $\mathbf{C}_{\mathbf{X}_{LT}}(m, n, p)$ by using the neighboring sites.
– For the likelihood PDF we need to estimate the noise covariance matrix $\mathbf{C}_{\mathbf{N}_{LT}}$, which does not depend on the site indices (m, n, p) as the noise is assumed to be homogeneous. This noise covariance matrix can be estimated in a similar way as the one proposed in Sect. 24.3.2 for the scalar case, but modified accordingly to deal with covariance matrices instead of variances.
– For the posterior PDF using the prior parameters $\boldsymbol{\mu}_{\mathbf{X}_{LT}}(m, n, p)$ and $\mathbf{C}_{\mathbf{X}_{LT}}(m, n, p)$, the noise covariance matrix $\mathbf{C}_{\mathbf{N}_{LT}}$ and the observed noisy field $\mathbf{Y}_{LT}(m, n, p)$ we can determine the posterior means $\boldsymbol{\mu}_{\mathbf{X}_{LT}|\mathbf{Y}_{LT}}(m, n, p)$ and the posterior covariances $\mathbf{C}_{\mathbf{X}_{LT}|\mathbf{Y}_{LT}}(m, n, p)$ by means of[4]

$$\boldsymbol{\mu}_{\mathbf{X}_{LT}|\mathbf{Y}_{LT}} = \mathbf{C}_{\mathbf{N}_{LT}}\left(\mathbf{C}_{\mathbf{X}_{LT}} + \mathbf{C}_{\mathbf{N}_{LT}}\right)^{-1}\boldsymbol{\mu}_{\mathbf{X}_{LT}} + \mathbf{C}_{\mathbf{X}_{LT}}\left(\mathbf{C}_{\mathbf{X}_{LT}} + \mathbf{C}_{\mathbf{N}_{LT}}\right)^{-1}\mathbf{Y}_{LT}$$
$$(24.29)$$

and

$$\mathbf{C}_{\mathbf{X}_{LT}|\mathbf{Y}_{LT}} = \mathbf{C}_{\mathbf{X}_{LT}}\left(\mathbf{C}_{\mathbf{X}_{LT}} + \mathbf{C}_{\mathbf{N}_{LT}}\right)^{-1}\mathbf{C}_{\mathbf{N}_{LT}} . \tag{24.30}$$

These equations are a vector generalization of the ones given by (24.25) in Sect. 24.3.3. In [5] we can also find some hints on how to prove that equations. In the vector case, special care has to be taken, however the procedure is similar to the scalar case.

For the SA algorithm we need to sample the posterior local characteristic, that is a 6-dimensional multivariate Gaussian distribution with parameters $\boldsymbol{\mu}_{\mathbf{X}_{LT}|\mathbf{Y}_{LT}}$ and $\mathbf{C}_{\mathbf{X}_{LT}|\mathbf{Y}_{LT}}$. This can be done by first generating a 6×1 sample vector $\mathbf{U}$ whose elements are independent and have Gaussian distribution with zero mean and unit standard deviation, and then transforming this sample according to

$$\mathbf{X}_{LT} = \sqrt{T}\,\mathbf{D}_{\mathbf{X}_{LT}|\mathbf{Y}_{LT}}\mathbf{U} + \boldsymbol{\mu}_{\mathbf{X}_{LT}|\mathbf{Y}_{LT}} \tag{24.31}$$

where $\mathbf{D}_{\mathbf{X}_{LT}|\mathbf{Y}_{LT}}$ is a matrix given by[5]

$$\mathbf{D}_{\mathbf{X}_{LT}|\mathbf{Y}_{LT}} = \mathbf{Q}_{\mathbf{X}_{LT}|\mathbf{Y}_{LT}}\sqrt{\boldsymbol{\Lambda}_{\mathbf{X}_{LT}|\mathbf{Y}_{LT}}} \tag{24.32}$$

---

[4] We omit the indices (m, n, p) to enhance the readability of the equations.
[5] The square root of a diagonal matrix is a diagonal matrix whose elements are the square root of the corresponding original matrix.

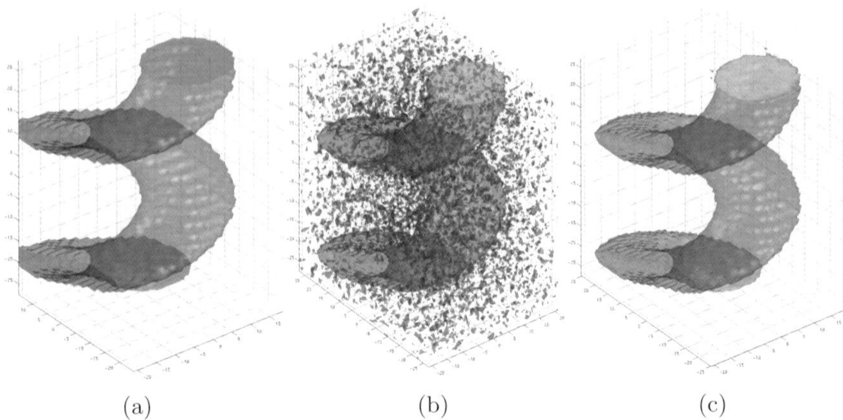

Fig. 24.7. Original synthetic tensor field (**a**), with noise added (**b**) and regularization result (**c**)

where the matrix $\mathbf{Q}_{\mathbf{X}_{LT}|\mathbf{Y}_{LT}}$ has in its columns the eigenvectors of the covariance matrix $\mathbf{C}_{\mathbf{X}_{LT}|\mathbf{Y}_{LT}}$. The matrix $\boldsymbol{\Lambda}_{\mathbf{X}_{LT}|\mathbf{Y}_{LT}}$ is diagonal having the corresponding eigenvalues in the principal diagonal.[6]

In order to assure the positive semidefinite condition of the diffusion tensors, the SA algorithm is modified as follows: after visiting a voxel, the condition is tested; if the test is not passed then the tensor is discarded and sampled again until the condition is satisfied.

We have generated a 3D helix synthetic tensor field for which the internal tensors are anisotropic and the external tensors are isotropic. Figure 24.7(a) shows the surface corresponding to the boundary separation between the two tensor classes. We have added noise to that tensor field and repeated the same visualization obtaining the Fig. 24.7(b). The random spots outside the helix surface correspond to anisotropic tensors and the internal random holes to isotropic tensors. After applying the proposed regularization method, although the field is not completely homogeneous, the two tensor classes are recovered as shown in Fig. 24.7(c). The regularization parameter λ was set to 0.5.

We have also regularized a DT-MRI data volume of a monkey brain. The results can be shown in Figs. 24.8, 24.9 and 24.10. The regularization parameter λ was set to 0.05. Figure 24.8(a) shows an axial view of the original noisy tensor described by the trace of the tensors, and Fig. 24.8(b) the result after regularization. Note that the main structures are maintained while the background noise in the flat regions have been removed. Figure 24.8(c) shows the fractional anisotropy (FA) measure [1] for the original data and Fig. 24.8(d)

---

[6] A real symmetric positive semidefinite matrix $\mathbf{C}$ can be factorized as $\mathbf{C} = \mathbf{Q}\boldsymbol{\Lambda}\mathbf{Q}^{T} = \mathbf{D}\mathbf{D}^{T}$, where $\mathbf{D} = \mathbf{Q}\sqrt{\boldsymbol{\Lambda}}$. A covariance matrix is always real, symmetric and positive semidefinite.

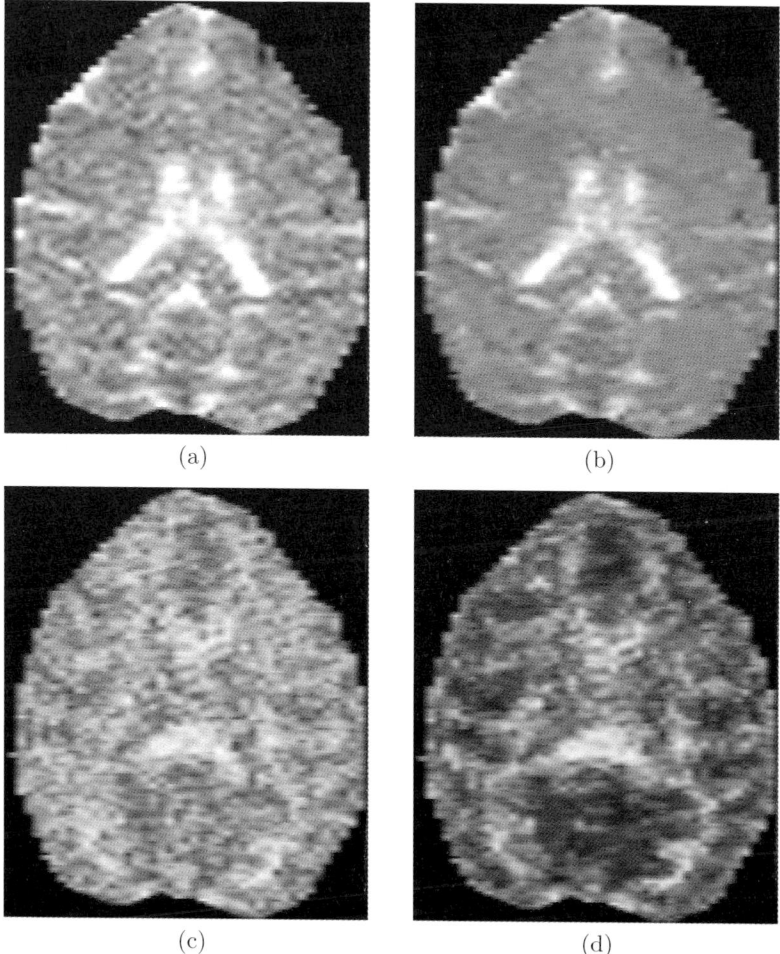

Fig. 24.8. Axial slice of the tensor trace for the original noisy DT-MRI data from a monkey brain (**a**), trace after regularization (**b**), axial slice of the FA measure for the original noise DT-MRI data (**c**) and FA measure after regularization (**d**)

after regularization. The higher the FA value, the more likely the presence of white matter fiber tracts. Notice that after regularization the white matter structures are better defined. In Fig. 24.9(a) a glyph visualization using superquadratics [6] for same data is shown. A description of these glyphs can be found in Chap. 7. Figure 24.9(b) shows the results after regularization. Notice that fiber tracts can be better distinguished in the filtered data set. To further explore the result of regularization we present results from tractography in the corpus callosum. Figure 24.10(a) displays the result of tractography in the original data and Fig. 24.10(b) in the regularized data. Notice that the fiber tracts are more continuous and better grouped in the filtered data.

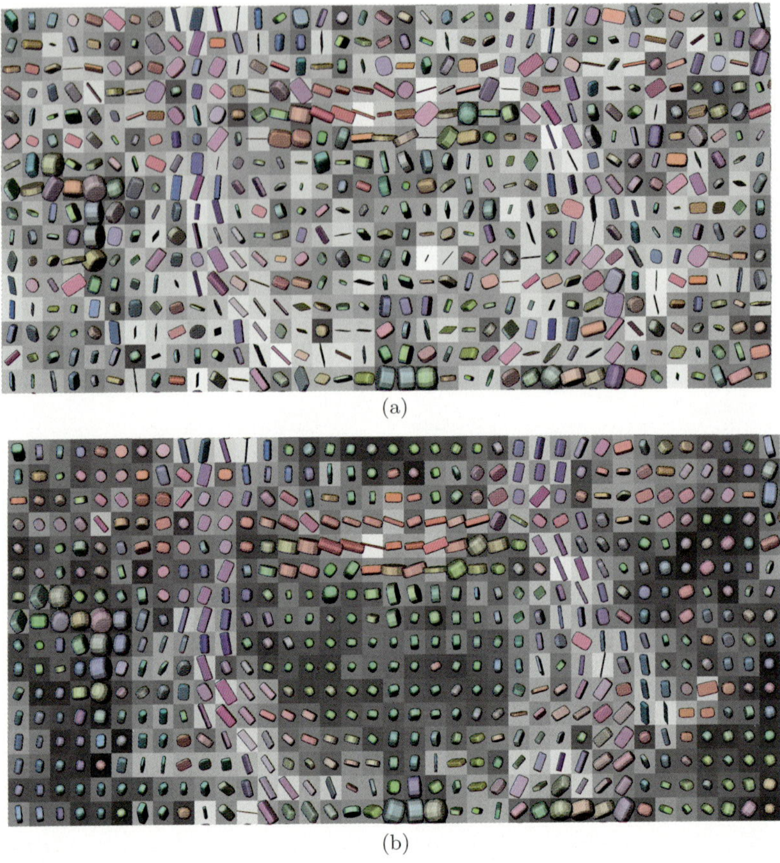

(a)

(b)

Fig. 24.9. Glyph visualization for a coronal slice for the original noisy DT-MRI data from a monkey brain (**a**) and the same visualization after regularization (**b**). See appendix for color plates

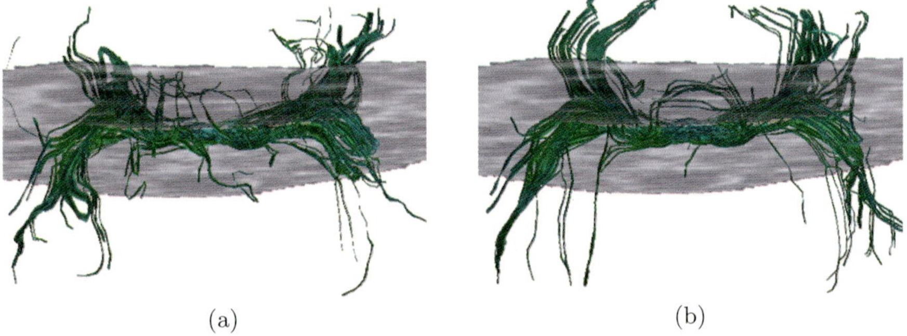

(a)   (b)

Fig. 24.10. Tractography in the corpus callosum for the original noise DT-MRI data from a monkey brain (**a**) and the same after regularization (**b**). See appendix for color plates

24.4 Conclusion

In this chapter we have described two different regularization methods. First we described NC, a general method for filtering missing and uncertain data. This filtering method solves a WLS problem by applying filters in a basis set which are assumed to span the signal locally. In NC, a certainty is defined for the signal, and localization of the basis functions is achieved by an applicability function, the corresponding certainty function for the basis filters. The effect of this is that spatial localization of the filter is achieved by a certainty window and not by changing the filter coefficients as in traditional windowing. The strengths of NC are the power of signals/certainty framework, and the use of basis functions that can be defined to span a subspace locally that fits the signal.

Second, we described a purely stochastic approach to regularization based on Gaussian MRF modeling of the signal. The strength of this approach is the Bayesian framework which enables an efficient control of the trade-off of applying the model (here the Gaussian model) where it fits, and not applying it in areas where it does not. The presented method can be improved by introducing boundary models for the prior at an expense of increasing the computational load.

Future work combining the best of the two approaches presented in this chapter will likely provide interesting and useful results.

Acknowledgments

This work was funded by NIH grants P41-RR13218 and R01-MH 50747, CIMIT, Spanish CICYT for the research grant TIC2001-3808-C02-02, the European Commission for the funding associated to the Network of Excellence SIMILAR FP6-5076609. The second author acknowledges the Fulbright Commission for the postdoctoral grant FU2003-0968.

References

1. P. J. Basser. Inferring microstructural features and the physiological state of tissues from diffusion-weighted images. *NMR in Biomedicine*, 8:333–344, 1995.
2. P. J. Basser and S. Pajevic. A normal distribution for tensor-valued random variables: Application to diffusion tensor MRI. *IEEE Trans. Medical Imaging*, 22:785–794, 2003.
3. S. Geman and D. Geman. Stochastic relaxation, gibbs distributions and the bayesian restoration of images. *IEEE Trans. Pattern Analysis and Machine Intelligence*, 6:721–741, 1984.
4. H. Gudbjartsson and S. Patz. The rician distribution of noisy msri data. *Magnetic Resonance in Medicine*, 24:910–914, 1995.

5. S. M. Kay. *Fundamentals of statistical signal processing: estimation theory.* Prentice-Hall, 1993.

6. G Kindlmann. Superquadric tensor glyphs. In *IEEE TVCG/EG Symposium on Visualization*, pp. 147–154, 2004.

7. H. Knutsson and C.-F. Westin. Normalized and differential convolution: Methods for interpolation and filtering of incomplete and uncertain data. In *Computer Vision and Pattern Recognition*, pp. 515–523, 1993.

8. M. Martin-Fernandez, C. Alberola-Lopez, J. Ruiz-Alzola, and C. F. Westin. Regularization of diffusion tensor maps using a non-gaussian markov random field approach. In *Medical Image Computing and Computer-Assisted Intervention*, volume 2879 of *Lecture Notes in Computer Science*, pp. 92–100, 2003.

9. M. Martin-Fernandez, R. San Jose-Estepar, C. F. Westin, and C. Alberola-Lopez. A novel gauss-markov random field approach for regularization of diffusion tensor map. In *Computer Aided Systems Theory*, volume 2809 of *Lecture Notes in Computer Science*, pp. 506–517, 2003.

10. M. Martin-Fernandez, C.-F. Westin, and C. Alberola-Lopez. 3d bayesian regularization of diffusion tensor mri using multivariate gaussian markov random fields. In *Medical Image Computing and Computer-Assisted Intervention*, volume 3216 of *Lecture Notes in Computer Science*, pp. 351–359, 2004.

11. J. M. F. Moura and S. Goswami. Gauss markov radom fields (gmrf) with continuous indices. *IEEE Trans. Information Theory*, 43:1560–1573, 1997.

12. C. Pierpaoli, P. Jezzard, P. J. Basser, A. Barnett, and G. Di Chiro. Diffusion tensor MR imaging of the human brain. *Radiology*, 201:637, 1996.

13. C. Poupon, C. A. Clark, F. Frouin, J. Régis, I. Bloch, D. Le Bihan, I. Bloch, and J.-F. Mangin. Regularization of diffusion-based direction maps for the tracking brain white matter fascicles. *NeuroImage*, 12:184–195, 2000.

14. C. Tomasi and R. Manduchi. Bilateral filtering for gray and color images. In *International Conference on Computer Vision*, pp. 839–846, 1998.

15. D. Tschumperlé and R. Deriche. Dt-mri images: Estimation, regularization and application. In *Computer Aided Systems Theory*, volume 2809 of *Lecture Notes in Computer Science*, pp. 530–541, 2003.

16. C.-F. Westin. *A Tensor Framework for Multidimensional Signal Processing.* PhD thesis, Linköping University, Sweden, 1994.

17. C.-F. Westin and H. Knutsson. Tensor field regularization using normalized convolution. In *Computer Aided Systems Theory*, volume 2809 of *Lecture Notes in Computer Science*, pp. 564–572, 2003.

18. C.-F. Westin, S. E. Maier, H. Mamata, A. Nabavi, F. A. Jolesz, and R. Kikinis. Processing and visualization of diffusion tensor MRI. *Medical Image Analysis*, 6:93–108, 2002.

19. G. Winkler. *Image Analysis, Random Fields and Markov Chain Monte Carlo Methods, Applications of Mathematics, Stochastic Modelling and Applied Probability.* Springer Verlag, 2003.

PDEs for Tensor Image Processing

Joachim Weickert, Christian Feddern, Martin Welk, Bernhard Burgeth, and Thomas Brox

Mathematical Image Analysis Group, Faculty of Mathematics and Computer Science, Saarland University, Building 27, 66041 Saarbrücken, Germany
`{weickert,feddern,welk,burgeth,brox}@mia.uni-saarland.de`

Summary. Methods based on partial differential equations (PDEs) belong to those image processing techniques that can be extended in a particularly elegant way to tensor fields. In this survey chapter the most important PDEs for discontinuity-preserving denoising of tensor fields are reviewed such that the underlying design principles becomes evident. We consider isotropic and anisotropic diffusion filters and their corresponding variational methods, mean curvature motion, and self-snakes. These filters preserve positive semidefiniteness of any positive semidefinite initial tensor field. Finally we discuss geodesic active contours for segmenting tensor fields. Experiments are presented that illustrate the behaviour of all these methods.

25.1 Introduction

In the last 15 years, partial differential equations (PDEs) have become increasingly popular in image processing. This has a number of reasons: PDE-based methods are mathematically well-understood techniques, they allow a reinterpretation of several classical methods under a unifying framework, they have led to novel methods with more invariances, and they are the natural framework for scale-space analysis. Moreover, the PDE formulation reflects the continuous structure of space. Thus, PDE approximations aim to be independent of the underlying grid and may reveal good rotational invariance. In a number of image processing and computer vision areas, PDE-based methods and related variational approaches and level-set techniques belong to the best performing methods; see e.g. the books [2, 4, 18, 20, 25, 30] and the references therein.

Interestingly, PDEs are also among the first image processing techniques that have been extended from scalar- and vector-valued images to matrix-valued data. One of the reasons for this is the fact that these extensions are not too difficult, once the scalar-valued processes are mastered.

In this chapter we give a survey on some of the most important PDE methods for discontinuity-preserving denoising of tensor images, namely nonlinear diffusion filters and their corresponding regularisation methods, mean curvature motion, and self-snakes. Moreover, we describe an extension of geodesic active contours for tensor images. In order to keep things as simple as possible, we focus on 2-D methods. It should be noted, however, that these concepts can be extended in a natural way to higher dimensions [13]. Parts of our description follow the original papers [12, 13, 31]. We would like to emphasise that we focus on methods for genuine tensor processing. Thus we do not consider scalar- or vector-valued PDE methods working on the eigensystem or filtering channels that are measured prior to computing tensors [10, 27, 28].

The chapter is organised as follows. In Sect. 25.2 we introduce a generalised structure tensor for matrix fields. It is used for steering all nonlinear PDE methods that are discussed in the course of this chapter. Section 25.3 describes nonlinear diffusion filters for tensor data, both in the isotropic case with a scalar diffusivity as well as in the anisotropic case with a diffusion tensor. Closely related regularisation methods are presented in Sect. 25.4. In Sect. 25.5 we design a mean curvature type evolution for tensor-valued data. Modifying tensor-valued mean curvature motion by a suitable edge stopping function leads us to tensor-valued self-snakes. They are discussed in Sect. 25.6. In Sect. 25.7 we use the self-snake model in order to derive geodesic active contours for tensor fields. The chapter is concluded with a summary in Sect. 25.8.

25.2 Structure Analysis of Tensor-Valued Data

In this section we generalise the concept of an image gradient to the tensor-valued setting [12]. This may be regarded as a tensor extension of Di Zenzo's method for vector-valued data [11].

Let us consider some rectangular image domain $\Omega \in \mathbb{R}^2$ and some tensor image $F = (f_{i,j}) : \Omega \to \mathbb{R}^{2\times 2}$, where the indices (i,j) specify the tensor channel. We intend to define an 'edge direction' for such a matrix-valued function. In the case of some scalar-valued image f, we would look for the direction v which is orthogonal to the gradient of a Gaussian-smoothed version of f:

$$0 = v^\top \nabla f_\sigma \tag{25.1}$$

where $f_\sigma := K_\sigma * f$ and K_σ denotes a Gaussian with standard deviation σ. Gaussian convolution makes the structure detection more robust against noise. The parameter σ is called *noise scale*.

In the general tensor-valued case, we cannot expect that all tensor channels yield the same edge direction. Therefore we proceed as follows. Let $F_\sigma = (f_{\sigma,i,j})$ be a Gaussian-smoothed version of $F = (f_{i,j})$, where the smoothing is performed componentwise. Then we define the edge direction as the unit vector v that minimises

$$E(v) := \sum_{i=1}^{2}\sum_{j=1}^{2}(v^\top \nabla f_{\sigma,i,j})^2 = v^\top \left(\sum_{i=1}^{2}\sum_{j=1}^{2} \nabla f_{\sigma,i,j} \nabla f_{\sigma,i,j}^\top \right) v \, .$$

This quadratic form is minimised when v is an eigenvector to the smallest eigenvalue of the *structure tensor*

$$J(F_\sigma) := \sum_{i=1}^{2} \sum_{j=1}^{2} \nabla f_{\sigma,i,j} \nabla f_{\sigma,i,j}^{\top} \,. \tag{25.2}$$

The eigenvalues of this positive semidefinite matrix measure the local contrast in the directions of the eigenvectors. Its trace

$$\mathrm{tr}\, J(F_\sigma) = \sum_{i=1}^{2} \sum_{j=1}^{2} |\nabla f_{\sigma,i,j}|^2 \tag{25.3}$$

sums up all eigenvalues. It can be regarded as a tensor-valued generalisation of the squared gradient magnitude. The matrix $J(F_\sigma)$ will allow us to generalise a number of PDE methods to the tensor-valued setting.

Figure 25.1 illustrates the concept of edge detection with the structure tensor. The test image we use for our experiments is obtained from a DT-MRI data set of a human brain. We have extracted a 2-D section from the 3-D data. The 2-D image consists of four quadrants which show the four tensor channels of a 2×2 matrix. The top right channel and bottom left channel are identical since the matrix is symmetric. To test the robustness under noise we have replaced 30% of all data by random matrices: The angles of their eigensystem obey a uniform distribution on $[0, \pi]$, while their eigenvalues are random numbers uniformly distributed in $[0, 127]$. Figure 25.1 shows the outcome of using $\mathrm{tr}\, J(F_\sigma)$ for detecting edges in tensor-valued images. We observe that this method gives good results for the original data set. When increasing the noise scale σ, it is also possible to handle situations where substantial noise is present.

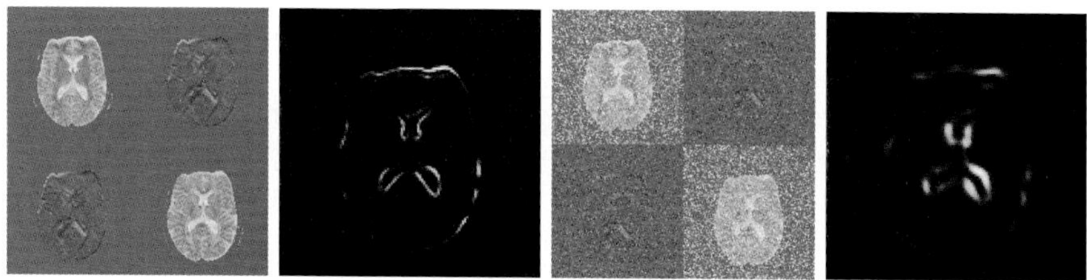

Fig. 25.1. Edge detection with a structure tensor for matrix-valued data. From *left* to *right*: (**a**) Original 2-D tensor field extracted from a 3-D DT-MRI data set by using the channels $(1,1)$, $(1,2)$, $(2,1)$ and $(2,2)$. Each channel is of size 128×128. The channels $(1,2)$ and $(2,1)$ are identical for symmetry reasons. (**b**) Trace of the structure tensor of (a) with $\sigma = 1$. (**c**) Noisy version of (a) with 30% noise. (**d**) Trace of the structure tensor from (**c**) with $\sigma = 3$. From [13]

25.3 Diffusion Filtering

25.3.1 Linear Diffusion

Linear diffusion filtering is the oldest PDE method for image denoising [15]. It creates a family of simplified images $\{u(x,t) \mid t \geq 0\}$ from some scalar initial image $f(x)$ by solving the PDE

$$\partial_t u = \Delta u \quad \text{on} \quad \Omega \times (0, \infty) , \tag{25.4}$$

with f as initial condition,

$$u(x,0) = f(x) \quad \text{on} \quad \Omega , \tag{25.5}$$

and reflecting (homogeneous Neumann) boundary conditions:

$$\partial_\nu u = 0 \quad \text{on} \quad \partial\Omega \times (0, \infty) . \tag{25.6}$$

Here ∂_ν denotes differentiation in the direction of the outer normal of the image boundary $\partial\Omega$. The diffusion time t determines the degree of simplification: For $t = 0$ the original image f is recovered, and larger values for t result in more pronounced smoothing. On an infinitely extended image domain, linear diffusion filtering with stopping time T is equivalent to Gaussian convolution with standard deviation $\sigma = \sqrt{2T}$.

It is straightforward to extend linear diffusion filtering to tensor images: All one has to do is to apply this process channelwise.

Figure 25.2 zooms into the corpus callosum region of Fig. 25.1(a),(c), and displays the evolution of this region under linear diffusion. The tensors are visualised by ellipses with colour-coded orientation. We observe that linear diffusion is well-suited for removing noise, but suffers from blurring important features such as discontinuities in the tensor field.

25.3.2 Isotropic Nonlinear Diffusion

The goal of nonlinear diffusion filtering is to smooth an image while respecting its discontinuities [6, 22]. Nonlinear diffusion filtering replaces the linear diffusion equation (25.4) by

$$\partial_t u = \operatorname{div} \left(g(|\nabla u_\sigma|^2) \nabla u \right) \quad \text{on} \quad \Omega \times (0, \infty) . \tag{25.7}$$

The *diffusivity function g* is a decreasing nonnegative function of the squared gradient magnitude of u_σ, a Gaussian smoothed version of u. One may choose e.g. [22]

$$g(|\nabla u_\sigma|^2) = \frac{1}{1 + |\nabla u_\sigma|^2/\lambda^2} \tag{25.8}$$

with some contrast parameter $\lambda > 0$. We observe that $|\nabla u_\sigma|^2$ serves as an edge detector: Locations where $|\nabla u_\sigma| \gg \lambda$ are regarded as edges where diffusion

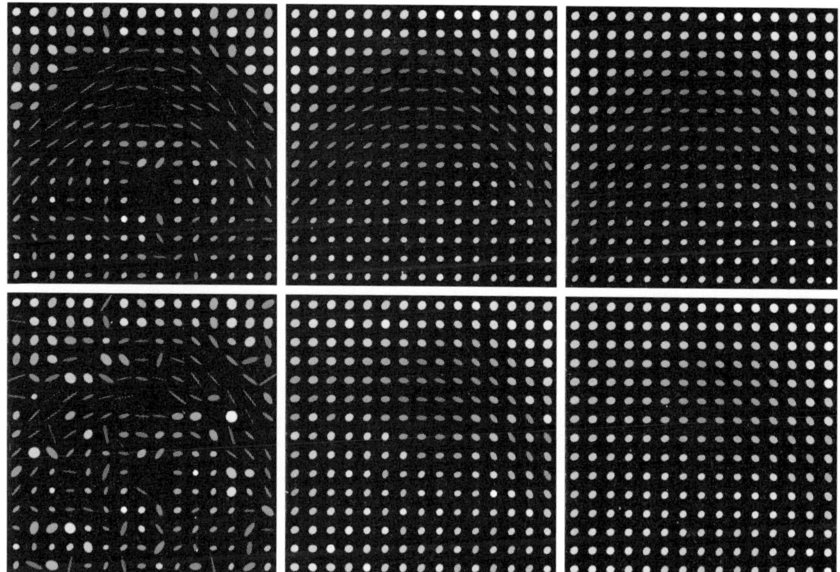

Fig. 25.2. Tensor-valued linear diffusion. *Top row*, from *left* to *right*: Detail from a DT-MR image (size 15×15), at time $t = 0.96$, at time $t = 2.4$. *Bottom row*, from *left* to *right*: Same experiment with 30% noise. See colour plates

is inhibited, while locations with $|\nabla u_\sigma| \ll \lambda$ are considered to belong to the interior of a segment, where full diffusion is performed.

This scalar-valued diffusion scheme can also be generalised for smoothing a matrix field $F = (f_{i,j}) : \Omega \to \mathbb{R}^{2 \times 2}$. Tschumperlé and Deriche [27] have proposed a PDE system for matrix-valued diffusion where a joint diffusivity function is used that depends on the trace of the structure tensor (in their case with $\sigma = 0$):

$$\partial_t u_{i,j} = \operatorname{div}\left(g(\operatorname{tr} J(U_\sigma)) \nabla u_{i,j}\right) \qquad (i, j \in \{1, 2\}) . \tag{25.9}$$

The synchronised channel evolution with a joint diffusivity avoids that edges are formed at different locations for the different tensor channels. This synchronisation of channel smoothing is also a frequently used strategy in vector-valued diffusion filtering [14].

Figure 25.3 illustrates the evolution under isotropic nonlinear diffusion. Discontinuities are well-preserved, but noise at discontinuities is removed rather slowly.

25.3.3 Anisotropic Nonlinear Diffusion

Besides isotropic diffusion schemes with a scalar-valued diffusivity, there exist also anisotropic counterparts. In the anisotropic case not only the amount of

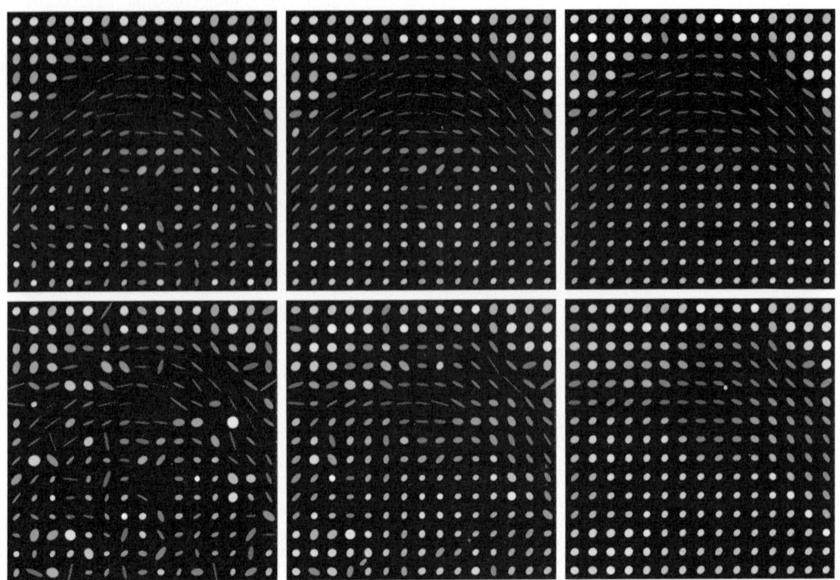

Fig. 25.3. Tensor-valued isotropic nonlinear diffusion. *Top row*, from *left* to *right*: Detail from a DT-MR image (size 15×15), at time $t = 4.8$, and at $t = 12.0$ ($\lambda = 0.5$, $\sigma = 0.5$). *Bottom row*, from *left* to *right*: Same experiment with 30% noise ($\lambda = 0.5$, $\sigma = 1$). See colour plates

diffusion is adapted locally to the data but also the direction of smoothing. It allows to encourage smoothing along discontinuities rather than across them. This can be achieved by replacing the scalar-valued diffusivity function by a matrix-valued diffusion tensor.[1]

Tensor-valued anisotropic diffusion regards the original image $F(x) = (f_{i,j}(x))$ as initial value for the coupled PDE system [31]

$$\partial_t u_{i,j} = \operatorname{div}\left(g(J(U_\sigma))\,\nabla u_{i,j}\right) \qquad (i,j \in \{1,2\}) \tag{25.10}$$

subject to the reflecting boundary conditions

$$\partial_\nu\left(g(J(U_\sigma))\,\nabla u_{i,j}\right) = 0 \qquad (i,j \in \{1,2\})\,. \tag{25.11}$$

Here the scalar-valued function g is generalised to a matrix-valued function in the following way: Let $J(U_\sigma) = Q\,\operatorname{diag}(\lambda_i)Q^\top$ denote the principal axis decomposition of $J(U_\sigma)$, with the eigenvalues λ_i as the elements of the diagonal matrix $\operatorname{diag}(\lambda_i)$, and the normalised eigenvectors as the columns of the orthogonal matrix Q. Then it is common to set $g(J(U_\sigma)) := Q\,\operatorname{diag}(g(\lambda_i))Q^\top$, where the scalar diffusivity g is the same decreasing function as in the isotropic case.

---

[1] In the diffusion filtering literature, the word anisotropic is often already used for space-variant diffusion processes with a scalar diffusivity function.

Anisotropic diffusion offers the advantage of smoothing in a direction-specific way: Along the i-th eigenvector of $J(U_\sigma)$ with corresponding eigenvalue λ_i, the eigenvalue of the diffusion tensor is given by $g(\lambda_i)$. In eigendirections with large variation of local structure, λ_i is large and $g(\lambda_i)$ is small. This avoids smoothing across discontinuities. Along discontinuities, λ_i is small. Hence, $g(\lambda_i)$ is large and full diffusion is performed. For more information about anisotropic diffusion in general, we refer to [30].

Interestingly, the bare coupling of the tensor channels via a joint diffusion tensor guarantees – without additional projection steps – that the evolving matrix field $U(x,t) = (u_{i,j}(x,t))$ remains positive semidefinite if its initial value $F(x) = (f_{i,j}(x))$ is positive semidefinite. In the discrete case, this follows from the fact that convex combinations of positive semidefinite matrices are computed [31]. In the continuous case, going from matrices to their quadratic forms allows to prove preservation of positive semidefiniteness by means of a scalar-valued maximum-minimum principle [3]. This reasoning also holds for linear and isotropic nonlinear diffusion. Hence one does not have to consider more sophisticated constrained flows [8] if one is only interested in preserving positive semidefiniteness.

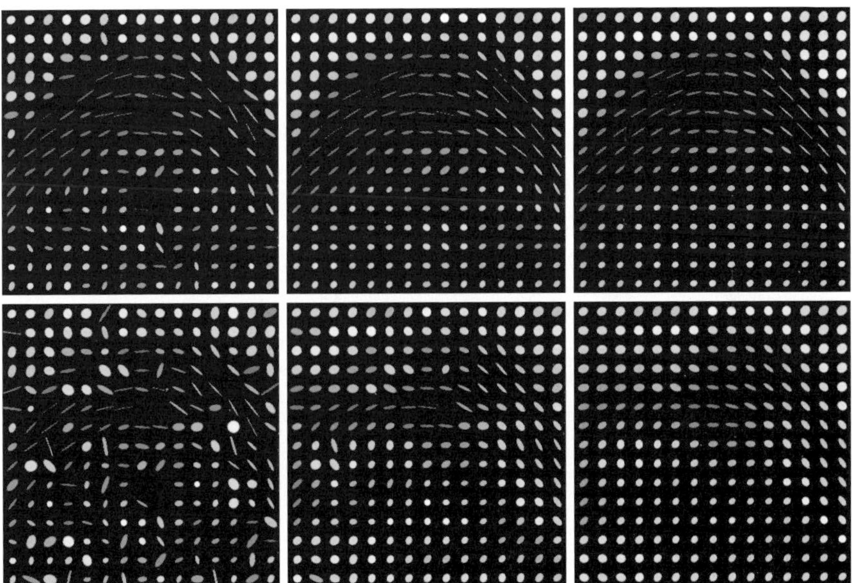

Fig. 25.4. Tensor-valued anisotropic nonlinear diffusion. *Top row*, from *left* to *right*: Detail from a DT-MR image (size 15×15), at time $t = 1.92$, and at $t = 4.8$ ($\lambda = 0.5$, $\sigma = 0.5$). *Bottom row*, from *left* to *right*: Same experiment with 30 % noise, at time $t = 1.92$ and $t = 4.8$ ($\lambda = 0.5$, $\sigma = 1$). See colour plates

The effects of anisotropic nonlinear diffusion are illustrated in Fig. 25.4. It seems to combine the advantages of linear and isotropic nonlinear diffusion: Noise is removed efficiently while discontinuities are preserved for a long time.

Tensor-valued nonlinear diffusion has also led to nonlinear structure tensors, a refinement of the structure tensor concept itself, see [3] and Chap. 2 of this book. They offer advantages for optic flow estimation, texture analysis, and corner detection.

25.4 Regularisation Methods

Regularisation methods belong to the class of variational approaches for image restoration. Typically one calculates a restoration of some degraded scalar-valued image f as the minimiser of an energy functional

$$E(u) := \int_\Omega \left(|u - f|^2 + \alpha \, \Psi(|\nabla u|^2) \right) \, dx \qquad (25.12)$$

where the penaliser $\Psi : [0, \infty) \to \mathrm{I\!R}$ is an increasing function [19]. The first summand encourages similarity between the restored image and the original one, while the second one rewards smoothness. The smoothness weight $\alpha > 0$ is called *regularisation parameter*. From variational calculus it follows that a minimiser of $E(u)$ satisfies the Euler–Lagrange equation

$$\frac{u - f}{\alpha} = \mathrm{div}\left(\Psi'(|\nabla u|^2)\, \nabla u \right) \qquad (25.13)$$

with homogeneous Neumann boundary conditions. This elliptic PDE can be regarded as a fully implicit time discretisation of the diffusion filter

$$\partial_t u = \mathrm{div}\left(\Psi'(|\nabla u|^2)\, \nabla u \right) \qquad (25.14)$$

with initial image f and stopping time α; see [26] for more details.

In the tensor case, Deriche and Tschumperlé [27] consider the energy

$$E(U) = \int_\Omega \left(\|U - F\|^2 + \alpha \, \Psi(\mathrm{tr}\, J(U)) \right) \, dx \qquad (25.15)$$

where $\| \cdot \|$ is the Frobenius norm for matrices. Then the corresponding Euler–Lagrange equations are given by

$$\frac{u_{i,j} - f_{i,j}}{\alpha} = \mathrm{div}\left(\Psi'(\mathrm{tr}\, J(U))\, \nabla u_{i,j} \right) \qquad (i, j \in \{1, 2\}) \, . \qquad (25.16)$$

They can be regarded as an approximation to the isotropic nonlinear diffusion filter (25.9) if one chooses $\Psi' := g$ and $\sigma := 0$.

Weickert and Brox [31], on the other hand, consider

$$E(U) = \int_\Omega \left(\|U - F\|^2 + \alpha \operatorname{tr} \Psi(J(U)) \right) dx \, . \tag{25.17}$$

It leads to the Euler–Lagrange equation

$$\frac{u_{i,j} - f_{i,j}}{\alpha} = \operatorname{div} \left(\Psi'(J(U)) \nabla u_{i,j} \right) \qquad (i,j \in \{1,2\}) \tag{25.18}$$

which is an approximation to the anisotropic nonlinear diffusion filter (25.10).

These considerations show that regularisation methods are closely related to nonlinear diffusion filtering. In practise they can lead to results that are hardly distinguishable from diffusion results [26]. For this reason we refrain from presenting specific experiments for this filter class.

25.5 Mean Curvature Motion

In this section we describe tensor-valued mean curvature motion [12]. To this end, we first have to sketch some basic ideas behind scalar-valued mean curvature motion.

We start with the observation that the Laplacian Δu of an isotropic linear diffusion model may be decomposed into two orthogonal directions $\xi \perp \nabla u$ and $\eta \parallel \nabla u$:

$$\partial_t u = \Delta u = \partial_{\xi\xi} u + \partial_{\eta\eta} u \tag{25.19}$$

where $\partial_{\xi\xi} u$ describes smoothing parallel to edges and $\partial_{\eta\eta}$ smoothes perpendicular to edges. *Mean curvature motion (MCM)* uses an anisotropic variant of this smoothing process by permitting only smoothing along the level lines:

$$\partial_t u = \partial_{\xi\xi} u \, . \tag{25.20}$$

This can be rewritten as

$$\partial_t u = |\nabla u| \operatorname{div} \left(\frac{\nabla u}{|\nabla u|} \right) . \tag{25.21}$$

Alvarez et al. have used this evolution equation for denoising highly degraded images [1]. It is well-known from the mathematical literature that under MCM convex level lines remain convex, nonconvex ones become convex, and in finite time they vanish by approximating circular shapes while converging to points.

If we want to use an MCM-like process for processing tensor-valued data $F = (f_{i,j})$, it is natural to replace the second directional derivative $\partial_{\xi\xi} u$ in (25.20) by $\partial_{vv} u$, where v is the eigenvector to the smallest eigenvalue of the structure tensor $J(U)$. This leads us to the evolution

$$\partial_t u_{i,j} = \partial_{vv} u_{i,j} \quad \text{on} \quad \Omega \times (0, \infty) \tag{25.22}$$

$$u_{i,j}(x,0) = f_{i,j}(x) \quad \text{on} \quad \Omega, \tag{25.23}$$

$$\partial_\nu u_{i,j} = 0 \quad \text{on} \quad \partial\Omega \times (0, \infty) \tag{25.24}$$

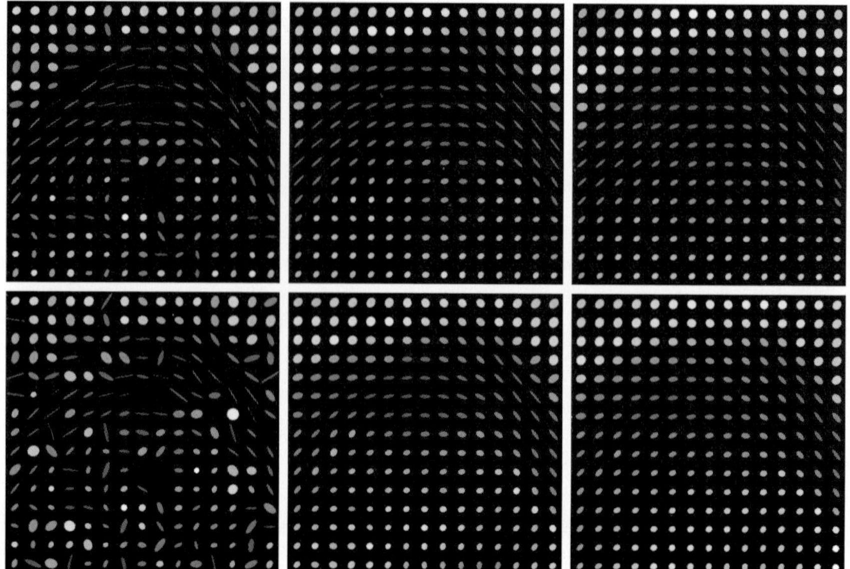

Fig. 25.5. Tensor-valued mean curvature motion. *Top row*, from *left* to *right*: Detail of size 15×15 from a DT-MR image; at time $t = 2.4$, at time $t = 6$. *Bottom row*, from *left* to *right*: Same experiment with 30% noise. See colour plates

for all tensor channels (i, j). Note that this process synchronises the smoothing direction in all channels. It may be regarded as a tensor-valued generalisation of the vector-valued mean curvature motion by Chambolle [7].

Our notion of edge directions as eigenvectors of the structure tensor is equivalent to the generalised level lines in [9]. Hence, tensor-valued MCM can be regarded as smoothing along these lines. Reinterpreting the concept of curve evolution in the same spirit allows even to gain a theoretical foundation of MCM as shortening flow for its level lines [13]. It is also possible to show that tensor MCM preserves positive semidefiniteness [13].

Figure 25.5 illustrates the tensor-valued mean curvature model. As can be seen in the first row, this process regularises the tensor field while it is capable of respecting anisotropies in a better way than linear diffusion. The second row of Fig. 25.5 shows the same algorithm applied to the noisy image. It displays a fairly high robustness to noise: For increasing evolution times the results for the original and the noisy images approach each other.

25.6 Self-Snakes

In [24], Sapiro has proposed a specific variant of MCM that is well-suited for image enhancement. This process – which he names *self-snakes* – introduces an edge-stopping function into mean curvature motion in order to prevent further shrinkage of the level lines once they have reached important image edges. In the scalar-valued setting, a self-snake $u(x, t)$ of some image $f(x)$ is generated by the evolution process

$$\partial_t u = |\nabla u| \operatorname{div} \left(g(|\nabla u_\sigma|^2) \frac{\nabla u}{|\nabla u|} \right) \quad \text{on} \quad \Omega \times (0, \infty) \,, \qquad (25.25)$$

$$u(x, 0) = f(x) \quad \text{on} \quad \Omega \,, \qquad (25.26)$$

$$\partial_\nu u = 0 \quad \text{on} \quad \partial\Omega \times (0, \infty) \,, \qquad (25.27)$$

where g is a decreasing function such as the diffusivity (25.8). Self-snakes have been advocated as alternatives to nonlinear diffusion filters [32], they can be used for vector-valued images [24], and related processes have also been proposed for filtering 3-D images [23].

Using the product rule of differentiation, we may rewrite (25.25) as

$$\partial_t u \;=\; g(|\nabla u_\sigma|^2) \, \partial_{\xi\xi} u + \nabla^\top (g(|\nabla u_\sigma|^2)) \, \nabla u \qquad (25.28)$$

with $\nabla^\top := (\partial_x, \partial_y)$. This formulation suggests a straightforward generalisation to the tensor-valued setting. All we have to do is to replace $|\nabla u_\sigma|^2$ by $\operatorname{tr} J(U_\sigma)$, and $\partial_{\xi\xi}$ by ∂_{vv}, where v is the eigenvector to the smallest eigenvalue of $J(U)$. This leads us to the following tensor-valued PDE:

$$\partial_t u_{i,j} \;=\; g(\operatorname{tr} J(U_\sigma)) \, \partial_{vv} u_{i,j} + \nabla^\top (g(\operatorname{tr} J(U_\sigma))) \, \nabla u_{i,j} \,. \qquad (25.29)$$

We observe that the main difference to tensor-valued MCM consists in the additional term $\nabla^\top (g(\operatorname{tr} J(U_\sigma))) \, \nabla u_{i,j}$. It can be regarded as a shock term [21] that is responsible for the edge-enhancing properties of self-snakes.

With only minor modifications, it is possible to extend the semidefiniteness preservation proof for tensor-valued MCM also to the case of tensor-valued self-snakes.

Experimental results for the tensor-valued self-snake technique are shown in Fig. 25.6. Compared to tensor-valued MCM, self-snakes offer increased sharpness at discontinuities due to the additional shock term. The filtered tensor fields look segmentation-like.

25.7 Geodesic Active Contour Models

Active contours go back to Kass et al. [16]. They play an important role in interactive image segmentation, in particular for medical applications. The underlying idea is that the user specifies an initial guess of an interesting contour (organ, tumour, ...). Then this contour is moved by image-driven forces to the edges of the object in question.

So-called geodesic active contour models [5, 17] achieve this by applying a specific kind of level set ideas. In its simplest form, a geodesic active contour model consists of the following steps. One embeds the user-specified initial

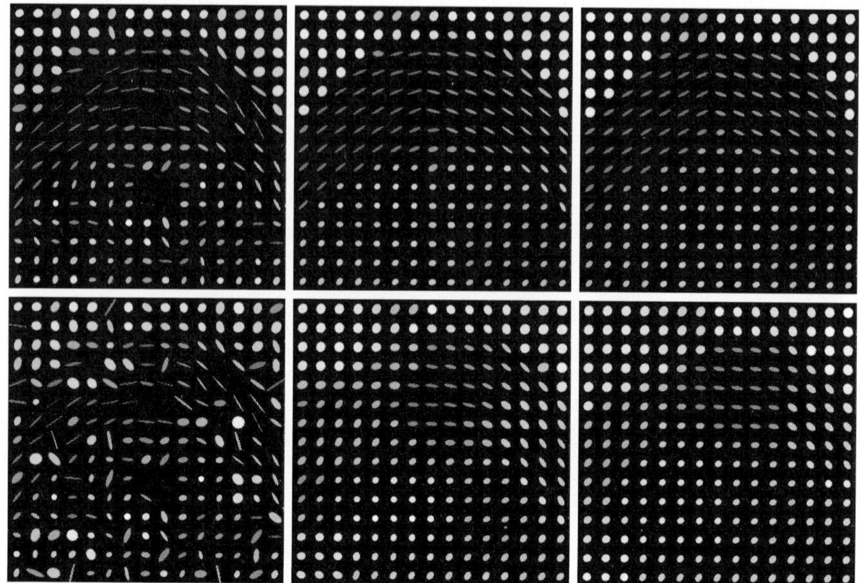

Fig. 25.6. Tensor-valued self-snakes. *Top row*, from *left* to *right*: Detail of size 15×15 from a DT-MR image; at time $t = 2.4$, at time $t = 6$ ($\sigma = 0.5$, $\lambda = 2$). *Bottom row*, from *left* to *right*: Same experiment with 30% noise ($\sigma = 1$, $\lambda = 2$). See colour plates

curve $C_0(s)$ as a zero level curve into a function $f(x)$, for instance by using the distance transformation. Then f is evolved under a PDE that includes knowledge about the original image h:

$$\partial_t u = |\nabla u| \operatorname{div} \left(g(|\nabla h_\sigma|^2) \frac{\nabla u}{|\nabla u|} \right) \quad \text{on} \quad \Omega \times (0, \infty), \qquad (25.30)$$

$$u(x, 0) = f(x), \quad \text{on} \quad \Omega, \qquad (25.31)$$

$$\partial_\nu u = 0 \quad \text{on} \quad \partial\Omega \times (0, \infty), \qquad (25.32)$$

where g inhibits evolution at edges of f. One may choose decreasing functions such as the diffusivity (25.8). Experiments indicate that, in general, (25.30) will have nontrivial steady states. The evolution is stopped at some time T, when the process does hardly alter anymore, and the final contour C is extracted as the zero level curve of $u(x, T)$. This contour turns out to be a shortest path with respect to an image-induced metric which motivates the notion of *geodesic* active contours.

In [12] geodesic active contours have been extended to tensor valued data $H = (h_{i,j})$ by using $\operatorname{tr}(J(H_\sigma))$ as argument of the stopping function g:

$$\partial_t u = |\nabla u| \operatorname{div} \left(g(\operatorname{tr} J(H_\sigma)) \frac{\nabla u}{|\nabla u|} \right). \qquad (25.33)$$

Note that, in contrast to the processes in the previous section, this equation is still scalar-valued, since the goal is to find a contour that segments all channels simultaneously. In [13] it is shown that the final contour is a geodesic in a metric that now depends on $J(H_\sigma)$. The PDE (25.33) may also be rewritten as

$$\partial_t u \ = \ g(\operatorname{tr} J(H_\sigma))\, \partial_{\xi\xi} u \ + \ \nabla^\top (g(\operatorname{tr} J(H_\sigma)))\, \nabla u \ . \tag{25.34}$$

Since a tensor-valued image involves more channels than a scalar-valued one, we can expect that this additional information stabilises the process when noise is present.

Figure 25.7 shows the temporal evolution of the active contour model for tensor fields. The goal was to extract the contour of the human brain shown in the original image. First one notices that the evolution is slower in the noisy case. The reason is that noise creates large values in the trace of the structure tensor. As a consequence, the evolution is slowed down. For larger times, however, both results become very similar. This shows the high noise robustness of the active contour model for tensor-valued data sets. A comparison with an uncoupled active contour model in Fig. 25.8 demonstrates the crucial role of channel coupling.

Alternative active contour models based on the Mumford–Shah functional have been considered recently in [29].

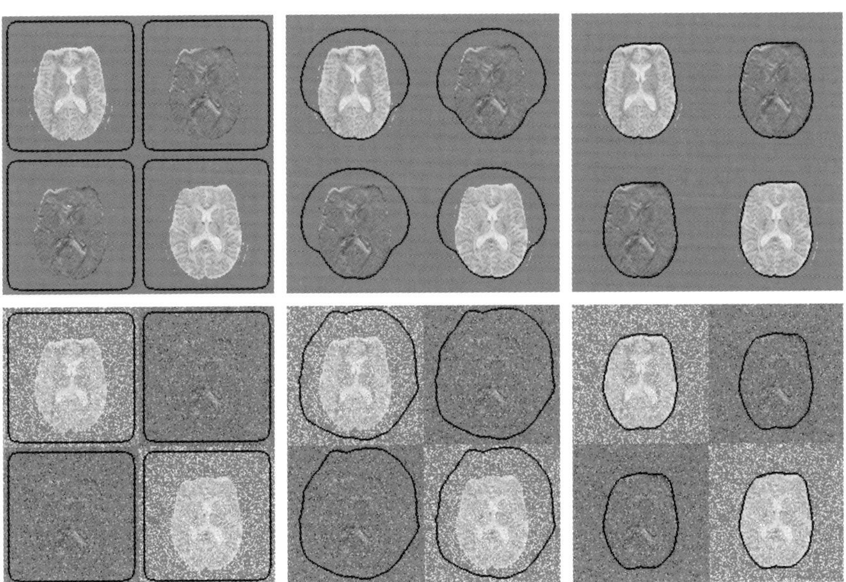

Fig. 25.7. Tensor-valued geodesic active contours ($\sigma = 3$, $\lambda = 1$). *Top row*, from *left* to *right*: Tensor image of size 128×128 including contour at time $t = 0$, $t = 960$ and $t = 9600$. *Bottom row*, from *left* to *right*: Same experiment with 30% noise. From [13]

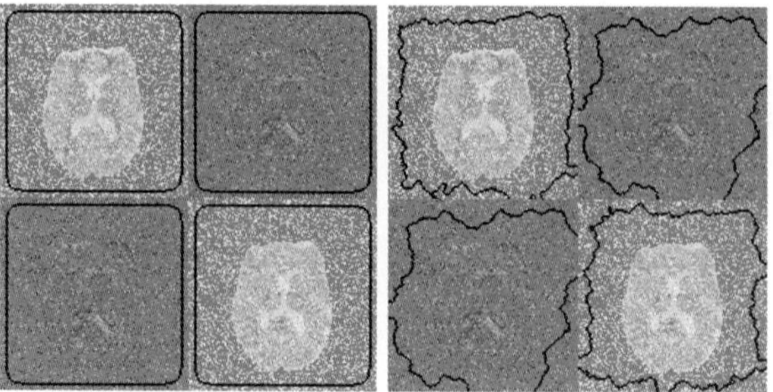

Fig. 25.8. *Left*: Noisy tensor image from Fig. 25.7 with initial contour. *Right*: Result when no channel coupling is used. ($\sigma = 3$, $\lambda = 1$, $t = 9600$). From [13]

25.8 Summary and Conclusions

We have surveyed a number of discontinuity-preserving PDEs for denoising or segmenting tensor fields. They include isotropic and anisotropic nonlinear diffusion and their corresponding regularisation methods, mean curvature motion, self-snakes, and geodesic active contours. We have seen that they arise as natural extensions of their scalar-valued predecessors provided that uniform design principles are obeyed: The evolution of the different channels has to be coupled by a joint diffusivity, diffusion tensor or smoothing direction. Instead of adapting the nonlinear PDEs to the evolving image structure via the squared gradient magnitude, the trace of a structure tensor is used. In those cases where the edge direction is required, it is replaced by the eigenvector direction for the smallest eigenvalue of the structure tensor. Apart from these natural design principles, PDEs for tensor fields offer additional qualities: Their continuous nature supports rotationally invariant models. Last but not least, by virtue of the channel coupling a maximum–minimum principle for the scalar-valued PDEs translates into preservation of positive semidefiniteness in the tensor setting.

Acknowledgements

We are grateful to Anna Vilanova i Bartrolí (Eindhoven Institute of Technology) and Carola van Pul (Maxima Medical Center, Eindhoven) for providing us with the DT-MRI dataset and for discussing questions concerning data conversion. Our research is partly funded by the *DFG* under the projects We2602/1-1 and We2602/1-2.

References

1. L. Alvarez, P.-L. Lions, and J.-M. Morel. Image selective smoothing and edge detection by nonlinear diffusion. II. *SIAM Journal on Numerical Analysis*, 29:845–866, 1992.

2. G. Aubert and P. Kornprobst. *Mathematical Problems in Image Processing: Partial Differential Equations and the Calculus of Variations*, volume 147 of *Applied Mathematical Sciences*. Springer, New York, 2002.

3. T. Brox, J. Weickert, B. Burgeth, and P. Mrázek. Nonlinear structure tensors. Technical Report 113, Dept. of Mathematics, Saarland University, Saarbrücken, Germany, October 2004.

4. F. Cao. *Geometric Curve Evolution and Image Processing*, volume 1805 of *Lecture Notes in Mathematics*. Springer, Berlin, 2003.

5. V. Caselles, R. Kimmel, and G. Sapiro. Geodesic active contours. *International Journal of Computer Vision*, 22:61–79, 1997.

6. F. Catté, P.-L. Lions, J.-M. Morel, and T. Coll. Image selective smoothing and edge detection by nonlinear diffusion. *SIAM Journal on Numerical Analysis*, 32:1895–1909, 1992.

7. A. Chambolle. Partial differential equations and image processing. In *Proc. 1994 IEEE International Conference on Image Processing*, volume 1, pp. 16–20, Austin, TX, November 1994. IEEE Computer Society Press.

8. C. Chefd'Hotel, D. Tschumperlé, R. Deriche, and O. Faugeras. Constrained flows of matrix-valued functions: Application to diffusion tensor regularization. In A. Heyden, G. Sparr, M. Nielsen, and P. Johansen, editors, *Computer Vision – ECCV 2002*, volume 2350 of *Lecture Notes in Computer Science*, pp. 251–265. Springer, Berlin, 2002.

9. D. H. Chung and G. Sapiro. On the level lines and geometry of vector-valued images. *IEEE Signal Processing Letters*, 7(9):241–243, 2000.

10. O. Coulon, D. C. Alexander, and S. A. Arridge. Diffusion tensor magnetic resonance image regularisation. *Medical Image Analysis*, 8(1):47–67, 2004.

11. S. Di Zenzo. A note on the gradient of a multi-image. *Computer Vision, Graphics and Image Processing*, 33:116–125, 1986.

12. C. Feddern, J. Weickert, and B. Burgeth. Level-set methods for tensor-valued images. In O. Faugeras and N. Paragios, editors, *Proc. Second IEEE Workshop on Geometric and Level Set Methods in Computer Vision*, pp. 65–72, Nice, France, October 2003. INRIA.

13. C. Feddern, J. Weickert, B. Burgeth, and M. Welk. Curvature-driven PDE methods for matrix-valued images. *International Journal of Computer Vision*, 2005. In press.

14. G. Gerig, O. Kübler, R. Kikinis, and F. A. Jolesz. Nonlinear anisotropic filtering of MRI data. *IEEE Transactions on Medical Imaging*, 11:221–232, 1992.

15. T. Iijima. Basic theory on normalization of pattern (in case of typical one-dimensional pattern). *Bulletin of the Electrotechnical Laboratory*, 26:368–388, 1962. In Japanese.

16. M. Kass, A. Witkin, and D. Terzopoulos. Snakes: Active contour models. *International Journal of Computer Vision*, 1:321–331, 1988.

17. S. Kichenassamy, A. Kumar, P. Olver, A. Tannenbaum, and A. Yezzi. Conformal curvature flows: from phase transitions to active vision. *Archive for Rational Mechanics and Analysis*, 134:275–301, 1996.

18. R. Kimmel. *Numerical Geometry of Images: Theory, Algorithms, and Applications*. Springer, New York, 2003.

19. N. Nordström. Biased anisotropic diffusion – a unified regularization and diffusion approach to edge detection. *Image and Vision Computing*, 8:318–327, 1990.

20. S. Osher and N. Paragios, editors. *Geometric Level Set Methods in Imaging, Vision and Graphics*. Springer, New York, 2003.

21. S. Osher and L. I. Rudin. Feature-oriented image enhancement using shock filters. *SIAM Journal on Numerical Analysis*, 27:919–940, 1990.

22. P. Perona and J. Malik. Scale space and edge detection using anisotropic diffusion. *IEEE Transactions on Pattern Analysis and Machine Intelligence*, 12:629–639, 1990.

23. T. Preußer and M. Rumpf. A level set method for anisotropic geometric diffusion in 3D image processing. *SIAM Journal on Applied Mathematics*, 62(5):1772–1793, 2002.

24. G. Sapiro. Vector (self) snakes: a geometric framework for color, texture and multiscale image segmentation. In *Proc. 1996 IEEE International Conference on Image Processing*, volume 1, pp. 817–820, Lausanne, Switzerland, September 1996.

25. G. Sapiro. *Geometric Partial Differential Equations and Image Analysis*. Cambridge University Press, Cambridge, UK, 2001.

26. O. Scherzer and J. Weickert. Relations between regularization and diffusion filtering. *Journal of Mathematical Imaging and Vision*, 12(1):43–63, February 2000.

27. D. Tschumperlé and R. Deriche. Orthonormal vector sets regularization with PDE's and applications. *International Journal of Computer Vision*, 50(3):237–252, December 2002.

28. B. Vemuri, Y. Chen, M. Rao, T. McGraw, Z. Wang, and T. Mareci. Fiber tract mapping from diffusion tensor MRI. In *Proc. First IEEE Workshop on Variational and Level Set Methods in Computer Vision*, pp. 73–80, Vancouver, Canada, July 2001. IEEE Computer Society Press.

29. Z. Wang and B. C. Vemuri. An affine invariant tensor dissimilarity measure and its applications to tensor-valued image segmentation. In *Proc. 2004 IEEE Computer Society Conference on Computer Vision and Pattern Recognition*, volume 1, pp. 228–233, Washington, DC, June 2004. IEEE Computer Society Press.

30. J. Weickert. *Anisotropic Diffusion in Image Processing*. Teubner, Stuttgart, 1998.

31. J. Weickert and T. Brox. Diffusion and regularization of vector- and matrix-valued images. In M. Z. Nashed and O. Scherzer, editors, *Inverse Problems, Image Analysis, and Medical Imaging*, volume 313 of *Contemporary Mathematics*, pp. 251–268. AMS, Providence, 2002.

32. R. T. Whitaker and X. Xue. Variable-conductance, level-set curvature for image denoising. In *Proc. 2001 IEEE International Conference on Image Processing*, pp. 142–145, Thessaloniki, Greece, October 2001.

A

Color Plates

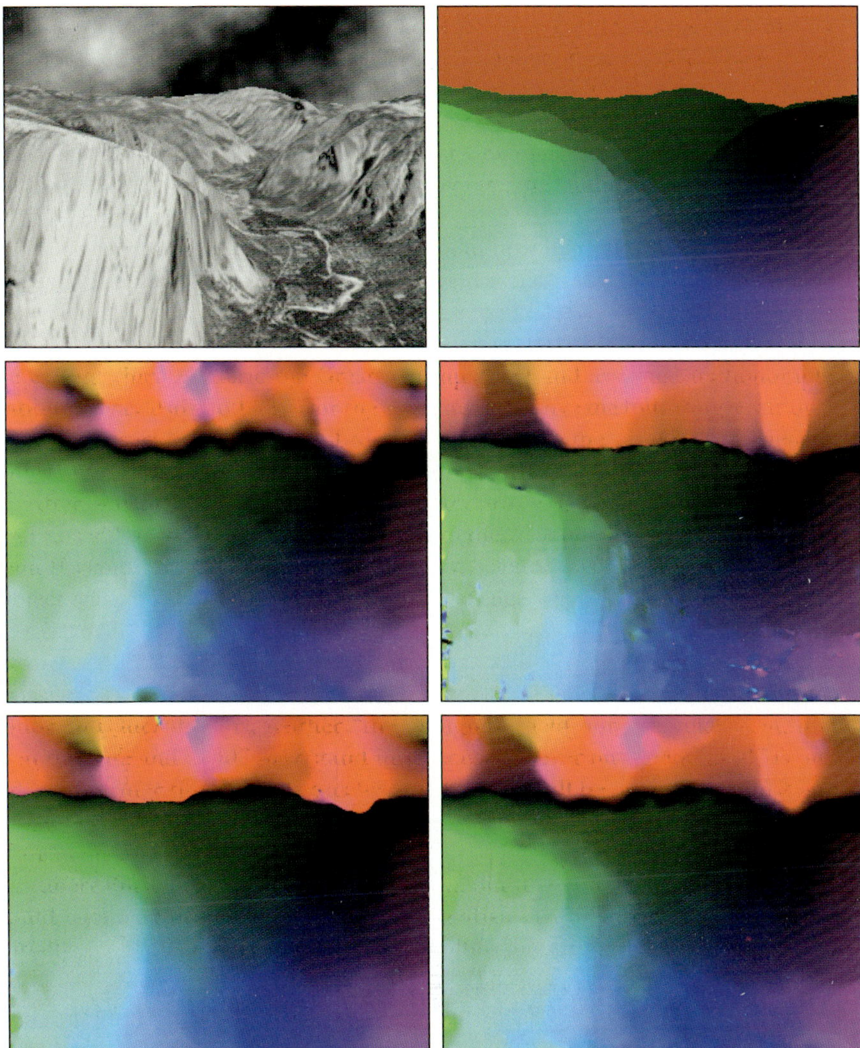

Fig. 2.6. Yosemite sequence ($316 \times 252 \times 15$). From *Left* to *Right, Top* to *Bottom:* (**a**) Frame 8. (**b**) Ground truth. (**c**) Classic structure tensor. (**d**) Nonlinear structure tensor. (**e**) Robust structure tensor. (**f**) Coherence based smoothing

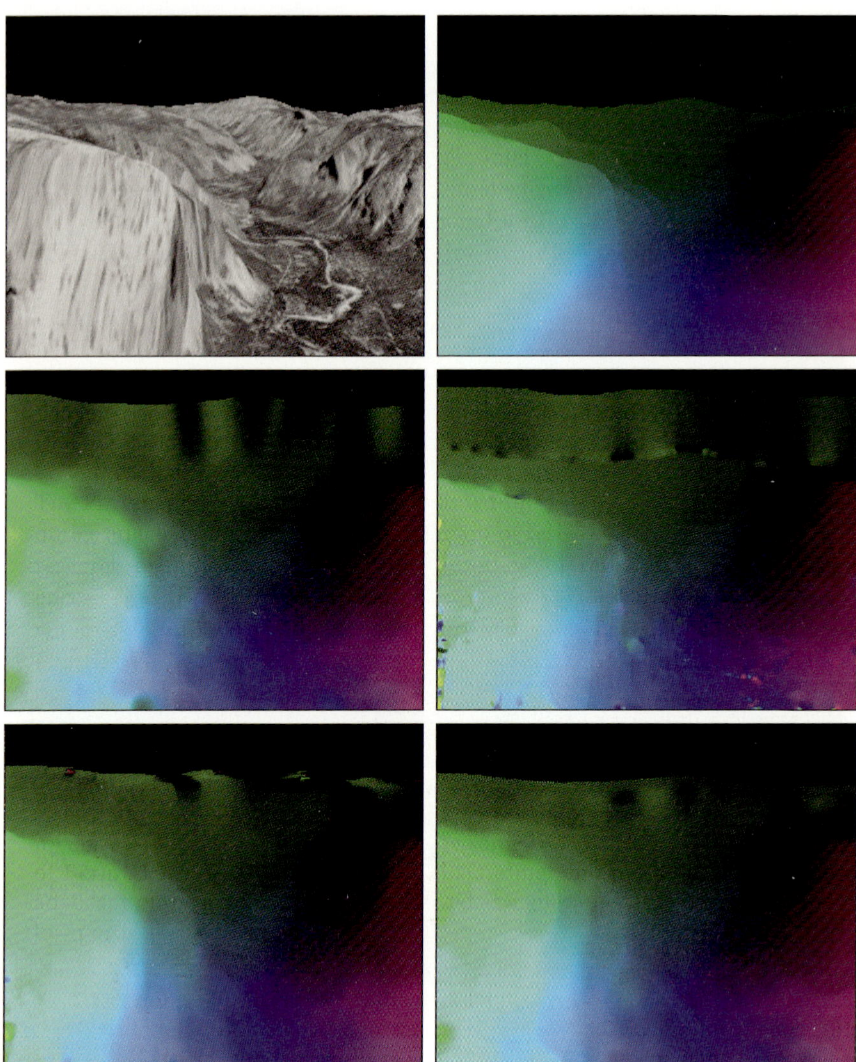

Fig. 2.7. Yosemite sequence without clouds ($316 \times 252 \times 15$). From *Left* to *Right*, *Top* to *Bottom*: (**a**) Frame 8. (**b**) Ground truth. (**c**) Classic structure tensor. (**d**) Nonlinear structure tensor. (**e**) Robust structure tensor. (**f**) Coherence based smoothing

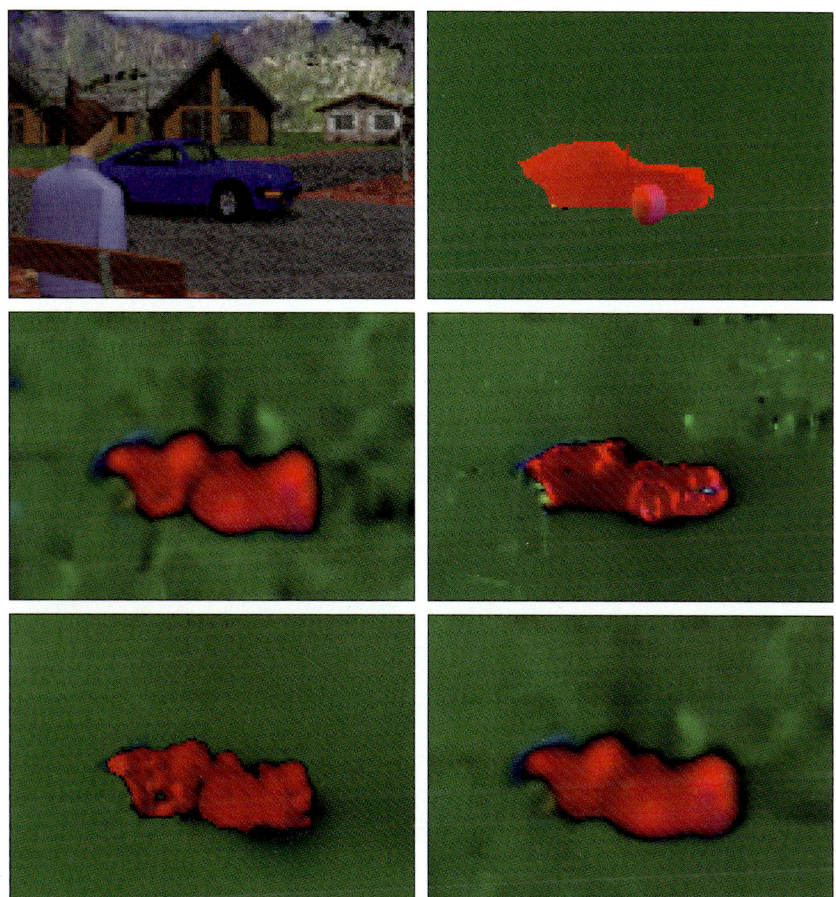

Fig. 2.8. Street sequence (cropped) ($145 \times 100 \times 20$). From *Left* to *Right*, *Top* to *Bottom*: (**a**) Frame 10. (**b**) Ground truth. (**c**) Classic structure tensor. (**d**) Nonlinear structure tensor. (**e**) Robust structure tensor. (**f**) Coherence based smoothing

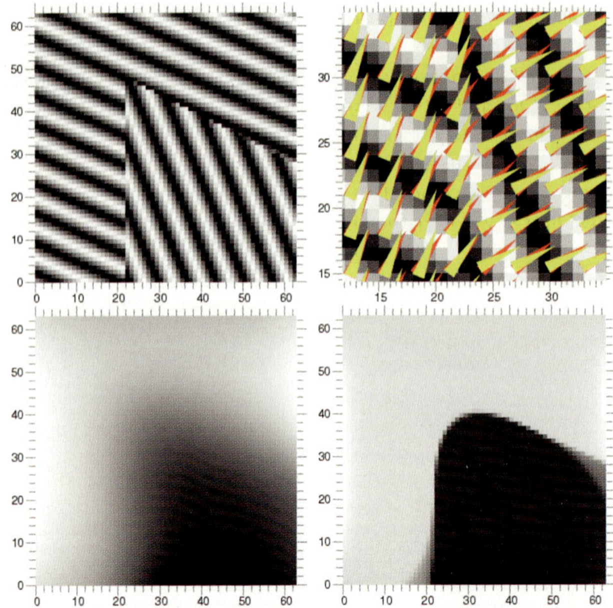

Fig. 2.10. Comparison between least squares and robust orientation estimation

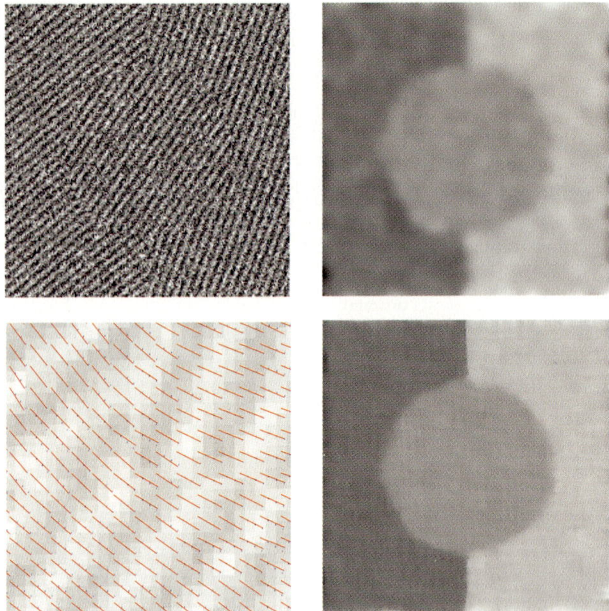

Fig. 2.11. Comparison between least squares and robust orientation estimation

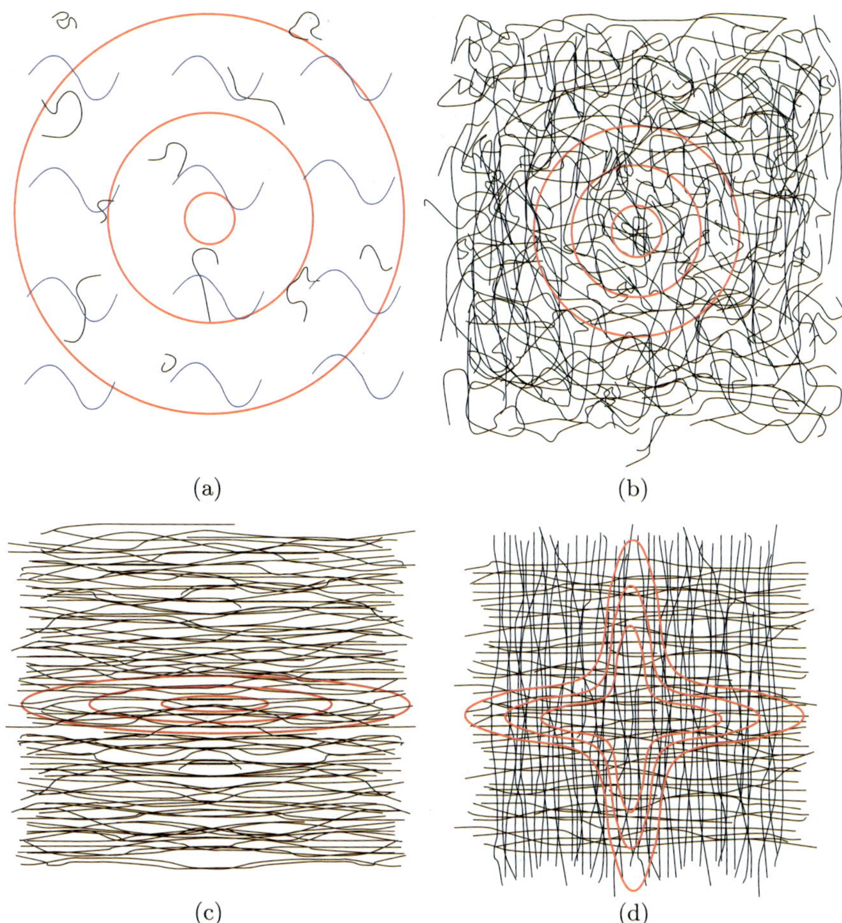

(a)   (b)

(c)   (d)

Fig. 5.1. Schematic diagrams four microstructures found in the brain. The black lines are barriers to the movement of water molecules. The red contours show the expected shape of p in each tissue. Panel (a) shows a fluid-filled region. Panel (b) shows isotropic grey matter. Panels (c) and (d) show white matter with one and two dominant fibre orientations, respectively

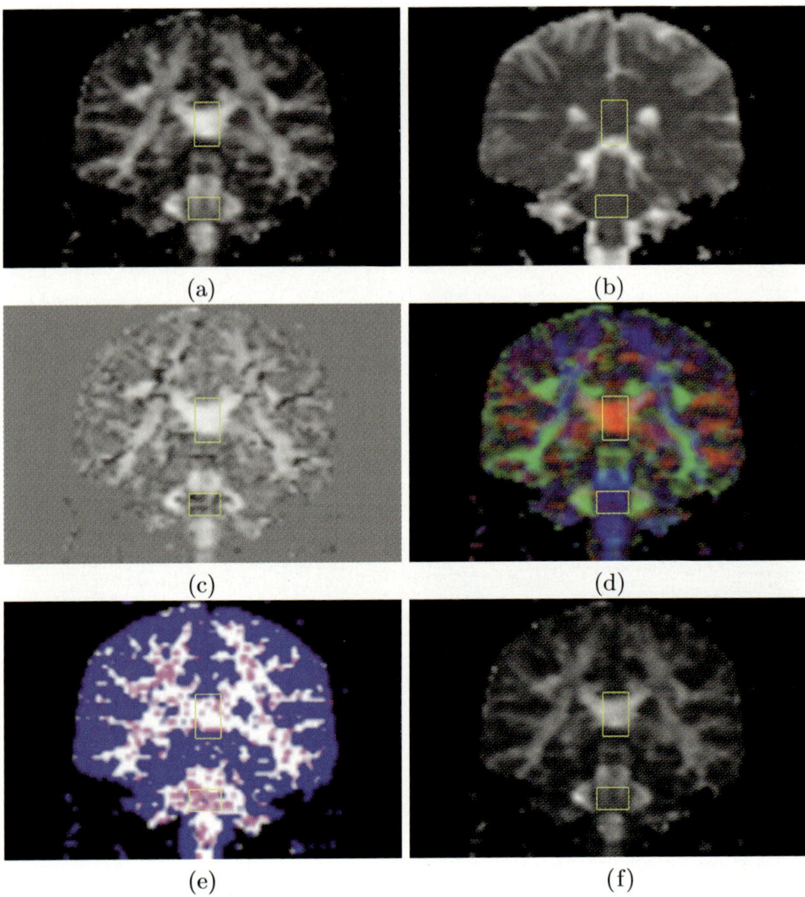

Fig. 5.3. Shows various features of p plotted over a coronal slice through a healthy human brain. Panel (a) shows the fractional anisotropy, ν. Panel (b) shows Tr(D). Panels (c) shows the skewness, μ. Panel (d) shows the colour coded principal direction, $\mathbf{e}_1$. Panel (e) shows the output of Alexander's voxel classification algorithm (Sect. 3.2); black is background, blue is order 0, white is order 2 and pink is order 4. Panel (f) shows the spherical-harmonic anisotropy (Sect. 3.2). In each panel, the upper region of interest contains some grey matter (*top*), part of the corpus callosum (*middle*) and some CSF (*bottom*). The lower region contains the fibre crossing in the pons

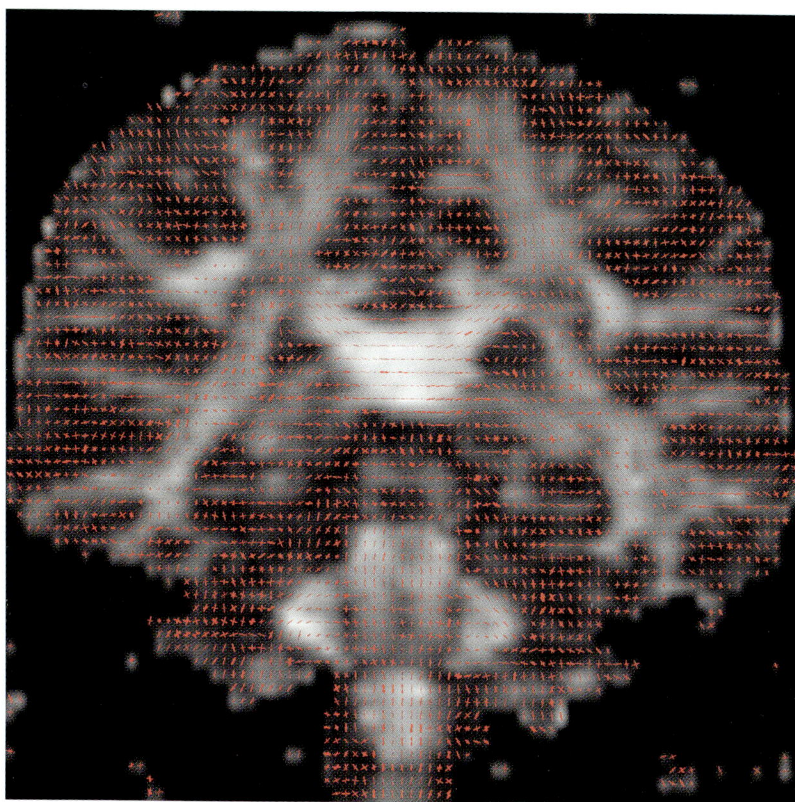

Fig. 5.4. Shows the PAS (*in red*) in brain voxels of the coronal slice in Fig. 5.3 superimposed on the fractional anisotropy map

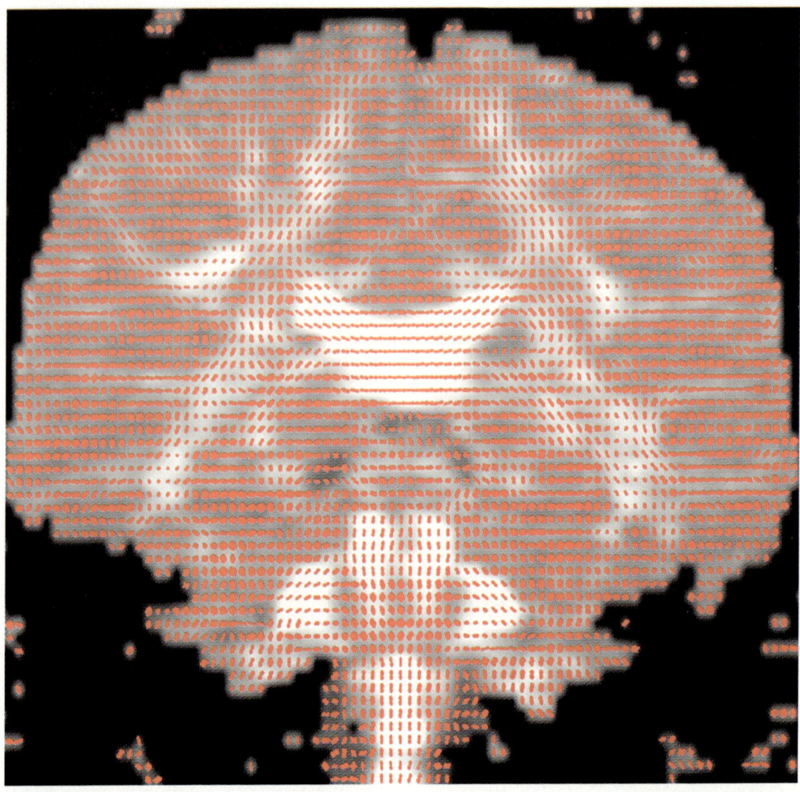

Fig. 5.5. Shows the ODF (*in red*) approximated using **q**-ball in brain voxels of the coronal slice in Fig. 5.3 superimposed on the fractional anisotropy map

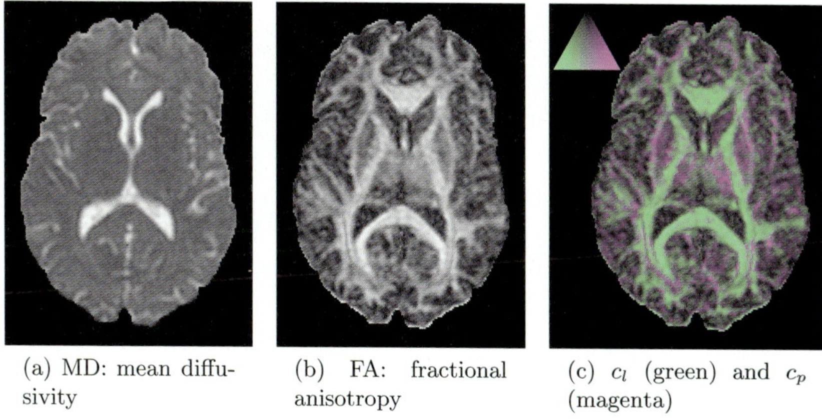

(a) MD: mean diffu-
sivity

(b) FA: fractional
anisotropy

(c) c_l (green) and c_p
(magenta)

Fig. 7.4. Different shape metrics applied to one slice of a brain DTI scan

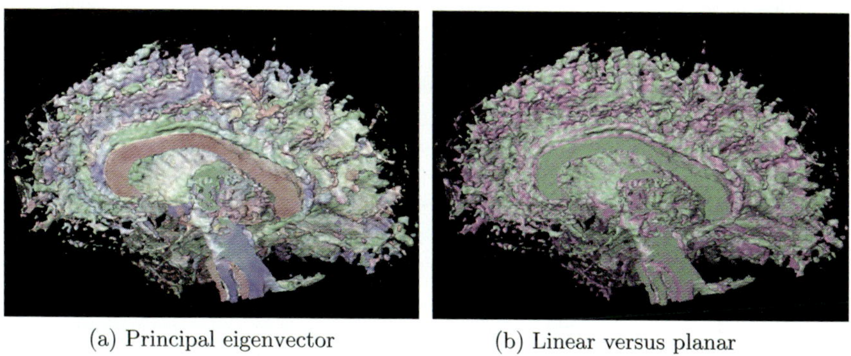

(a) Principal eigenvector

(b) Linear versus planar

Fig. 7.6. Volume renderings of half a brain scan, (**a**) colored according to orientation
of principal eigenvector; (**b**) the distribution of linear (*green*) and planar (*magenta*)
anisotropy. Surface is defined by FA = 0.4

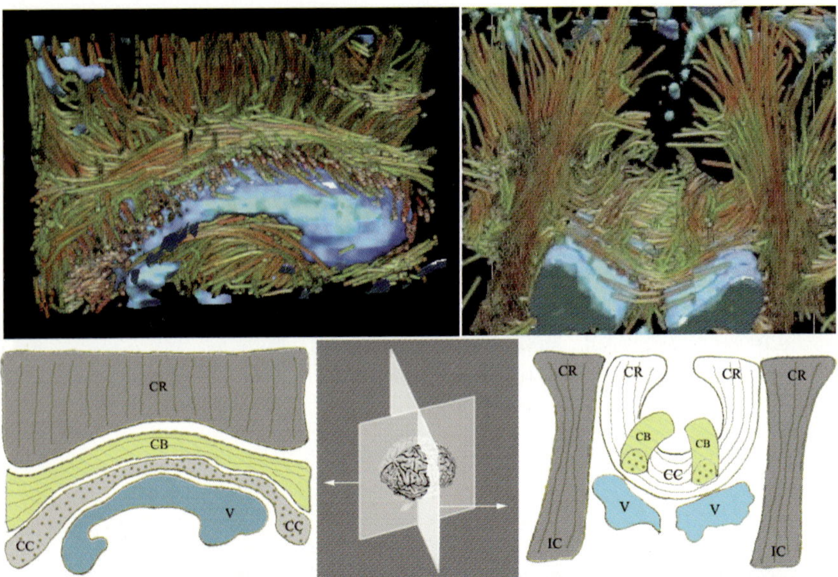

Fig. 7.7. Interactive volume renderings of a human brain data set. The volume renderings (*top*) show collections of threads consistent with major white-matter structures: IC = internal capsule, CR = corona radiata, CB = cingulum bundle, CC = corpus callosum diagrammed on the bottom. Components of the tensor-valued data control thread orientation, color, and density. Direct volume rendering simultaneously shows in blue the cerebral spinal fluid in the ventricles (labeled V) and some sulci for anatomical context

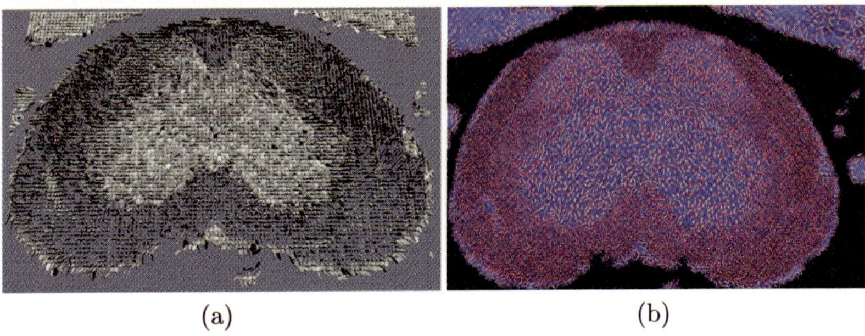

(a)   (b)

Fig. 7.8. Brush strokes illustrate the orientation and magnitude of the diffusion: background color and texture-map show additional information

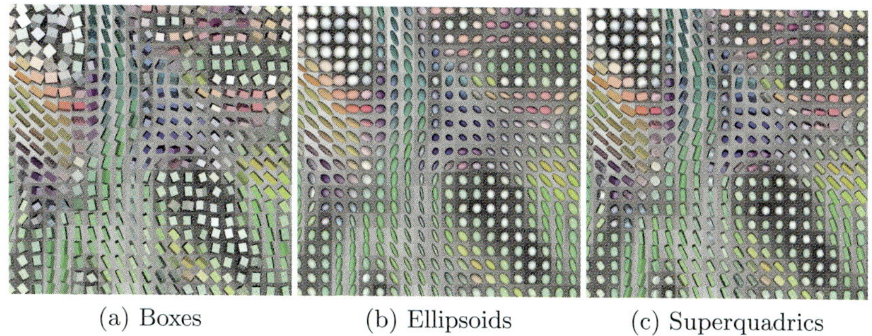

(a) Boxes   (b) Ellipsoids   (c) Superquadrics

Fig. 7.9. A portion of a brain DTI scan as visualized by three different glyph methods (overall glyph sizes have been normalized)

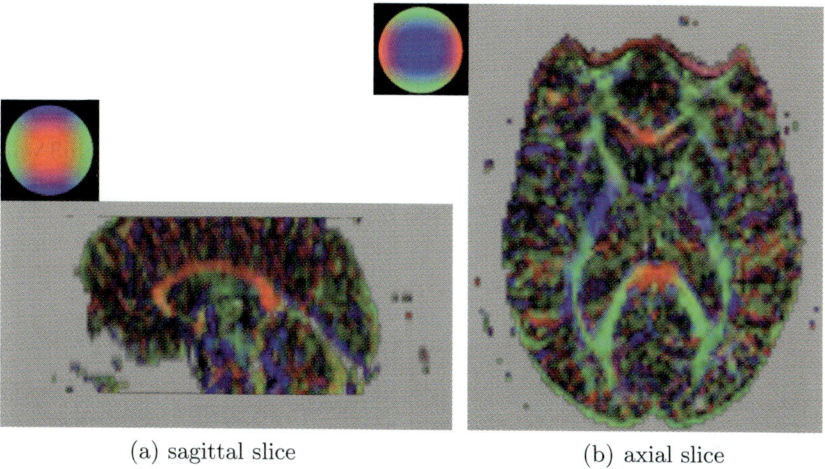

(a) sagittal slice   (b) axial slice

Fig. 7.11. Mapping of $\mathbf{e}_1$ to the RGB channel shown in 2D slices of a healthy volunteer brain

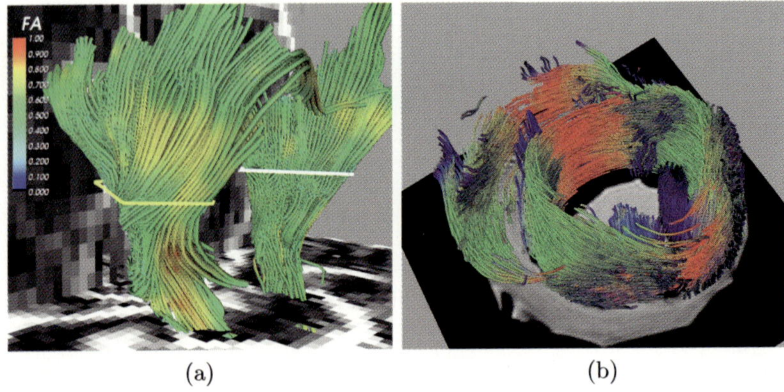

(a)   (b)

Fig. 7.12. (a) Streamline tracing using two ROIs to trace the corona radiata in a data set of a healthy volunteer brain. (b) Streamlines in a data set of a goat heart using the seeding technique of Vilanova et al. [38]

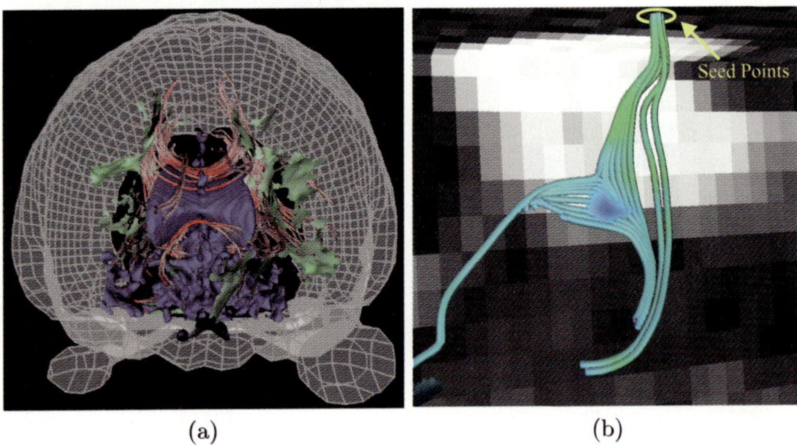

(a)   (b)

Fig. 7.13. Examples of streamsurfaces: (a) red streamlines (represented as cylinders) and green streamsurfaces generated using the method of Zhang et al. [40] show linear and planar anisotropy, respectively, together with anatomical landmarks for context; (b) Streamlines using seed points (yellow region) trace streamsurfaces and show the possible prolongation of the fiber bundle, generated using the algorithm of Vilanova et al. [38]

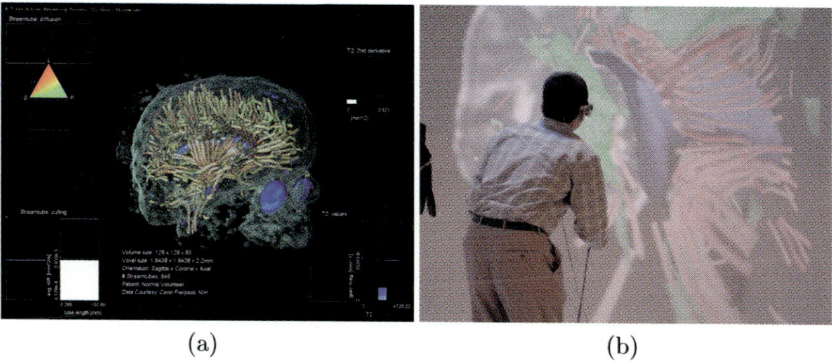

(a)   (b)

Fig. 7.14. (**a**) An interactive exploration tool for DTI volume rendering. Clockwise from upper left are a 2D barycentric widget, a 1D widget, a 2D Cartesian widget, and a 2D Cartesian culling widget. (**b**) A user explores a complex 3D model in a virtual reality CAVE

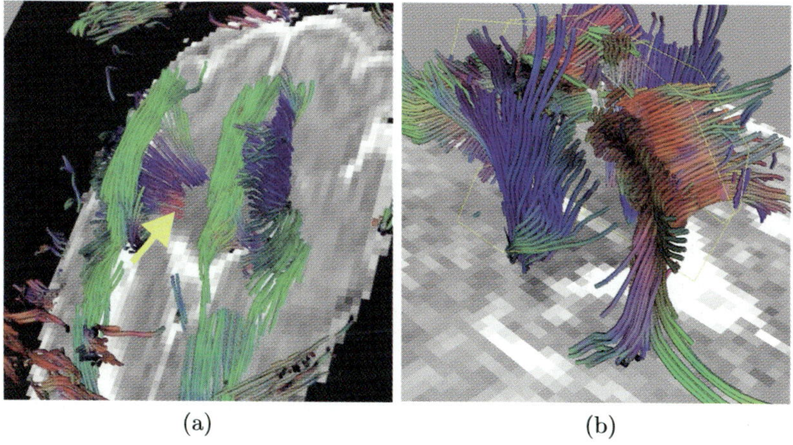

(a)   (b)

Fig. 7.15. Studies of white matter fibers in neonatal brains with different data sets. (**a**) Premature neonate lacking corpus callosum (*see arrow*), (**b**) full-term neonate where no fiber abnormalities were found. Corpus callosum and corona radiata are seen

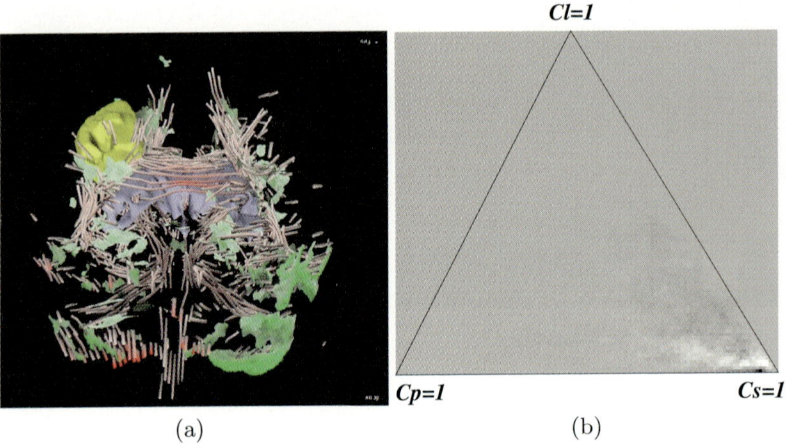

(a)   (b)

Fig. 7.16. Visual exploration and quantitative analysis of a cancerous brain. (a) A 3D visualization showing streamtubes and streamsurfaces as well as tumor and ventricles. (b) The difference histogram obtained by subtracting normalized barycentric histograms calculated from tumor-bearing and contralateral sections. Here zero maps to medium gray because the difference is signed. Note that the most striking difference occurs near the $c_s = 1$ vertex

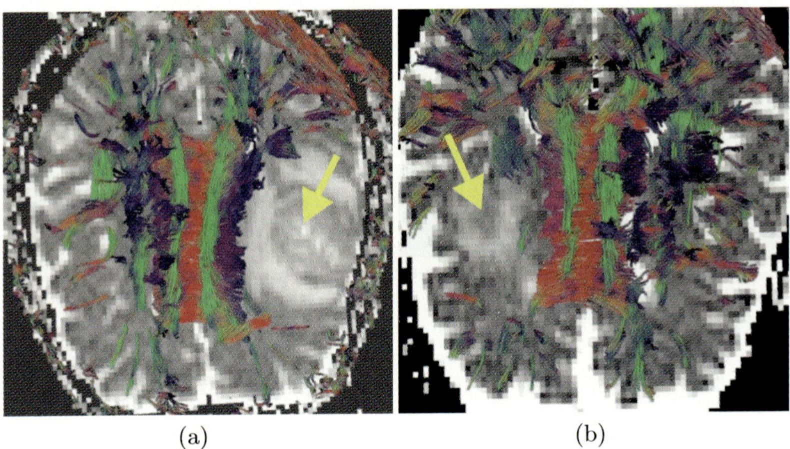

(a)   (b)

Fig. 7.17. Two cases of adult tumor brain. (a) Fibers are pushed by the tumor. (b) No fibers are in the tumor area, indicating the destruction of neural structures there

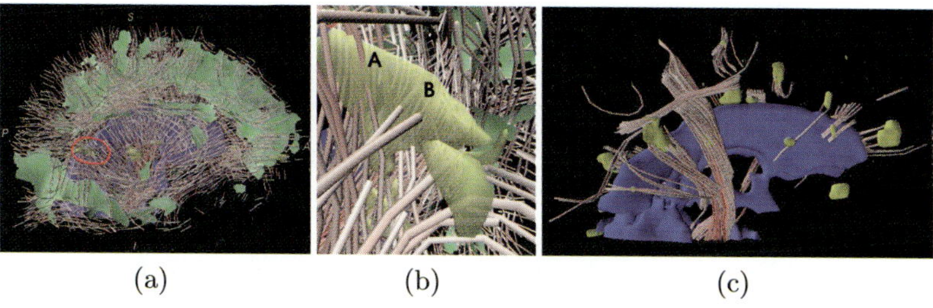

(a)   (b)   (c)

Fig. 7.18. Visualization of coregistered DTI and MS lesion models. (**a**) The whole brain with streamtubes, streamsurfaces, lesion masks and ventricles. (**b**) A closeup view of white matter fibers near the MS lesions. The streamtubes around the lesion area give some clues about white matter structural changes there. (**c**) The same brain and view as (a) but showing only streamtubes that contact the lesions, thus clarifying the white matter structures involved

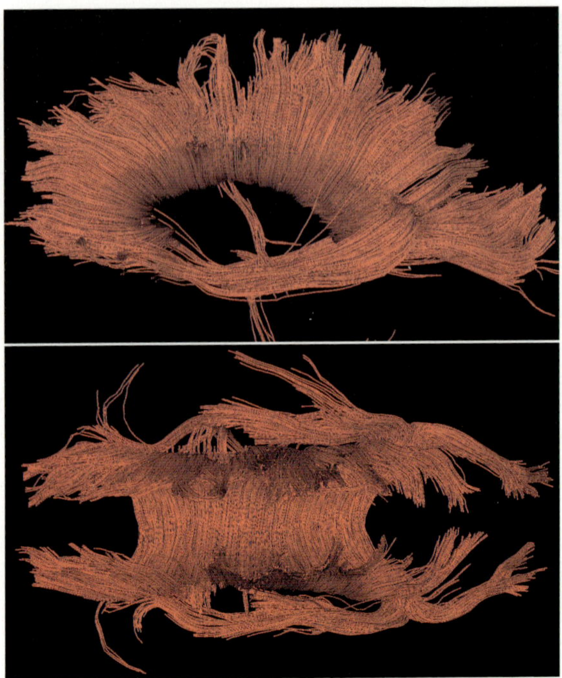

Fig. 8.1. Visualization of the corpus callosum as extracted via fiber tractography [5] from the diffusion tensor MR image of a female human brain. Views are from the side (*top*) and top (*bottom*) of the brain, with the head facing toward the left. The corpus callosum is the connecting band of white matter fibers that provide the primary means of communication between the two cerebral hemispheres

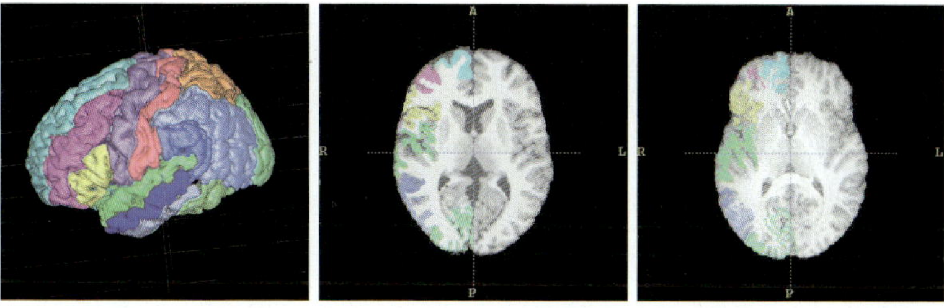

Fig. 8.2. Atlas-based brain image segmentation. (*Left*) A surface rendering of
the labeled atlas used in this work. (*Middle*) The gray matter labels for one hemisphere are shown superimposed on the underlying structural image of the brain atlas.
(*Right*) The atlas is registered to the corresponding T1-weighted structural image
of the female subject whose corpus callosum is depicted in Fig. 8.1, and the warped
gray matter labels for one hemisphere are shown superimposed on the subject's
structural image. The following brain regions are delineated in the atlas, further
details of which can be found in [6]: precentral gyrus; superior temporal gyrus; middle temporal gyrus; inferior temporal gyrus; superior frontal gyrus; middle frontal
gyrus; inferior frontal gyrus; supramarginal gyrus; postcentral gyrus; parahippocampal gyrus; occipitotemporal gyrus; superior parietal lobule; inferior parietal lobule;
occipital lobe

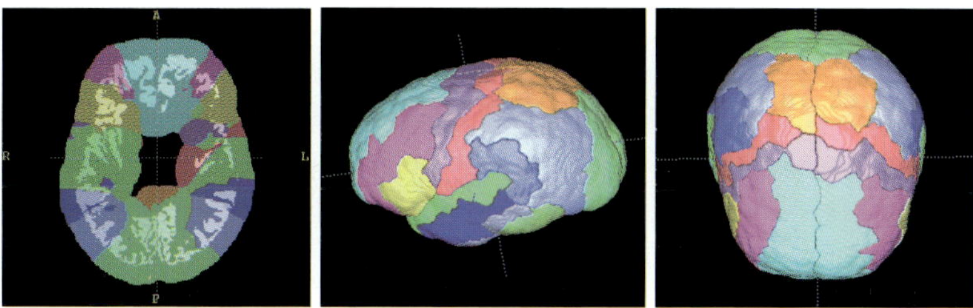

Fig. 8.3. Voronoi partition derived from the individualized atlas. (*Left*) The
distance-constrained Voronoi tessellation superimposed on the individualized gray
matter labels on which the tessellation is based. (*Middle* and *Right*) Surface renderings of the same three-dimensional Voronoi partition

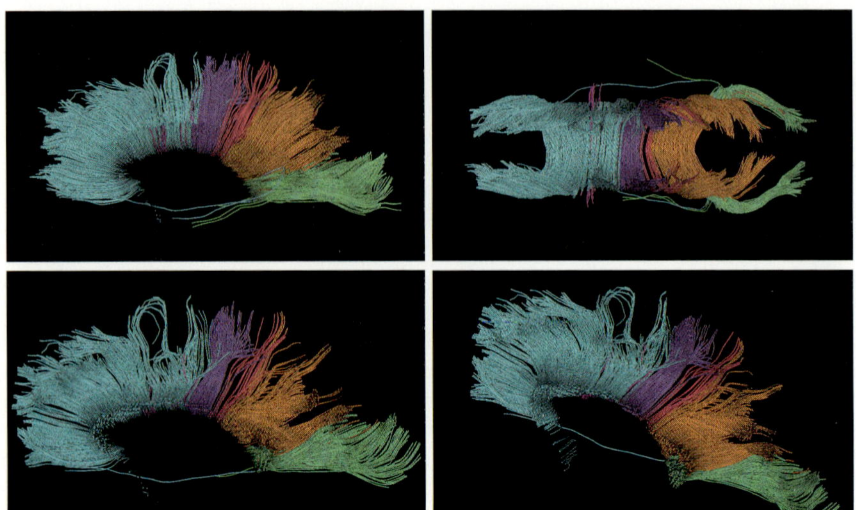

Fig. 8.5. Visualization of the anatomically labeled version of the callosal tract depicted in Fig. 8.1. The color legend is the same as that for the atlas in Fig. 8.2. The bottom row shows the tract within one hemisphere (*oblique view*) and its appearance at the midsagittal plane (*bottom left*)

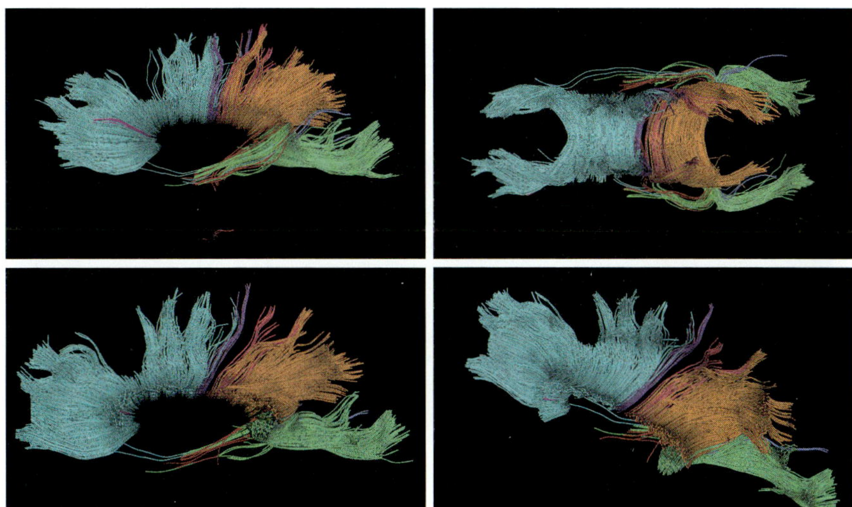

Fig. 8.6. Visualization of the anatomically labeled version of the callosal tract from a male subject. The color legend is the same as that for the atlas in Fig. 8.2. The bottom row shows the tract within one hemisphere (*oblique view*) and its appearance at the midsagittal plane (*bottom left*)

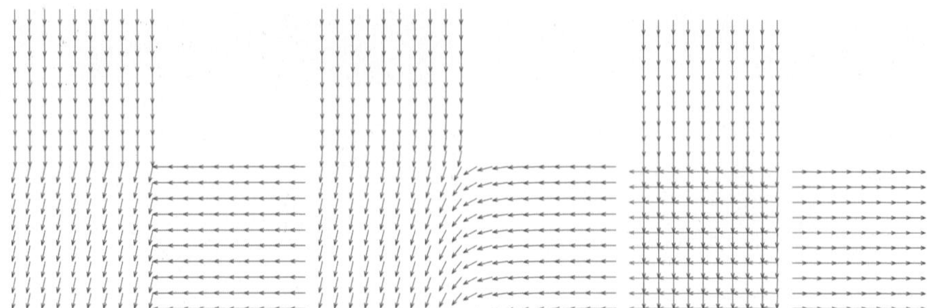

Fig. 9.1. Synthetic data. Computer simulation of crossing fibers. (a) *Left*: DTI results. *Middle*: (b) DTI variational regularization (VR) results. (c) *Right*: MTV results.Each arrow represents a voxel. Voxels represented by more than one arrow have multiple components. Only components with a considerable volume fraction are shown ($f_i > 0.3$)

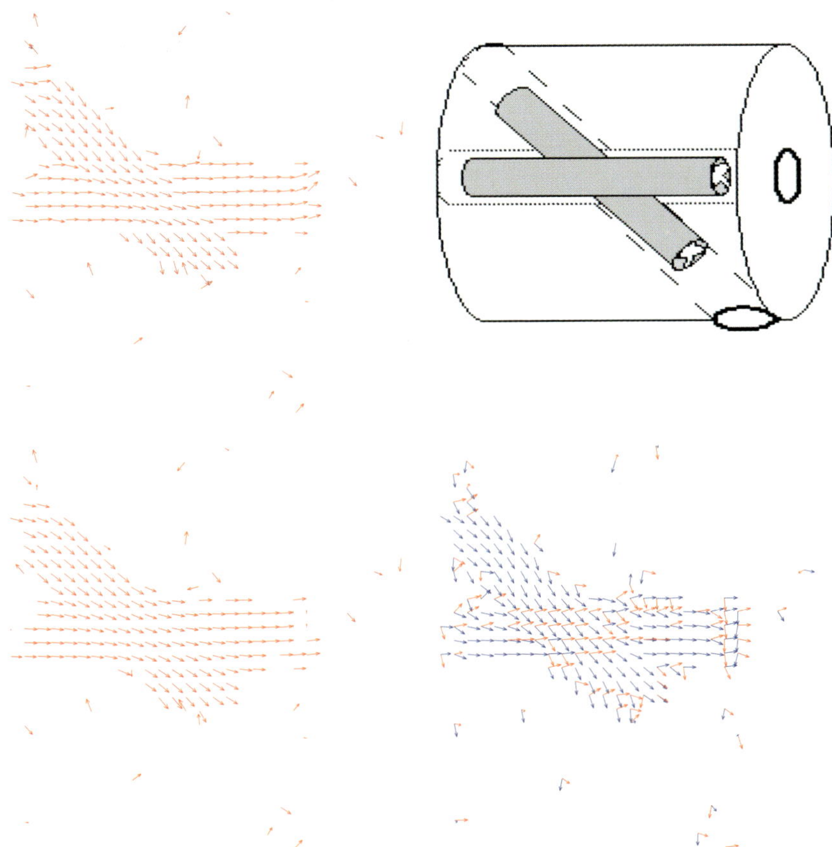

Fig. 9.2. Phantom. (a) *Top Right*: Excised spinal cords placed crossing at 45 degrees (illustration). (b) *Top Left*: DTI results. (c) *Bottom Left*: Regularization results. (d) *Bottom Right* MTV results. Only components with a considerable volume fraction are shown ($f_i > 0.3$) The directions supplied by MTV are parallel to the original fiber orientations

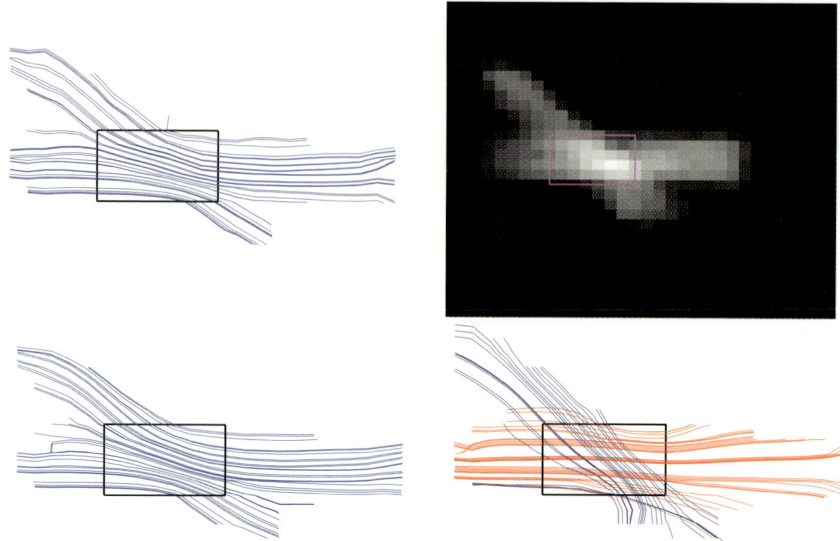

Fig. 9.3. Fiber Tracking. (**a**) *Top Right*: T_2 non diffusion weighted reference image. (**b**) *Top Left*: DTI resulted fiber tracking. (**c**) *Bottom Left*: Fiber tracking of a regularized tensor field. (**d**) *Bottom Right*: MTV resulted fiber tracking. The tracking originated from the ROI, marked with a rectangle

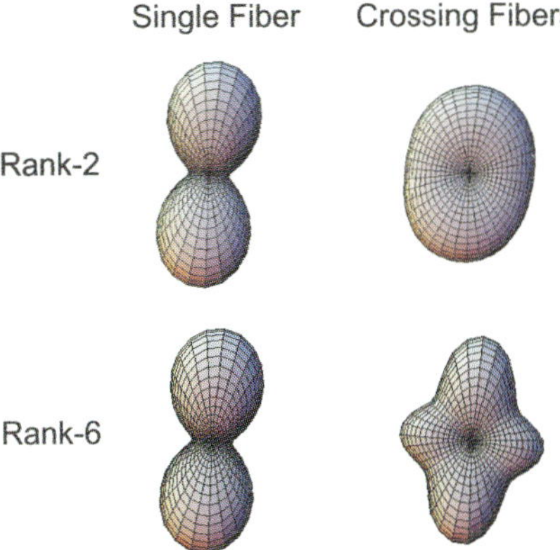

Fig. 10.1. Simulations of the diffusivity profiles from rank-2 (*top*) and rank-6 (*bottom*) tensors from a unidirectional voxel (*left*) and a voxel with two different fiber orientations (*right*)

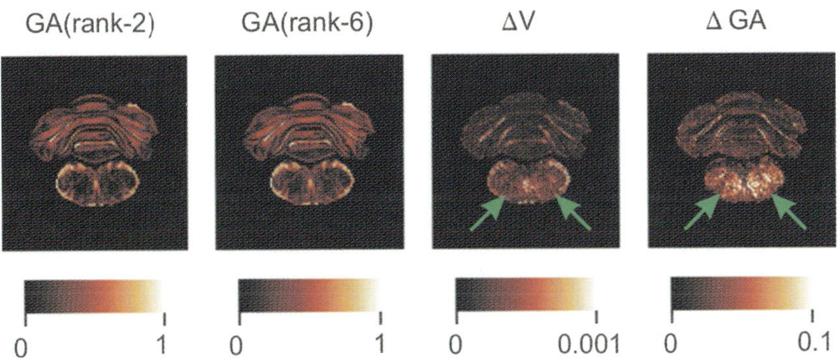

Fig. 10.2. GA values from rank-2 (left column) and rank-6 (second column) tensors from a coronal slice of an excised rat brain image. The right two columns show the difference between the variance and GA values when these two tensor models were used

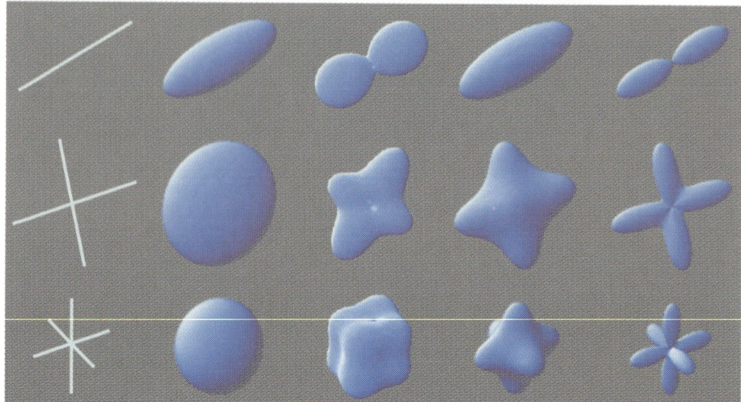

Fig. 10.3. The simulation results. The three rows show the 1, 2 and 3 fiber systems from top to bottom. The different columns show the orientations of the cylinders, probability isosurfaces obtained using rank-2 DTI, diffusivity profiles, equiprobability surfaces from rank-6 DTI, and these probability surfaces after a sharpening transformation (from *left* to *right*)

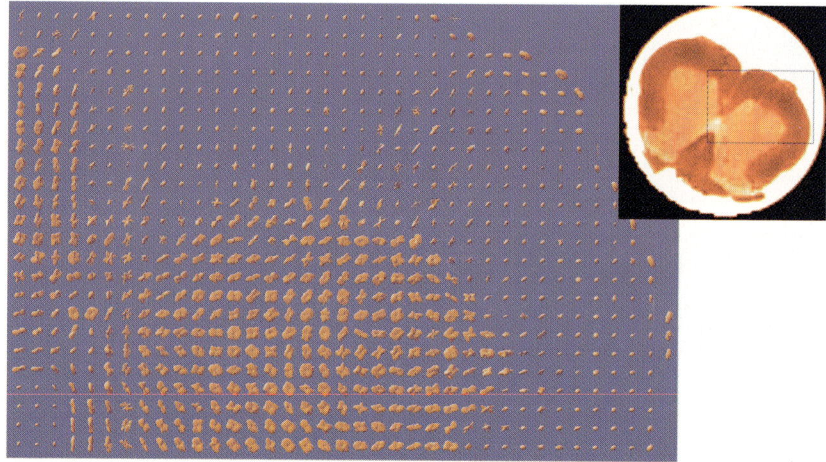

Fig. 10.4. Isosurfaces of displacement probability functions implied by a rank-6 tensor model from a selected region of interest (ROI) in an excised rat spinal cord image. The top right image is from a non-diffusion weighted dataset showing the ROI where the probability isosurfaces were calculated

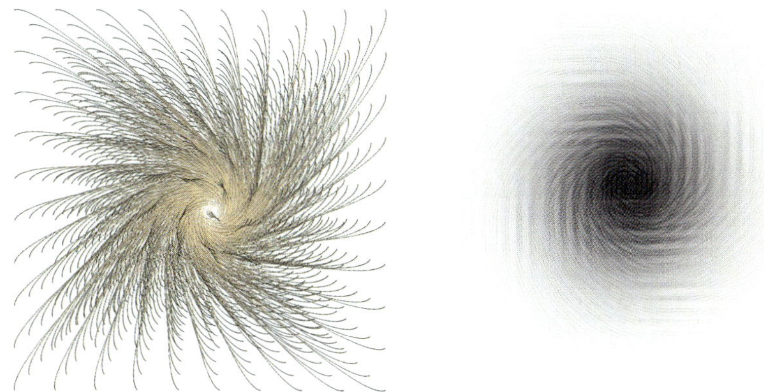

Fig. 11.1. Maelstrom of spacetime around a rotating black hole, visualized via integral lines (*left*) and vertex-based glyphs (*right*)

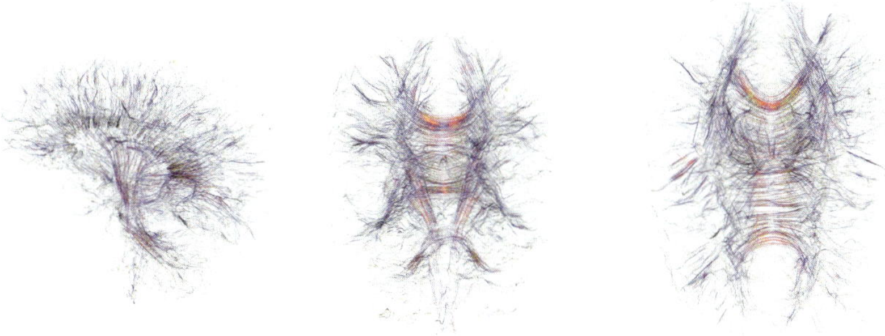

Fig. 11.2. Front, side and top view of stream lines along the maximum eigenvector in linear regions of a human brain data set

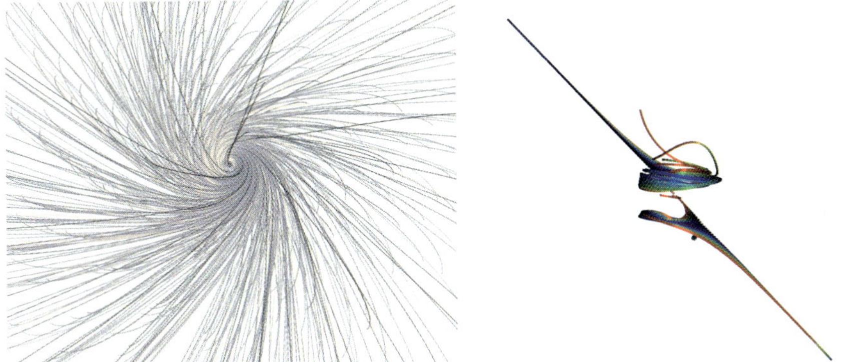

Fig. 11.4. Particle geodesics in the vicinity of a rotating black hole

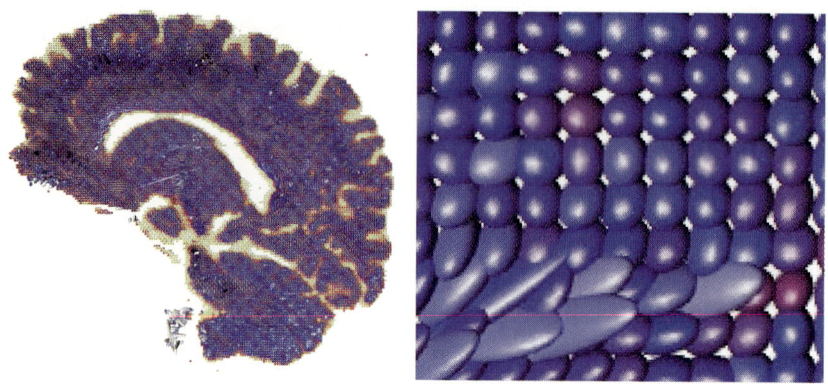

Fig. 11.5. Metric ellipsoids applied to a slice of the human brain – overview (*left*) and enlargement (*right*)

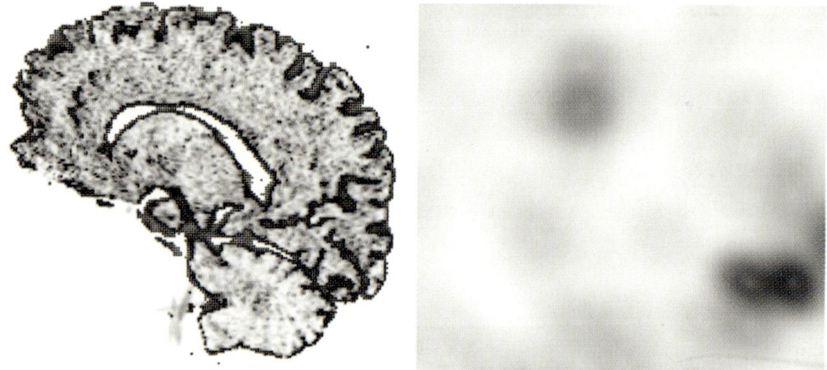

Fig. 11.6. Tensor glow technique applied to a slice of the human brain – overview (*left*) and enlargement (*right*)

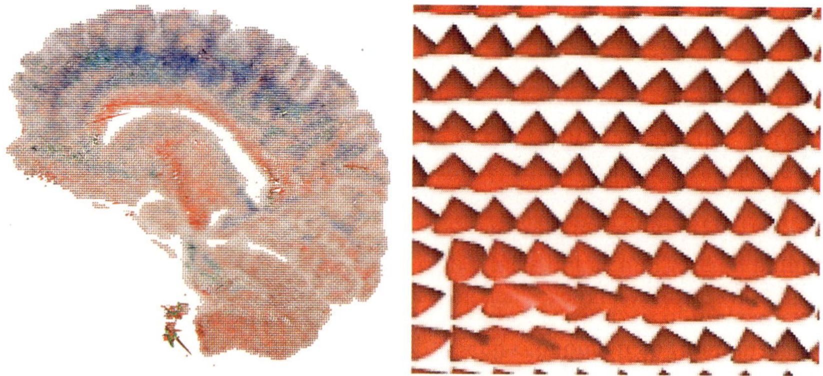

Fig. 11.7. Tensor cones applied to a slice of the human brain – overview (*left*) and enlargement (*right*)

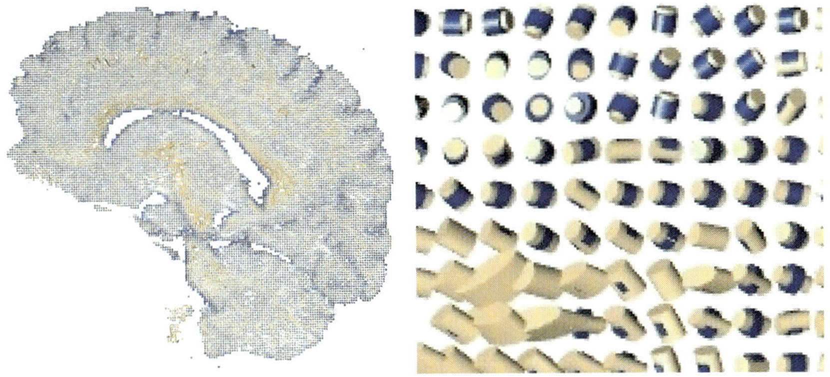

Fig. 11.8. Haber glyphs applied to a slice of a human brain – overview (*left*) and enlargement (*right*)

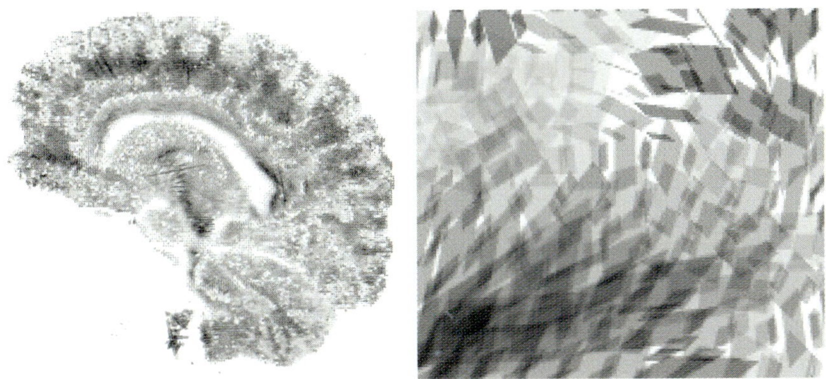

Fig. 11.9. Tensor schlieren applied to a slice of a human brain – overview (*left*) and enlargement (*right*)

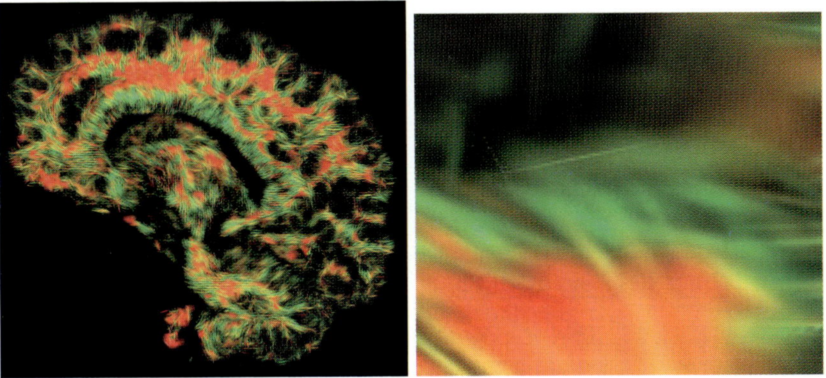

Fig. 11.10. Tensor splats applied to a slice of a human brain – overview (*left*) and enlargement (*right*)

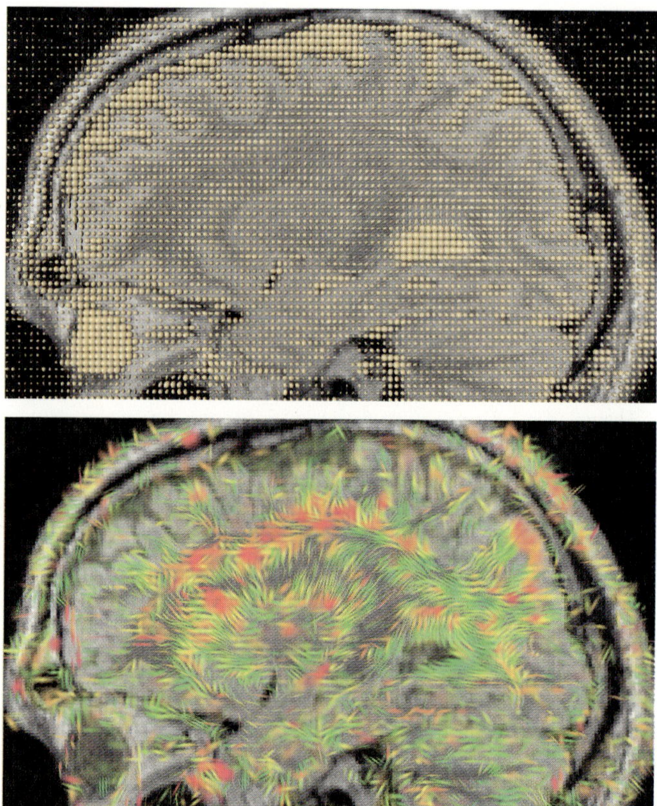

Fig. 11.11. Comparison of metric ellipsoids with tensor splats technique applied to a slice through a diffusion tensor field acquired from a human brain

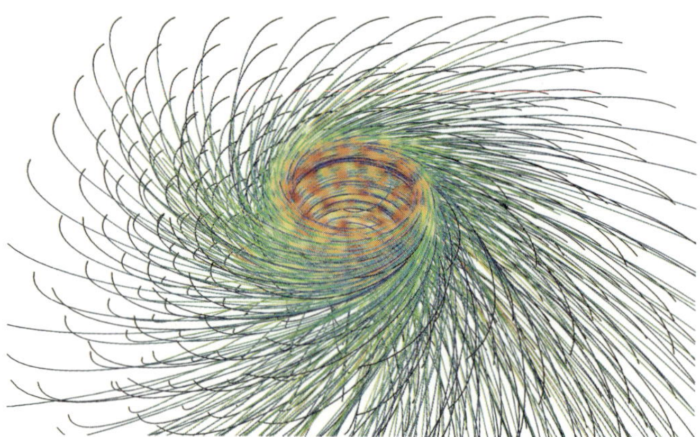

Fig. 11.12. Geodesics in the spacetime of a rotating black hole, indicating the 'event horizon' of the black hole at the location of their congruence

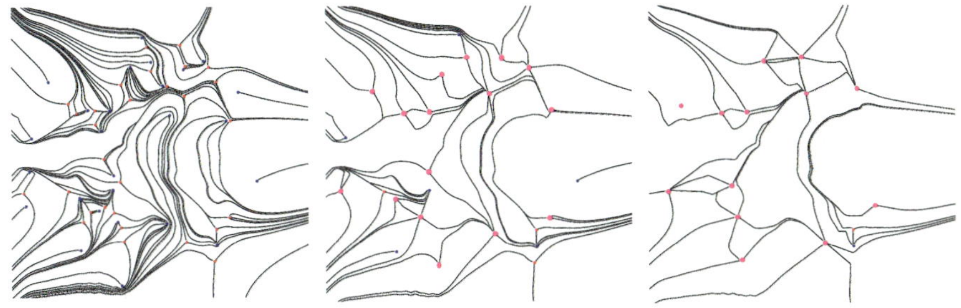

Fig. 13.11. Original and scaled topology

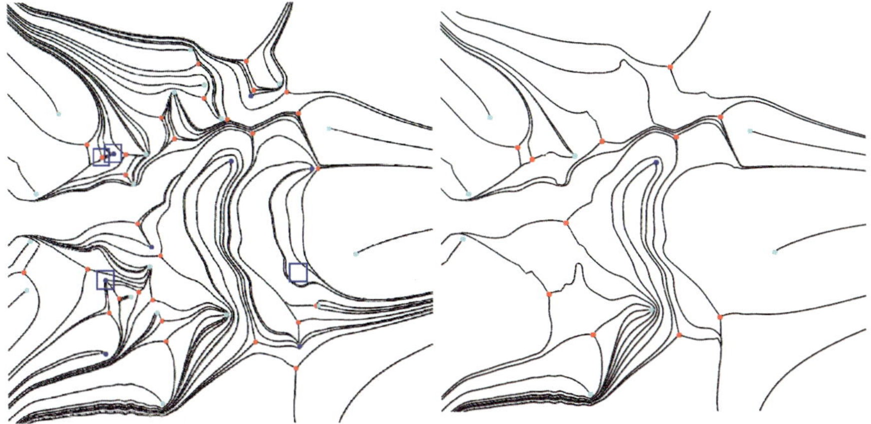

Fig. 13.12. Progressive topology simplification by enforced bifurcations

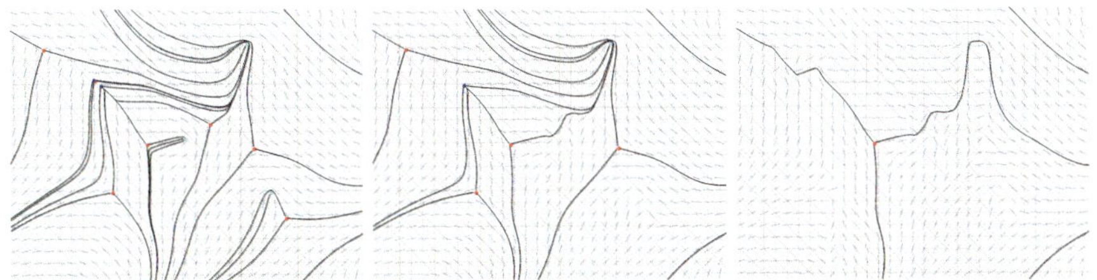

Fig. 13.13. Local topology simplification

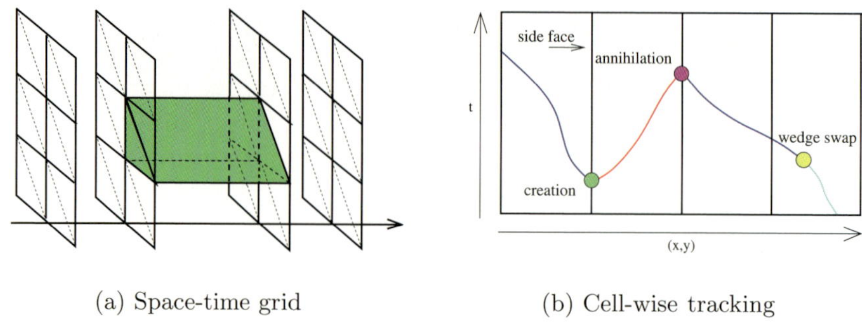

(a) Space-time grid   (b) Cell-wise tracking

Fig. 13.14. Local topology simplification

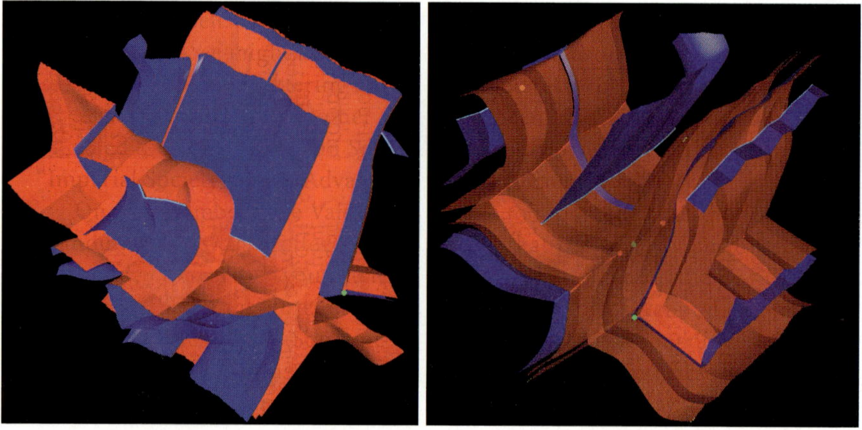

Fig. 13.15. Visualization of the complete topology evolution

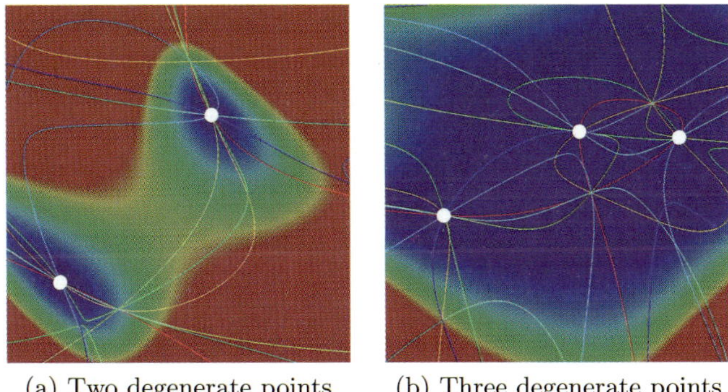

(a) Two degenerate points   (b) Three degenerate points

Fig. 14.2. White dots are degenerate points indicating places where all seven constraint functions are zero. Each colored curve corresponds to a constraint function being equal to zero. Places where multiple curves intersect are where multiple constraint functions are satisfied simultaneously. The background is pseudo-colored by the discriminant functions. The data is a 2D slice of a randomly generated 3D tensor field

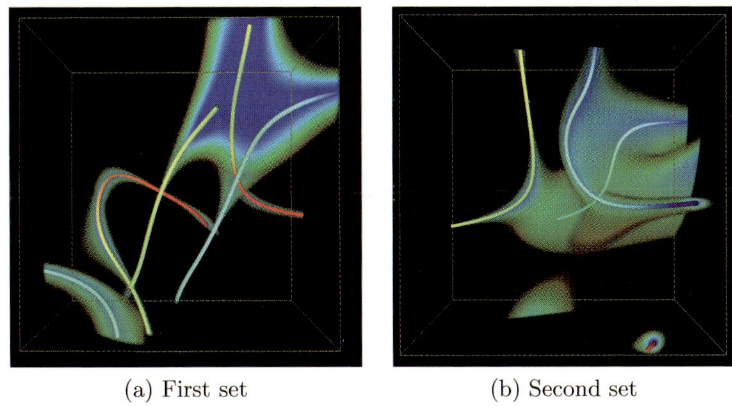

(a) First set   (b) Second set

Fig. 14.4. Randomly generated 3D tensors. Warmer line colors are closer to type P degenerate points where major and medium hyperstreamlines intersect, while cooler line colors are closer to type L degenerate points where medium and minor hyperstreamlines intersect. The rest of the volume is pseudo-colored by the discriminant using cool colors for low discriminant values (closer to feature lines) and warm transparent colors for distant values

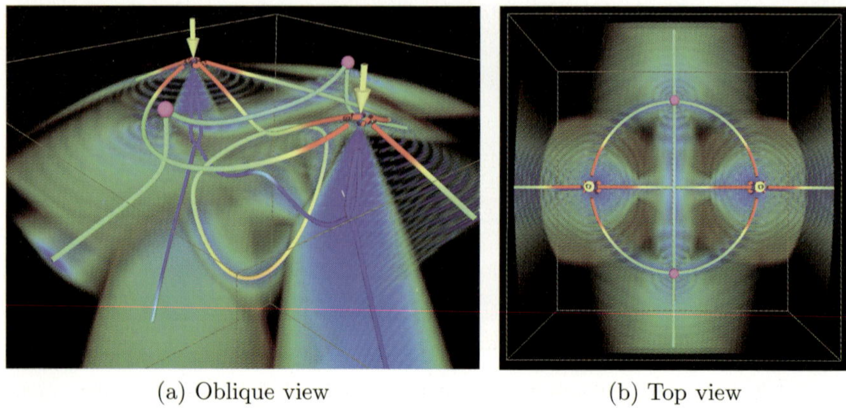

(a) Oblique view   (b) Top view

Fig. 14.5. Double point load data. Yellow arrows indicate point load, while the 2 magenta spheres show the location of the triple degenerate points. Color scheme is the same as Fig. 14.4

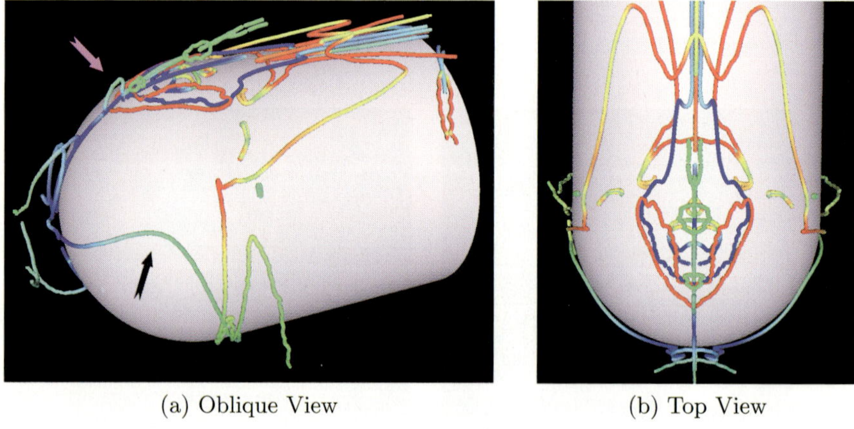

(a) Oblique View   (b) Top View

Fig. 14.6. Degenerate lines in deformation tensors of flow past a cylinder with a hemispherical cap. Feature lines are colored as in Fig. 14.4

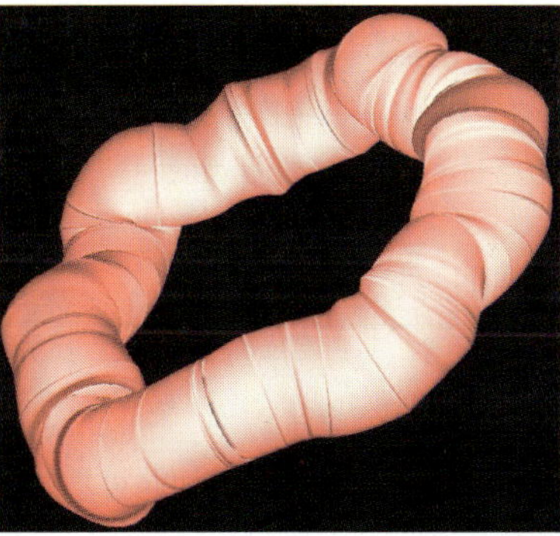

Fig. 15.1. Example of a closed hyperstreamline in a 3D tensor field

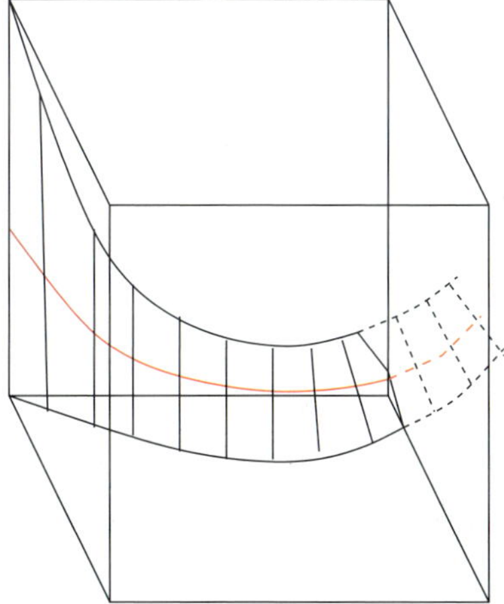

Fig. 15.2. Backward integrated hyperstreamsurface

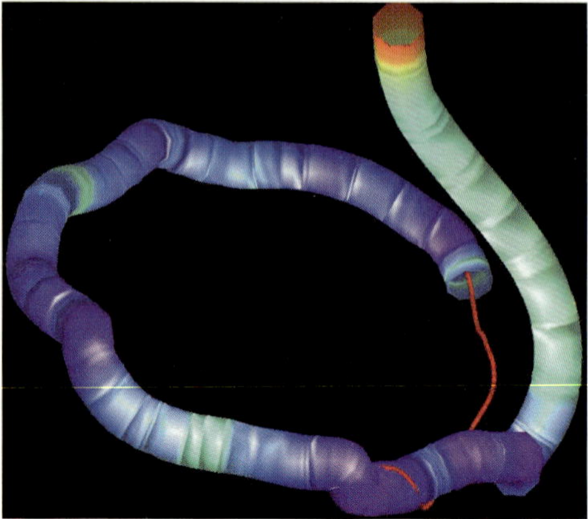

Fig. 15.3. Closed hyperstreamline (minor eigenvector field) in combination with a regular hyperstreamline

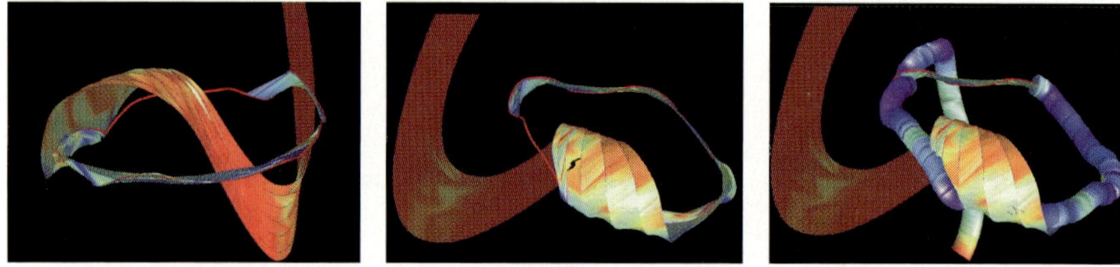

Fig. 15.4. Closed hyperstreamline including hyperstreamsurfaces exposing the surrounding tensor field (minor eigenvector field)

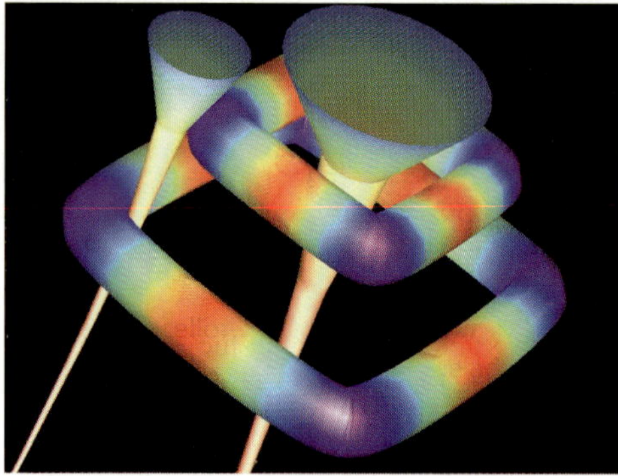

Fig. 15.5. Closed hyperstreamlines in single point load data set

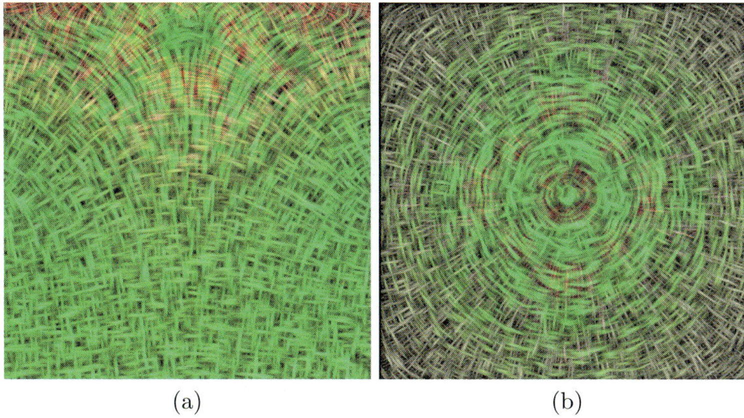

(a)   (b)

Fig. 16.7. This figure shows a single-top-load. Spot size and density of the input images are adapted to the corresponding eigenvectors. Red shows regions of compression, green expansion according the respective eigenvector field: the images are planar slices along the (**a**) yz-plane and (**b**) xy-plane slice orthogonal to the force

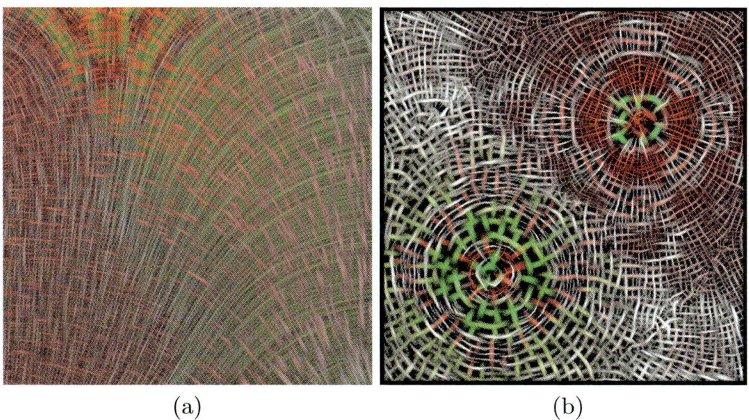

(a)   (b)

Fig. 16.8. The images represents a yz-plane (a) and xz-plane (b) slice of a two-force dataset. (**a**): In the lower-left corner we see a region of compression, a result mainly due to the pushing force on the left; in the upper-right corner expansion dominates as a result of the right pulling force. (**b**): The left circle corresponds to the pushing and the right to the pulling force. The fluctuation of the color is a result of the low resolution of the simulation

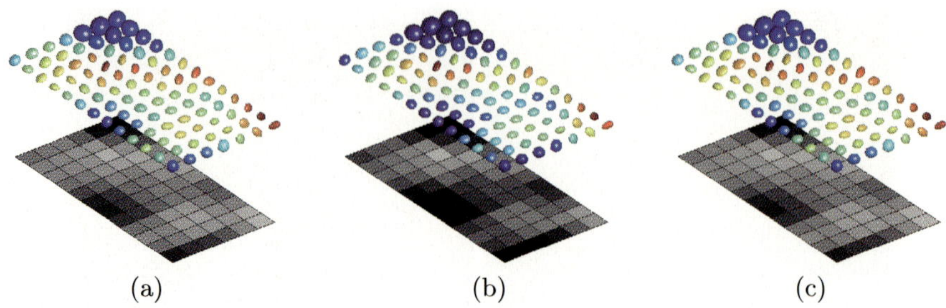

Fig. 17.4. *Anisotropies:* Diffusion ellipsoids of a brain region colored by the FA (**a**), the GA (**b**) and the KLA (**c**)

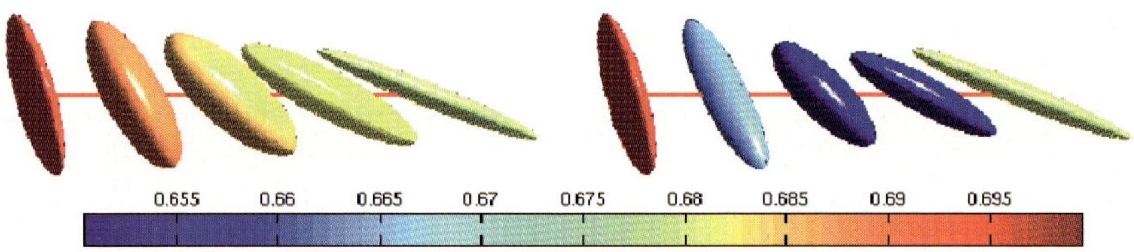

Fig. 17.5. *Univariate interpolation:* Ellipsoidal representation of linear interpolation (*left*) and geodesic interpolation (*right*) between two SPD tensors. In both cases, the colors are based on the values of the geodesic anisotropy index

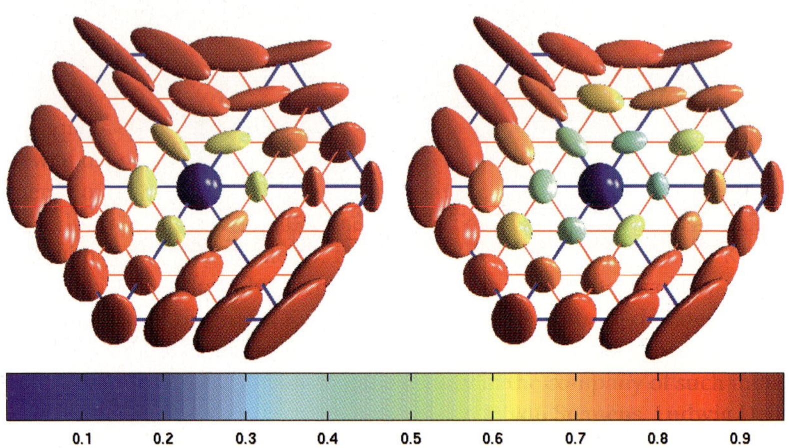

Fig. 17.6. *Bivariate interpolation:* Ellipsoidal representation of the interpolation of a 3D tensor field over a 2-dimensional hexagonal region: Euclidean interpolation (*left*) and geodesic interpolation (*right*). In both cases, the colors correspond to the values of the geodesic anisotropy index

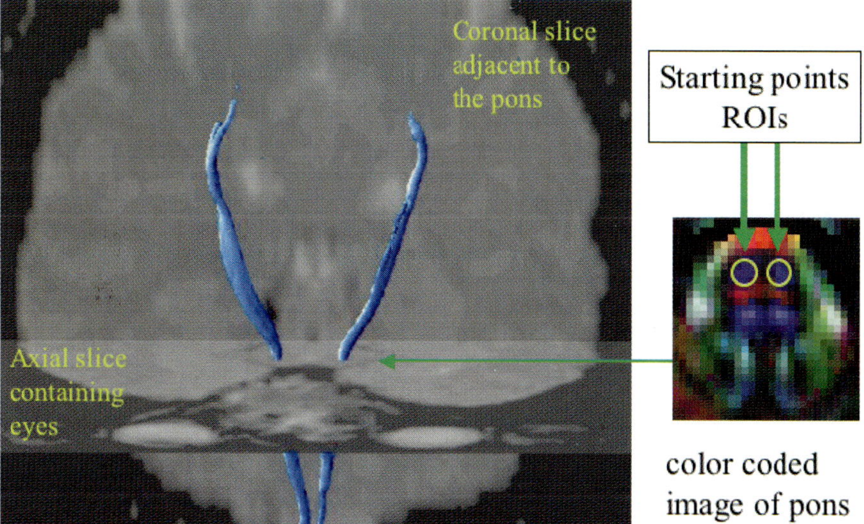

Fig. 18.2. Fiber tracts result from integrating along the tangent direction of the B-spline approximated tensor field, and with starting points chosen from the two circular regions in the area of pons. The obtained result agrees well with known anatomical data

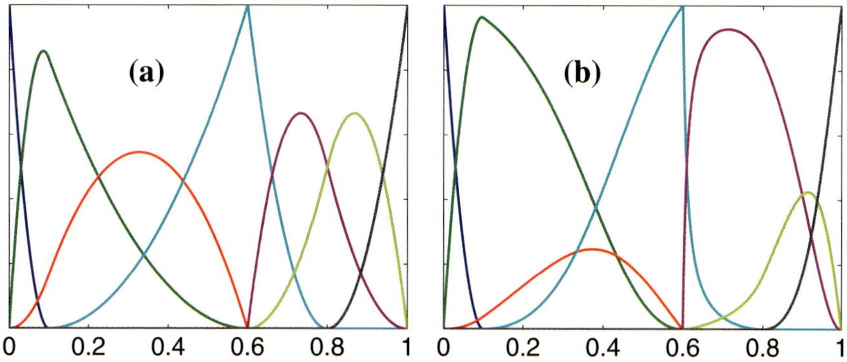

Fig. 18.3. (a) A set of 1-D NUB-basis functions with $p = 2$ and the knot vector $U = [0\ 0\ 0\ 0.1\ 0.6\ 0.6\ 0.8\ 1\ 1\ 1]$. (b) A set of rational basis functions (NURBS) obtained using the NUBs in (a) and by changing the weights for the 3rd, 4th and 5th basis function to 0.2, 0.5 and 5, respectively. The remaining NUBs had weights $w = 1$

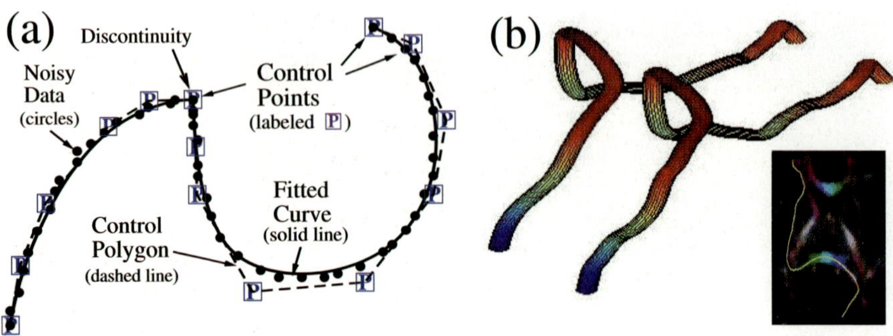

Fig. 18.4. (a) 2-D curve NURBS model fit to noisy data (b) 3-D curve NURBS model fit to fiber tracking data, indicated on the inset image

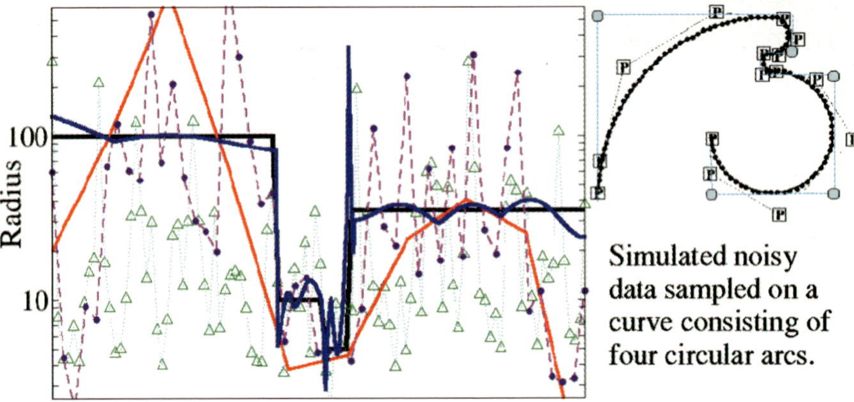

Fig. 18.5. Radii of curvature obtained from a noisy data set of points sampled from a curve consisting of four circular arcs (see the inset in upper right corner) with radii 100,10,5,35. The sampling error was 1%. The *solid black line* indicates the true radius (at inflection points the radius is infinite). The *solid blue line* indicates the NURBS fit, while B-spline approximation estimates are labeled as follows: $\Delta = 1$, i.e., interpolation (green triangles), $\Delta = 0.5$ (purple dots), or $\Delta = 0.2$ (*red solid line*). Note that the original curve could have been described with only 10 control points (the *light blue circles*, not all shown)

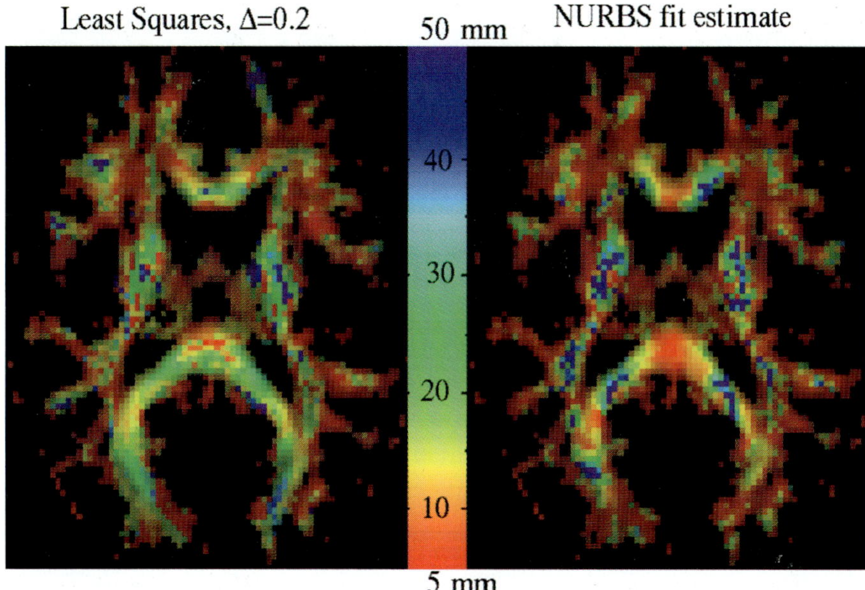

Fig. 18.6. Color coded images of the radius of curvature obtained at the center of each voxel for the given slice using B-spline approximation with $\Delta = 0.2$ (*left*) and NURBS (*right*), with colorbar indicating the scales. We see that the NURBS estimates are capable of showing the spatial variation of the fiber curvature. Note, that although the models are continuous, the estimates obtained from them are not necessarily smooth. The pixelization in the image, however, is arbitrary and we could have obtained the estimates at any point in space with the continuous models

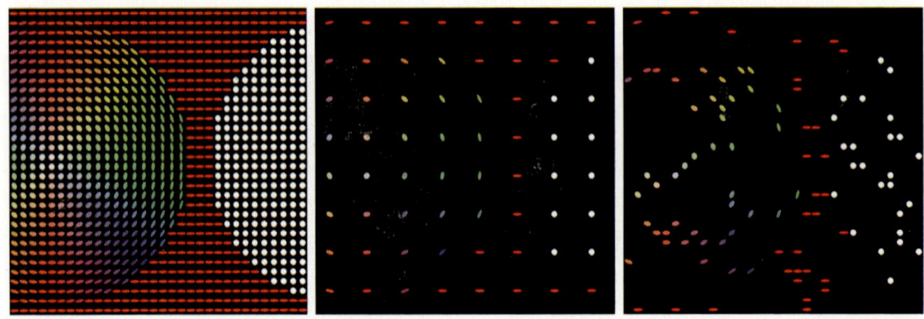

Fig. 19.3. (a) *Left*: Synthetic 2-D tensor test image, 32×32 pixels. (b) *Middle*: Regular interpolation data where every fourth pixel in each direction is given. (c) *Right*: Scattered interpolation data where 10 percent of all pixels have been selected randomly

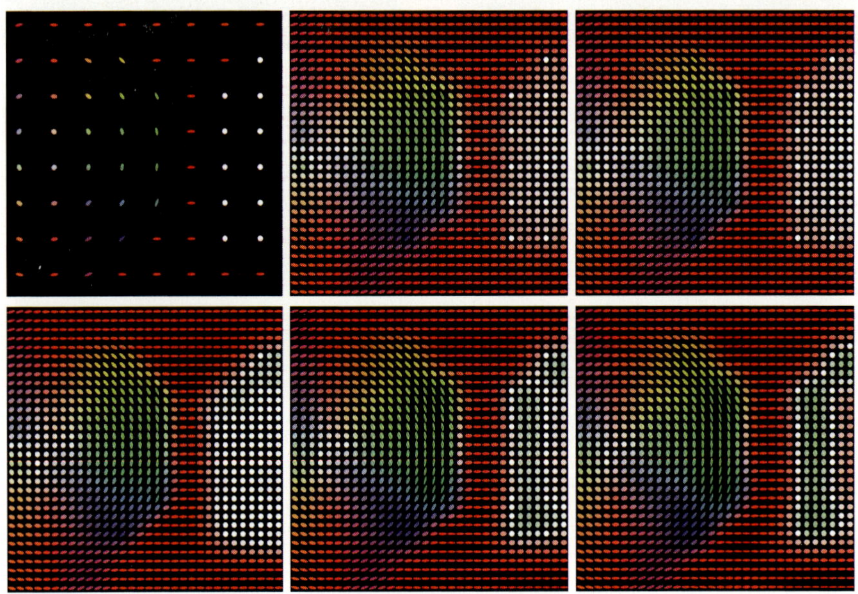

Fig. 19.4. Tensor-valued interpolation of Fig. 19.3(b). (a) *Top Left*: Interpolation data. (b) *Top Middle*: Interpolation with linear diffusion. (c) *Top Right*: Isotropic nonlinear diffusion. (d) *Bottom Left*: Anisotropic nonlinear diffusion. (e) *Bottom Middle*: Biharmonic smoothing. (f) *Bottom Right*: Triharmonic smoothing

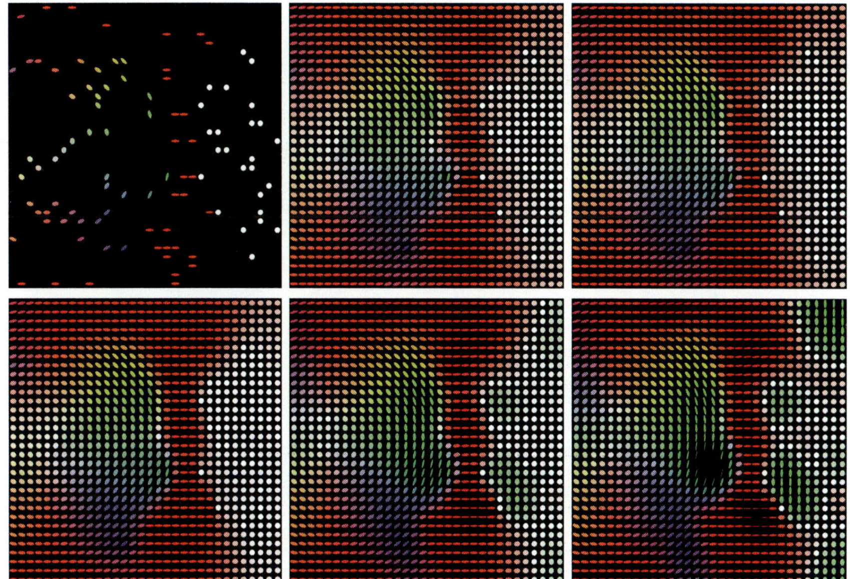

Fig. 19.5. Tensor-valued scattered data interpolation of Fig. 19.3(c). (**a**) *Top Left*: Interpolation data. (**b**) *Top Middle*: Interpolation with linear diffusion. (**c**) *Top Right*: Isotropic nonlinear diffusion. (**d**) *Bottom Left*: Anisotropic nonlinear diffusion. (**e**) *Bottom Middle*: Biharmonic smoothing. (**f**) *Bottom Right*: Triharmonic smoothing

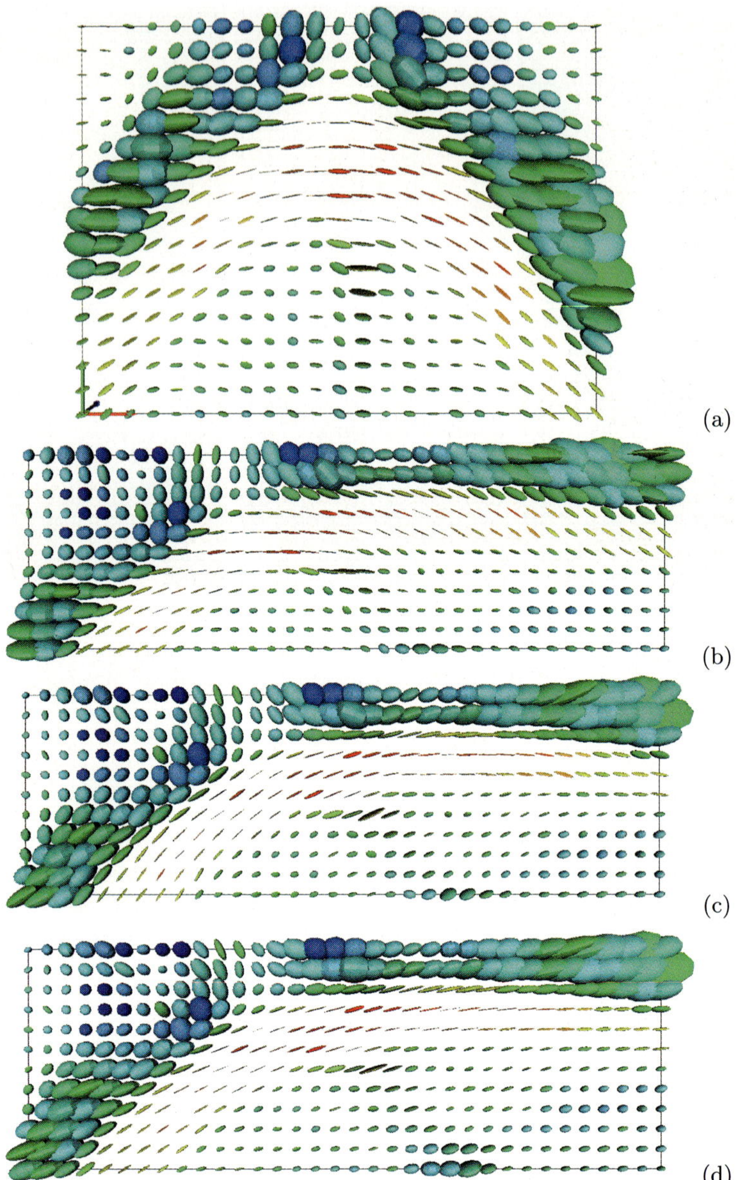

Fig. 20.4. Compares the results of Alexander's reorientation strategies. (See color plates.) Panel (**a**) shows the apparent diffusion tensors in the region of interest in Fig. 1(a). Panels (**b**), (**c**) and (**d**) show the apparent diffusion tensors in the same region after a shear along the left-hand arm of the corpus callosum fiber in the region, as highlighted in Fig. 1(d), using no reorientation, finite-strain reorientation and PPD, respectively

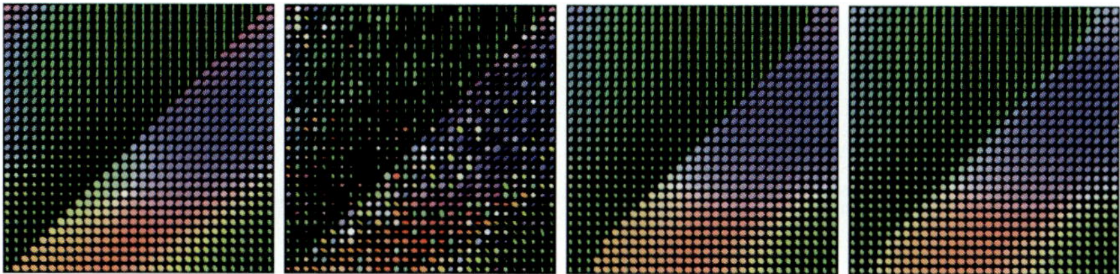

Fig. 21.1. Edge preserving tensor denoising. *Left* to *right:* (**a**) Positive semidefinite matrix field, 29 × 30. (**b**) Eigenvalues perturbed by Gaussian noise. (**c**) Median filtering of (**a**), 5×5 stencil, Frobenius norm, 5 iterations. (**d**) Same for (b). Adapted from [19]

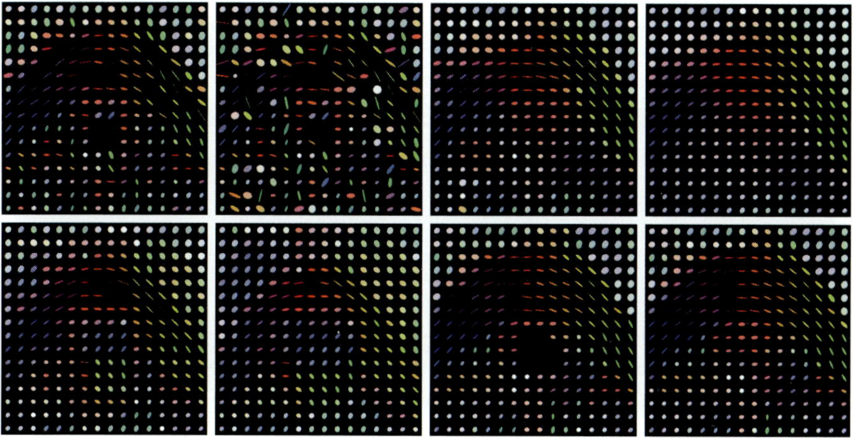

Fig. 21.4. Filtering of 2D DT-MRI data. *Top, left* to *right:* (**a**) Corpus callosum detail, cf. Fig. 3(b), represented by ellipses. Missing ellipses result from outliers with negative eigenvalues. (**b**) Same with noise, cf. Fig. 2(b). (**c**) Median filtering of noisy image, 3 × 3 stencil, Frobenius norm, 1 iteration. (**d**) Same as (c) but 5 iterations. *Bottom, left to right:* (**e**) Mid-range filtering of the original image, 3 × 3 stencil, Frobenius norm. (**f**) Same but with 5 × 5 stencil. (**g**) M-smoothed ($p = 0.1$, 3 × 3 stencil, Frobenius norm) using grid search. (**h**) Same with focussing strategy

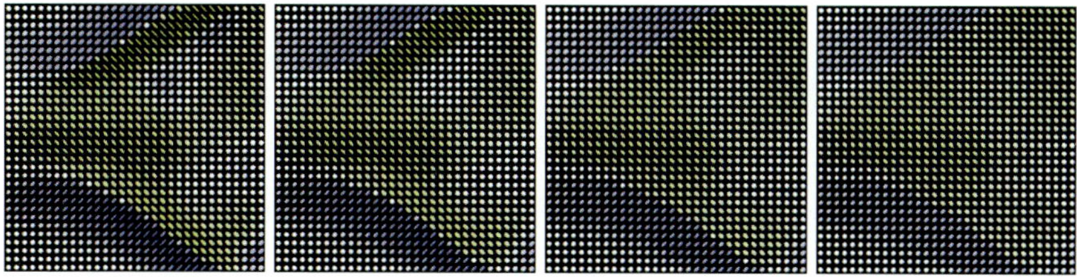

Fig. 21.6. Median filtering of fluid dynamics data. *Left* to *right:* (**a**) Detail (32 × 32) from Fig. 5(a). (**b**) Median filtering, 3 × 3 stencil, Frobenius norm, 10 iterations. (**c**) 100 iterations. (**d**) 1000 iterations

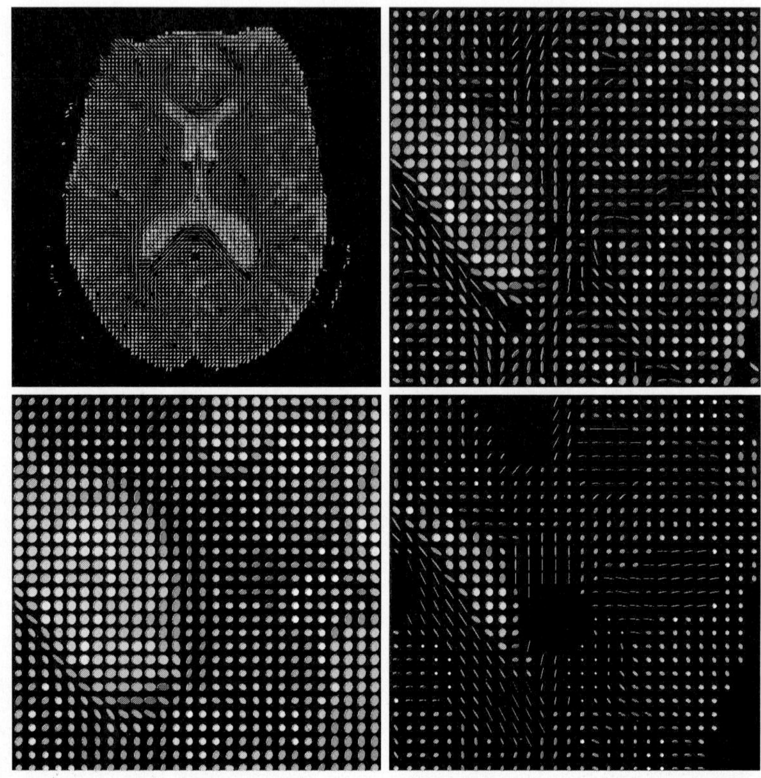

Fig. 22.2. (a) *Top left*: 2-D tensor field extracted from a DT-MRI data set of a human head. (b) *Top right*: enlarged section of left image. (c) *Bottom left*: dilation with DSE($\sqrt{5}$). (d) *Bottom right*: erosion with DSE($\sqrt{5}$)

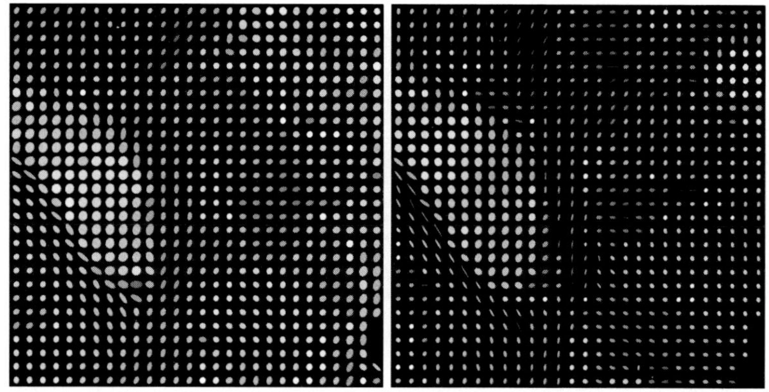

Fig. 22.3. (a) *Left*: closing with DSE($\sqrt{5}$). (b) *Right*: opening with DSE($\sqrt{5}$)

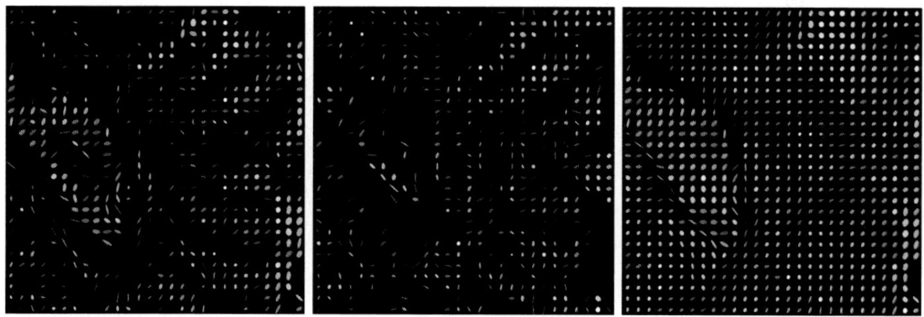

Fig. 22.4. (a) *Left*: white top hat with DSE($\sqrt{5}$). (b) *Middle*: black top hat with DSE($\sqrt{5}$). (c) *Right*: self-dual top hat with DSE($\sqrt{5}$)

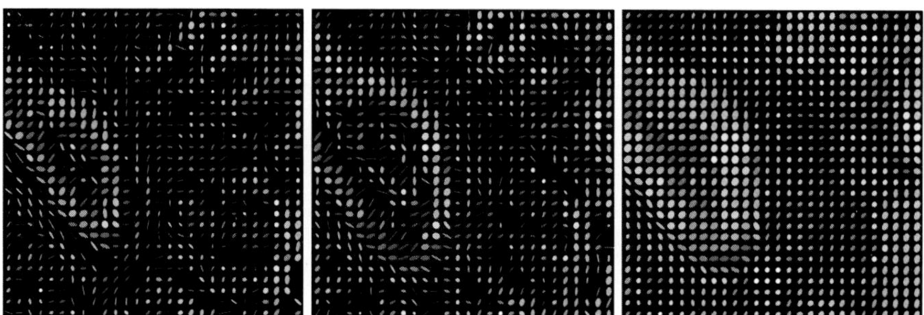

Fig. 22.5. (a) *Left*: external gradient with DSE($\sqrt{5}$). (b) *Middle*: internal gradient with DSE($\sqrt{5}$). (c) *Right*: Beucher gradient with DSE($\sqrt{5}$)

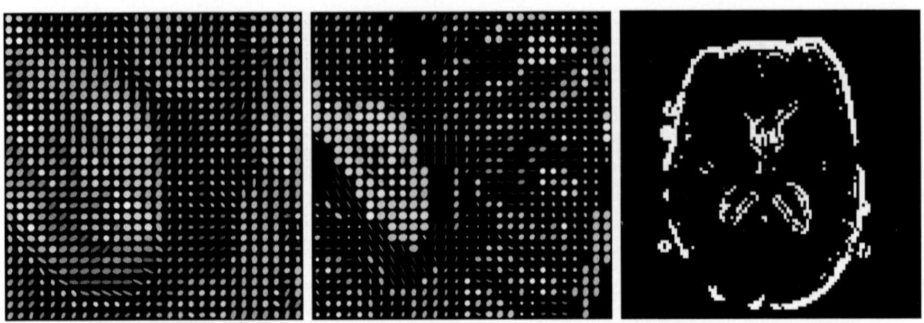

Fig. 22.6. (a) *Left*: morphological Laplacian with DSE($\sqrt{5}$). (b) *Middle*: result of shock filtering with DSE($\sqrt{5}$). (c) *Right*: edge map derived from zero crossings of the morphological Laplacian with DSE($\sqrt{5}$)

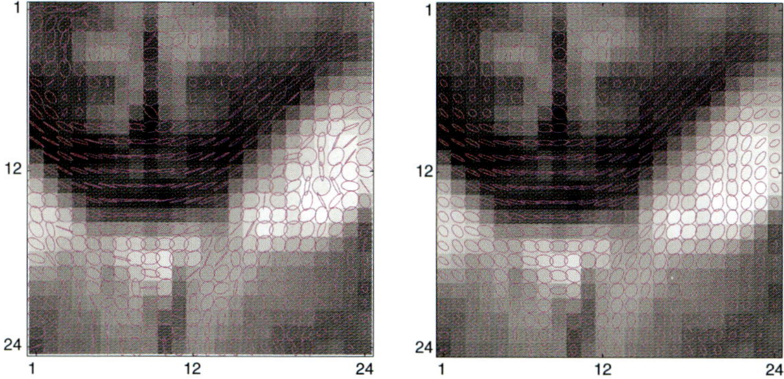

Fig. 23.2. *Left*: A 25×25 zoomed corpus callosum region of a slice in a DT-MRI dataset, overlapped by the 2D projections of the diffusion tensor (ellipses) in every point; *right*: the result after our filtering approach

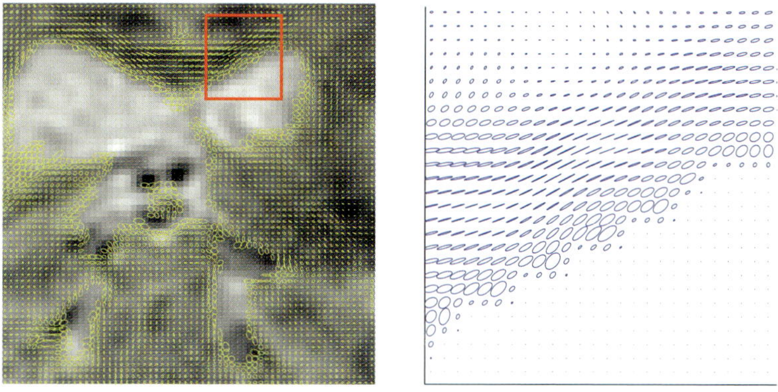

Fig. 23.4. *Left*: DT-MRI section of the *corpus callosum*; *right*: upsampling of the framed region

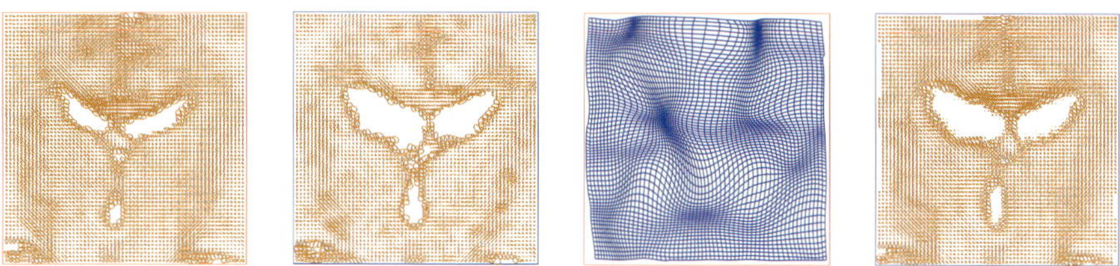

Fig. 23.6. Registration of two DT-MR images. (**a**) source tensor image; (**b**) target tensor image; (**c**) estimated deformation field, shown as a warping, from target to source; (**d**) source deformed

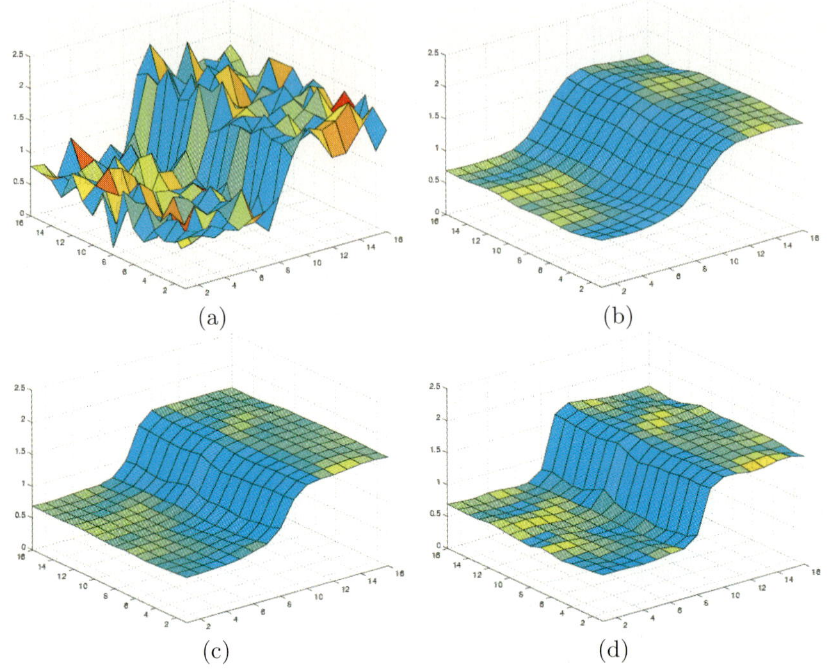

Fig. 24.1. Original scalar field (step edge) with added noise (**a**), the result without using the magnitude certainty measurement c_m (**b**), results using c_m with $\sigma = 1$ (**c**) and with $\sigma = 0.5$ (**d**)

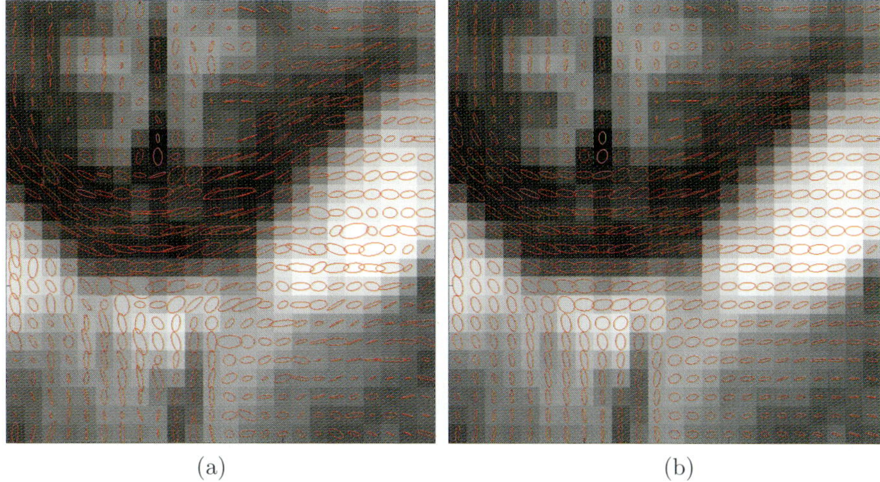

(a)   (b)

Fig. 24.3. Tensor field generated from noisy DT-MRI data (**a**) and result of filtering the tensor field using the NC method (**b**). The ROI is the corpus callosum, the dark bow-shaped region

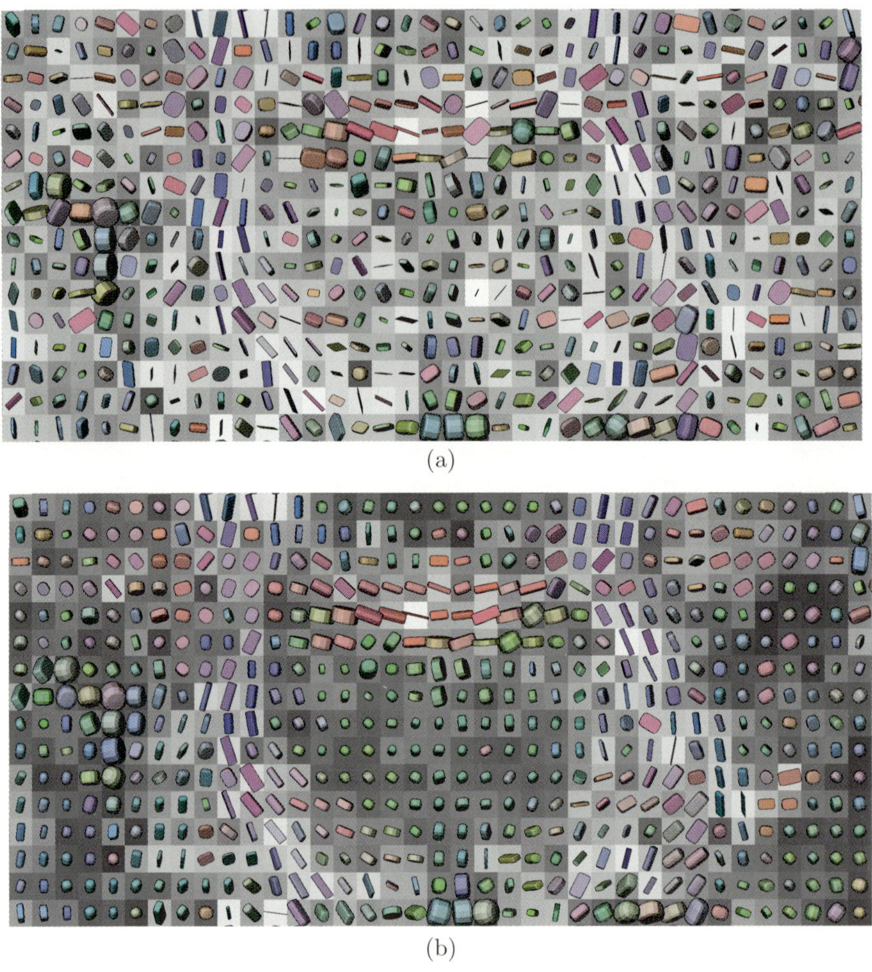

(a)

(b)

Fig. 24.9. Glyph visualization for a coronal slice for the original noisy DT-MRI data from a monkey brain (**a**) and the same visualization after regularization (**b**)

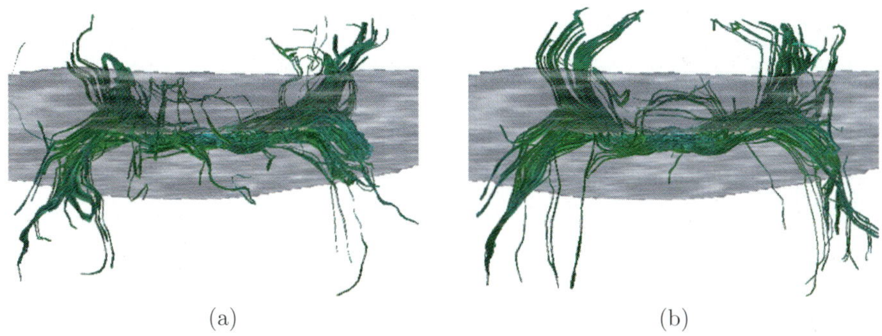

(a)   (b)

Fig. 24.10. Tractography in the corpus callosum for the original noise DT-MRI data from a monkey brain (**a**) and the same after regularization (**b**)

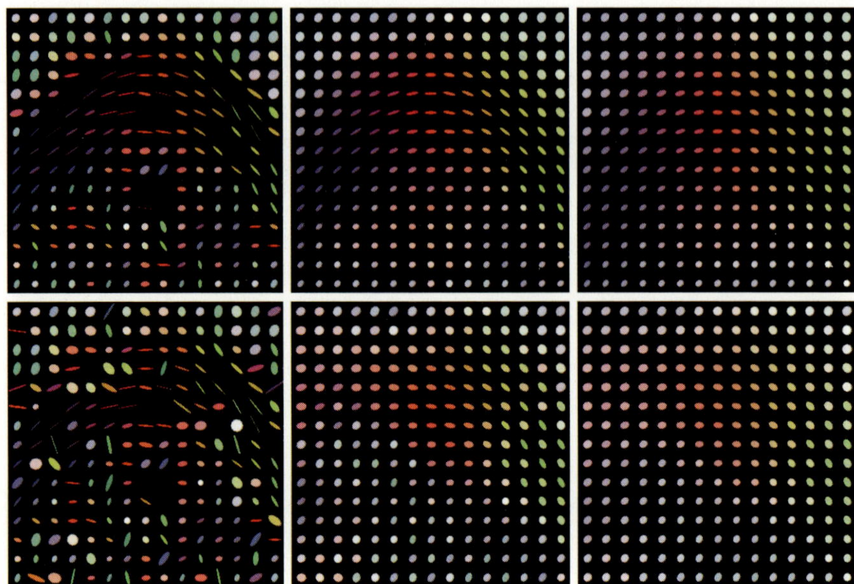

Fig. 25.2. Tensor-valued linear diffusion. *Top row*, from *left* to *right*: Detail from a DT-MR image (size 15×15), at time $t = 0.96$, at time $t = 2.4$. *Bottom row*, from *left* to *right*: Same experiment with 30% noise

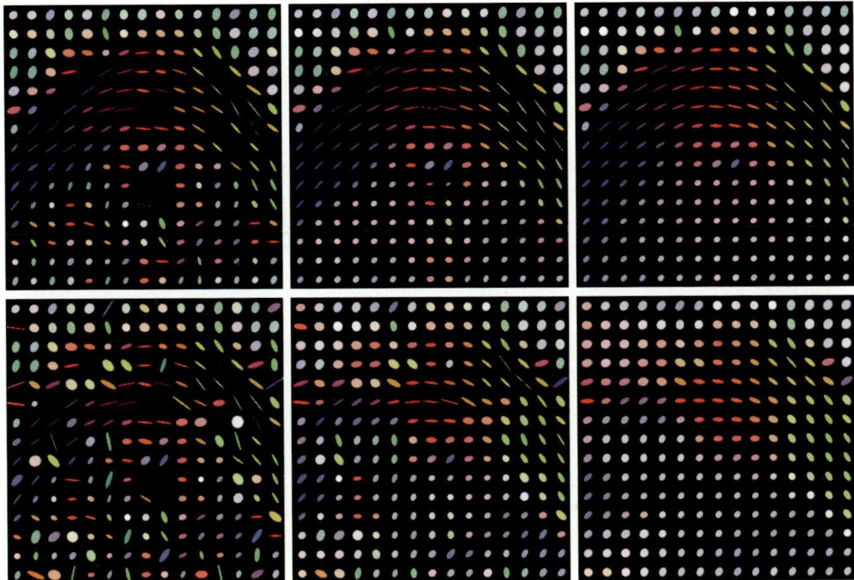

Fig. 25.3. Tensor-valued isotropic nonlinear diffusion. *Top row*, from *left* to *right*: Detail from a DT-MR image (size 15×15), at time $t = 4.8$, and at $t = 12.0$ ($\lambda = 0.5$, $\sigma = 0.5$). *Bottom row*, from *left* to *right*: Same experiment with 30% noise ($\lambda = 0.5$, $\sigma = 1$)

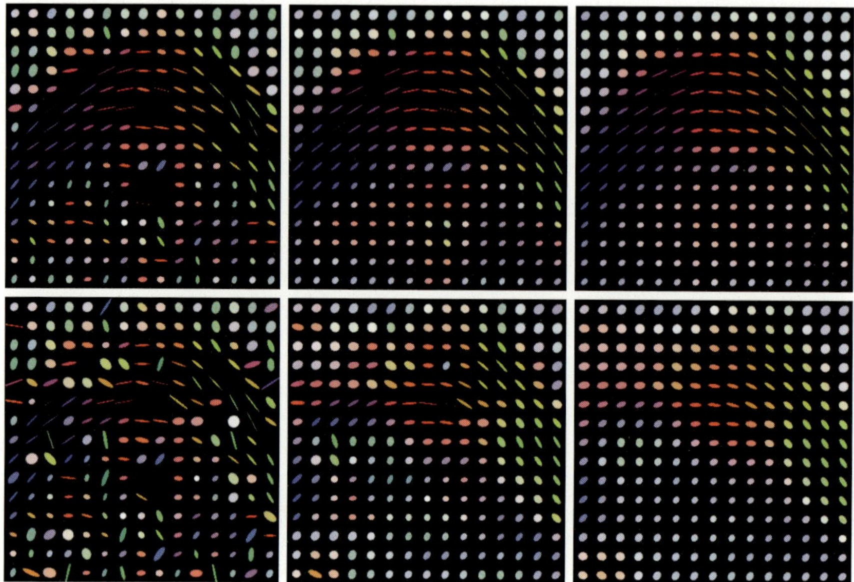

Fig. 25.4. Tensor-valued anisotropic nonlinear diffusion. *Top row*, from *left* to *right*: Detail from a DT-MR image (size 15×15), at time $t = 1.92$, and at $t = 4.8$ ($\lambda = 0.5$, $\sigma = 0.5$). *Bottom row*, from *left* to *right*: Same experiment with 30% noise, at time $t = 1.92$ and $t = 4.8$ ($\lambda = 0.5$, $\sigma = 1$)

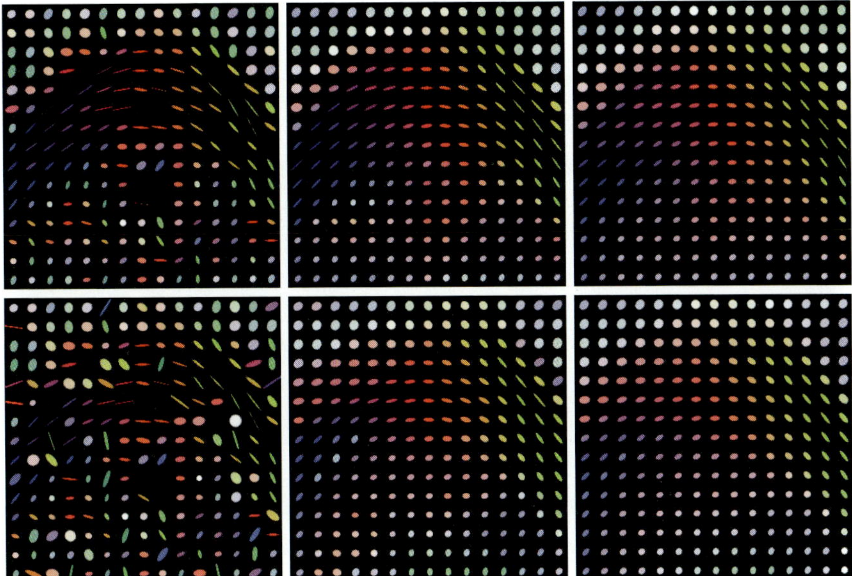

Fig. 25.5. Tensor-valued mean curvature motion. *Top row*, from *left* to *right*: Detail of size 15×15 from a DT-MR image; at time $t = 2.4$, at time $t = 6$. *Bottom row*, from *left* to *right*: Same experiment with 30% noise

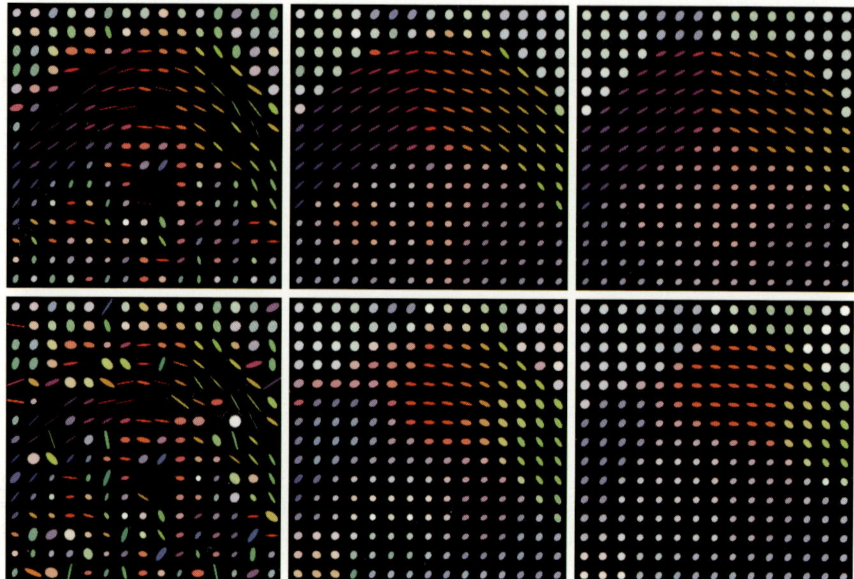

Fig. 25.6. Tensor-valued self-snakes. *Top row*, from *left* to *right*: Detail of size 15×15 from a DT-MR image; at time $t = 2.4$, at time $t = 6$ ($\sigma = 0.5$, $\lambda = 2$). *Bottom row*, from *left* to *right*: Same experiment with 30% noise ($\sigma = 1$, $\lambda = 2$)

Printing: Krips bv, Meppel
Binding: Stürtz, Würzburg